Manual of
Critical Care Nursing

Manual of
Critical Care Nursing

NURSING INTERVENTIONS AND COLLABORATIVE MANAGEMENT

Fourth Edition

Edited by

Pamela L. Swearingen, RN
Special Project Editor

Janet Hicks Keen, RN, MS(N), CIC, CCRN
Critical Care Nursing Consultant
Infection Control Specialist
Saint Joseph's Hospital of Atlanta
Atlanta, Georgia

Consultant to the Fourth Edition

Marianne Saunorus Baird, RN, MN
Case Manager for Pulmonary and Nephrology
Saint Joseph's Hospital of Atlanta
Atlanta, Georgia

 Mosby

A Harcourt Health Sciences Company

St. Louis   London   Philadelphia   Sydney   Toronto

Mosby

A Harcourt Health Sciences Company

Vice-President and Nursing Editorial Director: Sally Schrefer
Executive Editor: Barbara Nelson Cullen
Developmental Editor: Cindi Anderson
Project Manager: John Rogers
Project Specialist: Betty Hazelwood
Designer: Kathi Gosche

Mosby, Inc.
A Harcourt Health Sciences Company
11830 Westline Industrial Drive
St. Louis, MO 63146

Printed in the United States of America

International Standard Book Number 0-323-00998-0

01   02   03   04   GW/RDC   9   8   7   6   5   4   3   2

Contributors

PATRICE C. AL-SADEN, RN
Liver Study Unit
University of Chicago
Chicago, Illinois

LINDA S. BAAS, RN, PhD, CS-CANP, CCNS
Assistant Professor and Acute Care Nurse Practitioner Program Coordinator
University of Cincinnati College of Nursing
Cincinnati, Ohio

MARIANNE SAUNORUS BAIRD, RN, MN
Case Manager for Pulmonary and Nephrology
Saint Joseph's Hospital of Atlanta
Atlanta, Georgia

CAROL A. BARCH, RN, MN, CRNP, CNRN
University of Pennsylvania Medical Center Stroke Institute
Program Director
Pittsburgh, Pennsylvania

CHERYL L. BITTEL, RN, MSN, CCRN
Clinical Nurse Specialist
Saint Joseph's Hospital of Atlanta
Atlanta, Georgia

MIMI CALLANAN, RN, MSN
Epilepsy Clinical Nurse Specialist
Stanford Comprehensive Epilepsy Center
Department of Neurology and Neurological Sciences
Stanford, California

ALICE DAVIS, RN, PhD, CNRN, CGNP
Assistant Professor
University of Michigan School of Nursing
Ann Arbor, Michigan

BEVERLY GEORGE-GAY, RN, MSN
Assistant Professor
Medical College of Georgia
School of Nursing;
Clinical Nurse Specialist
Surgical Intensive Care Unit
Medical College of Georgia Hospital and Clinics
Augusta, Georgia

CHERI A. GOLL, RN, MSN
Director
St. Vincent's Hospital
Indianapolis, Indiana

PATRICIA HALL, RN, PHD
Director of Clinical Research
Cardiology Associates of Mobile
Mobile, Alabama

MIMA M. HORNE, RN, MS, CDE
Diabetes/Renal Clinical Nurse Specialist
New Hanover Regional Medical Center;
Adjunct Lecturer, School of Nursing
University of North Carolina—Wilmington
Wilmington, North Carolina

MARGUERITE McMILLAN JACKSON, RN, PHD, CIC, FAAN
Administrative Director
Nursing Research and Education and Epidemiology Unit
Associate Clinical Professor of Family and Preventive Medicine
University of California, San Diego Medical Center
San Diego, California

JOYCE YOUNG JOHNSON, RN, PHD
Resource Nurse
Crawford Long Hospital of Emory University;
Adjunct Faculty, School of Nursing
Georgia University
Atlanta, Georgia

JENNI JORDAN, RN, CME
Staff Nurse
Surgical Intensive Care
Preceptor
Critical Care Residency Program
University of Colorado Hospital
Denver, Colorado

JANET HICKS KEEN, RN, MS(N), CIC, CCRN
Critical Care Nursing Consultant
Infection Control Specialist
Saint Joseph's Hospital of Atlanta
Atlanta, Georgia

CHERYL McKAY, RN, MSN, CNS
President, Medical Outcomes Management;
Clinical Nurse Specialist
Select Specialty Corporation
Oklahoma City, Oklahoma

BARBARA McLEAN, RN, MN, CCRN, CFNP
Critical Care Clinical Specialist Consultant
Grady Memorial Hospital
Atlanta, Georgia

MARGUERITE J. MURPHY, RN, MS
Assistant Professor—Adult Health
School of Nursing
Medical College of Georgia
Barnesville, Georgia

†DENNIS ROSS, RN, MAE, PHD
Professor of Nursing
Castleton State College
Castleton, Vermont

SUSAN L. SCHROEDER, RN, MS
Clinical Nurse Specialist
Department of Nursing
University of Wisconsin Hospital and Clinics
Madison, Wisconsin

MARILYN SAWYER SOMMERS, RN, PHD, CCRN, FAAN
Professor, College of Nursing
University of Cincinnati
Cincinnati, Ohio

JOHANNA K. STIESMEYER, RN, MS
Consultant, Nursing Education Services
Placitas, New Mexico

NANCY A. STOTTS, RN, EDD
Professor
University of California, San Francisco
San Francisco, California

ANN COGHLAN STOWE, RN, MSN, DNSC(C)
Chairperson and Assistant Professor
Department of Nursing
West Chester University
West Chester, Pennsylvania

KAREN S. WEBBER, RN, MN
Assistant Professor
Memorial University of Newfoundland
School of Nursing
St. Johns, Newfoundland
Canada

PATRICIA D. WEISKITTEL, RN, MS, CNN, CS
Clinical Nurse Specialist
Renal Transplant
University Hospital Inc.
Cincinnati, Ohio

LAURA D. WILLIAMS, RN, BSN, CCRN
Cardiac and Vascular Surgery Case Manager
Saint Joseph's Hospital of Atlanta
Atlanta, Georgia

†Deceased.

Reviewers

ARLENE M. AIRHART, RN, BSN, MSN, PhD
Professor
Graduate Studies and Research in Nursing
College of Nursing
Northwestern State University of Louisiana
Shreveport, Louisiana

REITHA CABANISS, RN, MSN, POST-MASTER CERTIFICATE—GERONTOLOGY
Cardiovascular Clinical Specialist
Nursing Faculty
Bevill State Community College
Sumiton, Alabama

GRETCHEN CARROUGHER, RN, MNS, CNS
Research Coordinator
Department of Rehabilitative Medicine
University of Washington Burn Center
Harborview Medical Center
Seattle, Washington

CHERYL GATTI, RN, BSN, CCRN
Independent Nurse Consultant;
Staff Nurse, Overlook Hospital
Summit, New Jersey

BARBARA HABERMANN, RN, PhD
Chronic Care Clinical Nurse Specialist/Nurse Researcher
Kaiser Permanente Medical Center
Walnut Creek, California

JUDE LARK, RN, BSN, CCRN
Independent Nurse Consultant;
Staff Nurse, St. Barnabas Hospital
Livingston, New Jersey

STEPHEN M. SETTER, PharmD, DVM
Washington State University
College of Pharmacy
Spokane, Washington

Preface

Manual of Critical Care Nursing: Nursing Interventions and Collaborative Management was developed to provide nurses with a portable compendium of more than 80 clinical phenomena seen in critical care. This updated, two-color fourth edition includes new sections on Ethics, Septic Shock, Systemic Inflammatory Response Syndrome (SIRS) and Multiple Organ Dysfunction Syndrome (MODS), Anaphylactic Shock, and Cardiac Transplantation. Also new to this edition is the inclusion of Research Boxes to illustrate important or interesting results of critical care–related clinical research. In this edition we have included age-specific information when applicable. Content that applies to older adults is easily recognizable by elder icons in the margin.

Focusing on nursing diagnoses and interventions that are specific to each critical disorder, the book also provides a brief review of pathophysiology and discusses assessment data, diagnostic testing, and collaborative management. The order of presentation provides a hierarchy of information that enables the nurse to make nursing diagnoses and determine interventions specific to the individual patient. Although patient teaching in critical care may, by necessity, be concentrated on immediate learning needs, ideally the information provided in this text should be incorporated before discharge from the intensive care or step-down unit, verbally or via written instructions.

This edition has been thoroughly revised and updated. The outcome criteria are specific, positive statements that facilitate evaluation of care. Suggested time frames for the outcome criteria are included with each outcome statement. Time frames are provided as guidelines, since patients have their own unique response times, and to serve as reminders that Medicare and other third-party payors monitor the fine line between quality, cost-effective care, and premature discharge, enabling nurses to set more realistic goals for nursing outcomes.

For clarity and consistency throughout the book, normal values are given for hemodynamic monitoring and other measurements. However, all values should be individualized to correspond to the patient's normal range of measurements. Although the book offers a host of interventions for each critical disorder, not all interventions are appropriate for every patient. It is our intent that interventions that do apply to the individual patient be used in the development of a personalized plan of care.

Only NANDA-approved nursing diagnoses are used in this manual. To promote consistency in the wording of nursing diagnoses among all nurses, we have followed closely the wording used by NANDA for its related factors. New to this edition is the inclusion of Nursing Interventions Classification (NIC) labels. This feature provides nurses with a convenient grouping of suggested interventions and related activities. For additional information on NIC, readers should refer to McCloskey JC, Bulechek GM: *Nursing Interventions Classification (NIC),* ed 3, St. Louis, 2000, Mosby.

Readers who desire more information on disorders traditionally seen in the medical-surgical setting (e.g., chronic obstructive pulmonary disease, renal calculi, diverticulosis, cancer) are encouraged to read *Manual of Medical-Surgical Nursing Care: Nursing Interventions and Collaborative Management,* fourth edition, edited by Pamela L. Swearingen and Dennis G. Ross (Mosby).

Manual of Critical Care Nursing was written to supplement critical care textbooks and assumes that the reader has a background in critical care pathophysiology and assessment parameters. The book can serve as a resource not only for clinicians but for academicians and students as well. The textual information and numerous tables will stimulate the clinician's recall of previously learned concepts. Academicians can use the book in teaching students to apply theoretical concepts to clinical practice. Students will find the book an excellent tool in helping them assess the patient systematically, as well as in setting priorities in nursing interventions. Our primary goal is to provide staff and students in critical care a wealth of clinical information in a quick and easy-to-use format. Our reviewers believe that we have achieved this objective. We welcome comments from nurses who consult the book on a daily basis so that we can enhance its usefulness in future editions.

Pamela L. Swearingen
Janet Hicks Keen

Acknowledgments

We would like to thank the many individuals whose input was valuable in the development of this manuscript. In particular, we are grateful for the expertise and many contributions of Marianne Baird, RN, MN, to this fourth edition. In addition, we would like to thank the following third edition contributors: Robert Aucker, PharmD, BCPS; Barbara Tueller Steuble, RN, MS; and Ursula Easterday Heitz, RN, MSN.

We are deeply appreciative of the tremendous direction and support from our developmental editor, Cindi Anderson. We would also like to acknowledge our production editor, Betty Hazelwood, whose attention to detail and terrific suggestions made substantial contributions to this edition.

P.L.S.
J.H.K.

I would like to acknowledge the patience and loving encouragement of my family: Laura, Glenna, and Raymond.

J.H.K.

Contents

CHAPTER 1

General Concepts in Caring for the Critically Ill

Nutritional support

The body adapts to starvation through a series of hormonal changes that compensate for the decreased intake of nutrients. If starvation is prolonged, the body uses its own substrate to optimize survival, with a resulting loss of skeletal muscle and adipose tissue. This state of protein-calorie malnutrition, marasmus, when complicated with severe stress, such as burns, serious injury, or sepsis, generates a neuroendocrine response—hypermetabolism, hypercatabolism, insulin resistance with hyperglycemia, and depletion of lean body mass. Studies indicate that patient outcomes for those with protein-calorie malnutrition are associated with an increased mortality and morbidity, including weakness, compromised immunity, decreased wound healing, infection, and organ failure. Consequently, the goal of therapy is to identify the preexisting malnutrition, prevent further protein-calorie deficiencies, optimize the patient's current state, and reduce further morbidity.

NUTRITIONAL ASSESSMENT

Multiple sources of information are used, including historical data, nutritional history, anthropometric data, biochemical analysis of blood and urine, and duration of the disease process. With a critically ill individual, the nutritional history may be obtained from significant others.

Nutritional history: A nutritional history identifies individuals who are or may be at risk for malnutrition during hospitalization. Investigate the adequacy of usual and recent food intake and, in particular, anything that has impaired adequate selection, preparation, ingestion, digestion, absorption, and excretion of nutrients before admission. Include the following in your history:

- Comprehensive review of usual dietary intake, including food allergies, food aversions, and use of nutritional supplements including vitamins and alternative therapies
- Recent unplanned weight loss or gain
- Chewing or swallowing difficulties
- Nausea, vomiting, or pain with eating
- Altered pattern of elimination (e.g., constipation, diarrhea)
- Chronic disease affecting utilization of nutrients (e.g., malabsorption, pancreatitis, diabetes mellitus)
- Recent trauma, surgery, or sepsis
- Use of medications (e.g., laxatives, antacids, antibiotics, antineoplastic drugs) and alcohol

Note excesses or deficiencies of nutrients and any special eating patterns (e.g., various vegetarian or prescribed diets), use of fad diets, or excessive supplementation.

Physical assessment: Most physical findings are not conclusive for particular nutritional deficiencies. Compare current assessment findings with past assessments, especially related to the following:

- Loss of muscle and adipose tissue
- Work and muscle endurance
- Changes in hair, skin, or neuromuscular function

Anthropometric data: Anthropometrics is the measurement of the body or its parts. It is helpful to remember that 1 liter (L) of fluid equals approximately 2 pounds (lb). Pounds and inches are converted to metric measurements using the following formulas:

   Divide pounds by 2.2 to convert to kilograms (kg).
   Divide inches by 39.37 to convert to meters (m).

- *Height:* Used to determine ideal weight and body mass index; if unavailable, obtain estimate from family or significant others or compare patient's recumbent length with known mattress length.
- *Weight:* A readily available and practical indicator of nutritional status that can be compared with previous weight and ideal weight or used to calculate body mass index. Changes may reflect fluid retention (edema, third spacing), diuresis, dehydration, surgical resections, traumatic amputations, or weight of dressings or equipment. Use actual body weight to avoid overfeeding in starved patients and ideal body weight in patients who weigh >120% of ideal body weight. See Table 1-1.
- *Body mass index (BMI):* Used to evaluate adult weight. One calculation and one set of standards are applicable for both men and women:

$$\text{BMI (kg/m)} = \frac{\text{Weight (kg)}}{\text{Height (m)} \times \text{Height (m)}}$$

BMI values of 20-25 are optimal; values >25 indicate obesity; and values <20 indicate underweight status.

- *Triceps skinfold thickness (TSF):* Measured at the midpoint of the upper arm, which is located by taking half the distance between the olecranon and acromion process and grasping the skin and subcutaneous tissue at the back of the arm approximately 1 cm from the midpoint. Surgical calipers are used to measure the skinfold. Because of the variation among clinicians, the site of measurement, and the patient's position, age, and fluid status, it is difficult to use these measurements as a basis for evaluating patient status. Specially trained clinicians and dietitians should perform this assessment for more accurate results. A TSF measurement of <3 mm signals severely depleted fat stores.

TABLE 1-1   Height and Weight Guidelines for Men and Women

Height	Men (weight in lb)			Women (weight in lb)		
	Small frame	Medium frame	Large frame	Small frame	Medium frame	Large frame
4 ft 10 in	—	—	—	102-111	109-121	118-131
4 ft 11 in	—	—	—	103-113	111-123	120-134
5 ft	—	—	—	104-115	113-126	122-137
5 ft 1 in	—	—	—	106-118	115-129	125-140
5 ft 2 in	128-134	131-141	138-150	108-121	118-132	128-143
5 ft 3 in	130-136	133-143	140-153	111-124	121-135	131-147
5 ft 4 in	132-138	135-145	142-156	114-127	124-138	134-151
5 ft 5 in	134-140	137-148	144-160	117-130	127-141	137-155
5 ft 6 in	136-142	139-151	146-164	120-133	130-144	140-159
5 ft 7 in	138-145	142-154	149-168	123-136	133-147	143-163
5 ft 8 in	140-148	145-157	152-172	126-139	136-150	146-167
5 ft 9 in	142-151	148-160	155-176	129-142	139-153	149-170
5 ft 10 in	144-154	151-163	158-180	132-145	142-156	152-173
5 ft 11 in	146-157	154-166	161-184	135-148	145-159	155-176
6 ft	149-160	157-170	164-188	138-151	148-162	158-179
6 ft 1 in	152-164	160-174	168-192	—	—	—
6 ft 2 in	155-168	164-178	172-197	—	—	—
6 ft 3 in	158-172	167-182	176-202	—	—	—
6 ft 4 in	162-176	171-187	181-207	—	—	—

Data courtesy Metropolitan Life Insurance Company, 1983. For ages 25 through 59, based on lowest mortality. Includes 3 lb of indoor clothing for women and 5 lb for men, both with 1-in heels.

DIAGNOSTIC TESTS

No laboratory test specifically measures nutritional status. Status can be estimated, however, using the following:

Protein status: Evaluated in the following tests, with normal values in parentheses: serum albumin (3.5-5.5 g/dl), transferrin (180-260 mg/dl), thyroxine-binding prealbumin (20-30 mg/dl), and retinol-binding protein (4-5 mg/dl). Normal values vary somewhat with different laboratory procedures and standards. Albumin and transferrin have relatively long half-lives of 19 and 9 days, respectively, whereas thyroxine-binding prealbumin and retinol-binding protein have very short half-lives of 24-48 h and 10 h, respectively. If hydration status is normal and anemia is absent, albumin and transferrin levels can be used as baseline indicators of adequacy of protein intake and synthesis. During protein-calorie malnutrition, however, the plasma albumin level, an indicator of visceral protein, is unchanged. For evidence of response to nutritional therapy, values for the short turnover proteins (i.e., thyroxine-binding prealbumin [although very expensive] and retinol-binding protein) are the most useful.

Nitrogen balance: If more nitrogen is taken in than excreted, nitrogen is said to be positive and an anabolic state exists. If more nitrogen is excreted than taken in, nitrogen balance is said to be negative and a catabolic state exists. Most nitrogen loss occurs through the urine, with a small, constant amount lost via skin and feces. Nitrogen balance studies should be performed by specialists, because accurate measurement of 24-h food intake and urine output is required.

Creatinine-height index: Comparison of a patient's 24-h urinary creatinine excretion with a predicted urinary creatinine for individuals with the same height. This test evaluates body muscle mass. The quantity of creatinine produced is directly related to skeletal muscle wasting. The validity of results is affected by inaccuracies in the urine collection procedure and a lack of age-referenced norms.

ESTIMATING NUTRITIONAL REQUIREMENTS

The primary goal of nutritional support is to meet the needs for body temperature, metabolic processes, and tissue repair. Energy needs can be estimated using the following options:

Indirect calorimetry: Performed using a bedside metabolic cart. Specialized personnel are required to provide accurate results.

Harris and Benedict equations: Determine basal energy expenditure (BEE). BEE can be calculated using the following equations developed by Harris and Benedict:

$$\text{BEE (male)} = 66.5 + (13.8 \times W) + (5 \times H) - (6.8 \times A)$$
$$\text{BEE (female)} = 655.1 + (9.6 \times W) \, (1.9 \times H) - (4.7 \times A)$$
$$\text{when:}$$
$$W = \text{weight (kg)}; \ H = \text{height (cm)}; \ A = \text{age (yr)}$$

Then multiply the BEE by a stress factor that is estimated from the degree of stress and the need for weight maintenance or repletion. Multiplying the BEE by 1.2-1.5 provides a range appropriate for most patients. The lower factor is appropriate for patients without significant stress, whereas the higher factor is appropriate for patients with higher levels of stress, such as major trauma or sepsis. Individuals with burns may require an even higher stress factor (e.g., 2-3 times the caloric requirements of the BEE).

Distribution of calories: A relatively normal distribution of calories usually is adequate. Percentages of total calories from carbohydrates, protein, and fat should equal approximately 50%, 15%, and 35%, respectively. To avoid overfeeding, 30-35 kilocalories (kcal)/kg is appropriate for most critically ill patients.

- *Protein requirements:* Usually 1.5-2 g/kg/day.
- *Carbohydrate requirements:* Glucose administration of 5 mg/kg/min is a suitable amount. Carbohydrates provided in excess of this amount are not well utilized and may lead to hyperglycemia, excessive CO_2 production, hypophosphatemia, and fluid overload.
- *Fat requirements:* If protein and glucose are supplied as outlined, the remainder of needed calories can be supplied as fat. Fat can be administered in minimal quantities to satisfy needs for essential fatty acids, or it can be provided in larger quantities, as tolerated, to meet energy needs. Abnormal elevations in liver enzymes often occur in patients maintained on total parenteral nutrition (TPN) longer than 3 weeks. Usually the enzymes return to normal upon cessation of TPN. Giving cyclic TPN, in which the patient receives TPN for 12-16 h out of 24 h, may prevent enzyme elevation.

Vitamin and essential trace mineral requirements: In general, follow the Recommended Dietary Allowances (RDA) to provide minimum quantities of vitamins, minerals, and essential fatty acids. For specific patients, supplement specific vitamins or minerals needed in increased amounts for existing disease states (e.g., zinc and vitamins A and C for burns; thiamine, folate, and vitamin B_{12} for chronic alcohol ingestion).

Fluid requirements: Many factors affect fluid balance. All sources of intake (oral, enteral, intravenous, medications), as well as output (urine, stool, drainage, emesis, fluid shifts, respiratory and evaporative losses), must be considered.

Special diets for organ-specific pathology: Costly, and the metabolic advantages of some products remain unproven.

- *Hepatic failure:* Branched-chain amino acids in combination with reduced aromatic amino acid concentrations may help alleviate encephalopathy secondary to hepatic failure.
- *Renal disease:* High percentages of essential amino acids are used to improve nitrogen use and decrease urea formation.
- *Respiratory disease:* A low-protein and low-carbohydrate diet decreases CO_2 production and, consequently, the work of breathing.

NUTRITIONAL SUPPORT MODALITIES

Cost, safety, and convenience have been the rationale for enteral over parenteral nutritional support, but the potential physiologic benefits are a more compelling argument. The gastrointestinal (GI) system, believed by many to be dormant during stressful events, is metabolically, immunologically, and bacteriologically active. Studies indicate that enteral feedings prevent passage of bacteria from the GI tract into the lymphatic system and other organs, reducing a major source of sepsis and possible organ failure while fostering wound healing and immunocompetence.

Enteral formulas: Composed of a wide variety of standard and modular formulas. Also see Table 1-2.

- *Standard:* Include (1) blended whole food diets, which are less costly but have problems that include possible bacterial growth, solids that settle out, variation in nutrient composition, and the requirement of a large-bore tube for the viscous solution and (2) commercial formulas, which are sterile, homogenous, and suitable for small-bore feeding tubes and have a fixed nutrient composition.
- *Modular:* Consist of a single nutrient that may be combined with other modules (nutrients) to form a package tailor-made for an individual's specific deficits (e.g., carbohydrate, fat, protein, vitamin modules).

Nutritional composition

- *Carbohydrates:* The most easily digested and absorbed component in enteral formulas; 80% of all carbohydrates are broken down and absorbed as simple glucose in the normal intestine.

TABLE 1-2   Types of Enteral Formulations

Enteral formula	Description
Blenderized diet	
Compleat, Compleat Modified, Vitaneed	Nutritionally complete, requiring complete digestive capabilities; composed of natural foods, including meat, vegetables, milk, and fruit
Milk-based formula	
Meritene, Sustagen, Carnation Instant (if mixed with milk)	Nutritionally adequate diet for general nutritional support
Lactose-free formula	
Ensure, Entrition 1, Isocal, Osmolite	Nutritionally adequate, liquid preparation; used for general nutritional support; isoosmolar or hypoosmolar; all except Osmolite are low residue
Elemental or chemically defined	Nutrients tailored for specific needs
Criticare HN	Low-Na^+, lactose-free, high-N diet; 40% protein supplied as small peptides; nutritionally adequate; used for general nutritional support
Travasorb HN	Nutritionally adequate; used for general nutritional support; contains additional hydrolyzed protein that is readily digested and absorbed
Specialty formulas	
Hepatic failure	
Hepatic Travasorb	Nutritionally complete; has a greater ratio of branched chain to aromatic amino acids while restricting total amino acid concentrations and adding nonprotein calories

Modified from Webber KS. In Swearingen PL, Ross DG, editors: *Manual of medical-surgical nursing care: nursing interventions and collaborative management,* ed 4, St Louis, 1999, Mosby.

- ☐ *Lactase:* An enzyme that aids in the digestion of lactose and is deficient most commonly in African Americans, Asians, Native Americans, and Jews. A secondary form also may be found in individuals for whom large amounts of lactose are given in a milk-based diet. Symptoms include watery diarrhea, abdominal cramps, flatulence, fullness, nausea, stool with a pH of <6, and stool that tests positive for glucose.
- ☐ *Fiber:* Now included in many commercial preparations because it is claimed to be helpful in controlling blood glucose, reducing hyperlipidemia, and controlling bowel disorders, such as diverticula. These preparations are highly viscous and require a large-bore feeding tube, such as a 10 French (10 Fr) or an infusion pump. Begin the infusion slowly to reduce transient symptoms of gas and abdominal distention.
- • *Protein:* Three forms commonly are used:
  - ☐ *Polymeric:* Protein found in complete and original form (e.g., commercial and blenderized whole food diets that require normal levels of pancreatic enzyme).

TABLE 1-2   Types of Enteral Formulations—cont'd

Enteral formula	Description
Specialty formulas—cont'd	
Hepatic failure—cont'd	
Hepatic-Aid II	Nutritionally incomplete powder diet with essential nutrients in easily digestible form; high in branched chain amino acids; low in aromatic amino acids and methionines
Renal failure	
Renal Travasorb	Electrolyte, lactose, fat-soluble, vitamin-free; high in calories; contains mostly essential amino acids; restricted total protein content may reduce or postpone need for dialysis
Amin-Aid	Nutritionally incomplete supplement with essential nutrients in readily digestible form with minimal electrolytes
Respiratory insufficiency	
Pulmocare	Nutritionally complete; contains a higher proportion of fat to carbohydrates; reduces CO_2 production
Hypermetabolic and trauma states	
Trauma-Aid HB	High in branched chain amino acids; readily digestible essential nutrients
Trauma Cal	Nutritionally adequate with high proportions of protein and calories in a limited volume
Modular formulas	Offer highly flexible tailoring of nutrients (e.g., fat [Lipomul], protein [Pro Mod], and carbohydrates [Moducal]) for specific patient needs

□ *Hydrolyzed:* Protein that has broken down into smaller forms to assist absorption. It is helpful in short bowel syndrome or pancreatic insufficiency.
□ *Elemental:* Protein that requires no further digestion and is ready for absorption. It is most useful in hepatic and renal disorders.
- *Fat:* Two forms are the primary sources:
  □ *Long-chain triglycerides (LCT):* A major source of essential fatty acids, fat-soluble vitamins, and calories.
  □ *Medium-chain triglycerides (MCT):* Foster the absorption of fat but have fewer side effects of nausea and vomiting, abdominal distention, and diarrhea.

Types of feeding tubes and sites
- *Stomach:* Easiest for tube placement, simulates normal GI function, and may be used for intermittent or continuous feedings. The stomach is the site best reserved for patients who are alert, with intact gag and cough reflexes. Entry site is nasal, oral, or percutaneous.

- ☐ *Small bore:* Soft polyurethane or silicone with or without tungsten tip; designed for long-term use; size 6-12 Fr; length 36-45 in. Trade names include Keofeed, Dobbhoff. Some nasoenteric feeding tubes have a Y port added, allowing irrigation and medication administration without disconnecting the administration set. Examples include Flexiflow, Ross.
- ☐ *Large bore:* Stiff, polyvinyl chloride; size 10-18 Fr; used for short-term feeding of highly viscous fluids. One trade name is Levine.
- ☐ *Combination:* A soft silicone tube may be contained within a stiff outer tube that is removed, leaving the inner soft tube in place, or the tube may have a rigid guidewire that is removed after insertion. This tube is easier to place.
- ☐ *Gastrostomy:* A soft tube inserted directly into the stomach either temporarily or permanently. Problems include site difficulties, leakage, mobility, and catheter occlusion and expulsion.
- ☐ *Percutaneous endoscopic gastrostomy (PEG) tube:* Soft tube inserted into the stomach via the esophagus and then drawn through the abdominal skin using a stab incision.
- • **Small bowel:** Used for patients with diminished protective pharyngeal reflexes; the small bowel is less affected by postoperative ileus than the stomach and the colon. Tube placement is more difficult. Elemental formulas often are required for easier absorption. Continuous feedings are tolerated better inasmuch as the continuous drip approximates normal function. Entry sites are nasal, oral, duodenal, and jejunal.
  - ☐ *Small bore:* See "Stomach" on previous page. Some tubes have one port for feeding into the jejunum and a second port that allows for aspiration and decompression of the stomach.
  - ☐ *Duodenum/jejunum:* Minimizes risk of vomiting and aspiration compared with gastric feedings. A jejunostomy tube is soft, inserted into the jejunum, and not easily dislodged. Needle catheter (Witzel) jejunostomy is an alternative method of nutrient delivery and often is placed at the time of surgery. Percutaneous endoscopic jejunostomy (PEJ) is an additional means of placement.

Infusion rates: See Table 1-3.
Management of complications: See Table 1-4.
Parenteral nutrition (PN):   The postinjury metabolic stress response is said to peak at 3-4 days. Initiating nutritional support within 48 h can decrease morbidity in a previously well-nourished person who is critically ill. This is done by supplying nutrients to prevent catabolism of skeletal and visceral protein stores.

Parenteral nutrition provides some or all nutrients by peripheral venous catheter or central venous catheter (CVC) (1) to meet total nutritional needs in patients who cannot be given enteral support or (2) to supplement patients who cannot absorb enough calories using the GI tract.

- • **Parenteral solutions:** These solutions are derived from combinations of dextrose, amino acids, fat, electrolytes, vitamins, and trace elements. Total nutrient admixtures (TNA) are formulated by combining dextrose, fat, and amino acids in one container; or, alternately, dextrose and amino acids are combined and a separate delivery device is used for fat. An in-line filter cannot be used with TNA because it would trap lipid molecules.
  - ☐ *Carbohydrates:* Dextrose solutions 5%-50% are used to meet part of the patient's energy needs. With higher concentrations of dextrose the solution becomese hypertonic. Insulin demand and CO_2 and O_2 consumption are increased, which may lead to respiratory distress and hypermetabolism.
  - ☐ *Protein:* Synthetic crystalline essential and nonessential amino acid formulations are available in concentrations of 3%-15%. Special amino acid formulations for specific disorders are available (see "Estimating Nutritional Requirements," p. 4).
  - ☐ *Fat:* Lipid 10%-20% is an isotonic solution providing essential fatty acids and a source of concentrated calories. For best use and tolerance, lipids

TABLE 1-3	Methods and Rates of Administration for Enteral Products	
Type	Typical rate of administration	Comments
Bolus	250-400 ml 4-6×/day	May cause cramping, bloating, nausea, diarrhea, aspiration; not recommended for critically ill patients
Intermittent	120 ml isotonic formula with 30-50 ml H$_2$O; flush over 30-60 min	Starting regimen
	Advancement: Increase formula q8-12h by 60 ml if residual <½ volume of previous feeding	Should not exceed 30 ml/min; may cause cramping, nausea, bloating, diarrhea, aspiration
Continuous	40-50 ml/h, full strength, isotonic formula	Starting regimen
	Advancement: If serum albumin levels <2.5 g/dl or initial loose stools, dilute formula to 150 mOsm	Allows more time for absorption of nutrients

Modified from Webber KS: Providing nutritional support. In Swearingen PL, Ross DG, editors: *Manual of medical-surgical nursing care,* ed 4, St Louis, 1999, Mosby.

should be infused with carbohydrates and protein over no less than 8 h. The most common symptoms of an adverse reaction include febrile response, chills and shivering, and pain in the chest and back. A second type of adverse reaction occurs with prolonged use of IV fat emulsions and may result in a transient increase in liver enzymes, kernicterus, eosinophilia, and thrombophlebitis. Maintain the infusion rate at 1 ml/min for the first 15-30 min, and then increase it to 80-100 ml/h for the remainder of the first infusion.

Selection of feeding site

CVC: Used for infusion of large amounts of nutrients or electrolytes with smaller fluid volumes (hypertonic solutions) than with peripheral parenteral nutrition. The solution usually is delivered through a large-diameter vein (e.g., superior vena cava via the subclavian or jugular vein). The volume of blood flow rapidly dilutes the hypertonic solutions and decreases the irritation of vein walls. However, there are more complications with CVC than with the peripheral route. (See Table 1-6.)

Peripheral venous catheter: The need for low osmolality of solutions (<800 milliosmole [mOsm]/L) can limit usefulness. However, combining solutions of dextrose, amino acids, and lipids lowers the osmolality, providing a concentrated energy source that can be delivered through a peripheral vein, usually of the hand or forearm. This method is usually reserved for individuals who need partial or total nutritional support for short periods and for whom CVC access is unavailable.

Types of catheters: See Table 1-5.

TABLE 1-4   Management of Complications in the Tube-Fed Patient

Complication/possible causes	Suggested management strategy
Nausea and vomiting	
Fast rate	Decrease rate
Fat intolerance	Fat should compose no more than 30%-40% of total intake
Lactose intolerance	As prescribed, change to lactose-free product
Delayed gastric emptying	See **Risk for aspiration,** p. 15
Product odor	Mask with flavoring
Blocked tube	
Viscous formula/ medications: inadequate flushing	Flush tube with 50-150 ml water after each feeding/medication administration. Flush q4h with 30 ml water.
Instillation of crushed medications	Do not instill crushed medications in small-bore tubes. Substitute liquid preparations after consulting a pharmacist and prescriber. Some medications may be crushed into a fine powder and dissolved. Check with pharmacist, since crushing can alter medication characteristics. Never crush time-released medications. Incompatibilities between drugs and feeding formulas are possible.

TABLE 1-5   Catheters Used in Parenteral Nutrition

Catheter	Description
Subclavian/jugular	
Single lumen	Inserted at bedside. Multiple uses for specimen retrieval, feeding, and medication administration increase the risk of infection, especially in compromised patients
Multilumen	Inserted at bedside. Dedication of one lumen in this catheter is common practice, enabling other lumen(s) to be used for medication administration and laboratory monitoring
Right atrial (e.g., Hickman, Broviac)	Composed of silicone rubber with plastic external segment, which is implanted in OR. Its safety enables use by home care patients
Implantable (e.g., Infuse-a-Port, Port-a-Cath)	Implanted in OR. Designed for repeated access, making the need for repeated venipuncture unnecessary

Modified from Webber KS. In Swearingen PL, Ross DG: *Manual of medical-surgical nursing care,* ed 4, St Louis, 1999, Mosby.

TABLE 1-6 **Management of Complications in Patients Receiving Parenteral Nutrition**

Potential complications	Management strategy
Pneumothorax	Ensure that x-ray is done immediately after insertion. Determine placement of catheter before initiating feeding by monitoring for diminished or unequal breath sounds, tachypnea, dyspnea, and labored breathing.
Subclavian artery injury	If pulsatile, bright red blood returns into the syringe, assist with immediate removal of the needle and apply pressure for 10 min anteriorly and posteriorly at the point of penetration.
Catheter occlusion	If solution is infusing sluggishly, flush line with heparinized saline. check to see if line or tubing is kinked. If line is occluded, try to aspirate clot and contact health care provider, who may prescribe a thrombolytic agent.

Monitoring infusion rates: Using an infusion pump, PN is given at a consistent rate, with gradual acceleration of the infusion rate on initiation or deceleration on cessation over a 3-day period to avoid wide fluctuations in blood glucose. A typical rate is 50-100 ml/h, which increases 25-50 ml/h/day, depending on the patient's status.

Managing complications: See Table 1-6.

Electrolyte imbalances occurring in both enteral and parenteral nutrition: See Table 1-7.

TRANSITIONAL FEEDING

A period of adjustment is needed before discontinuing nutritional support. Taper enteral and parenteral nutrition as oral intake increases. Patients receiving parenteral nutrition may have some mucosal atrophy of the bowel and need a period of adjustment before the bowel can fully resume its usual functions.

NURSING DIAGNOSES AND INTERVENTIONS (FOR PATIENTS RECEIVING ENTERAL AND PARENTERAL NUTRITION)

Altered nutrition: less than body requirements, related to inability to ingest, digest, or absorb nutrients

Desired outcome: Within 7 days of initiating parenteral/enteral nutrition, patient has adequate nutrition as evidenced by level weight or steady weight gain of ¼-½ lb/day; improved or normal measures of protein stores (serum albumin 3.5 g/dl, transferrin 180-260 mg/dl, thyroxine-binding prealbumin 20-30 mg/dl, and retinol-binding protein 4-5 mg/dl); state of nitrogen balance as measured by nitrogen balance studies; presence of wound granulation; and absence of infection (see **Risk for infection,** p. 16).

- Ensure nutritional screening and assessment of patient within 72 h of admission; document. See "Nutritional Assessment," p. 1. Reassess weekly.
- Monitor electrolytes, blood urea nitrogen (BUN), and blood sugar daily until stabilized. Ensure that serum albumin, transferrin, or prealbumin and trace elements are monitored weekly. Document.
- Weigh patient daily.

T A B L E 1 - 7 Possible Electrolyte Imbalances Occurring in Enteral and Parenteral Nutrition

Sodium: Daily requirement is 60-150 mEq. Sodium is the primary extracellular cation in maintaining concentration and volume of extracellular fluid.

Complication	Pathophysiology/strategy
Hypernatremia	In PCM, patients have increased sodium because of extravascular volume expansion and intravascular volume depletion. Monitor sodium levels as depletion resolves, edema decreases, and diuresis occurs. Hypernatremia also occurs in patients receiving hypertonic tube feedings without adequate water supplements. **Sources:** Amino acid solutions contain varying amounts of sodium (up to 70 mEq/L); some antibiotics (e.g., sodium penicillin) also have a high sodium content (31-200 mEq/dl). Corticosteroids may cause sodium retention, and blood products can contain increased levels 130-160 mEq/L).
Hyponatremia	Can be a problem in patients with gastric suctioning and in those receiving diuretic agents or those with SIADH. **Replacement:** TPN solutions can replace sodium by using acetate, phosphate, or chloride salt form, depending on underlying disease state. The phosphate form should not be used in patients with renal failure. In acidemia, the acetate form is preferred to correct the imbalance.

Potassium: Daily requirement is 50-100 mEq. Potassium is the major intracellular cation required for neurotransmission, protein synthesis, cardiac and renal function, and carbohydrate metabolism.

Complication	Pathophysiology/strategy
Hyperkalemia	May be caused by excessive parenteral or enteral potassium supplementation or increased tissue catabolism, especially in renal insufficiency. **Sources:** Amino acid solutions contain potassium. Elevated potassium levels occur in patients receiving ACE inhibitors, heparin, cyclosporine, and potassium-sparing diuretics.

Hypokalemia	May occur during anabolism (tissue synthesis) in patients being refed. Potassium shifts into intracellular space, and patients require supplementation. It also may occur in patients with high GI losses or increased loss from diuretics. Potassium levels in patients with acid-base disorders may be misleading; potassium decreases by 0.4-1.5 mEq/L for every 0.1 increase in pH. **Replacement:** In daily TPN solutions, 80-120 mEq may be given to patients without renal problems. Potassium can be replaced using acetate, phosphate, and chloride forms, depending on the underlying disease state, but it should be titrated separately to avoid wasting TPN solutions. Infusion rates >0.5 mEq/kg/h are associated with cardiac irregularities.

Phosphorus: Daily requirement is 2.5-4.5 mg/dl. Phosphorus is required for release of oxygen from hemoglobin in the form of 2,3-diphosphoglycerate and for bone deposition, calcium regulation, and synthesis of carbohydrates, fats, and protein.

Complication	Pathophysiology/strategy
Hyperphosphatemia	Occurs in catabolic stress, renal failure, and hypocalcemia. Treatment involves ingestion of aluminum antacids, which bind phosphate in the intestine. **Sources:** Phosphorus-rich solutions, antacids, diuretic agents, and steroids.
Hypophosphatemia	A complication with a high mortality, often found in malnourished patients on refeeding. As the patient receives fluids containing dextrose, phosphorus shifts rapidly into the intracellular space, causing hypophosphatemia. **Replacement:** Phosphate-rich TPN solutions.

PCM, Protein-calorie malnutrition; *SIADH,* syndrome of inappropriate antidiuretic hormone; *TPN,* total parenteral nutrition; *ACE,* angiotensin-converting enzyme; *GI,* gastrointestinal.

Continued

T A B L E 1 - 7   Possible Electrolyte Imbalances Occurring in Enteral and Parenteral Nutrition—cont'd

Magnesium: Daily requirement is 18-30 mEq. Magnesium is required for carbohydrate and protein metabolism and enzymatic reactions.

Complication	Pathophysiology/strategy
Hypermagnesemia	Transient elevations can occur with use of diuretics or extracellular volume depletion. **Source:** Magnesium-containing antacids.
Hypomagnesemia	Low levels commonly occur in patients with severe malnutrition or lower GI losses and in those given insulin for hyperglycemia. For anabolism to occur, the body requires 2 mEq of magnesium per gram of nitrogen. **Replacement:** Parenteral magnesium.

Calcium: Daily requirement is 1000-1500 mg. Calcium is a necessary ingredient of the cells that play a major role in neurotransmission and bone formation.

Complication	Pathophysiology/strategy
Hypercalcemia	Occurs in thiazide diuretic use, prolonged immobilization, and decreased excretion. **Source:** Side effect of diuretic use.
Hypocalcemia	May occur from reduced total body calcium or reduced ionized calcium. It also occurs with hyperphosphatemia. A deficit can be misleading, inasmuch as serum calcium is bound to protein and varies with changing albumin levels. Also, in acidosis, a lower pH results in release of more calcium from protein, which elevates serum calcium levels. The opposite is true as pH rises. **Replacement:** Calcium-rich parenteral solutions.

- Record intake and output (I&O) carefully, tracking fluid balance trends.
- Administer formula within 10% of prescribed rate. Check volume infused and rate of infusion hourly.
- Ensure that patient receives the prescribed amount of calories.

Risk for aspiration related to GI bleeding; delayed gastric emptying; site of feeding tube

Desired outcome: Patient is free of aspiration problems as evidenced by auscultation of clear lung sounds; vital signs (VS) within patient's baseline; and absence of signs of respiratory distress.

- Check x-ray film for position of feeding tube before each feeding. Insufflation with air and aspiration of stomach contents do not confirm placement of feeding tubes. Mark and secure tubing for future reference.
- Assess respiratory status q4h, observing respiratory rate and effort and presence of adventitious breath sounds.
- Monitor for fever of unexplained origin q4h.
- Auscultate bowel sounds, percuss abdomen, and assess abdominal contour and girth q8h. Consult physician if bowel sounds are absent, the abdomen becomes distended, or nausea and vomiting occur.
- Elevate head of bed (HOB) ≥30 degrees during and for 1 h after feeding. If this is not possible or comfortable for patient, turn patient into a slightly elevated right side-lying position to enhance gravity flow from the greater stomach curve to the pylorus.
- Consult physician if residual feeding is >50% of the hourly feed. Hold the feeding for 1 h, and recheck residual.
- Stop tube feeding ½-1 h before chest physical therapy, suctioning, or placing patient supine.
- Discuss with physician the possibility of placing feeding tube well beyond the pylorus.
- As prescribed, administer metoclopramide HCl or other agents that promote gastric motility.

Diarrhea (or risk for same) related to bolus feeding; lactose intolerance; bacterial contamination; osmolality intolerance; medications; low fiber content
Desired outcome: Patient has formed stools within 24-48 h of intervention.

General
- Assess abdomen and GI status, including bowel sounds, distention, consistency and frequency of bowel movements, cramping, skin turgor, and other indicators of hydration.
- Monitor I&O status carefully.

Specific problems
- Bolus feeding: Switch to intermittent or continuous feeding method.
- Lactose intolerance: As prescribed, switch to lactose-free products.
- Bacterial contamination
  - ☐ Obtain stool sample for culture and sensitivity.
  - ☐ Use clean technique in handling feeding tube, enteral products, and feeding sets.
  - ☐ Change all equipment q24h.
  - ☐ Refrigerate all opened products but discard after 24 h.
  - ☐ Discard feedings hanging for >8 h.
- Osmolality intolerance
  - ☐ Determine osmolality of feeding formula. Most are isotonic (plasma osmolality 300 mOsm). If hypertonic, reduce rate. If problem continues, dilute to ½ formula and ½ water but maintain rate.
- Medications
  - ☐ Monitor use of antibiotics, antacids, antidysrhythmics, aminophylline, H_2-receptor blocker, potassium chloride, and use of sorbitol in liquid medications.

☐ As prescribed, administer *Lactobacillus acidophilus* to restore GI flora or use tincture of opium to decrease GI motility.
- Low fiber content: Add bulk-forming agents (psyllium or fiber preparations).

Impaired tissue integrity (or risk for same) related to mechanical irritant (presence of enteral tube)

Desired outcome: At time of discharge from critical care, patient's tissue is intact with absence of erosion around orifices, excoriation, skin rash, or mucous membrane breakdown.

Gastric/enteral tube
- Assess skin for irritation or tenderness q8h.
- Use a small-bore tube if possible.
- If long-term support is needed, discuss potential for using gastrostomy or jejunostomy tube with physician.
- Give ice chips, chewing gun, or hard candies prn if permitted.
- Apply petroleum jelly to lips q2h.
- Brush teeth and tongue q4h.
- Alter position of tube daily to avoid pressure on underlying tissue. Use hypoallergenic tape to anchor tube.

Gastrostomy tube/PEG
- Assess site for erythema, drainage, tenderness, and odor q4h.
- Monitor placement of tube q4h.
- Secure tube so there is no tension on patient's tissue and skin.
- Wash skin with soap and water daily; pat dry.

Jejunostomy tube/PEJ
- Assess site for erythema, drainage, tenderness, and odor q4h.
- Secure tube so there is no tension. Coil tube on top of dressing if necessary.
- Cleanse skin with half-strength solution of hydrogen peroxide and water; rinse hydrogen peroxide from skin; dry. Apply povidone-iodine ointment around insertion site daily and prn.
- Dress site with split 4×4s, and tape with paper or hypoallergenic tape.

Risk for infection related to invasive procedures or malnutrition

Desired outcome: Patient is free of infection as evidenced by temperature and VS within normal limits; total lymphocytes 25%-40% (1500-4500 µl); white blood cell (WBC) count ≤11,000/mm^3; and absence of the clinical signs of sepsis, including erythema and swelling at insertion site, chills, fever, and glucose intolerance.
- Ensure adequate nutritional support, based on individual needs. See "Nutritional Assessment," p. 1.
- Twice weekly and prn, monitor total lymphocyte count, WBC count, and differential for values outside normal range.
- Check blood glucose q6h for values outside normal range.
- Examine catheter insertion site(s) q8h for erythema, swelling, or purulent drainage.
- Use meticulous sterile technique when changing central line dressing, containers, or lines.
- Avoid using central line that is being used for nutritional support for blood drawing, pressure monitoring, or administration of medications or other fluids.
- Change all administration sets within the time frame established by agency. Rotate central insertion sites on a regular basis within agency recommendation.
- Culture specimens from the catheter tip and exit site prn.
- If sepsis is suspected, take blood specimens for culture and administer antibiotics as prescribed.

- Administer fat emulsion for the prescribed time period or period established by agency.

Altered cardiopulmonary tissue perfusion (or risk for same) related to interruption of arterial flow (air embolus)

Desired outcome: Patient has adequate cardiopulmonary tissue perfusion as evidenced by VS, arterial blood gas (ABG) values, and arterial oximetry within normal limits; and absence of dyspnea, tachypnea, cyanosis, chest pain, tachycardia, and hypotension.

- Check chest x-ray film to determine catheter position.
- Position patient in Trendelenburg position when changing tubing or when neck vein catheters are inserted or removed.
- Teach patient Valsalva maneuver (if possible) for implementation during tubing changes.
- Use Luer-Lok connectors on all connections.
- Use occlusive dressing over insertion site for 24 h after catheter is removed to prevent air entry via catheter-sinus tract.
- Monitor patient for chest pain, tachycardia, tachypnea, cyanosis, and hypotension.
- If air embolus is suspected, clamp the catheter and turn patient to left side-lying Trendelenburg position to trap air in the right ventricle. Administer high-flow oxygen and consult physician immediately.

Risk for fluid volume deficit related to failure of regulatory mechanisms; hyperglycemia; hyperglycemic hyperosmolar nonketotic syndrome (HHNS)

Desired outcome: Patient's hydration status is adequate as evidenced by baseline VS; glucose <300 mg/dl; balanced I&O; urine specific gravity 1.010-1.025; and electrolytes within normal limits.

- Weigh patient daily; monitor I&O hourly.
- Consult physician for urine output <1 ml/kg/h.
- Check urine specific gravity; consult physician for value >1.035.
- Monitor serum osmolality and electrolytes daily and prn; consult physician for abnormalities.
- Monitor for circulatory overload during fluid replacement.
- Monitor for indicators of hyperglycemia. Perform finger stick q6h prn until blood glucose is stable. Administer insulin as prescribed to keep blood glucose levels <200 mg/dl.
- Assess rate and volume of nutritional support hourly. Reset to prescribed rate as indicated.
- Provide 1 ml free water for each calorie of enteral formula provided (or 30-50 ml/kg body weight).

ADDITIONAL NURSING DIAGNOSES

For other nursing diagnoses and interventions, see "Fluid and Electrolyte Disturbances," p. 636, which includes discussion of the electrolyte abnormalities listed in Table 1-7.

Mechanical ventilation

To ensure optimal care of the patient who requires mechanical ventilation, the practitioner must have adequate knowledge of the equipment and processes involved in mechanical ventilation. An in-depth discussion of the entire process is beyond the scope of this book; therefore it is assumed that the reader has basic knowledge on which to build.

TYPES OF VENTILATORS

Three categories of ventilators are used to deliver oxygen and artificial respiration.

Volume cycled: Most widely used ventilator. It is designed to deliver a preset volume of gas (tidal volume). The machine continues to deliver the predetermined tidal volume independent of changes in airway resistance or lung compliance. The ventilator is equipped with safety valves that can be set to terminate inspiration when peak inspiratory pressures are excessive. Generally these pressure limits are set at 10-20 cm H_2O pressure over the patient's normal delivery pressure. The sophisticated design permits variable modes of delivery (see below).

Pressure cycled: Terminates inspiration once a preset pressure is reached, at which time the patient exhales passively. When airway resistance increases because of mucus secretions or bronchospasm, the inspiratory cycle may terminate before adequate tidal volume is delivered. This ventilator is used only for stable patients with normal lung compliance.

Negative pressure: Intrapleural pressure ranges from −2 to −10 cm H_2O. The positive pressure ventilators already discussed generate 5-10 cm H_2O pressure to deliver a breath. Negative pressure ventilators generate subatmospheric pressure to the thorax and trunk to initiate respiration and do not require intubation for use. The iron lung, chest cuirass shell, and poncho chest shell are examples. There has been a resurgence of interest in and use of these devices for long-term home therapy.

MODES OF MECHANICAL VENTILATION

Controlled mechanical ventilation (CMV):   Delivers a preset tidal volume at a preset rate, ignoring the patient's own ventilatory drive (the patient cannot trigger this machine). Its use is restricted to patients with central nervous system (CNS) dysfunction, drug-induced paralysis or sedation, or severe chest trauma for whom negative pressure–driven respiratory effort is contraindicated. This is the simplest but least frequently used mode.

Assist-control ventilation (ACV):   Delivers a preset tidal volume when the patient initiates a negative pressure respiratory effort (inspiration) or independently of the patient's effort if the preset time limit is reached. With adequate tidal volume delivery, work of breathing is decreased and alveolar ventilation improves. Machine sensitivity can be adjusted to prevent hyperventilation in patients whose respiratory rate increases because of mild anxiety or neurologic factors. If hyperventilation cannot be controlled, the patient may need to be changed to the mode that follows.

Synchronized intermittent mandatory ventilation (SIMV):   Delivers a preset tidal volume at a preset rate. In addition, between ventilator breaths the patient can breathe spontaneously (at his or her own rate and tidal volume) from an oxygen reservoir that is attached to the machine. The ventilator is synchronized to deliver the mandatory breath when the patient initiates inspiratory effort. Optimally, this mode prevents breath stacking caused by exhaling against machine-delivered inspirations. This is considered the standard mode of ventilation.

Positive end-expiratory pressure (PEEP):   Frequently used in conjunction with mechanical ventilation to improve ventilatory function of the lungs, thereby increasing partial pressure of oxygen in arterial blood (Pao_2). PEEP increases functional residual capacity (FRC) and compliance and decreases dead space ventilation and shunt fraction by applying a given pressure at the end of expiration. This pressure counteracts small airway collapse and keeps alveoli open to optimize gas exchange across the alveolar-capillary membrane, thereby decreasing shunting. This mechanism is effective for atelectatic alveoli, as well as for alveoli that are filled with fluid, but it does not improve lung function if the problem is one of poor perfusion. Generally, PEEP pressures range from 2.5 to 10 cm H_2O. Higher pressures (>35 cm H_2O) may be used if the patient can tolerate the increase and if the condition warrants. Application of PEEP increases intrathoracic pressure and compromises the patient's hemodynamic status by decreasing venous return, right ventricular filling pressures, and cardiac output. These mechanisms may cause or potentiate hypotension and shock, particularly in patients with volume depletion. PEEP also can cause pneumothorax if used at levels >10 cm H_2O or if lung compliance is diminished.

> **Note:** Continuous positive airway pressure (CPAP) functions in the same manner as PEEP but is a mode used independently of mechanically delivered breaths and is continuous throughout the respiratory cycle.

Pressure support ventilation (PSV):   Augments or supports a patient's spontaneous inspiration with a preselected pressure level. This pressure is applied beginning with the initiation of inspiration and ends when a minimum inspiratory flow rate is reached. The volume of inspired gas varies with the patient's inspiratory effort. The flow of gas begins once the patient's inspiratory pressure decreases to a preset level. Each breath must be triggered by the patient. The patient retains control over inspiratory time and flow rate, expiratory time, frequency, tidal volume, and minute ventilation. PSV creates less dyssynchrony than assist-control or SIMV and decreases inspiratory work by compensating for resistance from the demand valve or endotracheal tube size. PSV may be combined with SIMV to improve patient tolerance to mechanical ventilation and to decrease the work of breathing through the endotracheal tube. PSV may also be used alone for patients ready to attempt weaning.

High-frequency ventilation: Jet ventilation and high-frequency oscillation are alternative modes of ventilation in which small tidal volumes are delivered at high rates. The resulting lower airway and intrathoracic pressures may reduce the risk of complications secondary to barotrauma and circulatory depression, which are associated with the high peak airway pressures of conventional ventilatory modes. Tidal volume is low and minute ventilation is high, making this the ideal mode for ventilation of patients with major airway disruption. High-frequency ventilation requires the use of special ventilators and a specially designed endotracheal (ET) tube. The three basic mechanisms that are used are discussed in Table 1-8.

Inverse ratio ventilation (IRV):   Technique in which the inspiratory phase is prolonged and the expiratory phase is shortened. Normal inspiration/expiration (I/E) ratio is 1:2-4. During IRV the I/E ratio is increased to >1:1 (e.g., 2:1), thereby promoting alveolar recruitment, which improves oxygenation at lower levels of PEEP. The patient may require administration of a paralyzing agent and sedation to minimize the discomfort associated with this unusual breathing pattern.

COMPLICATIONS RELATED TO MECHANICAL VENTILATION

Barotrauma: Can occur when ventilatory pressures increase intrathoracic pressure, causing damage to major vessels or organs in the thorax and referring damage to the abdomen.

Tension pneumothorax: Develops when pressurized air enters the thoracic cavity. The high pressure of positive-pressure ventilation may blow a hole in diseased or fragile lung tissue, leading to this life-threatening complication. Symptoms include the usual indicators of pneumothorax, as well as sudden and sustained increases in peak inspiratory pressure.

> *Caution:*   If it is suspected that a pneumothorax has developed, disconnect the ventilator and manually ventilate using 100% oxygen while an assistant notifies physician. Prepare for immediate emergency chest tube placement.

Gastrointestinal complications: Peptic ulcers with profound hemorrhage may develop as a result of physiologic pressures and stress. Histamine H_2-receptor antagonists (e.g., cimetidine), and sucralfate (Carafate) routinely

TABLE 1-8   High-Frequency Jet Ventilation

Mode	Rate	Tidal volume	Mechanism
High-frequency positive pressure ventilation (HFPPV)	60-100 cpm	3-6 ml/kg	Pneumatically controlled valve connected to high-pressure gas source; pulses gas into airway while additional gases are entrained into the airway via a humidification circuit
High-frequency jet ventilation (HFJV)	100-200 cpm	50-400 ml	Gas under pressure is propelled through a narrow cannula (inserted in ET tube) while additional gases are entrained through a humidifier
High-frequency oscillations (HFO)	>200 cpm (800-3000 vibrations/ min)	50-80 ml	Gas is oscillated through ET tube via a piston; gas flows over the connection, and PEEP is created via resistant tubing on the outflow port; gas exchange occurs primarily by diffusion

cpm, Cycles per minute; *ET,* endotracheal; *PEEP,* positive end-expiratory pressure.

are administered to prevent these ulcers from developing. In addition, gastric dilation can occur as a result of the large amounts of air swallowed in the presence of an artificial airway. If gastric dilation is left untreated, paralytic ileus, vomiting, and aspiration may develop. Extreme dilation can compromise respiratory effort because of the restriction of diaphragmatic movement. Treatment includes insertion of a gastric tube and application of intermittent suction to the GI tract.

Hypotension with decreased cardiac output: Develops as a result of decreased venous return secondary to increased intrathoracic pressure. Generally, this phenomenon is transient and is seen immediately after the patient has been placed on mechanical ventilation. PEEP, especially at levels >20 cm H_2O, may increase the incidence and severity of this phenomenon because of the significant increase in intrathoracic pressure that occurs with its use. The goal for fluid therapy when PEEP is used is to maintain the least intravascular volume that allows for sufficient cardiac output to perfuse vital organs. Monitor heart rate (HR) and blood pressure (BP) hourly or more frequently if the patient is unstable. Monitor cardiac output as prescribed via flow-directed pulmonary artery (Swan-Ganz) catheter. See "Hemodynamic Monitoring," p. 28, for details regarding cardiac output.

Increased intracranial pressure: Occurs as a result of decreased venous return, which causes pooling of blood in the head. See "Traumatic Brain Injury," p. 118, for additional information.

Research Brief 1-1 A prospective observational cohort study of 242 ICU patients requiring mechanical ventilation compared duration of mechanical ventilation, ICU length of stay, hospital length of stay, hospital mortality, and acquired organ system derangements between two groups of patients: those receiving continuous IV sedation and those receiving intermittent bolus or no IV sedation. Analysis of data indicated adjusted duration of mechanical ventilation was significantly longer for patients receiving continuous IV sedation. Also, ICU stay was longer. The authors concluded that the use of continuous IV sedation may be associated with prolongation of mechanical ventilation.

From Kollef M et al: The use of continuous IV sedation is associated with prolongation of mechanical ventilation, *Chest* 114(2):541-548, 1998.

Fluid imbalance: Increased production of antidiuretic hormone (ADH) occurs as a result of increased pressure on baroreceptors in the thoracic aorta, which causes the system to react as if the body were volume depleted. ADH stimulates the renal system to retain water. Patients may need diuretics if signs of hypervolemia are present. Be alert to new symptoms of dependent edema or adventitious breath sounds.

Ventilator-acquired pneumonia: Studies indicate 70%-90% of mechanically ventilated patients have been colonized by hospital-acquired bacteria in the oropharynx, trachea, or digestive tract. Aspiration of bacteria from the oropharynx may be the leading cause of ventilator-acquired pneumonia. The onset of infection may have several mechanisms:

- Presence of an endotracheal/tracheostomy tube bypasses upper respiratory tract defense mechanisms of cough and mucociliary clearance action.
- Contaminated secretions pool above the endotracheal/tracheostomy tube cuff and leak into the lower respiratory tract.
- Supine positioning, the presence of a nasogastric tube, or reflux of bacteria from the stomach contribute to oropharyngeal colonization. Mechanically ventilated patients often receive prophylaxis for gastrointestinal bleeding, which alters the gastric pH. Use of sucralfate, which does not increase gastric pH, decreases the incidence of pneumonia when compared with antacids alone or in combination with hydrogen ion antagonists.
- Use of contaminated equipment/supplies, inadequate hand washing, or poor infection control practices may directly inoculate the tracheobronchial tree with pathogens.

Anxiety: Many individuals experience anxiety related to discomfort associated with loss of control over their ventilatory process and the perception that their health status is threatened. Hypoxemia and air hunger, if present, contribute to anxiety and prompt rapid, shallow, and often irregular respiratory efforts. Coordinated and effective ventilation may not be possible with severe anxiety and agitation. For these patients, aggressive sedation with potent pharmacologic agents may be necessary to reduce the work of breathing and facilitate effective mechanical ventilation. See "Sedating and Paralytic Agents," p. 38.

WEANING THE PATIENT FROM MECHANICAL VENTILATION

The weaning process can involve any of the following: oxygen, PEEP, mechanical ventilation, and the artificial airway. Successful weaning depends more on the patient's overall condition than on the technique used. Physiologic factors (cardiovascular status, levels of fluids and electrolytes, acid-base and nutritional status, as well as comfort and sleep pattern) and emotional factors (fear, anxiety, coping skills, general emotional state, ability to cooperate) are important and must be evaluated both before and during the weaning process.

T A B L E 1 - 9   Pulmonary Function Parameters for the Patient Being Weaned from Mechanical Ventilation

Pulmonary function	Optimal parameters	Definition
Minute ventilation	$\leq$10 L/min	Tidal volume $\times$ respiratory rate; if adequate, means patient is breathing at a stable rate with adequate tidal volume
Negative inspiratory force	$\geq$-20 cm H_2O	Measures respiratory muscle strength; maximum negative pressure that patient is able to generate to initiate spontaneous respirations; indicative of patient's ability to initiate inspiration independently
Maximum voluntary ventilation	$\geq$2 $\times$ resting minute ventilation	Measures respiratory muscle endurance; indicates patient's ability to sustain maximal respiratory effort
Tidal volume	5-10 ml/kg	Indicates patient's ability to ventilate lungs adequately
Arterial blood gases	Pao_2 $\geq$60 mm Hg $Paco_2$ $\leq$45 mm Hg pH 7.35-7.45 **or** patient's baseline	
Fractional concentration of inspired oxygen (Fio_2)	$\leq$0.40	

In addition, pulmonary function parameters must be met before the weaning process is begun (Table 1-9). Goals for the weaning process are listed in Table 1-10. Traditionally, three methods are employed for weaning the patient from mechanical ventilation.

Intermittent mandatory ventilation (IMV):   Ventilator-generated breaths are decreased gradually while the patient builds strength and endurance. This is the most widely accepted method for patients receiving long-term ventilatory support. If multiple failures at weaning occur, the T-piece method may be used (see p. 23), starting with 1-2 min off the ventilator, followed by 58-59 min on, with a gradual reversal of this ratio until the patient breathes independently.

PSV: Assists the patient's normal breathing pattern with positive airway pressure applied during inspiration; 3-5 cm H_2O pressure support is added to SIMV (see p. 18), which significantly decreases the work of breathing through the demand flow system and overcomes resistance of the endotracheal tube. Patients control their rate, inspiratory time, tidal volume, and inspiratory flow

TABLE 1-10 Goals for Weaning	
RR	<25 breaths/min
Tidal volume (V_T)	At least 3-5 ml/kg
HR/BP	Within 15% of baseline
Arterial pH	≥7.35
Pao_2	≥60 mm Hg and stable
$Paco_2$	≤45 mm Hg and stable
O_2 saturation	≥90%
Cardiac dysrhythmias	None
Use of accessory muscles of respiration	None

RR, Respiratory rate; *HR,* heart rate; *BP,* blood pressure.

rate. When the patient stops inspiring, the positive pressure stops. The amount of pressure support is gradually decreased as the patient is weaned from the ventilator.

T-piece method: A "T"-shape adapter is placed at the end of the ET tube. Patient is taken off the ventilator and initiates spontaneous respiratory effort for increasingly longer periods. In this manner the patient builds strength and endurance for independent respiratory effort. CPAP may be added to prevent alveolar collapse, thus allowing for more efficient gas exchange.

TROUBLESHOOTING MECHANICAL VENTILATOR PROBLEMS

The most important assessment factor in troubleshooting a mechanical ventilator is the effect on the patient. Regardless of which alarm sounds, always assess the patient first to evaluate his or her physiologic response to the problem. (See Tables 1-11 and 1-12 for processes that contribute to high-pressure and low-pressure alarm situations.)

NURSING DIAGNOSES AND INTERVENTIONS

Impaired gas exchange (or risk for same) related to altered oxygen supply secondary to nonphysiologic tidal volume distribution associated with mechanical ventilation

Desired outcome: Patient has adequate gas exchange as evidenced by Pao_2 >60 mm Hg; $Paco_2$ 35-45 mm Hg; Spo_2 ≥92%; Svo_2 ≥60%; and respiratory rate (RR) 12-20 breaths/min.

- Observe for, document, and report any changes in patient's condition consistent with increasing respiratory distress. (See "Clinical Presentation," in "Acute Respiratory Failure," p. 244.)
- Position patient to allow for maximal alveolar ventilation and comfort. Remember that in normal situations the dependent lung receives more ventilation and more blood flow than the nondependent lung; however, during mechanical ventilation the dependent portion of the lung receives less distribution of tidal volume than do the nondependent areas. Follow body positioning protocol.
  - ☐ Analyze Spo_2, Svo_2, and ABG results with patient in different positions to determine adequacy of ventilation.
  - ☐ Use postural drainage principles where appropriate.
  - ☐ In unilateral lung disease, position patient with healthy lung down.
  - ☐ In bilateral lung disease, position patient in right lateral decubitus position, inasmuch as the right lung has more surface area. If ABG results show that the patient tolerates left lateral decubitus position, alternate between the two positions.

TABLE 1-11   Processes Contributing to High-Pressure Alarm Situations

Increased airway resistance	Decreased lung compliance
Patient requires suctioning	Pneumothorax
Kinks in ventilator circuitry	Pulmonary edema
Water or expectorated secretions in circuitry	Atelectasis
Patient coughs or exhales against ventilator breaths	Worsening of underlying disease process
Patient biting ET tube	ARDS
Bronchospasm	
Herniation of airway cuff over end of artificial airway	
Change in patient position that restricts chest wall movement	
Breath stacking	

ET, Endotracheal.

TABLE 1-12   Processes Contributing to Low-Pressure Alarm Situations

Patient disconnected from machine
Leak in airway cuff
   Insufficient air in cuff
   Hole or tear in cuff
   Leak in one-way valve of inflation port
Leak in circuitry
   Poor fittings on water reservoirs
   Dislodged temperature-sensing device
   Hole or tear in tubing
   Poor seal in circuitry connections
Displacement of airway above vocal cords
Loss of compressed air source

- Turn patient q2h or more frequently if signs of deteriorating pulmonary status occur.
- Auscultate over artificial airway to assess for leaks.
- Assess ventilator for proper functioning and parameter settings, including Fio_2, tidal volume, rate, mode, peak inspiratory pressure, sigh volume and rate, and temperature of inspired gases. In addition, ensure that circuits are tight and alarms are set.
- Keep ventilator circuitry free of condensed water and expectorated secretions because these fluids may obstruct the flow of gases to and from the patient.
- Monitor serial ABG results. Be alert for decreases in Pao_2 or increases in $Paco_2$ with concomitant decrease in pH (<7.35), which can signal inadequate gas exchange. Also observe for decreased $Paco_2$ (<35 mm Hg) with increased pH (>7.45), which may signal mechanical hyperventilation. Notify physician of dysrhythmias, which can occur even with modest alkalosis if the patient

has heart disease or is receiving inotropic medications (see Appendix 7). Arrange for ABG analysis when change in patient's condition warrants.

- Keep manual resuscitator at bedside for ventilation in case of malfunctioning equipment.

Ineffective airway clearance (or risk for same) related to altered anatomic structure secondary to presence of ET or tracheostomy tube
Desired outcome: Patient maintains a patent airway as evidenced by absence of adventitious breath sounds or signs of respiratory distress such as restlessness and anxiety.

- Assess and document breath sounds in all lung fields at least q2h. Note quality and presence or absence of adventitious sounds.
- Monitor patient for restlessness and anxiety, which can signal early airway obstruction.
- Using sterile technique, suction patient's secretions, based on assessment findings, to maintain patency of airway. Document amount, color, and consistency of tracheobronchial secretions. Report significant changes (e.g., increase in production of secretions, tenacious secretions, bloody sputum) to physician. In addition, document patient's tolerance to suctioning procedure.
- Maintain artificial airway in a secure and proper alignment.
- Maintain correct temperature (32°-36° C [89.6°-96.8° F]) of inspired gas. Cold air irritates airways, and hot air may burn fragile lung tissue.
- Maintain humidification of inspired gas to prevent drying of tracheal mucosa. In addition, without humidification, tracheobronchial secretions may become thick and tenacious, creating mucous plugs that place patient at risk for development of atelectasis and infection.

Ineffective breathing pattern (or risk for same) related to anxiety secondary to use of mechanical ventilation
Desired outcomes: Patient exhibits stable RR of 12-20 breaths/min (synchronized with ventilator) and absence of restlessness, anxiety, lethargy, and/or sounding of high-pressure alarm.

- Monitor for evidence that patient is fighting ventilator: frequent sounding of high-pressure alarm when patient breathes against mechanical inspiration or mismatch of patient's respiratory rate and ventilator cycle.
- Monitor respiratory rate and quality, and monitor for signs of respiratory distress (e.g., tachypnea, hyperventilation, anxiety, restlessness, lethargy, and cyanosis, which is a late sign).
- Teach patient technique for progressive muscle relaxation (see **Health-seeking behavior**, p. 302). Stay with patient until the respirations are under control. Reassure patient that he or she will be able to synchronize respirations with the ventilator once he or she relaxes.
- Administer prescribed pain medication or sedation when prescribed for restlessness; restlessness increases O_2 demand and consumption, thus interfering with adequate ventilation.

Risk for infection related to increased environmental exposure (contaminated respiratory equipment); tissue destruction (during intubation or suctioning); invasive procedures (intubation, suctioning, presence of ET tube)
Desired outcome: Patient is free of infection as evidenced by normothermia; WBC count ≤11,000/mm^3; clear sputum; and negative sputum culture results.

- Assess patient for signs and symptoms of infection, including temperature >38° C (100.4° F), tachycardia (HR >100 beats per minute [bpm]), erythema of tracheostomy, and foul-smelling sputum. Document all significant findings.
- To minimize the risk of cross-contamination, wash hands before and after contact with the respiratory secretions of any patient (even though gloves were worn) and before and after contact with patient who is undergoing intubation.
- Maintain appropriate seal on artificial airway cuff to prevent aspiration of oral secretions.

- Keep cuff sealed and, unless contraindicated, HOB elevated 30-45 degrees, especially for patients receiving continuous gastric feedings. Monitor patient for reflux of feedings, as well as for signs of intolerance to feedings (absence of bowel sounds, abdominal distention, residual feedings >100 ml), which can precipitate vomiting and result in pulmonary aspiration of gastric contents.
- Recognize that bacteria and spores can be introduced easily during suctioning. Follow standard techniques:
  □ Use aseptic technique during suctioning process, including use of sterile catheter, gloves, and suctioning or lavage solutions.
  □ Suction tracheobronchial tree before suctioning the oropharynx to avoid introducing oral pathogens into tracheobronchial tree.
  □ Never store or reuse a single-use suction catheter. Consider use of closed system for suctioning.
  □ Change suction canisters and tubing within the time frame established by agency. Change canisters and tubing between patients.
  □ Tightly recap saline bottle used for suctioning. Be sure bottle is marked with date and time; dispose of unused portion within the time frame established by agency.
- To reduce the risk of infection caused by trauma or cross-contamination, suction on an "as needed" basis rather than routinely.
- Wash hand thoroughly and use sterile gloves when performing tracheostomy care to prevent colonization of stoma with bacteria from practitioner's hands.
- Provide oral hygiene at least q4-8h to prevent overgrowth of normal flora and aerobic gram-negative bacilli. Suction oropharynx to prevent pooling of secretions.
- Recognize ways that water reservoirs and ventilator equipment can be potential sources of contamination by following these precautions:
  □ Use sterile fluids in all humidifiers and nebulizers.
  □ Change all ventilatory circuitry within the time frame established by agency or sooner if soiled with secretions.
  □ Empty condensed water or expectorated secretions in tubes into attached traps. Avoid disconnecting tubing, and do not allow secretions to drain back into patient.
  □ Empty water traps on tubing during each ventilator check.
  □ When disconnecting patient from ventilatory circuits, keep ends of connectors sterile by placing them on opened sterile gauze pads. Avoid unnecessary disconnection.
  □ Keep connectors on manual resuscitator bags clean and free of secretions between use. Although no data suggest that bags be changed with any frequency when used for only one patient, they should not be used between patients without sterilization.
- Be aware of special risk factors for patients with tracheostomy tubes, and intervene accordingly:
  □ Maintain tracheostomy tube in a secure and proper alignment to avoid irritation of stoma from too much movement.
  □ Change tracheostomy ties q24h or more frequently if heavily soiled with secretions or wound exudate.
  □ Perform stoma care at least q8h, using aseptic technique until stoma is completely healed. Keep area around stoma dry at all times to prevent maceration and infection. Change stoma dressing as needed to keep it dry.
  □ Avoid use of cotton-filled gauze or other material that may shed small fibers. Patient may aspirate fibers, which in turn can lead to infection.
  □ Use aseptic technique (including use of sterile gloves and drapes) when changing tracheostomy tube.

- Culture secretions or wound drainage; administer antibiotics as prescribed.

Anxiety related to actual or perceived threat to health status as a result of need for or presence of mechanical ventilation

Desired outcomes: Within 12 h of initiation of mechanical ventilation, patient relates the presence of emotional comfort and exhibits a decrease in irritability, with a HR within patient's normal range.

- Because the general public equates ventilator placement with a hopelessly chronic, vegetative state, reassure patient and significant others that ventilatory support may be a temporary measure until the underlying pathophysiologic process has resolved. At that time the patient may be weaned from the ventilator.
- Reassure patient that he or she will not be left alone.
- Explain all procedures to patient and significant others before they are initiated. Inform patient of his or her progress.
- Describe and point out the alarm system, explaining that it will alert staff in the event of an accidental disconnection.
- Provide patient with mechanism for communication (e.g., picture board, erasable marker board, pen and paper). See **Impaired verbal communication** in "Psychosocial Support," p. 85.

Impaired gas exchange (or risk for same) related to altered oxygen supply secondary to weaning from mechanical ventilation

Desired outcome: Patient has adequate gas exchange as evidenced by Pao_2 >60 mm Hg; $Paco_2$ <45 mm Hg; Spo_2 ≥92%; Svo_2 ≥60%; and pH 7.35-7.45 (or values within 10% of patient's baseline).

- Maintain patient in a comfortable position to enhance ventilation. Many patients find that semi-Fowler's position promotes effective respirations.
- Observe for indicators of hypoxia, including tachycardia, tachypnea, cardiac dysrhythmias, anxiety, and restlessness.
- Assess and record VS q15min for the first hour of weaning, then hourly if patient is stable. Report significant findings to physician, such as increased respiratory effort, hyperventilation, anxiety, lethargy, cyanosis.
- Check patient's tidal volume after the first 15 min of weaning and as needed. Optimally, it will be within 5-10 ml/kg.
- Obtain specimen for ABG analysis 20 min after weaning has been initiated or as prescribed. As available, monitor Spo_2 and Svo_2 for values outside normal range.

Anxiety related to perceived threat to health status secondary to weaning process

Desired outcome: Within 4 h of initiation of weaning process, patient expresses the attainment of emotional comfort and is free of the signs of harmful anxiety as evidenced by HR ≤100 bpm; RR ≤20 breaths/min; and BP within patient's normal range.

- Before weaning process is initiated, discuss plans for weaning with patient and significant others. Explain that patient's condition will be assessed at frequent intervals during the weaning procedure. Provide time for questions and answers about the procedure.
- Stay with patient during the initial phase of weaning, keeping patient informed of progress being made. Provide positive feedback for positive efforts.
- Teach patient progressive muscle relaxation technique, which may reduce anxiety and fear and thus relax chest muscles. (See **Health-seeking behavior**, p. 302.)
- Instruct patient to take deep breaths if he or she is capable of doing so. This may provide the confidence of knowing that he or she can initiate and sustain respirations independently.
- Leave call light within patient's reach before leaving bedside. Reassure patient that help is nearby.

You may also wish to refer to the following interventions from the Nursing Interventions Classification (NIC):

NIC Acid-Base Management; Acid-Base Monitoring; Airway Management; Airway Suctioning; Anxiety Reduction; Aspiration Precautions; Bedside Laboratory Testing; Infection Control; Laboratory Data Interpretation; Mechanical Ventilation; Mechanical Ventilatory Weaning; Oxygen Therapy; Positioning; Respiratory Monitoring; Vital Signs Monitoring

ADDITIONAL NURSING DIAGNOSES

Also see nursing diagnoses and interventions under "Prolonged Immobility," p. 74; "Psychosocial Support," p. 83; and "Psychosocial Support for the Patient's Family and Significant Others," p. 95.

Hemodynamic monitoring

Many critically ill adults have cardiovascular disease or are at risk for cardiovascular complications; therefore it is important to be able to evaluate cardiac function and related factors. Four major cardiac mechanisms determine cardiac output (CO), which is the amount of blood ejected from the heart over 1 min. These mechanisms are preload, afterload, contractility, and heart rate.

Preload: Can be defined as the degree of myocardial fiber stretch at the end of diastole just before contraction. Starling's law of the heart describes the concept of preload: the greater the stretch of the myocardial muscle, the greater the force of contraction. However, if the stretch is excessive, contractility will diminish. This mechanism enables the heart to pump varying volumes of blood and to keep the output of the two ventricles matched. Preload is a function of the volume of blood delivered to the ventricle and the compliance (ability to stretch) of the ventricle at end diastole. Factors that affect ventricular volume include venous return, circulating blood volume, and atrial contractility. Factors that affect ventricular compliance include the stiffness and thickness of the cardiac muscle. Any problem that influences one of these factors will result in a change in preload, with a concomitant change in CO. Clinically, preload is described as ventricular end-diastolic pressure (VEDP), because pressure in the ventricle correlates closely with volume. Right ventricular diastolic (filling) pressure is reflected by the right atrial pressure (RAP) or the central venous pressure (CVP). Left ventricular diastolic (filling) pressure is reflected by the left atrial (LA), pulmonary artery diastolic (PAD), or pulmonary artery wedge (PAW) pressure measurements. Characteristics of preload are different in a diseased heart. A patient with biventricular heart failure cannot handle volume because of the low cardiac reserve. A stiff ventricle is very sensitive to volume changes. Diseased hearts will require greater fine tuning by the clinician.

Afterload: Refers to the pressure that develops within the ventricular myocardium during systole. For the heart to eject its contents, it must overcome any resistant forces. The pulmonary, aortic, and arterial pressures are the main impediments to flow for the right and left ventricles. Other resistant forces include blood viscosity, vascular resistance, distensibility of the vascular system, and the valves themselves. Because vascular resistance plays a major role in determining pressure, afterload is evaluated by calculating the pulmonary vascular resistance (PVR) for right ventricular afterload and systemic vascular resistance (SVR) for left ventricular afterload. The significance of these measures is that the higher the afterload, the greater the myocardial wall pressure and the greater the work of the heart to overcome resistance to flow. This work is achieved at the expense of oxygen utilization. When coronary blood flow (in a diseased heart) is diminished, an increased afterload may result in ischemic myocardial injury and possible infarction. Diseased ventricles are extremely sensitive to abrupt changes in afterload.

Contractility: Refers to the inherent capacity of the myocardium to contract. This mechanism functions independently of variations in preload and afterload. Although contractility cannot be measured directly, a change can be inferred when CO is decreased and other variables that affect CO (i.e., preload, afterload, heart rate) remain the same. Several factors positively influence contractility: sympathetic stimulation, calcium, positive inotropic agents such as digitalis and amrinone, and beta- (β-) adrenergic drugs. Factors such as acidemia, hypoxia, β-blocker drugs, and antidysrhythmic drugs decrease it.

Heart rate (HR): Alterations in HR affect myocardial functioning profoundly. Slight increases in HR with a constant stroke volume (SV) result in increased CO. Very rapid rates are associated with a reduction in CO as diastolic time is shortened, resulting in decreased coronary perfusion and reduced ventricular filling time. Bradycardia usually results in decreased CO unless there are increases in SV because of longer ventricular filling times. Increased heart rates require more oxygen but paradoxically may be receiving less oxygen. A heart rate of 100-130 bpm is often necessary to maintain a cardiac output appropriate to the oxygen demands of hypermetabolic states in the critically ill. Changes in any of the four components discussed produce significant hemodynamic deterioration and imbalance in myocardial oxygen supply and demand in patients with heart disease.

Hemodynamic monitoring refers to the specialized methods of evaluating cardiovascular performance. It provides information about cardiac performance, tissue perfusion, blood volume, tissue oxygenation, and vascular tone. Indirect methods of hemodynamic monitoring include measurement of arterial pressure via manual or automated BP cuff or Doppler test and measurement of CO with an echo Doppler device. Direct methods of measuring hemodynamic values include those obtained by arterial, central venous, and pulmonary artery catheters. This section focuses on direct methods of hemodynamic monitoring. Normal hemodynamic values with derived parameters are found in Table 1-13.

DIRECT HEMODYNAMIC MEASUREMENT

Arterial catheters: Generally inserted via the radial artery because this artery is readily accessible and collateral blood flow is usually adequate. Th arterial catheter may be inserted also in the femoral or brachial artery. The arterial pressure waveform is displayed on a bedside monitor for continuous observation of systolic, diastolic, and mean arterial pressures. The appearance of the arterial waveform is influenced by clinical conditions and mechanical factors. In hypertensive and hyperdynamic states, there is a steep rate of rise in the pressure waveform, as well as a high peak systolic pressure. In shock states or severe heart failure, the waveform is damped with a slow rate of rise. Dysrhythmias, such as premature ventricular complexes (PVCs), usually result in small, irregular waveforms associated with each abnormal contraction. Mechanical factors that influence the waveform include overdamping, catheter whip, and inaccurate calibration/zeroing (Table 1-14). Complications of arterial catheters include arterial thrombosis with ischemia, infection, infiltration, and blood loss caused by disconnection. Continuous observation of the arterial line insertion site for infection and leakage is an important nursing responsibility. Monitor and document pulses distal to the catheter site every 1 to 2 hours. It is important to know a patient's baseline blood pressure and to compare left and right cuff blood pressures with arterial blood pressures.

Systolic blood pressure: Determined by (1) the amount of blood ejected by the ventricle per beat (stroke volume), (2) wall compliance of the arterial system, and (3) peripheral resistance. Elevations in systolic pressure often reflect changes in vascular compliance, such as the hypertension seen in individuals with vascular atherosclerosis. A decrease in systolic pressure will be seen with heart disorders that result in decreased stroke volume or with the use of arterial vasodilators such as nitroprusside, nitroglycerin, and nifedipine.

TABLE 1-13   Hemodynamic Formulas

Parameter	Formula	Normal values
Cardiac output (CO)	$\dfrac{O_2 \text{ consumption}}{\text{A-V}o_2 \text{ difference}}$	4-7 L/min
Cardiac index (CI)	$\dfrac{CO}{\text{Body surface area (BSA)}}$	2.5-4 L/min/m^2
Coronary perfusion pressure (CPP)	Diastolic BP − PAWP	50-70 mm Hg
Stroke volume (SV)	$\dfrac{CO}{HR} \times 1000$	55-100 ml/beat
Stroke volume index (SVI)	$\dfrac{SV}{BSA}$	30-60 ml/beat/m^2
Arterial oxygen content (Cao_2)	(Hgb × 1.34) × Sao_2	18-20 ml/vol%
Venous oxygen content (Cvo_2)	(Hgb × 1.34) × Svo_2	15.5 ml/vol%
Oxygen delivery (Do_2)	Cao_2 × CO × 10	800-1000 ml/min
Oxygen delivery index (Do_2I)	Cao_2 × CI × 10	500-600 ml/min/m^2
Arteriovenous oxygen content difference (C[a-v]o_2)	Cao_2 − Cvo_2	4-6 ml/vol%
Oxygen consumption ($\dot{V}o_2$)	CO × 10 × C(a-v)o_2	200-250 ml/min
Oxygen consumption index ($\dot{V}o_2$I)	CI × 10 × C(a-v)o_2	115-165 ml/min/m^2
Systemic vascular resistance (SVR)	$\dfrac{MAP - RAP}{CO} \times 80$	900-1200 dynes/sec/cm^{-5}
Pulmonary vascular resistance (PVR)	$\dfrac{PAM - PAWP}{CO} \times 80$	60-100 dynes/sec/cm^{-5}

Diastolic blood pressure: Determined by (1) volume of blood within the arterial system, (2) compliance of the arterial wall, and (3) peripheral resistance. Because coronary artery blood flow occurs during diastole and a drop in diastolic pressure may result in ischemia of the subendocardium, diastolic BP is an important measure, particularly when vasodilating drugs are administered.

Mean arterial pressure (MAP):   The average pressure within the arterial tree throughout the cardiac cycle. It can be calculated by the following formula:

$$MAP = \frac{\text{Systolic BP} + 2(\text{Diastolic BP})}{3}$$

Normal value is 70-105 mm Hg. MAP reflects the average force that pushes blood through the systemic circulation throughout the cardiac cycle; therefore

TABLE 1-13 Hemodynamic Formulas—cont'd

Parameter	Formula	Normal values
Left ventricular stroke work index (LVSWI)	$SVI \times (MAP - PAWP) \times 0.136$	40-75 g/m²/ beat
Right ventricular stroke work index (RVSWI)	$SVI \times (MPAP - RAP) \times 0.136$	4-8 g/m²/beat
Mean arterial pressure (MAP)	$\dfrac{Systolic\ BP + 2(Diastolic\ BP)}{3}$	70-105 mm Hg
Mean pulmonary artery pressure (MPAP, PAM)	$\dfrac{PAS + 2(PAD)}{3}$	10-15 mm Hg
Mixed venous oxygen saturation (Svo_2)	$(CO \times Cao_2 \times 10) - \dot{V}o_2$	60%-80%
Central venous pressure (CVP)		2-6 mm Hg
Right atrial pressure (RAP)		4-6 mm Hg
Left atrial pressure (LAP)		8-12 mm Hg
Right ventricular pressure (RVP)		25/0-5 mm Hg
Pulmonary artery systolic pressure (PAS)		20-30 mm Hg
Pulmonary artery diastolic pressure (PAD)		8-15 mm Hg
Pulmonary artery wedge pressure (PAWP)		6-12 mm Hg

it is an important indicator of tissue blood flow. Because MAP is the product of $CO \times SVR$, an increase in CO or SVR will increase MAP and a decrease in either value will decrease MAP. Mean arterial pressure is the most accurate measurement of central aortic pressure, other than an intraaortic balloon pump (IABP).

Central venous catheters: CVP is the measurement of systemic venous pressure at the level of the right atrium (RA). CVP can be measured by a catheter that is threaded into the jugular, subclavian, or other large vein or by a separate port of a PA catheter. Normal value is 2-6 mm Hg. Because 60% of the blood volume is contained in the venous bed, the CVP is valuable in assessing fluid volume excess or deficit. In addition, it provides information regarding right ventricular (RV) function and venous tone. Disease processes that may increase CVP include right ventricular failure, cardiac tamponade, fluid volume overload, pulmonary hypertension, tricuspid valve disease, and chronic left ventricular failure. Usually, decreased CVP is caused by hypovolemia; however, venodilation caused by sepsis, drugs, or neurogenic causes also may decrease CVP. Complications of central venous catheters include venous

TABLE 1-14	Mechanical Problems Affecting Hemodynamic Measurements	
Problem	**Waveform appearance**	**Cause**
Overdamping*	Smaller than usual with a slow rise; diminished or absent dicrotic notch (arterial and pulmonary artery catheters)	Air bubbles in system Thrombus formation Lodging of catheter against vessel wall Kinking or knotting of catheter or tubing Loose connection in tubing or transducer Incorrect calibration Spontaneous catheter migration into a near-wedged position (PA catheter only)
Catheter whip	Erratic, "noisy" waveform with highly variable and inaccurate pressures	Spurious movement of the catheter tip within the vessel lumen (may require repositioning) Catheter too long for vessel (arterial)
No waveform	Complete absence of waveform	Large leak in the system, usually with blood backing up into the tubing Loose or cracked transducer or air in transducer Stopcock turned to wrong position Catheter tip or lumen totally occluded by clot Inadequate pressure (<300 mm Hg) on pressure bag Defective transducer or amplifier
Inability to obtain a wedged reading (PA catheter only)	Absence of wedge waveform after balloon inflation	Balloon rupture Retrograde catheter slippage

*Whenever the amplitude of an arterial or PA waveform decreases, the patient first should be assessed for hypovolemia or shock.

air embolism, dysrhythmias, hemorrhage, infection, vascular erosion, perforation of cardiac chambers, pneumothorax, and thromboembolic problems.
Pulmonary artery catheters: Inserted via the jugular, subclavian, or femoral vein and passed through the right side of the heart into the pulmonary artery, where the tip of the catheter is positioned in the pulmonary capillary bed. This catheter provides valuable information that can be used in the assessment or

TABLE 1-15 Abnormal Pulmonary Artery Pressures

Hemodynamic pressure	Normal range	Clinical conditions
PAS	20-30 mm Hg	*Increased:* right ventricular failure, chronic LV failure, constrictive pericarditis, cardiac tamponade, pulmonary hypertension (primary or related to lung disease) *Decreased:* hypovolemia, preload reduction
PAD*	8-15 mm Hg	*Increased:* left ventricular failure, mitral stenosis, left-to-right shunts, pulmonary hypertension (primary or related to lung disease) *Decreased:* hypovolemia, preload reduction
PAWP†	6-12 mm Hg	*Increased:* left ventricular failure, cardiac tamponade, mitral valve regurgitation, acute ventricular septal defect, fluid volume overload *Decreased:* hypovolemia, afterload reduction

PAS, Pulmonary artery systolic pressure; *PAD,* pulmonary artery diagnostic pressure; *PAWP,* pulmonary artery wedge pressure; *LV,* left ventricular.
*PAD may exceed PAWP by ≥5 mm Hg in patients with pulmonary hypertension, hypoxemia, acidosis, pulmonary emboli, and other lung disease.
†PAWP > PAD signals a mechanical problem (i.e., overwedging or improper identification of PAD).

treatment of life-threatening illness or injury during which assessment of blood volume, heart function, and tissue oxygenation is essential. Assessment data that may be derived from this catheter include RAP; right ventricular pressure (RVP); pulmonary artery mean (PAM); pulmonary artery systolic (PAS); pulmonary artery diastolic (PAD); PAWP; CO; core body temperature; and Svo_2. Other calculated hemodynamic and oxygen transport variables may be derived using PA catheter measurements (see Table 1-13). Abnormal pulmonary artery pressures are discussed in Table 1-15. Although the risk of major complications with this catheter is low (3%), it is important for the nurse to be familiar with the possibilities: ventricular or atrial dysrhythmias, pulmonary ischemia or infarction, pulmonic valve injury, endocarditis, tricuspid valve damage, pulmonary artery rupture, infection, and emboli (thrombotic, air, balloon) and pneumothorax.

Right atrial pressure: This is essentially the same as CVP. With the PA catheter, RAP can be monitored continuously and displayed on a bedside screen. In addition, the catheter lumen can be used for fluid or drug administration. Normal mean RAP is 4-6 mm Hg.

Right ventricular pressure: Measured during catheter insertion only and can provide information about the function of the right ventricle and the tricuspid and pulmonic valves. Normal RVP is 25/0-5 mm Hg. Elevation of right ventricular systolic pressure may be seen in pulmonic stenosis, pulmonary hypertension, or ventricular septal defect (VSD) with left-to-right shunt. Elevation of right ventricular diastolic pressure may occur with right ventricular failure, cardiac tamponade, or constrictive pericarditis. It is important for the nurse to identify the normal right ventricular waveform because a complication of the PA catheter is redirection of the catheter tip into the right ventricle, causing ventricular ectopy.

Pulmonary artery pressure: Used to evaluate left-sided heart function and pulmonary vascular disease. Normal pulmonary artery pressures are 20-30/8-15 mm Hg. In patients with healthy pulmonary vasculature, the PAD pressure corresponds closely to the PAWP and reflects the left ventricular end-diastolic pressure (LVEDP). A significant difference (i.e., >5 mm Hg) between the PAD and PAWP is seen with pulmonary disease or a pulmonary embolus. When this occurs, PA systolic and diastolic pressures are elevated, whereas the PAWP remains normal. Specific disease states that elevate PA pressures include pulmonary hypertension, pulmonary embolism, hypoxia, left ventricular failure because of valve disease, myocardial infarction (MI), cardiomyopathy, and left-to-right intracardiac shunt. Decreased PA pressures are seen with hypovolemia and pharmacologic preload reduction.

Pulmonary artery wedge pressure: Reflects the LVEDP and is used to evaluate cardiac performance. Normal mean PAWP is 6-12 mm Hg. An elevated PAWP may be seen with left ventricular failure, acute mitral regurgitation, acute VSD, and acute cardiac tamponade. A decreased PAWP is seen with hypovolemia and afterload reduction. PEEP/CPAP >10 cm H_2O may result in falsely elevated pulmonary artery pressures and PAWP. However, patients should not be disconnected from the ventilator to measure pulmonary artery pressures, because significant hypoxemia and inaccurate measurements can result. Correlation of measured pressures with the respiratory cycle improves the accuracy of these measurements.

Cardiac output: The volume of blood in liters ejected by the heart each minute and the product of the stroke volume (SV) and heart rate (HR). Normal value is 4-7 L/min. SV is the volume of blood ejected by the heart per beat. Normal SV is 55-100 ml/beat. To compare individual differences in CO in relation to body size, the CO is divided by the body surface area (BSA) to obtain the value known as the *cardiac index (CI).* Normal CI is 2.5-4 L/min/m^2. Continuous cardiac output monitoring is available. An average CO is recorded over 3-minute intervals and updated every 30-60 seconds. Continuous cardiac output monitoring provides a mechanism to closely and accurately monitor a patient's hemodynamic profile and respond quickly to changes demonstrated in 30-second intervals. Benefits of continuous cardiac output monitoring may outweigh the increased cost in select conditions (e.g., severe cardiomyopathy, ejection fractions [EFs] of less than 20 %), resulting in improved outcomes.

Systemic vascular resistance: The major factor that determines left ventricular afterload and therefore is the clinical measurement used to evaluate it. The formula for SVR is the following:

$$SVR = \frac{(MAP - RAP)}{CO} \times 80$$

Normal value for SVR is 900–1200 dynes/sec/cm^{-5}. Any factor that increases SVR will increase the workload of the heart; therefore other vasodilator therapy measures are taken to keep SVR within normal limits. Systemic vascular resistance should not be a sole determinant for treatment. SVR should be a part of the hemodynamic profile to determine the appropriate treatment.

Pulmonary vascular resistance: The clinical measure of right ventricular afterload. The formula for PVR is the following:

$$PVR = \frac{(PAM - PAWP)}{CO} \times 80$$

The normal value is 60-100 dynes/sec/cm^{-5} . PVR may be elevated as a result of mitral or aortic valve disease, congenital heart disease, long-standing left ventricular heart failure, hypoxia, chronic obstructive pulmonary disease (COPD), or pulmonary embolus. A number of drugs also may affect the PVR: norepinephrine and prostaglandins increase it, whereas isoproterenol, nifedipine, sodium nitroprusside, and acetylcholine decrease it.

Mixed venous oxygen saturation: Can be measured with the use of mixed venous blood samples from the distal port of the PA catheter or by continuous monitoring via a fiberoptic PA catheter. Svo_2 is the average percentage of Hgb bound with oxygen in the venous blood and is reflective of the patient's ability to balance oxygen supply and demand at tissue level. Normal range for Svo_2 is 60%-80%. Very low levels (<30%) usually are associated with lactic acidosis and a poor prognosis. Measurement of Svo_2 is valuable in the critical care setting because it can aid in the diagnosis and treatment of many life-threatening conditions. With continuous monitoring it can be used to evaluate the effects of medical and nursing interventions on tissue oxygen use. Four factors affect the oxygen supply-demand relationship and Svo_2 values: arterial oxygen saturation (Sao_2), CO, Hgb, and oxygen consumption ($\dot{V}o_2$). If the Svo_2 value changes by more than 10% and the change is sustained for more than 10 min, the nurse should evaluate each of the aforementioned factors and determine which are affecting Svo_2 (Table 1-16). Measurement of mixed venous oxygen saturation should not replace cardiac output measurement for treatment of patients with advanced heart failure.

Left atrial catheters: Inserted into the left atrium during cardiac surgery and brought through the chest wall or epigastric area. Left atrial pressure (LAP) is the most direct measure of LVEDP and may be indicated for the cardiac surgery patient with significant pulmonary hypertension. During connection to a transducer, a continuous display of left atrial pressure is possible. The normal value for LAP is 8-12 mm Hg. Because the catheter enters directly into the left atrium, the patient is at great risk for air or tissue emboli. An in-line air filter should be added to the flush system to reduce the risk of air emboli. If the waveform pattern dampens, aspirate until blood is seen. If there is no blood return, consult physician but do not flush.

NURSING DIAGNOSES AND INTERVENTIONS

Knowledge deficit: rationale for hemodynamic monitoring and procedure for catheter insertion

Desired outcome: Within 24 h of catheter placement, patient verbalizes knowledge of the rationale for hemodynamic monitoring; procedure for insertion of lines; and sensations that are experienced during and after the procedure.

- Assess patient's knowledge about hemodynamic monitoring. As indicated, explain to patient/family that hemodynamic monitoring is useful in guiding therapy and that the PA catheter can measure pressures in and near the heart.
- Teach patient about the insertion procedure, emphasizing that a local anesthetic agent will be used, he or she will not be able to move during the procedure, frequent x-rays will be taken, and a dressing will be applied to the insertion site. Explain to patient that a drape may be placed over patient's face for central or PA catheter insertion.
- Explain the sensations that may be felt during the procedure: a stick from injection of the local anesthetic, pressure as the catheter advances, coldness from the cleansing solution, burning from the injection of lidocaine, claustrophobia from drapes over the face, dull pushing and pulling sensations in the neck, and coldness from the injection of cardiac output iced solution (if used).
- Instruct patient to report any anxiety or discomfort that occurs during the procedure, because medications can be given as necessary.

TABLE 1-16   Factors Affecting Mixed Venous Oxygen Saturation

Factor	Effect on Svo_2	Clinical examples
Arterial oxygen saturation		
↑ Sao_2	↑ Svo_2	Supplemental oxygen
↓ Sao_2	↓ Svo_2	Reduced oxygen supply (e.g., ARDS, ET suctioning, removal of supplemental oxygen)
Cardiac output		
↑ CO	↑ Svo_2	Administration of inotropes to increase contractility
↓ CO	↓ Svo_2	Dysrhythmias, increased SVR, MI
Hemoglobin		
↓ Hgb	↓ Svo_2	Hemorrhage, hemolysis, severe anemia in patients with cardiovascular disease
Oxygen consumption		
↑ $\dot{V}o_2$	↓ Svo_2	States in which metabolic demand exceeds oxygen supply (e.g., shivering, seizures, hyperthermia, hyperdynamic states)
↓ $\dot{V}o_2$	↑ Svo_2	States in which there is failure of peripheral tissue to extract or use oxygen: • Significant peripheral arteriovenous shunting: cirrhosis, renal failure • Redistribution of blood away from beds where oxygen extraction occurs: sepsis, acute pancreatitis, major burns • Blockage of oxygen uptake or utilization: cyanide poisoning (including nitroprusside toxicity), carbon monoxide poisoning
Mechanical problems	Artifactitious ↑ Svo_2	Wedged PA catheter

ARDS, Acute respiratory distress syndrome; *ET,* endotracheal; *SVR,* systemic vascular resistance; *MI,* myocardial infarction; *CO,* cardiac output; *Hgb,* hemoglobin; *PA,* pulmonary artery.

Research Brief 1-2   The investigators examined the relationship between mixed venous oxygen saturation and cardiac output in patients with advanced heart failure and low ejection fractions. Simultaneous measurements of mixed venous saturation and cardiac output were compared in 42 patients. Similar correlations in the study groups suggest that changes in mixed venous oxygen saturation may not be reflected by concomitant changes in cardiac output. In patients with advanced heart failure and low ejection fractions, mixed venous saturation should not be substituted for measurement of cardiac output.

From Gawlinski A: Can measurement of mixed venous oxygen saturation replace measurement of cardiac output in patients with advanced heart failure? *Am J Crit Care* 7(5): 374-380, 1998.

Risk for infection related to presence of invasive hemodynamic catheters
Desired outcome: Patient is free of infection as evidenced by normothermia; WBC count ≤11,000/mm³; negative culture results; and absence of erythema, heat, swelling, or purulent drainage at the insertion site.

- Daily monitor temperature for elevations ≥37.7° C (100° F); WBC count for elevation; and catheter insertion site for erythema, tenderness to the touch, local warmth, and purulent drainage.
- As prescribed, obtain culture of any suspicious drainage and report positive findings.
- Use normal saline rather than D_5W for hemodynamic flush solution.
- Change hemodynamic tubing, transducer, and flush solution according to hospital protocol.
- Maintain closed system to transducer and for flush solution. Keep all external openings and stopcocks securely capped at all times.
- Use closed system for cardiac output injection fluid.
- Maintain occlusive, dry sterile dressing over insertion site.
- Change dressing per agency protocol, using aseptic technique.
- Record date of catheter insertion, and ensure that catheter is changed per agency protocol.
- If infection occurs, send catheter tip for culture and sensitivity test.

Altered cardiopulmonary tissue perfusion (or risk for same) related to interrupted blood flow secondary to migration of PA catheter into a wedged position, overwedging of balloon, continuous wedge position, or local vascular thrombosis
Desired outcome: Within 2 h of this diagnosis, patient has adequate pulmonary perfusion as evidenced by normal PA waveform and RR 12-20 breaths/min with normal depth and pattern (eupnea).

- Monitor PA waveform continuously. Report any change in configuration, particularly if the waveform becomes decreased in amplitude and flattened in appearance (see Table 1-14).
- Assess patient for interrupted pulmonary arterial blood flow as evidenced by acute onset of pleuritic chest pain, shortness of breath (SOB), tachypnea, and hemoptysis.
- Daily evaluate position of catheter via chest x-ray. Look for wedge-shaped infiltrate, which could signal impaired pulmonary tissue perfusion.
- Exercise care in taking PAWP measurements. Prolonged and repeated readings can cause trauma to the vessel wall. Another common problem is overwedging the catheter. Monitor PA waveform when wedging balloon. Inject enough air to obtain a wedge configuration but no more than the amount recommended by catheter manufacturer. Never pull back on plunger of syringe to remove air; disconnect syringe and allow passive deflation of balloon.
- Consider following trends of PAD pressures rather than those of PAWP. Verify correlation of PAD to PAWP q4-8h. Be aware that PAD may exceed PAWP by ≥5 mm Hg in patients with acidosis, hypoxemia, pulmonary emboli, lung disease, and pulmonary hypertension.
- Consult physician if PA waveform remains in wedged position after balloon deflation.
- Pay special attention to PA waveform when patient moves about (e.g., when being taken to x-ray department; getting into a chair).

Altered peripheral tissue perfusion (involved extremity) related to interrupted blood flow secondary to presence of arterial catheter or thrombosis caused by catheter
Desired outcome: Within 2 h of this diagnosis, patient has adequate perfusion to affected extremity as evidenced by brisk capillary refill (<2 sec); natural color; warm skin; normal sensation; and the ability to move the fingers.

- Continuously monitor capillary refill, color, temperature, sensation, pulses,

and movement. Be alert to indicators of ischemia, and teach them to the patient, stressing the importance of notifying staff members promptly if they occur.
- Maintain arterial line on continuous flush at 3 ml/h with heparinized normal saline (1 U heparin/ml saline or flush solution recommended by agency); ensure that pressure bag remains inflated at 300 mm Hg.
- Ensure tight connections of tubing throughout the system.
- Support patient's wrist or appropriate extremity with armboard or other supportive device to prevent flexion and movement of the catheter.

Risk for injury related to potential for insertion complications secondary to ventricular irritability, patient movement during insertion procedure, or difficult anatomy

> **Note:**   With PA or CVP catheter insertion, the following complications may occur: carotid artery puncture, air embolism, right ventricular perforation, hemorrhage, thoracic duct injury, pneumothorax, and cardiac tamponade. With PA catheter insertion, ventricular dysrhythmias may occur.

Desired outcome: Patient has no complications from PA or CVP catheter insertion as evidenced by normal sinus rhythm on ECG; BP within patient's normal range; HR ≤100 bpm; RR ≤20 breaths/min with normal pattern and depth (eupnea); normal breath sounds; and absence of adventitious breath sounds or muffled heart sounds.
- During preprocedure teaching, caution patient about the importance of remaining still during insertion of catheter. Provide sedation as prescribed.
- Perform a baseline assessment, monitoring BP, HR, RR, breath sounds, heart sounds, and ECG. Perform a postprocedure assessment, comparing it with baseline findings. Be alert to decreased BP, pulsus paradoxus (see Table 2-7, p. 145), increased HR or RR, diminished or absent breath sounds, and muffled heart sounds, as well as dysrhythmias on ECG. Report significant findings.
- After the procedure, obtain a chest x-ray as prescribed.
- Keep lidocaine at bedside for immediate IV injection if patient has sustained ventricular dysrhythmias.

Sedating and paralytic agents

Most, if not all, critically ill patients experience some degree of anxiety. Patients requiring critical care are severely ill or injured, and this realization alone promotes symptoms of anxiety in all but those who are deeply obtunded. Extreme anxiety, when outwardly expressed as agitation, restlessness, and increased random motor movement, may be termed *agitation syndrome.*

Anxiety and agitation in critically ill patients are prompted by emotional factors, including fear, loss of physical control, life-threatening illness, inability to communicate (e.g., mechanical ventilation), and feelings of helplessness. Common pathophysiologic factors contributing to agitation syndrome include hypoxemia, impaired cerebral perfusion, infection, alcohol withdrawal, and encephalopathy (Table 1-17). Inadequate pain control can often manifest as agitation. Environmental factors such as noise, temperature extremes, and sleep deprivation add to anxiety and agitation. Unrelieved stress, manifested in the form of anxiety or agitation, retards healing and can increase mortality.

Optimally, potential causes of agitation syndrome will be identified and alleviated or appropriately managed using nonpharmacologic methods. However, administration of potent drugs sometimes is necessary to relieve anxiety or agitation that is refractory to nonpharmacologic measures. See "Psychosocial Support," p. 83, for nonpharmacologic nursing interventions that should be used along with pharmacotherapy. The remainder of this section discusses use

TABLE 1-17　Pathologic Conditions Contributing to Agitation

Addison's crisis
Alzheimer disease
Anxiety disorder
Delirium tremens
Developmental disability
Drug intoxication
Fear
Encephalopathy
　Hepatic
　Metabolic
　Uremic
Hypercarbia
Hyperthyroidism
Hypoglycemia
Hyponatremia
Hypoxemia
Impaired cerebral perfusion
　Cerebral thrombosis
　Subarachnoid hemorrhage
　Intracranial bleeding
　Cerebral vasospasm
　Cerebral edema
Infection
　Meningitis
　Encephalitis
　Brain abscess
　Sepsis syndrome
Opiate withdrawal
Pain, inadequately controlled
Partial drug-induced paralysis
　Antibiotic (e.g., aminoglycosides)
　Electrolyte disorders (e.g., hypophosphatemia)
Sedative withdrawal
Sleep deprivation
Steroid psychosis

of sedatives in situations in which nonpharmacologic interventions are not entirely effective.

When pharmacologic sedation is necessary, the ultimate goal is to reduce anxiety and produce a calm but communicative state. This is best accomplished by administering frequent, incremental doses of sedatives just until the desired effects are achieved. Close monitoring, individualized dosing, and titration to desired effect are essential in avoiding oversedation and toxicity in critically ill patients. Major organ dysfunction, use of multiple medications, tissue catabolism, and other factors render critically ill patients particularly vulnerable to the toxic effects of many sedatives. Excessive sedation has been associated with delayed recognition of neurologic events, muscle wasting, and nosocomial complications, such as deep vein thrombosis, compression injury, and pneumonia.

ASSESSMENT

Anxiety: Subjective characteristics include increased tension, apprehension, fear, shakiness, uncertainty, distress, and feelings of helplessness. Objective findings include cardiovascular excitation, superficial vasoconstriction, pupil dilation, increased perspiration, restlessness, poor eye contact, tremors, extraneous motor movement, and facial tension.

Pain: Subjective description of pain by the patient. Use visual analog scale, numeric scale, and "happy faces" or other coded method to establish baseline and evaluate pain control. Objective findings include autonomic responses such as changes in BP and HR, increased or decreased RR, pupil dilation, increased perspiration, guarding, moaning, crying, restlessness, facial grimace, and rigid muscle tone.

Neuromuscular blockade: The level or depth of paralysis may be quantified using a device called a *peripheral nerve stimulator.* Typically a technique called the *train-of-four (TOF)* is chosen because it imposes the least discomfort. The TOF setting on the peripheral nerve stimulator will deliver four signals along the nerve path. The muscle response is then measured to evaluate how many signals are blocked compared with the number actually delivered. In the absence of neuromuscular blockade, the muscle should move four times equally in response to four signals. As receptors are loaded with neuromuscular blocking agents (NMBAs), fewer muscle contractions are seen (Table 1-18).

COLLABORATIVE MANAGEMENT

A variety of therapeutic options are available to produce sedation in critically ill patients. Alleviation of pain as a stimulus for anxiety/agitation is essential. Appropriate analgesics must be used for patients in whom pain is a component of agitation.

Opiate analgesics: Reliably relieve pain, are easily titrated, and have significant sedative effects. Morphine is widely used in intermittent bolus dosing and as a continuous infusion. Morphine has an active metabolite that accumulates in renal failure and should be reduced by fifty percent in these patients. Other opiates commonly used include meperidine (Demerol), hydromorphone (Dilaudid), and fentanyl citrate (Sublimaze). Demerol can accumulate with repeated doses, causing an increased risk of neurotoxicity, particularly in patients with renal failure. Demerol should not be used for more than 3 days, especially in elders. Fentanyl and hydromorphone are more rapidly taken up by the central nervous system and therefore are more potent than morphine.

Benzodiazepines: Relieve anxiety, promote sleep, and produce sedation by specific depressant effect on gamma (γ)-aminobutyric acid (GABA) and other nonspecific CNS depressant effects. Benzodiazepines produce muscle relaxation, which has the beneficial effect of reducing dosage requirements when NMBAs are used to induce paralysis. Dose-related effects on mental status range from relief of anxiety to sedation and coma. All benzodiazepines promote

TABLE 1-18   **Nerve Stimulation in Relationship to Percent Blockage**

Number of twitches	Percent blockage
4	0-50%
3	60%-70%
2	70%-80%
1	80%-90%
None	>90%

amnesia by preventing memory consolidation. This effect is particularly useful in patients undergoing unpleasant procedures. Midazolam (Versed) is reported to be superior to other benzodiazepines in preventing recall. Safety, ease of use, lack of paradoxic agitation, and lack of recall make benzodiazepines attractive choices for sedation in many critical care situations. They are the primary drugs used to alleviate symptoms of acute alcohol withdrawal. Table 1-19 describes specific characteristics of the widely used benzodiazepines.

- *Lorazepam (Ativan):* Most commonly given as an intermittent bolus but sometimes used as a continuous infusion. Lorazepam has no active metabolites; therefore in patients with advanced age or hepatic failure, drug effects do not seem to accumulate. Lorazepam has the slowest onset and the longest duration of action. Extreme caution should be used when administering lorazepam to the elderly, severely ill, and those with limited pulmonary reserve.

- *Diazepam (Valium):* Inexpensive but has a long half-life, which causes prolonged sedation. An active metabolite may result in prolonged sedative effects (up to 200 h after a given dose). Diazepam should be avoided in patients with liver dysfunction or severe heart failure because of reduced hepatic clearance. Limited solubility in water restricts use of standard formulation to intermittent IV bolus injections. A lipid suspension form of diazepam is now available. This formulation is less irritating to veins and may be used as a continuous IV infusion.

- *Midazolam (Versed):* Short acting and rapidly metabolized, which makes this drug particularly useful for short procedures, such as bronchoscopies and endoscopies. Because of its short half-life, continuous infusions are required to maintain sedation for longer periods. Delayed drug metabolism in some critically ill patients may lead to extended sedation, particularly with sepsis or hepatic impairment.

- *Chlordiazepoxide (Librium):* Sometimes used to manage agitation associated with alcohol withdrawal, which commonly contributes to agitation in the critically ill. When physiologically unstable patients are admitted to critical care, it is not always possible to obtain a clear history of alcohol use. The first clue may come 24-48 h later, when the patient becomes agitated and restless. However, because of chlordiazepoxide's relatively long half-life and several long-lived active metabolites, it is a poor choice for sedation and delirium tremens prophylaxis when compared with newer benzodiazepines that are safer and easier to titrate. Lorazepam (Ativan) generally is preferred because of its relatively short duration and simple metabolism.

TABLE 1-19 Benzodiazepine Characteristics

Benzodiazepines		Lorazepam (Ativan)	Diazepam (Valium)	Midazolam (Versed)
Dosage	**Intermittent**	0.5-1 mg, q1-2h	2.5-5 mg, q3-4h	0.15-0.35 mg/kg, q1-2h
	Continuous	0.25-2 mg/h 4-35 µg/min	N/A	0.03-0.22 mg/kg/h 0.5-4 µg/kg/min
Pharma-cokinetics	**Metabolism**	Hepatic	Hepatic	Hepatic
	Active metabolites	None	Yes	Yes
	Excretion	Renal	Renal	Renal

Anesthetic agents: Although there is no absolute definition of anesthesia, there are four general components: analgesia, amnesia, absence of pathologic reflexes (e.g., vagal response to pain), and lack of purposeful movement. Once restricted to surgical settings, forms of anesthesia increasingly are employed in critical care areas. Anesthesia can be accomplished via use of a single agent or by several combinations of drugs. Many anesthetics are restricted to use by or with the direct supervision of an anesthesiologist; however, one anesthetic, propofol (Diprivan), has been approved for sedation in mechanically ventilated patients. Propofol is often used in ICU for short-term sedation (several hours to 5 days).

- *Propofol:* A lipid suspension that is administered as a titratable, continuous infusion to provide a desired level of sedation to mechanically ventilated patients (Table 1-20). Patients usually awaken readily with prompt return to baseline mental function after sedation with propofol. Recovery time after prolonged infusion is not increased, in contrast to some benzodiazepines. Hemodynamic changes (e.g., vasodilation, decreased MAP) can be minimized by adequate hydration and slow increases in the infusion rate. This agent is particularly useful for patients with neurologic impairment, since the short action allows daily awakening to evaluate the underlying mental status. Propofol is not an analgesic, so pain medications should be considered. It is a lipid-base emulsion and is considered a caloric supplement. This should be taken into account when patients are receiving TPN in addition to propofol. Propofol accumulates more readily in obese patients; therefore dosing should be based on ideal body weight in the obese patient.

Antipsychotics: Have been used to reduce agitation in disoriented and agitated patients. Patients should be well hydrated to avoid hypotension associated with parenteral use of these drugs.

- *Haloperidol lactate (Haldol):* A butyrophenone antipsychotic that is especially helpful in managing psychosis and during withdrawal of sedatives. Incremental bolus doses or continuous infusions are used. IV route is considered investigational but has been widely used in critically ill patients because onset of action is rapid and extrapyramidal side effects occur less frequently than with the IM route. Haldol should be given cautiously to patients with severe cardiovascular disorders because of the possibility of transient hypotension and QT prolongation.

- *Chlorpromazine (Thorazine):* A phenothiazine sometimes used as a sedative, particularly if the patient also displays evidence, of psychosis.

TABLE 1-20   Propofol (Diprivan) Characteristics

*Dosage**		1-3 mg/kg/h
		5-50 µg/kg/min
Pharmacokinetics	**Metabolism**	Hepatic
	Metabolites	None
	Excretion	Renal
	Half-life	1.5-2h
Cardiovascular effects		Minimal: 15% ↓BP and
		MAP
		(short lived ≈ 15 min)
		(cause: ↓SVR and [−]
		inotrope)

*Propofol is a sedative-hypnotic at the above recommended dosages but is classified chemically as an anesthetic.

Chlorpromazine produces alpha (α)-receptor blockade, and hypotension is likely. For this reason and because it generally is less potent than haloperidol, chlorpromazine is not used frequently in critically ill patients.

Neuromuscular blocking agents: Used when longer periods of complete paralysis are necessary in mechanically ventilated patients. All possible causes of agitation (e.g., pain, fear, suctioning, hypoxemia) must be investigated thoroughly before neuromuscular blockade is initiated. Seek alternative means of management if feasible. NMBAs generally are used in the following situations: (1) to decrease oxygen consumption in patients who otherwise cannot obtain satisfactory oxygen saturation; (2) to alleviate specific medical conditions (e.g., status asthmaticus, tetanus, malignant hyperthermia, status epilepticus, acute respiratory distress syndrome [ARDS]); (3) to immobilize patients for surgical and invasive procedures; and (4) to manage increased intracranial pressure.

- *Depolarizing NMBAs:* Succinylcholine (Anectine) is the only depolarizing NMBA with widespread clinical use. It is used to produce rapid, brief paralysis, most often during emergent intubation. Long-term blockade is not practical because of rapid tachyphylaxis and desensitization of receptors to blocking effects.

- *Nondepolarizing NMBAs:* The class of NMBAs most commonly used in the critically ill patient. The most common agents used are pancuronium (Pavulon), vecuronium (Norcuron), and cisatracurium (Nimbex) (Table 1-21). Many drugs and certain physiologic states can augment or antagonize neuromuscular blockage in the critically ill patient (Table 1-22). These should be assessed continuously throughout the course of therapy.

Clinicians should determine a therapeutic endpoint or goal for paralysis and titrate neuromuscular blockade to achieve that goal. Examples of such therapeutic endpoints are decreases in peak inspiratory pressure, decreases in oxygen consumption, and inability to move. Monitoring the degree of neuromuscular blockade is essential. This can be done by using a peripheral nerve stimulator (see "Assessment," p. 40). Another commonly used method is providing a "drug holiday," to enable return of neuromuscular function to assess muscle strength. NMBAs provide no analgesia or anxiolysis. All patients receiving NMBAs must also have therapy with continuously dosed opiates and anxiolytics.

NURSING DIAGNOSES AND INTERVENTIONS

Anxiety related to actual or perceived threat of death; change in health status; threat to self-concept or role; unfamiliar people or environment; the unknown
Desired outcome: Within 4-6 h of initiating therapy, patient's anxiety is diminished as evidenced by verbalization of same; HR $\leq$100 bpm; RR $\leq$20 breaths/min; and decrease in restlessness and extraneous motor movement.

- Carefully assess for and correct factors contributing to anxiety (see Table 1-17).
- Evaluate adequacy of pain control. Administer opiate or other analgesics in small doses at frequent intervals.
- Initiate nonpharmacologic measures to reduce anxiety (see Table 1-35).
- Administer short-acting benzodiazepine in small doses at frequent intervals. Monitor carefully for excessive sedation and respiratory depression. Have flumazenil (Romazicon) immediately available for reversal of drug effects.
- If anxiety is profound and associated with sensory/perceptual alterations (e.g., hallucinations), consider use of antipsychotic agent. Ensure adequate hydration before use, and monitor closely for hypotension.

Impaired gas exchange (or risk for same) related to decreased oxygen supply secondary to decreased ventilatory drive occurring with sedative use and CNS depression or secondary to decreased chest wall movement occurring with residual neuromuscular blockade

TABLE 1-21 Neuromuscular Blocking Agent Characteristics

Neuromuscular blocking agents		Pancuronium (Pavulon)	Vecuronium (Norcuron)	Cisatracurium (Nimbex)
Dosage	**Intermittent**	0.04-0.1 mg/kg q1h prn	0.01-0.015 mg/kg q15min	.03 m/kg q15min
	Continuous	1-1.6 µg/kg/min	0.8-1.2 µg/kg/min	.5-10 µg/kg/min
Pharmacokinetics	**Metabolism**	Renal > Hepatic	Hepatic > Renal	Hoffman (organ independent) Elimination
	Excretion	Renal	Renal (15%) Biliary (30%-50%)	
	Metabolites (active or toxic)	Yes	Yes	No
	Half-life (elimination)	132-257 min (2-4h)	80-97 min	22-29 min
Cardiovascular effects		Moderate ↑HR, ↓BP, ↑CO	Minimal <1% ↑HR, ↓BP	None on HR and MAP

Important comments:
1. Pancuronium is by far the most cost-effective paralytic agent, followed by vecuronium.
2. Norcuron is 24× as expensive as Pavulon. Nimbex is 53× as expensive as Pavulon.
3. Nimbex is preferred in patients with hepatic or renal dysfunction.

TABLE 1-22 Drugs and Physiologic Conditions That Affect NMBAs

Drugs that augment neuromuscular blockade

Aminoglycoside antibiotics	Lidocaine
Bretylium	Procainamide
Calcium channel blockers	Propranolol
Clindamycin	Quinidine
Cyclosporine	Vancomycin

Drugs that antagonize neuromuscular blockade

Anticholinesterase agents	Phenytoin
Azathioprine	Ranitidine
Carbamazepine	Theophylline
Corticosteroids	

Physiologic conditions that increase neuromuscular blockade

Acidosis	Hypokalemia
Dehydration	Hyponatremia
Hypercalcemia	Hypothermia
Hypermagnesemia	Myasthenia gravis
Hypocalcemia	

Physiologic conditions that decrease neuromuscular blockade

Alkalosis	Hypernatremia
Hyperkalemia	Decreased peripheral perfusion

Research Brief 1-3 The effect of drug administration on cerebrovascular response to endotracheal suctioning in adults with severe head injuries was studied. The study involved three groups: those who received no drugs, those treated with opiates, and those treated with neuromuscular blocking agents plus opiates. Changes in intracranial pressure were significantly smaller in those who received neuromuscular blocking agent plus opiates than in subjects who did not receive a drug or those who received opiates only. The authors of the study support the use of NMBAs in patients with head trauma and call for additional research in this area.

From Kerr M et al: *Am J Crit Care* 7(3):205-217, 1998.

Desired outcome: Within 1 h of intervention, patient has adequate gas exchange as evidenced by orientation to time, place, and person; Pao_2 ≥80 mm Hg; $Paco_2$ 24-30 mm Hg; Spo_2 ≥90; and RR 12-20 breaths/min with normal depth and pattern (eupnea).

- Assess patient's respiratory rate, depth, and rhythm at least qh when heavily sedated. Fully sedated patients require continuous direct monitoring until VS are stable and protective reflexes (e.g., gag reflexes) are present.
- If NMBAs are used, assess depth of paralysis using peripheral nerve stimulator. Titrate dose to maintain desired level of paralysis (see Table 1-18).
- Continuously monitor Spo_2 via pulse oximetry. Alternatively, monitor chest wall movement via apnea monitor. Have appropriate antidote (e.g., naloxone for opiates, flumazenil for benzodiazepines, and pyridostigmine and atropine for NMBAs) and airway management equipment immediately available.
- Position patient to promote full lung expansion, and turn patient to mobilize sputum. Encourage deep breathing at frequent intervals.

Knowledge deficit: lack of recall, related to interrupted memory consolidation secondary to benzodiazepine use

Desired outcome: Within 12 h of cessation of benzodiazepine therapy, patient recalls information essential to self-protection and self-care.

- Remind patient and family that recall of unpleasant procedures (e.g., cardioversion, endoscopy) will be diminished and that this is a desired effect of the medication.
- Reinforce necessary information (e.g., NPO instructions, need to call for assistance when changing positions, need for deep breathing) with patient and family at frequent intervals until comprehension is demonstrated.
- Review outcome or findings of procedure with patient as necessary until patient expresses satisfactory understanding.

Alterations in consciousness

Consciousness is a state of awareness of self and the environment that consists of three components: arousal (appearance of wakefulness), ability to detect and encode internal and external perceptions, and the ability to perform goal-directed behavior. Changes in any of the three components caused by physiologic, psychologic, or environmental factors are considered alterations in the state of consciousness and result in a broad spectrum of syndromes including coma, delirium, and agitation. Factors precipitating various alterations in consciousness are listed in Table 1-23. Because of the many complications and safety issues surrounding it, impaired consciousness in the hospitalized patient is associated with longer hospital stays and higher morbidity and mortality.

ASSESSMENT

History and risk factors

- *Age:* Elders more prone to alterations in consciousness especially with changes in environment or for those who have sundowner's syndrome.
- *Brain injury:* Lesions of the cortex, subcortex, and brainstem caused by global or focal ischemia, stroke, or traumatic brain injury.
- *Cerebral disorders:* Deteriorating brain condition, such as an expanding lesion.
- *Cardiovascular status:* Disorders that lower cardiac output, procedures that cause postcardiotomy delirium, intraaortic balloon pump sequelae, states of lowered perfusion (lowered MAP), and dysrhythmias.
- *Pulmonary disorders:* Those causing hypoxia and hypoxemia.
- *Drug therapy:* Sedation, analgesia, drug toxicity, drug interactions, and drug sensitivity.
- *Surgical factors:* Nature and extent of surgery and anesthesia time.
- *Perceptual/sensory factors:* Sleep deprivation, sensory overload, sensory deprivation, impaired sensation (hypesthesia, decreased hearing or vision), impaired perception (inability to identify environmental stimuli), and impaired integration (inability to integrate environmental stimuli).
- *Metabolic factors:* Changes in glucose level, hypermetabolism, hypometabolism, and endocrine crises.
- *Fluid and electrolyte disturbances:* Sodium and potassium imbalances, hypovolemia.

Clinical presentation

- *Delirium/acute confusional state:* A state of disordered attention that reflects an underlying acute or subacute process. A usually transient condition that may be persistently prolonged that develops along the continuum of clouding of consciousness, attention deficit, global cognitive impairment, and psychosis. Defining characteristics include disorientation to time, place, and person;

TABLE 1-23 Factors Precipitating Alterations in Consciousness

Confusion
>   Age
>   Aggressive and dominant personality
>   Anesthesia time
>   Cardiac dysrhythmia
>   Body temperature
>   Cerebral disorders
>   Fluid and electrolyte imbalances
>   Drugs
>   Metabolic disturbances
>   Pulmonary disorders
>   Number of intensive care days
>   Sleep deprivation

Delirium
>   Cerebral disorders
>   Metabolic disorders
>   Toxins
>   Electrolyte imbalances
>   End-stage disease (renal, liver)
>   Pulmonary disorders
>   Impaired communication
>   Withdrawal syndromes
>   Drugs
>   Neuropsychiatric disorders

Stupor
>   Diffuse organic cerebral dysfunction
>   Confused with the catatonic behavior of schizophrenia or severe depressive reaction

Coma
>   Central nervous system dysfunction
>   Cerebral structural changes (brain injury)
>   Cerebrovascular impairment (hemorrhage, ischemia, or edema)
>   Metabolic conditions

Vegetative state (coma vigil)
>   Coma related to cerebral or metabolic disorders

Locked-in syndrome
>   Supranuclear motor deefferentation related to brainstem injury

disorganized thinking; fear; irritability; misinterpretation of sensory stimuli (e.g., pulling at tubes and dressings); appears distracted; altered psychomotor activity; altered sleep-wake cycles; memory impairment; hallucinations; inappropriate communication (e.g., yelling, swearing, nonsensical speech); and dreamlike delusions. Lucid intervals alternate with episodes of delirium. Patients may have difficulty following commands. Daytime drowsiness is contrasted with nighttime agitation. Clinical variants of delirium include the quiet form, hyperactive-hyperalert form, hypoactive-hypoalert form, and a combination form that includes lethargy and agitation.

- *Stupor:* Characterized by deep sleep with responsiveness only to vigorous and repeated stimuli with return to unresponsiveness when the stimulus is removed. Stupor usually is related to diffuse organic cerebral dysfunction but may be confused with the catatonic behavior of schizophrenia or the behavior associated with a severe depressive reaction.
- *Coma:* Manifestation of an alteration in arousal and diminished awareness of self and environment to such an extent that no understandable response to external stimuli or inner need is elicited. There is no language spoken, no covert or overt attempt to communicate, and no eye opening; there is no spontaneous purposeful movement or localizing movements. Motor responses to noxious stimuli do not result in recognizable defensive movements but are entirely reflexive. Sleep-wake cycles are absent on the electroencephalogram (EEG). The extent of coma, however, is difficult to quantify because limits of consciousness are difficult to define and self-awareness can only be inferred from appearance and actions. Coma occurs when normal central nervous system (CNS) function is disrupted by cerebral structural changes (brain injury), cerebrovascular impairment (hemorrhage, ischemia, or edema), or metabolic conditions (hepatic encephalopathy). If coma persists for longer than 4 weeks, it is defined as transitioning to a vegetative state.
- *Minimally conscious state (MCS):* MCS is a term used to describe patients who demonstrate inconsistent but reproducible behavior indicating awareness of self and environment. Generally they cannot reliably follow commands or communicate but show visual fixation and tracking, and emotional and behavioral responses to external stimuli. Once the patient consistently follows commands, uses a reliable communication method, and uses objects in a functional way, the minimal conscious state ends. Although the etiology is uncertain, MCS seems to be related to diffuse, bilateral, subcortical, and hemispheric damage.
- *Akinetic mutism (AM):* A subcategory of MCS, AM is characterized by a decrease in spontaneity and initiation of actions, thoughts, speech, or emotion despite sparing of sensory motor function. Visual tracking and eye movements are intact, and there is occasional speech and movement to commands. However, internally guided behavior is absent because cortical activation is inadequate. AM is associated with orbito-mesial frontal cortex, limbic system, and reticular formation lesions.
- *Vegetative state (VS):* Vegetative state is a subacute or chronic condition that either follows the coma of brain injury or occurs independently of coma as in dementia. Transition from coma to VS occurs if coma persists for longer than 4 weeks. Onset of VS is signaled by a return of wakefulness (eyes are open and sleep patterns may be observed) and return of spontaneous control of autonomic function but there is no observable signs of cognitive function. The patient cannot follow commands, offers no comprehensible sounds, and displays no localization to stimuli. There is complete loss of meaningful interaction with the environment. The vegetative state may exist for many years because the autonomic and vegetative functions necessary for life have been preserved.
- *Locked-in syndrome (LIS):* Characterized by paralysis of all four extremities and the lower cranial nerves but with preservation of cognition. Associated with deefferentation (disruption of the pathways of the brainstem motor neurons), this condition prevents the patient from communicating with a full range of language and body movement. Generally, consciousness, vertical eye movement, and eyelid blinking are intact and provide a mechanism for communication. LIS is classified by the degree of voluntary speech and motor function preservation. In complete LIS there is total immobility and anarthria. In incomplete LIS there is vertical eye movement and blinking function. LIS can be distinguished from a vegetative state because patients

TABLE 1-24   Mental Status Component of the Neurologic Examination

1. General appearance
2. Behavior (with and without stimulation)
3. Language and speech characteristics (organization, coherence, and relevance)
4. Mood and affect
5. Judgment
6. Abstract thinking
7. Orientation (time, place, person)
8. Attention and concentration
9. Memory (recent, remote)
10. Cognition (following commands, fund of knowledge, interpretation of information, problem solving)

give appropriate signs of being aware of themselves and their environment. Often, sleep patterns are disrupted.

Physical assessment: Requires a thorough evaluation of mental/emotional status, cranial nerve function, motor function, sensory function, and reflex activity. Baseline neurologic findings elicited from each component of the examination must be documented. When alterations in consciousness are manifested, the mental/emotional component of the examination is of particular importance. However, in patients who are unconscious or demonstrate low-level function, assessment techniques that do not require patient participation must be used. These may include coma and cognitive functioning scales. Minimally, the purpose of the assessment is to determine the extent of wakefulness and cognition through observed responses, such as eye opening, movement of the head and body, verbalization, and ability to follow commands. However, these observations alone will not fully discriminate the subtle differences in altered states of arousal and should be accompanied by an in-depth history focusing on the possible etiology of the change in cognition. Extensive cognitive testing including attention and concentration and memory and learning assessments will be performed when the patient has manifested arousal and awareness behavior.

- *Mental status testing:* A subjective assessment requiring patient cooperation for maximal results. See Table 1-24.
- *Mini mental status examination:* Objective neuropsychologic tool that measures orientation, recall, attention, calculation, and language. Scores less than 23 (total 25) indicate cognitive dysfunction. Patient participation is necessary to complete this examination. See Table 1-25.
- *Glasgow coma scale:* Quantitative, three-part scale that assesses the best eye opening, motor, and verbal responses. Scores range from 3 to 15, with 3 being unresponsive and 15 being awake, alert, and oriented. Patients who are unable to cooperate can be evaluated using this scale. See Appendix 3.
- *Coma recovery scale:* Quantitative 35-item scale that assesses the presence or absence of a physical sign that represents brain function at four levels (generalized, localized, emergent, cognitively mediated). Seven responses are evaluated: arousal and attention, auditory perception, visual perception, motor function, oromotor ability, communication, and initiative. Patients who are unable to cooperate can be evaluated using this scale.
- *Confusion assessment method:* A four-part scale that evaluates confusion related to onset and course, inattention, disorganized thinking, and level of consciousness.

TABLE 1-25   Mini Mental Status Examination

1. What is the year, season, date, day, month (5 points)
2. Where are we: state, county, town, hospital, room (5 points)
3. Name three objects (3)
4. Count backward by sevens (e.g., 100, 93, 86, 79, 72) (5 points)
5. Repeat same three objects from number 3 above (3 points)
6. Name a pencil and watch (2 points)
7. Follow a three-step command (3 points)
8. Write a sentence (1 point)
9. Follow the command "close your eyes" (1 point)
10. Copy a design (e.g., two hexagons) (1 point)

- *Rancho Los Amigos (RLA) cognitive functioning scale:* An eight-level scale that describes levels of cognitive functioning from unresponsive to sensory stimuli to purposeful/appropriate actions. Patients who cannot cooperate can be evaluated using this scale. See Table 1-26.

DIAGNOSTIC TESTS

Neurodiagnostic testing: See "Traumatic Brain Injury," p. 118.

Neuropsychologic testing: Although not a routine part of critical care, neuropsychologic testing should be anticipated and planned for during the recovery phase for patients with brain injury or alterations in consciousness. This testing serves as a comprehensive baseline for rehabilitation by evaluating higher cortical function, such as memory, learning, and language.

COLLABORATIVE MANAGEMENT

For confusion: Underlying physiologic imbalances or drug interactions are determined and corrected. Once these are eliminated, care should focus on any sensory/perceptual deficits (e.g., use of hearing aid, eyeglasses) and reorientation techniques that include orientation to self and environment.

For delirium: Underlying physiologic imbalances, drug interactions, and sensory/perceptual impairment are determined and corrected. Reorientation techniques to self and environment also are instituted. Neuropsychologic evaluation should be performed and appropriate drug therapy initiated (see "Sedating and Paralytic Agents," p. 38).

For coma: Determination of cognitive function based on the RLA score or coma recovery score should guide interventions. Low-level cognitive function (RLA I, II, and III or low coma recovery score) requires initiation of a sensory stimulation program (see box, p. 54), whereas higher scores such as an RLA IV (confused/agitated) require a structured program that minimizes stimulation. A rehabilitation consultation that includes physical, occupational, and speech therapy evaluations enables a plan of care that prevents or minimizes problems related to the injury, such as spasticity or swallowing disorders, or complications of immobility, such as disuse syndrome, contractures, and pressure ulcers.

For locked-in syndrome: Establishment of a communication pattern is a critical element. A mental health consultation should be obtained to assist in intervening with the psychologic sequelae that could accompany this syndrome. A rehabilitation consultation (see "Coma," above) also is indicated. Providing a normal day/night routine will help minimize sleep-wake cycle disturbances.

For vegetative state: Neurodiagnostic and neuropsychologic testing should confirm this diagnosis. Although the long-term prognosis is not optimistic for the majority of these patients, supportive care, which minimizes such complications as pressure ulcers and aspiration, is essential. A stimulation

TABLE 1-26 Cognitive Rehabilitation Goals

Level	Response	Goal/intervention
I	None	*Goal:* Provide sensory input to elicit responses of increased quality, frequency, duration, and variety.
II	Generalized	
III	Localized	*Intervention:* Give brief but frequent stimulation sessions, and present stimuli in an organized manner, focusing on one sensory channel at a time; for example:
		Visual: Intermittent television, family pictures, bright objects
		Auditory: Tape recordings of family or favorite song, talking to patient, intermittent TV or radio
		Olfactory: Favorite perfume, shaving lotion, coffee, lemon, orange
		Cutaneous: Touch or rub skin with different textures such as velvet, ice bag, warm cloth
		Movement: Turn, ROM exercises, up in chair
		Oral: Oral care, lemon swabs, ice, sugar on tongue, peppermint, chocolate
IV	Confused, agitated	*Goal:* Decrease agitation, and increase awareness of environment. This stage usually lasts 2-4 wk.
		Intervention: Remove offending devices (e.g., NG tube, restraints), if possible. Do not demand patient follow-through with task. Provide human contact unless this increases agitation. Provide a quiet, controlled environment. Use a calm, soft voice and manner around patient.

Modified from Rancho Los Amigos Hospital, Inc, Levels of Cognitive Functioning (scale based on behavioral descriptions or responses to stimuli). From Swift CM: Neurologic disorders. In Swearingen PL, editor: *Manual of medical-surgical nursing care,* ed 4, St Louis, 1999, Mosby. *ROM,* Range of motion; *NG,* nasogastric. *Continued*

program for low-level cognitive function, including visual, auditory, tactile, gustatory, and vestibular stimuli, may be initiated (see box, p. 54).

NURSING DIAGNOSES AND INTERVENTIONS

Sensory/perceptual alterations related to physiologic changes; psychologic changes; environmental changes; sensory deprivation; sensory overload; drug interactions

TABLE 1-26 Cognitive Rehabilitation Goals—cont'd

Level	Response	Goal/intervention
V VI	Confused, inappropriate Confused, appropriate	*Goal:* Decrease confusion and incorporate improved cognitive abilities into functional activity. *Intervention:* Begin each interaction with introduction, orientation, and interaction purpose. List and number daily activity in the sequence in which it will be done throughout the day. Maintain a consistent environment. Provide memory aids (e.g., calendar, clock). Use gentle repetition, which aids learning. Provide supervision and structure. Reorient as needed.
VII VIII	Automatic, appropriate Purposeful	*Goal:* Integrate increased cognitive function into functional community activities with minimal structuring. *Intervention:* Enable practicing of activities. Reduce supervision and environmental structure. Help patient plan adaptation of ADL and home living skills to home environment.

ADL, Activities of daily living.

Desired outcomes

    Cognitive ability: Ability to execute complex mental processes

    Cognitive orientation: Ability to identify person, place, and time

    Communication ability: Ability to receive, interpret, and express spoken, written, and nonverbal messages

    Information processing: Ability to acquire, organize, and use information
If cause of alteration in consciousness is extracerebral event, within 72 hours of this diagnosis, patient's level of arousal and cognition improve and patient responds consistently and appropriately to stimuli. If cause is cerebral, increased arousal and improvements in cognition may take days to weeks.

NIC Electrolyte Management; Delirium Management; Confusion Management; Environment Management; Reality Orientation; Cognitive Stimulation

• Eliminate environmental causes of sensory/perceptual deficit.

    ☐ Assess patient for potential causes of sensory/perceptual deficits. For the hearing- or vision-impaired patient, wearing eyeglasses or hearing aids will decrease misinterpretation of visual and auditory stimuli.

    ☐ Assess environment for potential causes of disorientation and confusion. Maintain day/night environment as much as possible. Keep clocks and calendars within patient's field of vision.

- Develop a plan of care consistent with sensory/perceptual deficit.
  - ☐ Assess patient for sensory deprivation and sensory overload. Decrease or increase stimulation based on RLA assessment (see box, p. 54) and patient's needs. For example, agitated and confused individuals require structure and reorientation interventions, whereas those who are comatose or stuporous require stimulation techniques.
  - ☐ Orient patient to time, place, and person during all interactions. Explain procedures in terms patient can understand.
  - ☐ Teach significant others reorientation and sensory stimulation strategies, and provide liberal visitation to facilitate their assistance.
  - ☐ Assess underlying cause of confusion or delirium before using sedation, antianxiolytic, analgesic, or antipsychotic drug therapy (see "Sedating and Paralytic Agents," p. 38). Also see "Psychosocial Support," p. 83, for this nursing diagnosis.

▌NIC Cognitive Restructuring; Cognitive Stimulation; Environmental Management; Reality Orientation; Dementia Management

Impaired verbal communication related to neurologic deficits

Desired outcome: If cause of alteration in consciousness is extracerebral event, within 72 h of this diagnosis, patient communicates needs and feelings and exhibits decreased frustration and fear related to communication barriers. If cause is cerebral, improvement in communication may take days to weeks.

- Determine underlying cause of impaired communication, including physiologic (cortical, brainstem, or cranial nerve injury) or psychologic (depression, fear, or anger).
- When communicating with these patients, use their name, face them, use eye contact if they are awake, speak clearly, and use a normal tone of voice.
- Be alert to nonverbal messages, especially eye movement, blinking, facial expressions, and head and hand movements. Attempt to validate these signals with the patient.
- Assure patient that you are attempting to find methods that promote communication if patient's needs cannot always be understood.
- For the patient who does not respond to or acknowledge verbal stimulation, continue communication attempts.
- Teach significant others methods of communication, and encourage them to continue attempts at communication.
- Brainstem-evoked potentials and audiometry (hearing test) can provide useful information related to a patient's ability to receive and process auditory stimuli. Detection and treatment of otitis media in patients who have ET tubes will improve hearing.
- Obtain a speech therapy consultation to assess nature and severity of communication impairment and assist in developing a communication plan. Special attention is required for individuals with locked-in syndrome.
- Obtain a mental health consultation to assist with patient who is angry, frustrated, and fearful because of the communication impairment.

▌NIC Communication Enhancement: Speech Deficit; Support System Enhancement

Impaired physical mobility related to perceptual or cognitive impairment; imposed restrictions of movement

Desired outcome: By the time of discharge from the critical care unit, patient demonstrates ROM and muscle strength within 10% of baseline parameters.

- Assess muscle strength and tone to determine type of interventions required. Consult physical therapy and occupational therapy for evaluation and treatment plan.
- Manage decreased muscle tone (flaccidity):
  - ☐ Maintain body alignment and positioning.
  - ☐ Perform passive range-of-motion (ROM) and stretching exercises.
  - ☐ Avoid prolonged periods of limb flexion.
  - ☐ Apply splints and other adaptive devices to maintain functional position of the extremities.

SENSORY STIMULATION (SS) PROGRAMS AS AN INTERVENTION TECHNIQUE IN THE CRITICALLY ILL

STRONG EVIDENCE	INSUFFICIENT EVIDENCE	RECOMMENDATIONS
SS programs appear to be safe to administer.	There is still no clear evidence that increased arousal is brain injury recovery or SS program enhanced recovery.	SS programs can be initiated as an adjunct therapy.
SS programs do not increase ICP or CPP and do not affect HR or BP.	It is unclear how the time when SS was started (early or late) influences outcome.	SS program can be incorporated into daily nursing routine
A positive trajectory of recovery has been documented in all studies.	It is unclear how the type of program (multimodal or unimodal) influences outcome.	Use rest periods between sessions to diminish fatigue.
	It is unclear what type of stimulation is most useful for increasing arousal (e.g., novel, familiar music, voices).	Stop intervention if an unstable medical status develops, and resume when patient is stable.
	It is unclear how long daily stimulation should last (concentrated or multiple short sessions).	Include family in intervention program.

From Davis A, Gimenez A: *Auditory sensory stimulation in comatose brain-injured patients.* Manuscript in preparation,1998; Kater K: Response of head-injured patients to sensory stimulation, *West J Nurs Res* 11(1):20-33, 1989; Lewinn E, Dimancescu M: Environmental deprivation and enrichment in coma, *Lancet* 2:156-157, 1978; Mackay L et al: Early intervention in severe head injury: long-term benefits of a formalized program, *Arch Phys Med Rehabil* 73:635-641, 1992; Mitchell S et al: Coma arousal procedure: a therapeutic intervention in the treatment of head injury, *Brain Inj* 4:273-279, 1990; Schinner K et al: Effects of auditory stimuli on intracranial pressure and cerebral perfusion pressure in traumatic brain injury, *J Neurosci Nurs* 27(6):348-354, 1995; Sosnowski C, Ustik M: Early intervention: coma stimulation in the intensive care unit, *J Neurosci Nurs* 26(6):336-341, 1994; Wilson S et al: Vegetative state and responses to sensory stimulation: an analysis of 24 cases, *Brain Inj* 10(11):807-818, 1996.
ICP, Intracranial pressure; *CPP,* cerebral perfusion pressure; *HR,* heart rate; *BP,* blood pressure.

☐ Turn patient q2h.
☐ Consider chair sitting as the patient stabilizes.
- Manage increased muscle tone (spasticity):
    ☐ Avoid supine position; use side-lying, semiprone, prone, and high Fowler's positions.
    ☐ Position limbs opposite flexion posture.
    ☐ Use skeletal muscle relaxant, such as baclofen (Lioresal), as prescribed for decreasing tone.
- Monitor calcium and alkaline phosphatase levels. Increased levels can lead to the development of heterogenous ossification, which often is seen with states

of impaired mobility, such as spinal cord injury. See "Fluid and Electrolyte Disturbances," p. 636.
* Maintain patient's skin integrity. See "Wound and Skin Care," below.
* Prevent pulmonary complications in the following ways:
  ☐ Encourage coughing and deep breathing if patient is able, or suction as needed.
  ☐ Assess swallowing ability before initiating oral feedings. Obtain dysphagia consultation (usually from a speech therapist) if swallowing reflexes are impaired.
  ☐ Initiate enteral feeding protocol for patients with feeding tubes to prevent aspiration. See "Nutritional Support," p. 1.

NIC Bed Rest Care; Positioning; Exercise Promotion; Self-Care Assistance

ADDITIONAL NURSING DIAGNOSES

Also see nursing diagnoses and interventions under "Nutritional Support," p. 1; "Sedating and Paralytic Agents," p. 38; "Prolonged Immobility," p. 74; and **Risk for disuse syndrome,** in "Traumatic Brain Injury," p. 132.

Wound and skin care

A wound is a disruption of tissue integrity caused by trauma, surgery, or an underlying medical disorder. Wound management is directed at preventing infection and/or deterioration in wound status and promoting healing.

WOUNDS CLOSED BY PRIMARY INTENTION

Clean surgical or traumatic wounds whose edges are closed with sutures, clips, or sterile tape strips are referred to as wounds closed by *primary intention.* Impairment of healing most frequently manifests as dehiscence, evisceration, infection, or delayed healing. Individuals at high risk for disruption of wound healing include those who are obese, diabetic, elderly, malnourished, receiving steroids, immunosuppressed, or undergoing chemotherapy or radiation therapy. Coexistent infections at another body site and colonization with microorganisms such as methicillin-resistant *Staphylococcus aureus* (MRSA) are factors that may contribute to the development of infection.

ASSESSMENT

Optimal healing: Immediately after injury, the incision line is warm, reddened, indurated, and tender. Inflammation normally subsides in 3 to 5 days. A healing ridge, a palpable accumulation of scar tissue, forms by postinjury day 7 to 9. In patients who undergo cosmetic surgery, a healing ridge is purposely avoided to minimize scar formation. See Table 1-27.
Impaired healing: Lack of an adequate inflammatory response; continued drainage from the incision line 2 days after injury (when no drain is present); absence of a healing ridge by day 9 after injury; presence of purulent drainage. See Table 1-27.

DIAGNOSTIC TESTS

CBC with WBC differential: To assess for anemia and presence of infection. Low hematocrit (Hct) indicates anemia. For optimal healing, the Hct should be >20%. Increased white blood cell (WBC) count signals infection. The production of more immature WBCs (shift to the left) occurs with infection but will be less pronounced if patient is immunosuppressed.
Gram stain of wound fluid or tissue: If infection is suspected, to identify the presence of pathogenic organism and aid in initial antimicrobial therapy.
Culture and sensitivity: To determine optimal antibiotic. Infection is said to

be present when 10^5 organisms per gram of tissue are present or fever and drainage are present.

COLLABORATIVE MANAGEMENT

Application of a sterile dressing in surgery or at the time of injury: To protect wound from external contamination or trauma or to provide pressure. Usually, surgeon or advanced practice nurse changes the initial dressing.

Regular (house) diet: To provide nutrients for wound healing.

Multivitamins, especially C: To promote tissue healing.

Minerals, especially zinc and iron: To correct any deficits and support healing.

Pain control: To maximize subcutaneous blood flow to the wound to support healing.

Supplemental oxygen: Empirically, 2-4 L/min in high-risk patients. After injury, wound O_2 may be low and administration of oxygen supports healing.

Insulin: As needed to control glucose levels in individuals with diabetes mellitus (DM) or hyperglycemia from other causes (e.g., steroid therapy, TPN, enteral nutrition). Hyperglycemia may delay healing.

Local or systemic antibiotics: Given when infection is present and sometimes used prophylactically.

Incision and drainage: To drain pus when infection is present and localized. Healing occurs by secondary intention. The wound may be irrigated to flush out organisms.

NURSING DIAGNOSES AND INTERVENTIONS

Impaired tissue integrity: wound, related to altered circulation; metabolic disorders (e.g., DM); alterations in fluid volume and nutrition; medical therapy (chemotherapy, radiation therapy, steroid administration)

Desired outcome: Patient exhibits the following signs of wound healing: well-approximated wound edges; good initial postinjury inflammatory response (erythema, warmth, induration, pain); no inflammatory response after the fifth day postinjury; no drainage (without drain present) 48 h after closure; healing ridge present by postoperative day 7 to 9. Skin integrity is restored.

* Assess wound for indications of impaired healing, including absence of a healing ridge, presence of drainage or purulent exudate, and delayed or prolonged inflammatory response. Monitor VS for signs of infection, including elevated temperature and HR. Document findings.
* Use standard (universal) precautions and follow proper infection-control techniques when changing dressings. If a drain is present, keep it sterile, maintain patency, and handle it gently to prevent it from becoming dislodged.

TABLE 1-27   Assessment of Healing of Wounds Closed by Primary Intention

Expected findings	Abnormal findings
Edges well approximated	Edges not well approximated
Good inflammatory response (redness, warmth, induration, pain) lasting 3-5 days	Decreased inflammatory response or inflammatory response that lasts more than 5 days after injury
No drainage (without drain present) 2 days after closure	Drainage continues more than 2 days after injury
Healing ridge present by postinjury day 7-9	No healing ridge present by day 9
	Hypertrophic scar or keloid present

If wound care will be necessary after hospital discharge, teach the dressing change procedure to the patient and significant others.

- For persons with hyperglycemia, perform serial monitoring of blood glucose and administer insulin to keep glucose level in a normal range.
- Explain to patient that deep breathing promotes oxygenation, which enhances wound healing. If indicated, provide incentive spirometry. Stress the importance of position changes and activity as tolerated to promote ventilation. Splint incision as needed.
- Monitor volume status by checking BP, HR, and capillary refill time in the tissue adjacent to incision, moisture of mucous membranes, skin turgor, and I&O.
- For nonrestricted patients, ensure a fluid intake of at least 2-3 L/day.
- To provide nutrients for healing, provide a diet with adequate protein, vitamin C, and calories. Encourage between-meal supplements and give frequent small feedings as needed.

SURGICAL OR TRAUMATIC WOUNDS HEALING BY SECONDARY INTENTION

Wounds healing by *secondary intention* are those with tissue loss or heavy contamination that form granulation tissue and contract in order to heal. Most often, impairment of healing is caused by increased contamination and impairment of perfusion, oxygenation, and nutrition, which results in a delay in the healing process. Individuals at risk for impaired healing include those who are obese, diabetic, malnourished, elderly, taking steroids, immunosuppressed, or undergoing radiation therapy or chemotherapy.

ASSESSMENT

Optimal healing: Initially, the wound edges are inflamed, indurated, and tender. Pale granulation tissue on the floor and walls progresses to a deeper pink and then to a beefy red; it should be moist. Epithelial cells from the tissue surrounding the wound gradually migrate across the granulation tissue. As healing occurs, the wound edges become pink, the angle between surrounding tissue and the wound becomes less acute, and wound contraction occurs. When present, a tract or sinus gradually decreases in size as healing occurs. The time frame for healing depends on the size and location of the wound, as well as on the patient's physical and psychologic status. See Table 1-27.

Impaired healing: Exudate and necrotic material appear on the floor and walls of the wound and do not abate as healing progresses. Note their distribution, color, odor, volume, and adherence. The periwound skin is assessed for signs of tissue damage, including disruption, discoloration, and increasing pain. When a drain is in place, the volume, color, and odor of the drainage are evaluated. See Table 1-28.

TABLE 1-28 Assessment of Healing of Wounds Closing by Secondary Intention	
Expected findings	**Abnormal findings**
Granulation tissue initially pale and moist and then becomes pink and beefy red over time	Granulation tissue remains pale or is excessively dry or moist
No odor	Abnormal odor
No slough or necrotic tissue	Slough or necrotic tissue
No tunneling or undermining	Tunneling or undermining

DIAGNOSTIC TESTS

CBC with WBC differential; Gram stain, tissue biopsy or culture and sensitivity of drainage: See discussion, "Wound Closed by Primary Intention," p. 55.

COLLABORATIVE MANAGEMENT

Débride slough and necrotic tissue: To remove dead tissue. Use sharp débridement for rapid removal and enzymatic (e.g., Accuzyme) for slower removal.

Dressings: To keep healthy wound tissue moist, to provide antiseptic agent to decrease wound surface bacterial counts, or for débridement. See Table 1-29.

Warming dressing: To assist with controlling the ambient environment around the wound to enhance closure.

Wound irrigation: To dislodge and remove bacteria and loosen necrotic tissue, foreign bodies, and exudate.

Fluids (oral/IV):   To ensure adequate intravascular volume to support healing.

Topical or systemic vitamin A: As needed to reverse adverse effects of steroids on healing. Use is limited to 7 to 10 days.

Drain(s):   To remove excess tissue fluid or purulent drainage.

Vacuum-assisted closure: To draw the edges of the wound together, reduce edema, increase blood flow, and stimulate granulation tissue.

Skin graft/cultured keratinocytes/cultured skin substitute: To provide coverage of wound if necessary.

Tissue flap: To fill tissue defect and provide wound closure with its own blood supply.

Growth factors: Naturally occurring proteins that stimulate new cell formation (e.g., platelet-derived growth factor, Regranex, and insulin).

Hyperbaric oxygen: Used with difficult wounds to support oxidative processes in healing.

Regular diet, multivitamins and minerals, insulin, pain control, supplemental oxygen, antibiotics, and incision and drainage: See discussion, "Wounds Closed by Primary Intention," p. 55.

NURSING DIAGNOSES AND INTERVENTIONS

Impaired tissue integrity: wound, related to presence of contaminants; metabolic disorders (e.g., DM); medical therapy (e.g., chemotherapy, radiation therapy); altered perfusion; immunosuppression; malnutrition

Desired outcomes: Patient's wound exhibits the following signs of healing: initially postinjury wound edges are inflamed, indurated, and tender; with epithelialization, edges become pink within 1 wk of injury; granulation tissue develops (identified by pink tissue that becomes beefy red) within 1 wk of injury; and there is no odor, exudate, or necrotic tissue. Patient or significant other successfully demonstrates wound care procedure before hospital discharge, if appropriate.

- Monitor for the following signs of impaired healing: initially postinjury, decreased inflammatory response or inflammatory response that lasts >5 days; epithelialization slowed or mechanically disrupted and noncontinuous around the wound; granulation tissue remains pale or excessively dry or moist; presence of odor, exudate, and/or necrotic tissue.
- Apply prescribed dressings (see Table 1-29). Insert dressing into all tracts to promote gradual closure of those areas. Ensure good hand washing before and after dressing changes, and dispose of contaminated dressings appropriately.
- When a drain is used, maintain its patency, prevent kinking of the tubing, and secure the tubing to prevent the drain from becoming dislodged.
- To help prevent contamination, cleanse the skin surrounding the wound with soap and water. Use minimal friction with cleansing if tissue is friable.

TABLE 1-29 Dressings Used for Wound Care

Dressing	Advantages	Disadvantages
Transparent dressing (e.g., Op-Site, Tegaderm, Bioclusive)	Transparent so can view wound; prevents loss of wound fluid; protects from external contamination; protects from friction and shear.	Nonabsorptive, may result in maceration of periwound tissue.
Hydrocollold (e.g., Duoderm, Restore, Cutinova)	Maintains moist wound surface while minimizing pooling; facilitates autolytic débridement; easy to apply, reduces pain.	Cannot be used with heavily draining wounds; opaque; exudate present on removal may be confused with infection; some roll.
Hydrogel (e.g., Curasol, Nu-gel, Vigilon)	Nonadherent; rehydrates wound; minimizes pain; can be used with infected wounds.	Cannot be used with heavily draining wounds; may macerate periwound skin.
Foam (e.g., Allevyn, Hydrosorb, Lyofoam)	Absorptive; nontraumatic; easy to apply and remove.	Not intended for dry wounds; may require tape or secondary dressing to secure.
Alginates (e.g., Kaltostat, Sorbsan)	Highly absorbent; can use on infected wounds; remove without trauma to wound.	Cannot be used for dry wounds; requires secondary dressing; has foul odor when removed.
Gauze (e.g., 2 × 2, 4 × 4, roller gauze)	Inexpensive; easy to use; ideal for packing wound.	May result in tissue maceration if inserted too moist; may result in tissue dehydration if allowed to dry out.
Composites (e.g., Alldress, Telfa Plus)	Use for partial to full-thickness wounds.	Adhesive borders may disrupt surrounding skin.

- If irrigation is prescribed for reducing contaminants, apply high-pressure irrigation using a 35-ml syringe with an 18-gauge flexible intravenous catheter. If the tissue is friable or the wound is over a major organ or blood vessel, use extreme caution with the irrigation pressure. To remove contaminants effectively, use a large volume of irrigant (e.g., 100-150 ml).
- When topical enzymes are prescribed, follow package directions carefully.

Research Brief 1-4   The antibacterial effect of two forms of a silver dressing (a film dressing and a silver-coated absorbent dressing) were compared in vitro. Bacterial strains included common clinical bacterial, including antibiotic-resistant strains. Findings showed that the silver-coated absorbent dressing provided more silver availability in the wound and that the bactericidal effects were faster and included a broader spectrum of organisms. Additional in vitro work is needed to confirm these positive effects in humans.

From Wright JB, Hansen DL, Burrell RE: The comparative efficacy of two antimicrobial barrier dressings: in vitro examination of two controlled release of silver dressings, *WOUNDS: A Compendium of Clinical Research and Practice* 10(6):179-88, 1998.

Be aware that some agents, such as povidone-iodine, deactivate the enzymes. Protect undamaged skin with zinc oxide or aluminum hydroxide paste.
• Teach patient or significant other the prescribed wound care procedure, if indicated.

Pressure Ulcers

Pressure ulcers are a disruption in tissue integrity and are caused by excessive tissue pressure or shearing of blood vessels. High-risk patients include the elderly and those who have decreased mobility, decreased level of consciousness (LOC), impaired sensation, debilitation, incontinence, sepsis/elevated temperature, or malnutrition.

ASSESSMENT
High-risk individuals should be identified upon admission assessment, with daily assessments during hospitalization, using a standard assessment tool. When pressure ulcers are present, their severity can be graded on a scale of I to IV.
Grade I: Nonblanchable erythema of intact skin. In dark-skinned individuals, heat may be the only indication of a grade I pressure ulcer.
Grade II: Partial-thickness skin loss that involves epidermis and/or dermis; seen as an abrasion, blister, or shallow crater.
Grade III: Full-thickness skin loss that involves subcutaneous tissue but does not extend through fascia.
Grade IV: Full-thickness injury that involves muscle, bone, or supporting structures. See "Surgical or Traumatic Wounds Healing by Secondary Intention," p. 57, for other assessment data.

DIAGNOSTIC TESTS
See "Diagnostic Tests," p. 55, in " Wounds Closed by Primary Intention."

COLLABORATIVE MANAGEMENT
See "Collaborative Management," p. 56, in "Surgical Wounds Healing by Primary Intention" and "Collaborative Management," p. 58, in "Surgical or Traumatic Wounds Healing by Secondary Intention."

NURSING DIAGNOSES AND INTERVENTIONS
Impaired tissue integrity (or risk for same) related to excessive tissue pressure; shearing forces; altered circulation
Desired outcomes: If patient at risk: patient's tissue remains intact. After interventions/instructions, patient participates in preventive measures and verbalizes understanding of the rationale for these interventions. For those with ulcers, ulcer is clean and decreasing in size. There is no slough tissue, necrotic tissue, or odor present.

- Identify individuals at risk, and systematically assess skin over bony prominences daily; document.
- Establish and post a position-changing schedule.
- Assist patient with turning q1-2h. Use pillows or foam wedges to prevent direct pressure on bony prominences. In addition, patients with a history of previous tissue injury will require pressure relief measures more frequently. Because high Fowler's position results in increased shearing, use low Fowler's position and alternate supine position with prone and 30-degree elevated side-lying positions.
- For immobile patients, float the heels using pillows that are inserted under the length of the lower leg.
- Minimize friction on tissue during activity. Lift rather than drag patient during position changes and transferring; use a draw sheet to facilitate patient movement. Do not massage over bony prominences.
- Minimize skin exposure to moisture. Cleanse at the time of soiling and at routine intervals. Use moisture barriers and disposable briefs as needed.
- Use a mattress that reduces pressure, such as foam, alternating air, gel, or water.

Impaired tissue integrity: presence of pressure ulcer with increased risk for further breakdown, related to altered circulation; presence of contaminants or irritants (chemical, thermal, mechanical)

Desired outcomes: Stages I and II are healed within 7 to 10 days; stages III and IV may require months to heal. After intervention/instructions, patient verbalizes causes and preventive measures for pressure ulcers and successfully participates in the plan of care to promote healing and prevent further breakdown.

- Evaluate grade of pressure ulcer (see "Assessment," p. 60).
- Maintain a moist physiologic environment to promote tissue repair and minimize contaminants. Change dressings as prescribed.
- Be sure patient's skin is kept clean with regular bathing, and be especially conscientious about washing urine and feces from the skin. Soap should be used and then thoroughly rinsed from the skin.
- If the patient has excessive perspiration, ensure frequent bathing and change bedding as needed.
- To absorb moisture and prevent shearing when the patient is moved, apply heel and elbow covers as needed.
- Use lamb's wool to keep the areas between the toes dry.
- Do not use a heat lamp because it increases the metabolic rate of the tissues, resulting in increased ulcer diameter and depth
- Teach patient and significant others the importance of and measures for preventing excess pressure as a means of preventing pressure ulcers.
- Provide wound care as needed (described under "Surgical or Traumatic Wounds Healing by Secondary Intention," p. 57).

ADDITIONAL NURSING DIAGNOSES

Also see **Impaired tissue integrity** under "Surgical or Traumatic Wounds Healing by Secondary Intention," p. 58.

NIC Skin Surveillance; Incision Site Care; Wound Care; Pressure Ulcer Care; Pressure Ulcer Prevention; Wound Irrigation

Pain

PATHOPHYSIOLOGY

Critically ill patients endure substantial pain from pathologic conditions, injury, such therapeutic interventions as surgery, and multiple invasive diagnostic procedures. Even seemingly unconscious patients experience pain. The pain experience is compounded by fear, anxiety, and barriers to communication. In addition, pain control assumes a low priority when juxtaposed against respiratory or hemodynamic instability, either of which is common in critical care areas. The presence of pain is a significant stressor for critically ill patients and contributes to other problems such as confusion, inadequate ventilation, immobility, sleep deprivation, depression, and immunosuppression.

The subjective nature of pain adds to its complexity. Pain has been defined by the International Association for the Study of Pain as "an unpleasant sensory and emotional experience associated with actual or potential tissue damage or described in terms of such damage." Pain is a warning signal to which the body responds to prevent further injury. Noxious substances that are released in response to damaged tissue initiate the pain (nociceptive) nerve transmission. Afferent nerve fibers such as A delta (Aδ) and C fibers respond to pain stimuli peripherally and relay this information to the spinal cord entering through the dorsal horn. A delta fibers are small, myelinated, fast-conducting fibers that transmit pain sensation that is well localized. C fibers are small, unmyelinated, slow-conducting fibers that transmit poorly localized, dull, aching pain sensations.

In the dorsal horn, nociceptive neurotransmitters are released in response to the nociceptive input that activates the second-order dorsal horn neurons. The activation of the second-order neurons results in (1) spinal reflex responses such as vasoconstriction, muscle spasm, and increased sensitization and (2) activation of the ascending tracts, which transmits the nociceptive input to several regions within the brain. This is where several responses to pain occur, including the perception of pain and the emotional and behavioral responses.

The modulation of nociceptive input occurs at several sites, including the opioid receptors located in the dorsal horn and the opioid receptors located supraspinally in such areas as the cortex, hypothalamus, and periaqueductal areas. Neuropeptides such as enkephalin molecules (endogenous opioids) bind with the opioid receptors to modulate nociceptive input. Exogenous (administered) opioids work in a similar fashion.

Characteristic pain patterns develop according to the area affected and the underlying pathophysiologic process. Cutaneous injury, transmitted by A delta fibers, produces sharp, well-localized pain sensation. Somatic pain arising from muscles, tendons, fascia, and other deep structures is transmitted by C fibers, resulting in dull and diffusely localized pain sensation. Visceral pain, similar to somatic pain, is transmitted also by C fibers and arises from hollow organs. Ischemic pain is a nociceptive response to hypoxia involving muscular soft tissue and skin.

Despite the availability of effective analgesics and many new pain-control technologies, many critically ill patients continue to be treated inadequately for pain. Patients have also reported satisfaction with their pain control even though their reported pain levels are severe.

Professional and patient-related barriers have contributed to poor pain management. These barriers include (1) societal expectations concerning pain (e.g., unrelieved pain is expected and accepted in certain situations such as during surgical or invasive procedures, treatment for malignant conditions, or as a normal part of aging; (2) professionals' knowledge deficits regarding the pharmacokinetics and equianalgesic dosing; (3) patients' lack of knowledge concerning the side effects of unrelieved pain and the lack of knowledge of pain management in general; (4) inadequate pain assessment techniques by health care professionals; (5) inappropriate professional attitudes and beliefs (e.g., certain patients do not have pain [e.g., neonates], pain management is low priority); (6) inappropriate patients' attitudes and beliefs (e.g., pain builds character, pain is a part of procedures; and (7) fear of tolerance, addiction, and analgesic side effects by both professionals and patients.

Uncontrolled pain has multisystem effects. The cardiovascular effects of unrelieved pain are increased HR, BP, SVR; increased myocardial oxygen consumption; altered regional blood flow; and deep vein thrombosis. The pulmonary effects noted of uncontrolled pain are decreased lung volumes, atelectasis, decreased cough effort, increased sputum retention, and hypoxemia. Gastrointestinal and genitourinary effects are decreased gastric and bowel motility and urinary retention. The neuroendocrine response to uncontrolled pain is to release more of the stress hormones such as catecholamines, cortisol, and glucagon. Psychologic effects are anxiety, fear, and sleeplessness. Nurses have an ethical obligation to relieve pain and reduce associated physiologic and psychologic risks of untreated pain.

Pain management must be made a priority and a visible part of patient care. Ways in which to make pain management more visible and a priority are to (1) display pain assessment tools in patients' rooms; (2) designate pain as the fifth vital sign to signify its importance; and (3) incorporate pain assessment into documentation tools. Continuous assessment and documentation increase awareness and effectiveness of pain intervention.

ASSESSMENT

A thorough baseline assessment, whenever possible, is important in accurately evaluating and managing pain. Frequent, brief assessments are necessary postoperatively and during acute episodes of pain until the pain is well controlled. Health care professionals need to establish a good rapport with patients and use therapeutic communication skills.

History and risk factors: Question patient regarding previous or current pain; usual ways in which pain is described and expressed; previously used pharmacologic and nonpharmacologic methods of pain control; previous history of chemical dependence, including alcohol use; attitudes and beliefs toward pain and use of opioid, anxiolytic, or other medications; typical coping responses for pain or stress; and expectations regarding pain management.

Subjective presentation: Because pain is subjective, the mainstay of pain assessment should be patients' self-report. Patients should be asked to describe the nature of the pain (e.g., location, intensity, quality, the timing of the pain, aggravating/alleviating factors). One or more of several pain assessment tools should be used to assist the patient in rating pain. Comparisons of the patient's ratings before and after a given intervention are used to guide therapy.

Numeric rating scale (NRS): Patient ranks pain numerically, usually from 1 to 5 or 1 to 10.

Visual analog scale (VAS): Patient marks a 10-cm line to indicate pain intensity.

Adjective rating scale (ARS): Patient selects an adjective that best describes the pain intensity.

Objective presentation: Used to supplement self-reports or used exclusively if the patient is unconscious or has other profound communication barriers.

Physiologic: Responses to pain are related to autonomic nervous system stimulation, as seen in increases in HR, BP, and RR, all which are associated with untreated pain. Other physiologic responses associated with autonomic stimulation are listed in Table 1-30.

Behavioral: Social, cultural, ethnic, and environmental factors affect a patient's understanding of and attitudes toward pain. Patients respond according to learned attitudes and beliefs. A number of nonverbal indicators are listed in Table 1-31.

Vital signs and hemodynamics: With untreated pain, usually reflect autonomic stimulation (e.g., elevated HR, RR, BP, SVR). IV opiate analgesics promptly reduce SVR directly as a result of vasodilation and indirectly as a result of pain relief.

COLLABORATIVE MANAGEMENT

Opioid agonists: Centrally acting analgesics that bind with receptors in the CNS and other tissues, thus blocking pain sensation and causing various other effects, including feelings of well-being, peripheral vasodilation, and possibly

TABLE 1-30 Autonomic Indicators of Pain

Diaphoresis, pallor
Vasoconstriction
Increased systolic and diastolic BP
Increased pulse rate (>100 bpm)
Pupillary dilation
Change in respiratory rate (usually increased to >20 breaths/min)
Muscle tension or spasm
Decreased intestinal motility, evidenced by nausea, vomiting, abdominal distention, and possibly ileus
Endocrine imbalance, evidenced by sodium and water retention and mild hyperglycemia

bpm, Beats per minute.

TABLE 1-31 Nonverbal Indicators of Pain

Skeletal muscle tension	Psychic reactions
Facial grimace, tension	Short attention span
Guarding or splinting of the affected part	Irritability
Restlessness	Anxiety
Increase in motor activity	Sleep disturbances
Decrease in motor activity	Anger
	Crying
	Fearfulness
	Withdrawal

respiratory depression. They are used to manage moderate to severe acute pain. For the most effective therapy, titrate in small increments to produce the desired analgesia with minimal side effects. "As needed" dosing provides poor pain management because of delays in administration and fluctuations in the patient's analgesic blood levels. Patient-controlled analgesia (PCA) pumps, continuous peripheral or epidural infusions, and small, frequent IV bolus dosing are effective methods used for patients in critical care areas. Opioid tolerance, physiologic or psychologic dependence, and addiction are unusual when opioids are used to manage acute pain in patients without a history of chemical dependency. Parenteral opioids may cause hypotension in patients with hypovolemia. Restore fluid volume before or concurrent with administration. Some patients are at a greater risk for respiratory depression. Those at a greater risk are the opioid naïve, those with compromised pulmonary status or neuromuscular disease, the extremely young (neonates), and the elderly.

Elderly people are more sensitive to the therapeutic and toxic effects of analgesics.

The distribution of medications is altered by age. With aging, lean body mass decreases and body fat increases. Also, muscle and soft-tissue mass decrease, and body water declines. This results in water-soluble opioid analgesics such as morphine having a lower volume of distribution. This causes an increased speed of onset of action and raises peak concentration, which is associated with increased toxicity. Lipid-soluble opioid analgesics (e.g., fentanyl) may be more widely distributed, resulting in a delayed onset of action and accumulation with repeated doses. Because of age-related changes in metabolism and elimination, the elderly are also at risk for drug-accumulation toxicity. In treating the elderly, it is best to start at lower doses (50%-75% of recommended younger adult doses); increase the interval between doses; use opioids with shorter half-lives (morphine, hydromorphone, oxycodone); and closely observe for signs of toxicity.

With careful assessment, proper dosing and titration, knowledge of analgesic onset and peak times, and careful monitoring, the risk for respiratory depression is low. However, naloxone (Narcan), an opioid antagonist, should be immediately available to reverse respiratory depression. See Table 1-32 for equianalgesic doses of narcotic analgesics and Table 1-33 for uses of opioid and opioid agonist-antagonist analgesia.

* *Morphine:* Most frequently used opioid; considered "first-line" therapy for moderate to severe acute pain. With its vasodilatory effects and little effect on CO and HR, morphine is beneficial for patients with left ventricular failure, pulmonary hypertension, or pulmonary edema. Rapid IV injection may trigger histamine release with related vasodilation, decreased preload, and decreased BP. Continuous opioid infusion minimizes hemodynamic changes that can occur with bolus dosing. Epidural administration may result in reduced responsiveness of the respiratory center in the brainstem to carbon dioxide. This results in gradual decrease in the depth and rate of respiration, increase in $Paco_2$, increase in sedation level, and respiratory acidosis.
* *Hydromorphone (Dilaudid):* Highly effective opioid; substitute analgesic for patient with morphine allergy or intolerance.
* *Meperidine (Demerol):* Indicated for brief courses (i.e., <48 h) in patients with allergy or intolerance to morphine, hydromorphone, or other opiates. Its toxic metabolite, normeperidine, is a cerebral irritant and may cause seizures.
* *Fentanyl:* Potent synthetic opioid. IV preparation is especially useful in critical care because of minimal cardiovascular effects, short duration of action, and rapid onset of action. Duration of action increases with repeated doses. Caution must be taken if large doses of Fentanyl are given rapidly. This may cause chest wall muscle rigidity requiring ventilatory support and rapid-acting muscle relaxants.

Caution: A fentanyl patch may be used for continuous analgesia, usually with supplemental doses of morphine or other opiate titrated to produce analgesia for breakthrough pain, but should be used only for patients with opiate tolerance. A fentanyl patch is not recommended for mild pain, acute postoperative pain, or intermittent pain because of its slow onset and long duration and because it is difficult to reverse its side effects and adverse effects. Respiratory depression with hypoventilation occurs, as with morphine.

Opioid agonist-antagonists: Stimulate and antagonize opiate receptors to varying degrees, depending on agent and dose. They may precipitate withdrawal in patients receiving opiates on a regular basis. See Tables 1-32 and 1-33.

* *Pentazocine (Talwin):* Predominately agonist effects but with weak antagonist activity. It may cause increased MAP, LVEDP, and mean PAP, thus increasing myocardial workload.
* *Butorphanol (Stadol):* Adverse effects reported in patients with congestive heart failure (CHF) or acute myocardial infarction (MI). It may be useful in decreasing side effects associated with epidural morphine.

Nonsteroidal antiinflammatory drugs (NSAIDs): They are used to treat mild to moderate pain or are used in conjunction with opioids to treat moderate

TABLE 1-32   Equianalgesic Doses of Narcotic Analgesics

Class/name	Route	Equianalgesic dose (mg)*	Average duration (h)
Morphine-like agonists			
Codeine	IM, SC	130†	3
	PO	180†	3
Hydromorphone	IM, SC	1.5	4
(Dilaudid)	PO	6-7.5	4
Levorphanol	IM, SC	2	6
(Levo-Dromoran)	PO	4	6
Morphine	IM, SC	10	4
Oxycodone (Percodan)	PO	30†	4
Oxymorphone	IM, SC	1	4
(Numorphan)	Rectal	15-20	4
Meperidine-like agonists			
Fentanyl (Sublimaze)	IV, IM, SC	0.1	3-4‡
Meperidine (Demerol)	IM, SC	100	3
Methadone-like agonists			
Methadone	IM, SC	10	6
(Dolophine)	PO	10-20	6
Propoxyphene	PO	130-250†	4
(Darvon)			
Mixed agonist-antagonist			
Buprenorphine	IM	0.3-0.4	4
(Buprenex)			
Butorphanol (Stadol)	IM, SC	2	3
Nalbuphine (Nubain)	IM, SC	10	3-4
Pentazocine (Talwin)	IM	150	3
	PO	60	3

Modified from Hazard V, Hopfer DJ: *Davis' drug guide for nurses,* ed 5, Philadelphia, 1997, Davis; Macintyre PE, Ready LB: *Acute pain management: a practical guide,* London, 1996, Saunders; Salerno E: Pharmacologic approaches. In Salerno E, Willens JS, editors: *Pain management handbook: an interdisciplinary approach,* St Louis, 1996, Mosby.
IM, Intramuscular; *SC,* subcutaneous; *PO,* oral; *IV,* intravenous; *mg,* milligram; *h,* hour.
*Recommended starting dose; actual dose must be titrated to patient response.
†Starting doses lower (codeine 30 mg, oxycodone 5 mg, meperidine 50 mg, propoxyphene 65-130 mg, pentazocine 50 mg).
‡Respiratory depressant effects persist longer than analgesic effects.

to severe pain. NSAIDs inhibit the synthesis and release of prostaglandins peripherally, rendering afferent receptors less sensitive to bradykinin, histamine, and serotonin, which in turn decreases pain receptor stimulation. Most NSAIDs are given orally (e.g., ibuprofen, aspirin), but injectable NSAIDs such as ketorolac are available. Prostaglandin inhibition leads to decreased renal blood flow and acute renal failure; increased gastric irritation; and decreased platelet adhesiveness, which may result in bleeding complications. See Table 1-34.

TABLE 1-33 Use of Opioid and Opioid Agonist-Antagonist Analgesia

Route	Commonly prescribed medications	Advantages	Disadvantages
Continuous IV infusion	Morphine, fentanyl (Sublimaze), hydromorphone (Dilaudid)	• Useful for severe, predictable pain • Relieves pain with lower doses than IV bolus • Avoids peaks and valleys of pain present with IV bolus and IM injections	• Requires frequent observation to monitor flow rate • VS must be monitored often, especially respiratory status • Weaning necessary
IV bolus	Morphine, fentanyl, hydromorphone, meperidine (Demerol)	• Useful for severe, intermittent pain (i.e., for procedures, treatments) • Rapid onset of action	• Relatively short duration of pain relief • Fluctuating levels • Possibility of excessive sedation as drug levels peak
Patient-controlled analgesia (PCA); may be delivered IV or SC	Morphine, fentanyl, buprenorphine (Buprenex)	• Useful for moderate to severe pain • Enables titration by patient for effective analgesia without excessive sedation • Relief of pain with lower dosages of medication • Immediate delivery of medication	• Pumps necessary to deliver drug are expensive • Patient must have clear mental status • Health care provider resistance to self-administration by patient

Continued

IV, Intravenous; *IM,* intramuscular; *SC,* subcutaneous; *VS,* vital signs.

TABLE 1-33 Use of Opioid and Opioid Agonist-Antagonist Analgesia—cont'd

Route	Commonly prescribed medications	Advantages	Disadvantages
Patient-controlled analgesia (PCA); may be delivered IV or SC—cont'd		• Patient's sense of self-control lowers anxiety • Less nursing time spent preparing medications	• Difficult to assess patency and placement • Significant infection risk
Epidural and intrathecal	Morphine, fentanyl, local anesthetics (e.g., bupivacaine)	• Provides greater analgesia with less CNS depression than parenteral narcotics • Enables direct binding of narcotics to opioid receptor sites in the spinal cord, thereby minimizing CNS depression • Directly blocks pain impulse transmission to central cortex when anesthetics are used	
IM/SC injection	Meperidine, morphine, pentazocine (Talwin), nalbuphine (Nubain), butorphanol (Stadol), buprenorphine	• Useful for moderate to severe pain • Longer duration of action than with IV route • Faster pain relief than with oral medication • SC route useful for patients with poor IV access and little muscle mass	• Variable absorption and fluctuating levels, especially in hypotensive and edematous patients • Possibility of excessive sedation as drug levels peak • Potential delay in administration

IV, Intravenous; *IM,* intramuscular; *SC,* subcutaneous; *CNS,* central nervous system.

TABLE 1-34	Common Nonnarcotic and Nonsteroidal Antiinflammatory Analgesics

Acetaminophen (Tylenol, Tempra)
Acetylsalicylic acid (aspirin)
Ibuprofen (Motrin, Advil, Nuprin)
Indomethacin (Indocin)
Ketorolac (Toradol)
Naproxen (Naprosyn, Anaprox, Aleve)

- *Ketorolac (Toradol):* Effective for short-term use in relieving mild to moderate pain. Effect on ventilation is minimal, and the drug has been effective when given on an alternate schedule with morphine or other opiate analgesic during ventilator weaning of postoperative patients. Renal toxicity is possible, which limits use to patients with normal renal function. Bleeding complications are more likely with high-dose therapy and in older adults.

Other pharmacologic interventions: Sedatives and anxiolytics (e.g., midazolam [Versed]) often used to reduce anxiety associated with pain and to promote amnesia when painful procedures are planned. Spinal analgesia with a local anesthetic agent may be used with epidural opiates. Intermittent or continuous local neural blockade, such as intercostal nerve block, is used for specific localized pain.

Nonpharmacologic interventions: Include sensory, emotional, and cognitive interventions, such as massage, relaxation, distraction, and guided imagery, TENS unit. These interventions are used for mild pain and anxiety and as adjuncts to pharmacologic management of moderate to severe pain. See Table 1-35.

NURSING DIAGNOSES AND INTERVENTIONS

Pain related to biophysical injury secondary to pathology; surgical, diagnostic, or treatment interventions; or related to trauma

Desired outcomes: Within 2 h of initiating therapy, patient's subjective evaluation of discomfort improves, as documented by a pain scale. Patient does not exhibit nonverbal indicators of pain (see Table 1-31). Autonomic indicators (see Table 1-30) are diminished or absent. Verbal responses, such as crying or moaning, are absent.

- Develop a systematic approach to pain management for each patient. The primary nurse should collaborate with the surgeon, anesthesiologist, and patient for optimal management of pain. See Figures 1-1 and 1-2 for pain treatment flow charts for preoperative and postoperative patients.
- Monitor patient at frequent intervals for the presence of discomfort. Use a formal, patient-specific method of assessing pain. One method is to have the patient rate discomfort on a scale of 0 (no discomfort) to 10 (worst pain). Other methods may be used, but the method selected should be used consistently.
- Evaluate patients with acute and chronic pain for nonverbal indicators of discomfort (see Table 1-31).
- Evaluate patients with acute pain for autonomic indicators of discomfort (see Table 1-30). Be aware that patients with chronic pain (>6 mo duration) will not exhibit an autonomic response.
- Evaluate health history for evidence of alcohol and drug (prescribed and nonprescribed) use. Individuals with a history of chemical dependence may require a higher dose for effective analgesia. Persons with evidence of chronic or acute hepatic insufficiency require a reduced dose and careful selection of appropriate analgesics. Consult pain control team if available. All

TABLE 1-35   Common Nonpharmacologic Methods of Pain Control

Physical therapies/modalities
- *Massage:* To relax muscular tension and increase local circulation. Back and foot massage are especially relaxing.
- *ROM exercises (passive, assisted, or active):* To relax muscles, improve circulation, and prevent pain related to stiffness and immobility.
- *Heat/cold applications:* To alter pain threshold, reduce muscle spasm, and decrease vascular congestion, particularly in the area of injury. Cold decreases initial tissue injury response. Heat facilitates clearance of tissue toxins and fluids.
- *Transcutaneous electrical nerve stimulation (TENS):* A battery-operated device used to send weak electric impulse via electrodes placed on the body. The sensation of pain is reduced during and sometimes after treatment.

Emotional interventions
- *Prevention and control of anxiety:* Limiting anxiety reduces muscle tension and increases the patient's pain tolerance. Anxiety and fear contribute to autonomic stimulation and pain responses. Progressive relaxation exercises and encouraging slow, controlled breathing may be helpful.
- *Promoting self-control:* Feelings of helplessness and lack of control contribute to anxiety and pain. Techniques such as PCA and promoting self-helping behaviors contribute to feelings of self-control.

Cognitive interventions
- *Preparatory information:* Preparing the patient by explaining what can be expected, thereby reducing stress and anxiety. Preoperative teaching is an example of this technique.
- *Patient education:* Teaching methods for preventing or reducing pain. Examples include suggesting comfortable postoperative positions, methods of ambulation, and splinting of incisions when coughing.
- *Distraction:* Encouraging patient to focus on something unrelated to the pain. Examples include conversing, reading, watching television or videos, listening to music, relaxation techniques (see **Health-seeking behavior,** p. 302)
- *Humor:* Can be an excellent distraction and may help the patient cope with stress.
- *Guided imagery:* The patient employs a mental process that uses images to alter a physical or emotional state. This technique promotes relaxation and decreases pain sensations.
- *Biofeedback:* The patient learns conscious control of physiologic processes that normally are controlled unconsciously. Muscle tension and chronic or episodic pain may be reduced.

Many of these techniques may be taught to and implemented by the patient and significant others.
ROM, Range of motion; *PCA,* patient-controlled analgesia.

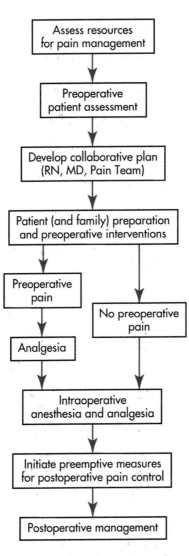

Figure 1-1: Pain treatment flow chart: preoperative and intraoperative phases.
Acute Pain Management Guideline Panel: *Acute pain management: operative and medical procedures and trauma, clinical practice guideline*, AHCPR Pub No 92-0032, Agency for Health Care Policy and Research, Public Health Service, Rockville, Md, 1992, US Department of Health and Human Services.

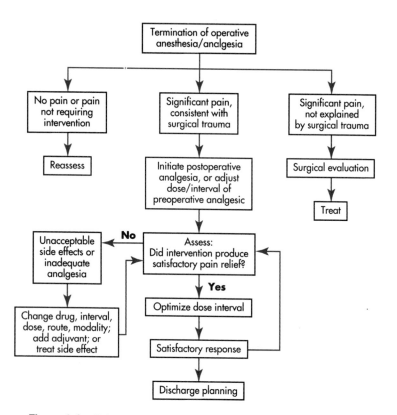

Figure 1-2:   Pain treatment flow chart: postoperative phase.
Acute Pain Management Guideline Panel: *Acute pain management: operative and medical procedures and trauma, clinical practice guideline*, AHCPR Pub No 92-0032, Agency for Health Care Policy and Research, Public Health Service, Rockville, Md, 1992, US Department of Health and Human Services.

care providers must be consistent in setting limits while providing effective pain control through pharmacologic and nonpharmacologic methods. Psychiatric or mental health consultation may be necessary. Be aware that some opioid agonist-antagonist analgesics (e.g., butorphanol, buprenorphine, pentazocine) have strong narcotic antagonist activity and may trigger withdrawal symptoms in individuals with opiate dependency.

• Administer opioid and related mixed agonist-antagonist analgesics as prescribed (see Table 1-33). Monitor for side effects, such as respiratory depression, excessive sedation, nausea, vomiting, and constipation. Be aware that meperidine (Demerol) may produce excitation, muscle twitching, and seizures, especially in conjunction with phenothiazines. Do not administer mixed agonist-antagonist analgesics concurrently with morphine or other pure agonists, because reversal of analgesic effects may occur.

- Assess patients receiving opioid analgesics at frequent intervals for evidence of excessive sedation when awake or respiratory depression (i.e., RR <10 breaths/min or Sao_2 <90%-92%). In the presence of respiratory depression, reduce the amount or frequency of the dose as prescribed. Have naloxone (Narcan) readily available to reverse severe respiratory depression.

> **Note:** Because of respiratory depression and excessive sedation, older adults and individuals with asthma, COPD, and other respiratory disorders should be monitored closely when receiving opiate analgesics.

- If the patient is receiving epidural or intrathecal narcotic, monitor closely for side effects and complications.
- Check patient's analgesia record for the last dose and amount of medication given during surgery and in the postanesthesia care unit. Be careful to coordinate timing and dose of postoperative analgesics with previously administered medication.
- Administer nonnarcotic and nonsteroidal antiinflammatory agents (see Table 1-34) as prescribed for relief of mild to moderate pain or on alternating schedule with opiate analgesics for moderate to severe pain. NSAIDs are especially effective when pain is associated with inflammation and soft-tissue injury. Ketorolac (Toradol) may be given IM or IV when oral agents are contraindicated. Monitor for excessive bleeding, gastric irritation, and renal compromise in patients receiving NSAIDs.
- Administer prn analgesics before pain becomes severe. Prolonged stimulation of pain receptors results in increased sensitivity to painful stimuli and will increase the amount of drug required to relieve pain.
- Administer intermittently scheduled or supplemental analgesics before painful procedures (e.g., suctioning, chest tube removal) and ambulation and at bedtime, scheduling them so that their peak effect is achieved at the inception of the activity or procedure.
- Augment analgesic therapy with sedatives and tranquilizers to prolong and enhance analgesia. Avoid substituting sedatives and tranquilizers for analgesics.
- Wean patient from opioid analgesics by decreasing dosage or frequency of the drug. When changing route of administration or medication, be certain to employ equianalgesic doses of the new drug (see Table 1-32).
- Augment action of medication by employing nonpharmacologic methods of pain control (see Table 1-35). Many of these techniques may be taught to and implemented by the patient and significant others.
- Maintain a quiet environment to promote rest. Plan nursing activities to enable long periods of uninterrupted rest at night.
- Evaluate for and correct nonoperative sources of discomfort (e.g., position, full bladder, infiltrated IV site).
- Position patient comfortably, and reposition at frequent intervals to relieve discomfort caused by pressure and to improve circulation.
- Sudden or unexpected changes in pain intensity can signal complications such as internal bleeding or leakage of visceral contents. Carefully evaluate the patient and consult the surgeon immediately.
- Document efficacy of analgesics and other pain control interventions, using the pain scale or other formalized method.

NIC Analgesic Administration; Pain Management; Analgesic Administration: Intraspinal; Patient-Controlled Anaglesia (PCA) Assistance

Ineffective breathing pattern related to neuromuscular impairment secondary to central respiratory depression; pain-induced splinting

Desired outcome: Patient exhibits effective ventilation within 30 min of this diagnosis as evidenced by relaxed breathing; RR 12-20 breaths/min with normal depth and pattern (eupnea); clear breath sounds; normal color; Pao_2 ≥80 mm Hg; pH 7.35-7.45; $Paco_2$ 35-45 mm Hg; HCO_3^- 22-26 mEq/L; and Spo_2 ≥92%.

- Assess and document respiratory rate and depth qh. Note signs of respiratory compromise, including RR <10 or >26; shallow or grunting respirations; use of accessory muscles of respiration; prolonged inspiratory/expiratory ratio; pallor or cyanosis; decreased vital capacity; and increased residual volume. Consult physician for evidence of respiratory compromise.
- Monitor Spo_2 and ABG values. Consult physician for decreased Spo_2 (<90%-92%) or increased $Paco_2$ (>45 mm Hg).
- Assess and document LOC q1-2h.
- Use apnea monitor as indicated.
- Keep naloxone (Narcan) at patient's bedside during and for 24 h after epidural or intrathecal administration.
- Maintain IV access for immediate administration of naloxone to reverse respiratory depression.
- Respiratory depression may persist for as long as 24 h after the last dose of epidural morphine. Monitor for respiratory depression during and for 24 h after patient's receipt of epidural or intrathecal opioids.

NIC Airway Management; Respiratory Monitoring; Oxygen Therapy; Aspiration Precautions

Urinary retention related to inhibition of reflex arc secondary to opioid action
Desired outcomes: Within 4 h of this diagnosis, complete bladder emptying is achieved. Overflow incontinence is absent.

- Monitor for symptoms of urinary retention: bladder distention, frequent voiding of small amounts of urine, sensation of bladder fullness, residual urine, dysuria, and overflow incontinence.
- Monitor I&O precisely.
- Catheterize bladder intermittently or insert indwelling catheter as prescribed.
- Administer IV naloxone as prescribed.

NIC Urinary Retention Care; Urinary Catheterization

Risk for impaired skin integrity related to itching secondary to alteration in sensory modulation from opioid effects
Desired outcome: Patient's skin remains intact.

- Administer diphenhydramine or hydroxyzine as prescribed.
- Maintain comfortably cool environment.
- Apply cool, moist compresses.
- If relief from the above measures is inadequate, administer small amounts of IV naloxone as prescribed.
- See also "Prolonged Immobility."

NIC Skin Surveillance; Positioning; Pressure Ulcer Prevention

Prolonged immobility

NURSING DIAGNOSES AND INTERVENTIONS

Activity intolerance related to prolonged bed rest; generalized weakness; an imbalance between oxygen supply and demand
Desired outcome: Within 48 h of discontinuing bed rest, patient exhibits cardiac tolerance to low-intensity exercise as evidenced by HR ≤20 bpm over resting HR; systolic BP ≤20 mm Hg over or under resting systolic BP; Sao_2 >90%; Svo_2 ≥60%; RR ≤20 breaths/min; normal sinus rhythm; warm and dry skin; and absence of crackles, murmurs, and chest pain.

- Perform ROM exercises bid to qid on each extremity. Individualize the exercise plan on the basis of the following guidelines:
  - □ *Mode or type of exercise:* Begin with passive exercises, moving the joints

through the motions of abduction, adduction, flexion, and extension. Progress to active-assisted exercises, in which you support the joints while the patient initiates muscle contraction. When the patient is able, supervise him or her in active isotonic exercises, during which the patient contracts a selected muscle group, moves the extremity at a slow pace, and then relaxes the muscle group. Have the patient repeat each exercise 3-10 times.

> *Caution:* Avoid isometric exercises in cardiac patients. Stop any exercise that causes muscular or skeletal pain. Consult with a physical therapist for necessary modifications.

☐ *Intensity:* Begin with 3-5 repetitions as tolerated by the patient. Assess exercise tolerance by measuring HR and BP at rest, peak exercise, and 5 min after exercise. If HR or systolic BP increases >20 bpm or >20 mm Hg over the resting level, decrease the number of repetitions. If HR or systolic BP decreases >10 bpm or >10 mm Hg at peak exercise, this could be a sign of left ventricular failure, denoting that the heart cannot meet this workload. For other adverse signs and symptoms, see "Assessment," which follows.

☐ *Duration:* Begin with 5 min or less of exercise. Gradually increase the exercise to 15 min as tolerated.

☐ *Frequency:* Begin exercises bid-qid. As the duration increases, the frequency can be reduced.

☐ *Assessment of exercise tolerance:* Be alert to signs and symptoms that the cardiovascular and respiratory systems cannot meet the demands of the low-level ROM exercises. Excessive SOB may occur if (1) transient pulmonary congestion occurs secondary to ischemia or left ventricular dysfunction; (2) lung volumes are decreased; (3) oxygen-carrying capacity of the blood is reduced; or (4) there is shunting of blood from the right to the left side of the heart without adequate oxygenation. If cardiac output does not increase to meet the body's needs during modest levels of exercise, systolic BP may fall; the skin may become cool, cyanotic, and diaphoretic; dysrhythmias may be noted; crackles may be auscultated; or a systolic murmur of mitral regurgitation may occur. If the patient tolerates the exercise, increase the intensity or number of repetitions each day. See Table 1-36 for physiologic effects of bed rest (deconditioning).

• Ask patient to rate perceived exertion (RPE) experienced during exercise, basing it on the following scale developed by Borg (1982):
   0 Nothing at all
   1 Very weak effort

TABLE 1-36 Physiologic Effects of Bed Rest (Deconditioning)

Increased heart rate and blood pressure for submaximal workload
Decrease in functional capacity
Decrease in circulating volume
Orthostatic hypotension
Reflex tachycardia
Modest decrease in pulmonary function
Increase in thromboemboli
Loss of muscle mass
Loss of muscle contractile strength
Deficient protein state
Negative nitrogen state

2 Weak (light) effort
3 Moderate
4 Somewhat stronger effort
5 Strong effort
6
7 Very strong effort
8
9 Very, very strong effort
10 Maximal effort

The patient should not experience an RPE >3 while performing ROM exercises. Reduce the intensity of the exercise and increase the frequency until an RPE of ≤3 is attained.

- As the patient's condition improves, increase activity as soon as possible to include sitting in a chair. Assess for orthostatic hypotension, which can occur as a result of decreased plasma volume and difficulty in adjusting immediately to postural change. Prepare the patient for this by increasing the amount of time spent in high Fowler's position and moving the patient slowly and in stages. (For additional information about activity progression, see Table 4-1, p. 258.)
- Increase activity level by having patient perform self-care activities such as eating, mouth care, and bathing as tolerated.
- Teach significant others the purpose and interventions for preventing deconditioning. Involve them in the patient's plan of care.
- To help allay fears of failure, pain, or medical setbacks, provide emotional support to patient and significant others as patient's activity level is increased.

NIC Exercise Therapy: Ambulation; Energy Management; Cardiac Care: Rehabilitative

Risk for disuse syndrome related to mechanical or prescribed immobilization; severe pain; altered LOC

Desired outcome: Patient displays full ROM without verbal or nonverbal indicators of pain.

> **Note:**   ROM exercises should be performed every day for all immobilized patients with *normal* joints. Modification may be required for patients with flaccidity (e.g., immediately after stroke or spinal cord injury) to prevent subluxation; or for patients with spasticity (e.g., during the recovery period for patients with stroke or spinal cord injury) to prevent an increase in spasticity. Consult with physical therapist or occupational therapist for assistance with modifying the exercise plan for these patients. In addition, be aware that ROM exercises are contraindicated during the inflammatory phase of rheumatologic disease and for dislocated or fractured joints.

- Be alert to the following areas that are especially prone to joint contracture: *shoulders,* which can become "frozen" to limit abduction and extension; *wrists,* which can "drop," prohibiting extension; *fingers,* which can develop flexion contractures that limit extension; *hips,* which can develop flexion contractures that affect the gait by shortening the limb or develop external rotation or adduction deformities that affect the gait; *knees,* which can develop flexion contractures that limit extension and alter the gait; and *feet,* which can "drop" as a result of plantar flexion, which limits dorsiflexion and alters the gait.
- Ensure that patient changes position at least q2h. Post a turning schedule at patient's bedside. Position changes not only will maintain correct body alignment, thereby reducing strain on the joints, but also will prevent contractures, minimize pressure on bony prominences, and promote maximal chest expansion.
  - ☐ Try to place patient in a position that achieves proper standing alignment: head neutral or slightly flexed on the neck, hips extended, knees extended

or minimally flexed, and feet at right angles to the legs. Maintain this position with pillows, towels, or other positioning aids.

☐ To prevent hip flexion contractures, ensure that the patient is prone or side-lying with the hips extended for the same amount of time patient spends in the supine position.

☐ When the HOB must be elevated 30 degrees, extend the patient's shoulders and arms, using pillows to support the position, and allow the fingertips to extend over the edge of the pillows to maintain normal arching of the hands.

> *Caution:* Because elevating the HOB promotes hip flexion, ensure that patient spends equal time with the hips in extension (see intervention, "To prevent hip flexion . . .," above).

☐ When patient is in the side-lying position, extend the lower leg from the hip to help prevent hip flexion contracture.

☐ When able to place patient in the prone position, use a special prone positioning device or move patient to the end of the bed and allow the feet to rest between the mattress and footboard. This not only will prevent plantarflexion and hip rotation, but also will prevent injury to the heels and toes. Place thin pads under the angles of the axillae and lateral aspects of the clavicles to prevent internal rotation of the shoulders and maintain anatomic position of the shoulder girdle. Ensure adequate lung expansion and padding to prevent pressure sores on the face. When using prone positioning for treatment of ARDS, be sure to establish a schedule that optimizes use of this position. Often the patient is prone for 6 hours, followed by 2 hours on the back.

> **Note:** Guidelines for the optimal use of prone positioning to improve oxygenation for the patient in ARDS are not well established.

- To maintain the joints in neutral position, use the following as indicated: pillows, rolled towels, blankets, sandbags, antirotation boots, splints, and orthotics. When using adjunctive devices, monitor the involved skin at frequent intervals for alterations in integrity and implement measures to prevent skin breakdown.
- Assess for footdrop by inspecting the feet for plantarflexion and evaluating patient's ability to pull the toes upward toward the nose. Although feet posture naturally in plantarflexion, be particularly alert to the patient's inability to pull the toes up. To prevent footdrop, foam boots or "high top" tennis shoes may be used to support the feet. Document this assessment daily. Teach patient the rationale and procedure for ROM exercises, and have patient return the demonstrations, if able. Review **Activity intolerance,** earlier, to ensure that patient does not exceed his or her tolerance. Provide passive exercises for patients unable to perform active or active-assistive exercises. In addition, incorporate movement patterns into care activities, such as position changes, bed baths, getting the patient on and off the bedpan, or changing the patient's gown. Ensure that joints especially prone to contracture are exercised more stringently.
- Perform and document limb girth measurements, dynamography (hand-grip device that measures muscle strength), ROM, and exercise baseline limits to assess patient's existing muscle mass and strength and joint motion.
- Explain to patient that muscle atrophy occurs because of disuse or failure to use the joint, often because of immediate or anticipated pain. Eventually, disuse may result in a decrease in muscle mass and blood supply and a loss of periarticular tissue elasticity, which in turn can lead to increased muscle fatigue and joint pain with use.
- Emphasize the importance of maintaining or increasing muscle strength and

periarticular tissue elasticity through exercise. If unsure about patient's complicating pathology, consult with physician about the appropriate form of exercise for patient.

- Explain the need to participate maximally in self-care as tolerated to help maintain muscle strength and enhance a sense of participation and control.
- For *non*cardiac patients needing greater help with muscle strength, assist with resistive exercises (e.g., moderate weightlifting to increase the size, endurance, and strength of the muscles). For patients in beds with Balkan frames, provide the means for resistive exercise by implementing a system of weights and pulleys. First, determine patient's baseline level of performance on a given set of exercises, and then set realistic goals with the patient for repetitions. For example, if the patient can do 5 repetitions of lifting a 5-lb weight with the biceps muscle, the goal may be to increase the repetitions to 10 within 1 wk, to an ultimate goal of 20 within 3 wk and then advance to 7½-lb weights.
- If the joints require rest, isometric exercises can be used. With these exercises, teach patient to contract a muscle group and hold the contraction for a count of 5 or 10. The sequence is repeated for increasing numbers or repetitions until an adequate level of endurance has been achieved. Thereafter, maintenance levels are performed.
- Provide a chart to show patient's progress, and combine this with large amounts of positive reinforcement. Post the exercise regimen at the bedside to ensure consistency by all health care personnel.
- Provide periods of uninterrupted rest between exercises/activities to enable patient to replenish energy stores.
- Seek a referral to a physical therapist (PT) or occupational therapist (OT) as appropriate.

NIC Positioning; Pressure Management; Exercise Therapy: Joint Mobility; Exercise Therapy: Muscle Control

Altered oral mucous membrane related to ineffective oral hygiene
Desired outcome: Patient's oral mucosa, lips, and tongue are intact within 24 h before discharge from intensive care unit.

- Assess patient's oral mucous membrane, lips, and tongue q2h, noting presence of dryness, exudate, swelling, blisters, and ulcers.
- If patient is alert and able to take oral fluids, offer frequent sips of water or ice chips to alleviate dryness.
- Perform mouth care q2-4h, using a soft-bristle toothbrush to cleanse the teeth and a moistened cloth or sponge-tip applicator to moisten crusty areas or exudate on tongue and oral mucosa. For patient who are intubated, suction mouth continuously during oral hygiene to remove fluid and debris.
- Apply lip balm q2h and prn to prevent cracking of lips.
- If indicated, use an artificial saliva preparation to assist in keeping mucous membrane moist.
- As appropriate, have patient wear dentures as soon as he or she is able, to improve communication and enhance comfort.

NIC Oral Health Maintenance

Self-care deficit related to cognitive, neuromuscular, or musculoskeletal impairment; activity intolerance secondary to prolonged bed rest
Desired outcome: Patient's physical needs are met by patient, nursing staff, or significant others.

- Assess patient's ability to perform self-care on the basis of functional status (e.g., comatose state, hemiplegia, sensory or motor deficit, alterations in vision).
- If patient is comatose, meet all patient's physical needs, including bathing, oral hygiene, feeding, and elimination. Involve significant others in the plan of care. Explain all procedures to patient and significant others before performing them.

- For patient who is not comatose, collaborate with him or her on a plan of care that promotes as much self-care as patient is capable of providing. Schedule care activities around the periods of time patient has the most energy to meet his or her needs. Use assessment criteria for activity tolerance, p. 75, to evaluate patient's tolerance of the activity.
- If patient is alert, keep toiletries and other necessary items within reach.
- Do not rush patient; allow adequate time for performance of self-care activities.
- Encourage patient; reinforce the value of progress that is made.
- As appropriate, consult with occupational therapy department regarding use of assistive devices such as long-handle tools.
- If visual impairment exists, place all objects within patient's field of vision. If diplopia is present, apply an eye patch and alternate it between patient's eyes q2-3h.

NIC Energy Management; Self-Care Assistance

Altered peripheral tissue perfusion related to interrupted arterial and venous flow secondary to prolonged immobility

Desired outcome: By discharge from the ICU, patient has adequate peripheral circulation as evidenced by normal skin color and temperature and adequate distal pulses (>2+ on a 0-4+ scale) in peripheral extremities.

- Identify patients at high risk for tissue impairment: individuals with altered LOC, immobility, hypothermia, hyperthermia, cachexia, hypoalbuminemia, inability to perform ADL, or advanced age.
- Identify patients at risk for deep vein thrombosis (DVT), including those with chronic infection, malignancy, and peripheral vascular disease, those with a history of smoking, and the aged, obese, and anemic.
- Teach patient that pain, redness, swelling, and warmth in the involved area and coolness, unnatural color or pallor, and superficial venous dilation distal to the involved area are all indicators of DVT and should be reported to a staff member promptly if they occur.
- Monitor for the same indicators listed earlier, along with routine VS checks. If patient is asymptomatic for DVT, consider assessing for a positive Homans sign. The Homans sign is not very sensitive or specific for DVT but can be elicited by flexing the knee 30 degrees and dorsiflexing the foot. Pain elicited with the dorsiflexion may be a sign of DVT, and patient should be referred to physician for further evaluation. Additional signs of DVT may include fever, tachycardia, and elevated sedimentation rate (ESR). Normal ESR (Westergren method) in males younger than 50 years is 0-15 mm/h, and older than 50 years it is 0-20 mm/h. In females younger than 50 years it is 0-20 mm/h, and older than 50 years it is 0-30 mm/h.
- Teach patient calf-pumping (ankle dorsiflexion-plantarflexion) and ankle-circling exercises. Instruct patient to repeat each movement 10 times, performing each exercise hourly during extended periods of immobility, provided that patient is free of symptoms of DVT. Help promote circulation by performing passive ROM or encouraging active ROM exercises.
- Encourage deep breathing, which increases negative pressure in the lungs and thorax to promote emptying of large veins.
- When not contraindicated by peripheral vascular disease, ensure that patient wears antiembolic hose or pneumatic sequential compression stockings. Remove them for 10-20 min q8h, and inspect underlying skin for evidence of irritation or breakdown. Reapply hose after elevating patient's legs at least 10 degrees for 10 min.
- Instruct patient not to cross the feet at the ankles or knees while in bed because doing so may cause venous stasis. If patient is at risk for DVT, elevate the foot of the bed 10 degrees to increase venous return.
- Patients at risk for DVT may require pharmacologic interventions such as heparin, low-molecular-weight heparin, aspirin, platelet inhibitors, or sodium

warfarin. Administer medication as prescribed, and monitor appropriate laboratory values (e.g., prothrombin time [PT], partial thromboplastin time [PTT]). Educate patient to self-monitor for and report bleeding (epistaxis, bleeding gums, hematemesis, hemoptysis, melena, hematuria, and ecchymoses). High-risk patients may have a vena cava filter placed to protect against pulmonary embolism.

- In patients prone to DVT, acquire bilateral baseline measurements of the midcalf, knee, and midthigh and record them on patient's initial assessment. Monitor these measurements daily and compare them with the baseline measurements to rule out extremity enlargement caused by DVT.

NIC Embolus Precautions; Circulatory Precautions

Altered cerebral tissue perfusion (orthostatic hypotension) related to interrupted arterial flow to the brain secondary to prolonged bed rest

Desired outcome: When getting out of bed, patient has adequate cerebral perfusion as evidenced by HR <120 bpm and BP ≥90/60 mm Hg immediately after position change (or within 20 mm Hg of patient's normal range); dry skin; normal skin color; and denial of vertigo and syncope, with return of HR and BP to resting levels within 3 min of position change.

- Assess patient for factors that increase the risk of orthostatic hypotension because of fluid volume changes (e.g., recent diuresis, diaphoresis, change in vasodilator therapy), altered autonomic control (e.g., diabetic cardiac neuropathy, denervation post heart transplant, advanced age), or severe left ventricular dysfunction.
- Explain the cause of orthostatic hypotension and measures for preventing it.
- Application of elastic stockings may be useful in preventing orthostatic hypotension once the patient is mobilized. For patients who continue to have difficulty with orthostatic hypotension, it may be necessary to supplement the hose with elastic wraps to the groin when the patient is out of bed. Ensure that these wraps encompass the entire surface of the legs.
- When patient is in bed, provide instructions for leg exercises as described under **Activity intolerance,** p. 74.
- Prepare patient for getting out of bed by encouraging position changes within necessary confines. It is sometimes possible and advisable to use a tilt table to reacclimate patient to upright positions.
- Follow these guidelines for mobilization:
  ☐ Check the BP of any high-risk patient for whom this will be the first time out of bed.
  ☐ Have the patient dangle legs at the bedside. Be alert to indicators of orthostatic hypotension, including diaphoresis, pallor, tachycardia, hypotension, and syncope. Question patient about the presence of lightheadedness or dizziness.
  ☐ If indicators of orthostatic hypotension occur, check the VS. A drop in systolic BP of 20 mm Hg and an increased pulse rate, combined with symptoms of vertigo and impending syncope, signal the need for return to a supine position.
  ☐ If leg dangling is tolerated, have patient stand at the bedside with two staff members in attendance. If no adverse signs or symptoms occur, have patient progress to ambulation as tolerated.

NIC Energy Management; Surveillance

Constipation related to less-than-adequate fluid or dietary intake and bulk; immobility; lack of privacy; positional restrictions; use of opioid analgesics

Desired outcomes: Within 24 h of this diagnosis, patient verbalizes knowledge of measures that promote bowel elimination. Patient relates the return of his or her normal pattern and character of bowel elimination within 3 to 5 days of this diagnosis.

- Assess patient's bowel history to determine normal bowel habits and interventions that are used successfully at home.
- Monitor and document patient's bowel movements, diet, and I&O. Be alert

> **Research Brief 1-5**   A structured interview of 51 experienced critical care and acute care nurses was conducted to describe the practices nurses employed to assist the patient to sit on the side of the bed (dangle). Most reported that nurses had authority to decide when and who to dangle. Many strategies were described that were performed to improve patient tolerance of the procedure and included premedication and breathing exercises. Indicators that the patient was not tolerating dangling included changes in heart rate, blood pressure, and level of consciousness. Results of this study will be used to test interventions in this common nursing activity.

Modified from Lane LD et al: Dangling practices of 51 nurses: a pilot project, *Am J Crit Care* 6:177-182, 1997.

to the following indications of constipation: fewer than patient's usual number of bowel movements, abdominal discomfort or distention, straining at stool, and patient complaints of rectal pressure or fullness. Fecal impaction may be manifested by oozing of liquid stool and confirmed via digital examination.
- Auscultate each abdominal quadrant for at least 1 min to determine the presence of bowel sounds. Normal sounds are clicks or gurgles occurring at a rate of 5-34/min.

> **Note:** Bowel sounds are decreased or absent with paralytic ileus. High-pitched rushing sounds may be heard during abdominal cramping, indicating an intestinal obstruction.

- If a rectal impaction is suspected, use a gloved, lubricated finger to remove stool from the rectum. This stimulation may be adequate to stimulate bowel movement. Oil-retention enemas may soften impacted stool.
- Unless contraindicated, encourage a high-roughage diet and a fluid intake of at least 2-3 L/day. Individualize fluid intake according to physiologic state for patients with renal, hepatic, or cardiac disorders.
- Maintain patient's normal bowel habits whenever possible by offering the bedpan; ensuring privacy; and timing medications, enemas, or suppositories so that they take effect at the time of day the patient normally has a bowel movement. Provide warm fluids before breakfast and encourage toileting to gain advantage of gastrocolic or duodenocolic reflexes.
- To promote peristalsis, maximize patient's activity level within the limitations of endurance, therapy, and pain.
- Consult physician for pharmacologic interventions as necessary. To help prevent rebound constipation, make a priority list of interventions to ensure minimal disruption of patient's normal bowel habits. The following is a suggested hierarchy of interventions:
  - ☐ Bulk-building additives (e.g., psyllium)
  - ☐ Mild laxatives (e.g., apple or prune juice, milk of magnesia)
  - ☐ Stool softeners (e.g., docusate sodium or docusate calcium)
  - ☐ Potent laxatives and cathartics (e.g., bisacodyl, cascara sagrada)
  - ☐ Medicated suppositories
  - ☐ Enemas
- Discuss the role narcotic agents and other medications have in constipation. Teach alternative methods of pain control (see Table 1-35, p. 70).

NIC Constipation/Impaction Management

Diversional activity deficit related to prolonged illness and hospitalization
Desired outcome: Within 24 h of intervention, patient engages in diversional activities and relates the absence of boredom.

- Be alert to patient indicators of boredom, including wishing for something to read or do, daytime napping, and expressed inability to perform usual hobbies because of hospitalization.
- Assess patient's activity tolerance as described on p. 75.
- Collect a data base by assessing patient's normal support systems and relationship patterns with significant others. Question patient about his or her interests, and explore diversional activities that may be suitable for the hospital setting and patient's level of activity tolerance.
- Personalize the patient's environment with favorite objects and photographs of significant others.
- Provide low-level activities commensurate with patient's tolerance. Examples include books or magazines pertaining to patient's recreational or other interests, television, or writing for short periods.
- Initiate activities that require little concentration, and proceed to more complicated tasks as patient's condition allows. For example, if reading requires more energy or concentration than patient is capable of, suggest that significant others read to patient or bring in audiotapes of books, such as those marketed for the visually impaired.
- Encourage discussion of past activities or reminiscence as a substitute for performing favorite activities during convalescence.
- As patient's endurance improves, obtain appropriate diversional activities, such as puzzles, model kits, handicrafts, and computerized games and activities; encourage patient to use them.
- Encourage significant others to visit within limits of patient's endurance and to involve patient in activities that are of interest to him or her, such as playing cards or backgammon. Encourage significant others to stagger their visits throughout the day.
- Spend extra time with patient.
- Suggest that significant others bring in a radio, or if appropriate, a TV, if not part of the standard room furnishings.
- If appropriate for patient, arrange for hospital volunteers to visit, play cards, read books, or play board games.
- As appropriate for patient who desires social interaction, consider relocation to a room in an area of high traffic.
- As patient's condition improves, assist him or her with sitting in a chair near a window so that outside activities can be viewed. When patients are able, provide opportunities to sit in a solarium so that they can visit with other patients. If the physical condition and weather permit, take patient outside for brief periods.
- Request consultation for interventions as appropriate from social services, occupational therapy, pastoral services, and psychiatric nurse.
- Increase patient's involvement in self-care to provide a sense of purpose, accomplishment, and control. Performing in-bed exercises (e.g., deep breathing, ankle circling, calf pumping), keeping track of I&O, and similar activities can and should be accomplished routinely by these patients.

NIC Energy Management; Activity Therapy; Art Therapy; Recreation Therapy; Self-Responsibility Facilitation

Altered sexuality patterns related to actual or perceived physiologic limitations on sexual performance secondary to disease, therapy, or prolonged hospitalization

Desired outcome: Within 72 h of this diagnosis, patient relates satisfaction with sexuality and/or understanding of the ability to resume sexual activity.

- Assess patient's normal sexual function, including the importance placed on sex in the relationship, frequency of interaction, normal positions used, and the couple's ability to adapt or change to meet requirements of patient's limitations.
- Identify patient's problem diplomatically, and clarify it with patient. Indicators of sexual dysfunction can include regression, acting-out with

inappropriate behavior such as grabbing or pinching, sexual overtures toward the hospital staff, self-enforced isolation, and other similar behaviors.
- Encourage patient and significant other to verbalize feelings and anxieties about sexual abstinence or hurting the patient. Develop strategies collaboratively among the patient, significant other, and yourself.
- Encourage acceptable expressions of sexuality by the patient. For example, a woman can wear makeup, jewelry, and her own clothing.
- Inform patient and significant other that it is possible to have time alone together for intimacy. Provide that time accordingly by putting a "Do Not Disturb" sign on the door, enforcing privacy by restricting staff and visitors from the room. Encourage caressing, touching, and kissing.

NIC Anxiety Reduction; Body Image Enhancement; Coping Enhancement; Counseling

Altered role performance: dependence versus independence
Desired outcomes: Within 48 h of this diagnosis, patient collaborates with caregivers in planning realistic goals for independence, participates in own care, and takes responsibility for self-care.
- Encourage patient to be as independent as possible within limitations of the endurance, therapy, and pain. Be aware, however, that temporary periods of dependence are appropriate, inasmuch as they enable the person to restore energy reserves needed for recovery.
- Ensure that all health care providers are consistent in conveying their expectations of eventual independence.
- Alert patient to areas of overdependence, and involve him or her in collaborative goal setting to achieve independence.
- Do not minimize patient's expressions of feelings of depression. Allow patient to express emotions, while providing support, understanding, and realistic hope for a positive role change.
- If indicated, provide self-help devices to increase patient's independence with self-care.
- Provide positive reinforcement when patient meets or advances toward goals.

NIC Normalization Promotion; Role Enhancement

Psychosocial support

Psychosocial support of patients and their families/significant others is an integral component of any care plan or care map. Founded on principles of holistic care, in which body, mind, and spirit operate in tandem, this section addresses psychosocial care within the context of the individual's primary social structure. Considerable overlap will be noted between nursing diagnoses for the patient and those for the family. Nursing interventions should occur simultaneously for both the patient and the family/significant others.

NURSING DIAGNOSES AND INTERVENTIONS

Knowledge deficit: current diet, disease process, health resources, medication, prescribed activity, treatment procedures, treatment regimen
Desired outcome: Before any medical or nursing intervention and within the 24-h period before discharge from the critical care unit, patient verbalizes understanding of current diet, disease process, health resources, medication, prescribed activity, treatment procedures, and treatment regimen.
- Assess current level of knowledge about diet, disease process, health resources, medication, prescribed activity, treatment procedures, and treatment regimen.
- Assess cognitive and emotional readiness to learn.
- Recognize barriers to learning, such as impaired verbal communication, altered thought processes, confusion, impaired memory, sensory alterations, fear, anxiety, and lack of motivation.

- Assess learning needs, and establish short- and long-term goals.
- Use individualized verbal or written information to promote learning and enhance understanding. Give simple, direct instructions. If indicated, use audiovisual tools to supplement information.
- Encourage significant others to reinforce correct information about diet, disease process, health resources, medication, prescribed activity, treatment procedures, and treatment regimen.
- As appropriate, facilitate referral of neurologically impaired patient to neurologic clinical nurse specialist or other specialist as appropriate.
- Encourage interest about health care information by involving patient in planning care. Explain rationale for care.
- Interact frequently with patient to evaluate comprehension of information given. Ask patient to repeat what has been explained. Individuals in crisis often need repeated explanations before information can be understood. Also be aware that many individuals may not understand seemingly simple medical terms (e.g., "terminal," "malignant," "constipation").
- As appropriate, assess understanding of informed consent. Assist patient to use information received to make informed health care decisions (e.g., about invasive procedures, surgery, resuscitation).
- Assess understanding of right to self-determination; provide information as indicated. If requested, assist patient with executing an advance directive for health care.

NIC Teaching: Disease Process; Teaching: Individual; Patient Rights Protection; Preparatory Sensory Information

Anxiety related to actual or perceived threat of death; change in health status; threat to self-concept or role; unfamiliar people and environment; the unknown
Desired outcomes: Within 1-2 h of intervention, anxiety is absent or reduced as evidenced by patient's verbalization of same; HR ≤100 bpm; RR ≤20 breaths/min; and an absence of or decrease in irritability and restlessness.

- Engage in honest communication; empathize. Actively listen, and establish an atmosphere that enables free expression.
- Assess level of anxiety. Be alert to verbal and nonverbal cues:
  - ☐ *Mild:* Restless, irritable, asks more questions, focuses on the environment
  - ☐ *Moderate:* Inattentive, expresses concern, narrowed perceptions, disturbed sleep pattern, increased HR
  - ☐ *Severe:* Expresses feelings of doom; rapid speech; tremors; poor eye contact; preoccupation with the past; inability to understand the present; possible presence of tachycardia, palpitations, nausea, and hyperventilation.
  - ☐ *Panic:* Cannot concentrate or communicate, distorts reality, increased motor activity, vomiting, tachypnea
- For severe anxiety or panic state, refer to psychiatric clinical nurse specialist, case manager, or other health-team members as appropriate.
- If hyperventilation occurs, encourage slow, deep breaths by having patient mimic your own breathing pattern.
- Validate the nursing assessment of anxiety with the patient. ("You seem distressed; are you feeling uncomfortable now?")
- After an episode of anxiety, review and discuss the thoughts and feelings that led to the episode.
- Identify coping behaviors currently being used (e.g., denial, anger, repression, withdrawal, daydreaming, drug or alcohol dependence). Review coping behaviors used in the past. Assist in using adaptive coping to manage anxiety.
- Encourage expression of fears, concerns, and questions. ("I know this room looks like a maze of wires and tubes; please let me know when you have any questions.")
- Reduce sensory overload by providing an organized, quiet environment. See **Sensory/perceptual alterations,** p. 51.

- Introduce self and other health care team members; explain each individual's role as it relates to the plan of care or care map.
- Teach relaxation and imagery techniques. See **Health-seeking behavior,** p. 302.
- Enable support persons to be in attendance whenever possible.
- Engage in and promote awareness of touch to significant others when appropriate. Kinds of touch are described in Table 1-37.

NIC Anxiety Reduction; Coping Enhancement; Calming Technique

Impaired verbal communication related to neurologic or anatomic deficit (e.g., hearing impairment, visual impairment); psychologic or physical barriers (e.g., tracheostomy, intubation); cultural or developmental differences

Desired outcome: At the time of intervention, patient communicates needs and feelings and relates decrease in or absence of frustration over communication barriers.

- Assess etiology of impaired communication (e.g., tracheostomy, stroke, cerebral tumor, Guillain-Barré syndrome).
- With patient and significant others, assess patient's ability to hear, see, speak, read, write, and comprehend English. If patient speaks a language other than English, collaborate with English-speaking family member or interpreter to establish effective communication.
- When communicating, use eye contact; speak in a clear, normal tone of voice; and face the patient.
- If patient cannot speak because of a physical barrier (e.g., tracheostomy, wired mandibles), provide reassurance and acknowledge frustration. ("I know this is frustrating for you, but please do not give up. I want to understand you.")
- Provide slate, word cards, pencil and paper, alphabet board, pictures, or other communication device to assist patient. Adapt the call system to meet the patient's needs. Document the meaning of the patient's signals in response to questions.
- Explain to significant others the source of the communication impairment; teach them effective communication alternatives (see preceding intervention).
- Be alert to nonverbal messages, such as facial expressions, hand movements, and nodding of the head. Validate meanings with the patient.

TABLE 1-37 Kinds of Touch

Instrumental touch
- Task or procedure related
- May be negatively perceived but accepted as impersonal

Affective touch
- Expressive, personal
- Caring
- Comforting
- May be positively or negatively perceived
- Influenced by cultural patterns

Therapeutic touch
- A deliberate intervention to accomplish a purpose
- Massage
- Acupressure
- Use of space around the individual to mobilize energy fields

- Recognize that the inability to speak may foster maladaptive behaviors. Encourage patient to communicate needs; reinforce independent behaviors.
- Be honest; do not relate understanding if you cannot interpret patient's communication.

NIC Active Listening; Communication Enhancement: Hearing Deficit, Speech Deficit, Visual Deficit

Sensory/perceptual alterations related to therapeutically or socially restricted environment; psychologic stress; altered sensory reception, transmission, or integration; chemical alteration

Desired outcomes: At the time of intervention, patient verbalizes orientation to time, place, and person; relates the ability to concentrate; and expresses satisfaction with the degree and type of sensory stimulation being received.

- Assess factors contributing to the sensory/perceptual alteration.
  - ☐ *Environmental:* Excessive noise in the environment; constant, monotonous noise; restricted environment (immobility, traction, isolation); social isolation (restricted visitors, impaired communication); therapies.
  - ☐ *Physiologic:* Altered organ function; sleep or rest pattern disturbance; medication; history of altered sensory perception.
- Determine the appropriate sensory stimulation needed; plan care accordingly.
- Control factors that contribute to environmental overload. For example, avoid constant lighting (maintain day/night patterns); reduce noise whenever possible (e.g., decrease alarm volumes, avoid loud talking, keep room door closed, provide ear plugs).
- Provide meaningful sensory stimulation:
  - ☐ Display clocks, large calendars, and meaningful photographs and objects from home.
  - ☐ Depending on patient's preferences, provide a radio, music, reading materials, and tape recordings of family and significant others. Earphones help block out external stimuli.
  - ☐ Position patient toward window when possible.
  - ☐ Discuss current events, time of day, holidays, and topics of interest during patient care activities.
  - ☐ As needed, orient patient to surroundings. Direct patient to reality as necessary.
  - ☐ Establish personal contact by touch to help promote and maintain contact with the real environment.
  - ☐ Encourage significant others to communicate with patient frequently, using a normal tone of voice.
  - ☐ Convey concern and respect. Introduce yourself, and call patient by name.
  - ☐ Stimulate vision with mirrors, colored decorations, and pictures.
  - ☐ Stimulate sense of taste with sweet, salty, and sour substances if appropriate.
  - ☐ Encourage use of eyeglasses and hearing aids.
- Inform patient before initiating interventions and using equipment.
- Encourage participation in health care planning and decision making whenever possible. Allow for choice when possible.
- Assess sleep-rest pattern to evaluate its contribution to the sensory/perceptual disorder. Ensure that patient attains at least 90 min of uninterrupted sleep as frequently as possible. For more information, see **Sleep Pattern Disturbance,** which follows.

NIC Environmental Management; Cognitive Restructuring; Cognitive Stimulation

Sleep pattern disturbance related to environmental changes; illness; therapeutic regimen; pain; immobility; psychologic stress

Desired outcomes: After discussion, patient identifies factors that promote sleep. Within 8 h of intervention, patient attains 90-min periods of uninterrupted sleep and verbalizes satisfaction with ability to rest.

- Assess usual sleeping patterns (e.g., bedtime routine, hours of sleep per night, sleeping position, use of pillows and blankets, napping during the day, nocturia).

- Explore relaxation techniques that promote rest/sleep (e.g., imagining relaxing scenes, listening to soothing music or taped stories, using muscle relaxation exercises).
- Identify causative factors and activities that contribute to sleep pattern disturbance, adversely affect sleep patterns, or awaken patient. Examples include pain, anxiety, depression, hallucinations, medications, underlying illness, sleep apnea, respiratory disorder, caffeine, fear, and medical and nursing interventions.
- Organize procedures and activities to allow for 90-min periods of uninterrupted rest/sleep. Limit visiting during these periods.
- Whenever possible, maintain a quiet environment by providing ear plugs or decreasing alarm levels. The use of "white noise" (e.g., low-pitched, monotonous sounds; electric fan; soft music) may facilitate sleep. Dim the lights for a period of time q24h by drawing the drapes or providing blindfolds.
- If appropriate, limit daytime sleeping. Attempt to establish regularly scheduled daytime activity (e.g., ambulation, sitting in chair, active ROM), which may promote nighttime sleep.
- Investigate and provide nonpharmacologic comfort measures that are known to promote sleep (Table 1-38).

NIC Environmental Management; Environmental Management: Comfort; Sleep Enhancement

Fear related to separation from support systems; unfamiliarity with environment or therapeutic regimen; loss of sense of control

Desired outcome: After intervention, patient communicates fears and concerns and relates the attainment of increased psychologic and physical comfort.

- Assess perceptions of the environment and health status, and determine contributing factors to feelings of fear. Evaluate verbal and nonverbal responses.
- Acknowledge fears. ("I understand that this equipment frightens you, but it is necessary to help you breathe.")
- Provide opportunities for expression of fears and concerns. ("You seem very concerned about receiving more blood today.") Listen actively. Recognize that anger, denial, occasional withdrawal, and demanding behaviors may be coping responses.
- Encourage asking questions and gathering information about the unknown. Provide ongoing information about equipment, therapies, and routines according to patient's ability to understand.
- To promote an increased sense of control, encourage participation in the plan of care whenever possible. Provide continuity of care by establishing a routine and arranging for consistent caregivers whenever possible. Appoint a primary nurse or care manager as appropriate.
- Discuss with health care team members the appropriateness of medication therapy for fear or anxiety that is disabling.
- Explore patient's desire for spiritual or psychologic counseling. Make referrals as appropriate.
- Collaborate with physician about a visit by another individual with the same disorder.

NIC Anxiety Reduction; Counseling; Crisis Intervention; Decision-Making Support; Security Enhancement

Ineffective individual coping and **ineffective denial** related to health crisis; sense of vulnerability; inadequate support systems

Desired outcomes: Within 24 h of this diagnosis, patient verbalizes feelings, identifies strengths, and begins using positive coping behaviors.

- Assess patient's perceptions and ability to understand current health status.

TABLE 1-38 Nonpharmacologic Measures to Promote Sleep	
Activity	**Example(s)**
Mask or eliminate environmental stimuli	Use eyeshields, ear plugs
	Play soothing music
	Dim lights at bedtime
	Mask odors from dressings/drainage; change dressing or drainage container as indicated
Promote muscle relaxation	Encourage ambulation as tolerated throughout the day
	Teach and encourage in-bed exercises and position changes
	Perform back massage at bedtime
	If not contraindicated, use a heating pad
Reduce anxiety	Ensure adequate pain control
	Keep patient informed of his or her progress and treatment measures
	Avoid overstimulation by visitors or other activities immediately before bedtime
	Avoid stimulant drugs (e.g., caffeine)
Promote comfort	Encourage patient to use own pillows, bedclothes if not contraindicated
	Adjust bed; rearrange linens
	Regulate room temperature
Promote usual presleep routine	Offer oral hygiene at bedtime
	Provide warm beverage at bedtime
	Encourage reading or other quiet activity
Minimize sleep disruption	Maintain quiet environment throughout the night
	Plan nursing activities to allow long periods (at least 90 min) of undisturbed sleep
	Use dim lights when checking on patient during the night

- Establish honest communication. ("Please tell me what I can do to help you.") Assist with identifying strengths, stressors, inappropriate behaviors, and personal needs.
- Support positive coping behaviors. ("I see that reading that book seems to help you relax.")
- Provide opportunities for expression of concerns; gather information from nurses and other support systems. Provide explanations about prescribed routine, therapies, and equipment. Acknowledge feelings and assessment of current health status and environment.
- Identify factors that inhibit ability to cope (e.g., unsatisfactory support system, knowledge deficit, grief, fear).
- Recognize defensive and maladaptive coping behaviors (e.g., severe depression, drug or alcohol dependence, hostility, violence, suicidal ideations). Confront these behaviors. ("You seem to be requiring more pain medication. Are you experiencing more physical pain, or does it help you to remove yourself from reality?") Refer patient to case manager, psychiatric liaison, clinical nurse specialist, or clergy, as appropriate.

TABLE 1-39   Stages of Grieving

Protest stage	Denial: "No, not me" Disbelief: "But I just saw her this morning" Anger Hostility Resentment Bargaining to postpone loss Appeal for help to recover loss Loud complaints Altered sleep and appetite
Disorganization	Depression Withdrawal Social isolation Psychomotor retardation Silence
Reorganization	Acceptance of loss Development of new interests and attachments Restructuring of life-style Return to preloss level of functioning

- As patient's condition allows, assist with reducing anxiety. See **Anxiety, p. 84.**
- Help reduce sensory overload by maintaining an organized, quiet environment. See **Sensory/perceptual alterations, p. 51.**
- Encourage regular visits by significant others. Encourage them to engage in conversation with patient to help minimize patient's emotional and social isolation.
- Assess significant others' interactions with patient. Attempt to mobilize support systems by involving them in patient care whenever possible.
- As appropriate, explain to significant others that increased dependency, anger, and denial may be adaptive coping behaviors used by patient in early stages of crisis until effective coping behaviors are learned.

NIC Emotional Support; Support System Enhancement

Anticipatory grieving related to perceived potential loss of physiologic well-being (e.g., expected loss of body function or body part, changes in self-concept or body image, terminal illness)

Desired outcomes: After interventions, patient and significant others/family express grief, participate in decisions about the future, and communicate concerns to health care team members and to one another.

- Assess whether perceived sense of loss is real or unreal.
- Assess factors contributing to anticipated loss.
- Assess and accept patient's behavioral response. Expect reactions such as disbelief, denial, guilt, anger, and depression. Determine stage of grieving as described in Table 1-39.
- Assess spiritual, religious, and sociocultural expectations related to loss. (Is religion an important part of your life? How do you and your family/significant others deal with serious health problems?") Refer to the clergy or community support groups as appropriate.
- Encourage patient and family/significant others to share their concerns. ("Is there anything you'd like to talk about today?") Also, respect their desire not to speak.

- Demonstrate empathy. ("This must be a very difficult time for you and your family.") Touch when appropriate (see Table 1-37).
- In selected circumstances, provide an explanation of the grieving process. This approach may assist in better understanding and acknowledging feelings.
- Assess grief reactions of patient and family/significant others, and identify a potential for dysfunctional grieving reactions (e.g., absence of emotion, hostility, avoidance). If the potential for dysfunctional grieving is present, refer to case manager, psychiatric clinical nurse specialist, clergy, or other as appropriate.
- When appropriate, assess patient's wishes about tissue donation.

NIC Active Listening; Dying Care; Grief Work Facilitation

Dysfunctional grieving related to loss of physiologic well-being; fatal illness
Desired outcomes: Within 24 h of this diagnosis, patient expresses grief, explains the meaning of the loss, and communicates concerns with family/ significant others. The patient completes necessary self-care activities.

- Assess grief stage (see Table 1-39) and previous coping abilities. Discuss patient's feelings, the meaning of loss, and goals. ("How do you feel about your condition/illness? What do you hope to accomplish in these next few days/weeks?")
- Acknowledge and permit anger; set limits on the expression of anger to discourage destructive behavior. ("I understand that you must feel very angry, but for the safety of others, you may not throw equipment.")
- Identify suicidal behavior (e.g., severe depression, statements of intent, suicide plan, previous history of suicide attempt). Ensure safety, and refer to case manager, psychiatric clinical nurse specialist, psychiatrist, clergy, or other support system.
- Encourage patient and family/significant others to participate in ADL and diversional activities. Identify physiologic problems related to loss (e.g., eating or sleeping disorders), and intervene accordingly.
- Collaborate with physician about a visit by another individual with the same disorder, if appropriate.

NIC Grief Work Facilitation; Anger Control Assistance

Powerlessness related to health care environment; treatment regimen
Desired outcome: Within 24 h of this diagnosis, patient makes decisions about self-care and therapies and relates an attitude of realistic hope and a sense of self-control.

- Assess personal preferences, needs, values, and attitudes.
- Before providing information, assess knowledge and understanding of the state of health and necessary interventions.
- Recognize expressions of fear, lack of response to events, and lack of interest in information, any of which may signal a sense of powerlessness.
- Evaluate medical and nursing interventions, and adjust them, as appropriate, to support patient's sense of control. For example, if the patient always bathes in the evening to promote relaxation before bedtime, modify the care plan or map to include an evening bath rather than follow the hospital routine of giving a morning bath.
- Assist patient to identify and demonstrate activities that can be performed independently.
- Whenever possible, offer alternatives related to routine hygiene, diet, diversional activities, visiting hours, or treatment times.
- Ensure privacy and preserve territorial rights whenever possible. For example, when distant relatives and casual acquaintances request information about the patient's status, refer them to the patient or a family member who can provide acceptable amounts of information.
- Discourage patient's dependency on staff. Avoid overprotection and parenting behaviors.

- Assess support systems; enable significant others to be involved in care whenever possible.
- Offer realistic hope for the future. If appropriate, encourage direction of thoughts beyond the present.
- Provide referrals to clergy and other support systems as appropriate.

NIC Emotional Support; Self-Responsibility Facilitation

Spiritual distress related to separation from spiritual/religious/cultural supports; challenged belief and value system

Desired outcomes: Within 24 h of this diagnosis, patient verbalizes spiritual or religious beliefs and expresses hope for the future, the attainment of spiritual or religious support, and the availability of the requisites for resolving conflicts.

- Assess spiritual or religious beliefs, values, and practices. ("Do you have a religious preference? How important is it to you? Are there any religious or spiritual practices you wish to participate in while in the hospital?")
- Inform patient and family/significant others of the availability of spiritual aids, such as a chapel or religious services.
- Present a nonjudgmental attitude toward patient's religious or spiritual beliefs and values. Attempt to create an environment that is conducive to free expression.
- Identify available support systems that may assist in meeting the patient's religious or spiritual needs (e.g., clergy, patient's fellow church members, support groups).
- Be alert to comments related to spiritual concerns or conflicts. ("I don't know why God is doing this to me." "I'm being punished for my sins.")
- Use active listening and open-ended questioning to assist in resolving conflicts related to spiritual issues. ("I understand that you want to be baptized. We can arrange to do that here.")
- Provide privacy and opportunities for religious practices, such as prayer and meditation.
- If spiritual beliefs and therapeutic regimens are in conflict, provide honest, concrete information to encourage informed decision making. ("I understand that your religion discourages receiving blood transfusions. Do you understand that by refusing blood your condition is more difficult to treat?")

NIC Spiritual Support; Hope Instillation; Coping Enhancement

Social isolation related to altered health status; inability to engage in satisfying personal relationships; altered mental status; altered physical appearance

Desired outcome: Within 24 h of this diagnosis, patient demonstrates interaction and communication with others.

- Assess factors contributing to social isolation.
  - ☐ Restricted visiting hours
  - ☐ Absence of or inadequate support system
  - ☐ Inability to communicate (e.g., presence of endotracheal tube/tracheostomy)
  - ☐ Physical changes that affect self-concept
  - ☐ Denial or withdrawal
  - ☐ Critical care environment
- Recognize patients at higher risk for social isolation: the older adult, disabled, chronically ill, economically disadvantaged.
- Assist with identification of feelings associated with loneliness and isolation. ("You seem very sad when your family leaves the room. Can you tell me more about your feelings?")
- Determine need for socialization, and identify available and potential support systems. Explore methods for increasing social contact (e.g., tapes of loved ones, more frequent visitations/hospital volunteers, scheduled interaction with nurse or support staff).

- Provide positive reinforcement for socialization that lessens feelings of isolation and loneliness. ("Please continue to call me when you need to talk to someone. Talking will help both of us to better understand your feelings.")
- Facilitate patient's ability to communicate with others (see **Impaired verbal communication,** p. 85).

NIC Socialization Enhancement

Body image disturbance related to loss of or change in body parts or function; physical trauma

Desired outcomes: Before hospital discharge, patient acknowledges body changes and demonstrates movement toward incorporating changes into self-concept. Maladaptive responses, such as severe depression, are absent.

- Establish open, honest communication. Promote an environment that is conducive to free expression. ("Please feel free to talk to me whenever you have any questions.") Assess indicators suggesting body image disturbance as listed in Table 1-40.
- When planning care, be aware of interventions that may influence body image (e.g., medications, procedures, monitoring).
- Assess knowledge of patient's pathophysiologic process and current health status. Clarify any misconceptions.
- Discuss the loss or change with the patient. Recognize that what may seem to be a small change may be of great significance to the patient (e.g., arm immobilizer, catheter, hair loss, ecchymoses, facial abrasions).
- Explore expressions of concern, fear, and guilt. ("I understand that you are frightened. Your face looks very different now, but you will see changes and it will improve. Gradually you will begin to look more like yourself.")
- Encourage patient and family/significant others to interact with one another. Help family/significant others to support the patient's feelings related to the changed body part or function. ("I know your son looks very different to you now, but it would help if you speak to him and touch him as you would normally.")
- Encourage gradual participation in self-care activities as the patient becomes physically and emotionally able. Allow for some initial withdrawal and denial behaviors. For example, when changing dressings over traumatized part, explain what you are doing but do not expect the patient to watch or participate initially.
- Discuss the potential for reconstruction of the loss or change (i.e., surgery, prosthesis, grafting, physical therapy, cosmetic therapies, organ transplant).
- Recognize manifestations of severe depression (e.g., sleep disturbances,

---

TABLE 1-40 **Indicators Suggesting Body Image Disturbance**

Nonverbal indicators

   Missing body part—internal or external (e.g., splenectomy, amputated extremity)

   Change in structure (e.g., open, draining wound)

   Change in function (e.g., colostomy)

   Avoiding looking at or touching body part

   Hiding or exposing body part

Verbal indicators

   Expression of negative feelings about body

   Expression of feelings of helplessness, hopelessness, or powerlessness

   Personalization or depersonalization of missing or mutilated part

   Refusal to acknowledge change in structure or function of body part

---

change in affect, change in communication pattern). As appropriate, refer to case manager, psychiatric clinical nurse specialist, clergy, or support group.

- Help patient attain a sense of autonomy and control by offering choices and alternatives whenever possible. Emphasize strengths, and encourage activities that interest patient.
- Offer realistic hope for the future.

NIC Body Image Enhancement; Emotional Support; Grief Work Facilitation

Risk for violence: self-directed or directed at others, related to sensory overload; suicidal behavior; rage reactions; neurologic disease; perceived threats; toxic reaction to medications; substance withdrawal

Desired outcome: Patient does not harm self or others.

- Assess factors that may contribute to or precipitate violent behavior (e.g., medication reactions, inability to cope, suicidal behavior, confusion, hypoxia, substance withdrawal, preictal and postictal states).
- Attempt to eliminate or treat causative factors. For example, provide patient teaching, reorient patient, ensure delivery of prescribed oxygen therapy, and reduce or prevent sensory overload (see **Sensory/perceptual alterations,** p. 51).
- Assess for history of physical aggression, family violence, and substance abuse as maladaptive coping behaviors.
- Monitor for early signs of increasing anxiety and agitation (e.g., restlessness, verbal aggressiveness, inability to concentrate). Assess for body language that is indicative of violent behavior: clenched fists, rigid posture, increased motor activity.
- Approach patient in a positive manner, and encourage verbalization of feelings and concerns. ("I understand that you are frightened. I will be here from 3 PM to 11 PM to care for you.")
- Offer as much personal and environmental control as the situation allows. ("Let's discuss the care you will need today. What fluids would you like to drink? Would you prefer a bath in the morning or evening?")
- Help patient distinguish reality from altered perceptions. Orient to time, place, and person. Alter the environment to promote reality-based thought processes (e.g., provide clocks, calendars, pictures of loved ones, familiar objects).
- For acute confusion that becomes aggressive, do not attempt to reorient patient and avoid arguing. Instead, provide support by stating "I believe that you (see, hear) that; however, I do not (see, hear) that." Use nonthreatening mannerisms, facial expressions, and tone of voice.
- Initiate measures that prevent or reduce excessive agitation:
  - ☐ Reduce environmental stimuli (e.g., alarms, loud or unnecessary talking).
  - ☐ Before touching patient, explain interventions, using short, concise statements.
  - ☐ Speak quietly (but firmly, as necessary), and project a caring attitude. ("We are very concerned for your comfort and safety. Can we do anything to help you feel more relaxed?")
  - ☐ Avoid crowding (e.g., of equipment, visitors, health care personnel) in patient's personal environment.
  - ☐ Avoid direct confrontation.
- Explain and discuss patient's behavior with family/significant others. Acknowledge frustration, concerns, fears, and questions. Review safety precautions with family/significant others (Table 1-41).

Hopelessness related to prolonged isolation or activity restriction; failing or deteriorating physiologic condition; long-term stress; loss of faith in God or belief system

Desired outcome: Before hospital discharge, patient verbalizes hopeful aspects of health status and relates that feelings of despair are absent or lessened.

- Develop open, honest communication with the patient. Actively listen, be

TABLE 1-41   Safety Precautions in the Event of Violent Behavior

Patient safety

- Remove harmful objects from the environment, such as heavy objects, scissors, tubing.
- Apply padding to side rails according to agency protocol.
- If available, use bed alarms.
- Use restraints as necessary and prescribed. Monitor patient's neurovascular status at frequent intervals.
- Set limits on patient's behavior, using clear and simple commands.
- As prescribed, consider chemical sedation when unable to control patient's behavior with other means.
- Explain safety precautions to patient and family/significant others.

Caregiver safety

- Place patient in bed closest to nursing station. Maintain visibility at all times by keeping door open.
- Alert hospital security department when risk of violence is present.
- Do not approach a violent patient without adequate assistance from others.
- Never turn your back on a violent patient.
- Maintain a calm, matter-of-fact tone of voice.
- Monitor security measures at frequent intervals.
- Remain alert.

---

empathetic about patient's fears and doubts, and promote an environment that is conducive to free expression.

- Assess patient's and family's/significant others' understanding of health status and prognosis; clarify any misperceptions.
- Assess for indicators of hopelessness: unwillingness to accept help, pessimism, withdrawal, lack of interest, silence, loss of gratification in roles, previous history of hopeless behavior, hypoactivity, inability to accomplish tasks, expressions of incompetence, closing eyes, and turning away.
- Provide opportunities for the patient to feel cared for, needed, and valued by others. For example, emphasize importance of relationships. ("Tell me about your grandchildren." "It seems that your family loves you very much.")
- Support significant others who seem to spark or maintain patient's feelings of hope. ("Your husband's mood seemed to improve after your visit.")
- Recognize factors that promote sense of hope (e.g., discussions about family members, reminiscing about better times).
- Explore patient's coping mechanisms; assist with expanding positive coping behavior (see **Ineffective individual coping,** p. 87).
- Assess spiritual foundation and needs (see **Spiritual distress,** p. 91).
- Promote anticipation of positive events (e.g., mealtime, grandchildren's visits, bath time, extubation, removal of traction).
- Help patient recognize that although there may be no hope for returning to original life-style, there *is* hope for a new but different life.
- Avoid insisting that the patient assume a positive attitude. Encourage hope for the future, even if it is the hope for a peaceful death.
- Set realistic, attainable goals, and reward achievement.

Psychosocial support for the patient's family and significant others

NURSING DIAGNOSES AND INTERVENTIONS

Altered family processes related to situational crisis (patient's illness)
Desired outcome: After intervention, family/significant others demonstrate effective adaptation to change/traumatic situation as evidenced by seeking external support when necessary and sharing concerns.

- Assess character of family/significant others: social, environmental, ethnic, and cultural factors; relationships; and role patterns. Identify developmental stage. Be aware that other situational or maturational crises may be ongoing, such as an elderly parent or teenager with a learning disability.
- Assess previous adaptive behaviors. ("How do you react in stressful situations?") Discuss observed conflicts and communication breakdown. ("I noticed that your brother would not visit your mother today. Has there been a problem we should be aware of? Knowing about it may help us better care for your mother.")
- Acknowledge the family's/significant others' involvement in patient care, and promote strengths. ("You were able to encourage your wife to turn and cough. That is very important to her recovery.") Encourage participation in patient care conferences. Promote frequent, regular patient visits.
- Provide information and guidance related to the patient. Discuss the stresses of hospitalization, and encourage discussions of feelings, such as anger, guilt, hostility, depression, fear, or sorrow. ("You seem to be upset since having been told that your husband is not leaving the hospital today.") Refer to clergy, case manager, clinical nurse specialist, or social services as appropriate.
- Evaluate interactions among patient and family/significant others. Encourage reorganization of roles and priority setting as appropriate. ("I know your husband is concerned about his insurance policy and seems to expect you to investigate it. I'll ask the financial counselor to talk with you.")
- Encourage family/significant others to schedule periods of rest and activity outside the critical care unit and to seek support when necessary. ("Your neighbor volunteered to stay in the waiting room this afternoon. Would you like to rest at home? I'll call you if *anything* changes.")

NIC Family Integrity Promotion; Family Process Maintenance; Normalization Promotion

Family coping: potential for growth, related to use of support systems and referrals; choosing experiences that optimize wellness
Desired outcomes: At the time of the patient's diagnosis, family/significant others express their intent to use support systems and resources and identify alternative behaviors that promote communication and strengths. Family/significant others express realistic expectations and do not demonstrate ineffective coping behaviors.

- Assess relationships, interactions, support systems, and individual coping behaviors. Permit movement through stages of adaptation. Encourage further positive coping.
- Acknowledge expressions of hope, future plans, and growth among family members/significant others.
- Encourage development of open, honest communication. Provide opportunities in a private setting for interactions, discussions, and questions. ("I know the waiting room is very crowded. Would you like some private time together?")
- Refer the family/significant others to community or support groups (e.g., ostomy support group, head injury rehabilitation group).

* Encourage exploration of outlets that foster positive feelings, for example, periods of time outside the hospital area, meaningful communication with the patient or support individuals, and relaxing activities (e.g., showering, eating, exercising).

Ineffective family coping: compromised, related to inadequate or incorrect information or misunderstanding; temporary family disorganization and role change; exhausted support systems; unrealistic expectations; fear; anxiety

Desired outcomes: After interventions, family/significant others verbalize feelings, identify ineffective coping patterns, identify strengths and positive coping behaviors, and seek information and support from the nurse or other support systems.

* Establish open, honest communication. Assist in identifying strengths, stressors, inappropriate behaviors, and personal needs. ("I understand your mother was very ill last year. How did you manage the situation?" "I know your loved one is very ill. How can I help you?")
* Assess for ineffective coping (e.g., depression, substance abuse, violence, withdrawal), and identify factors that inhibit effective coping (e.g., inadequate support system, grief, fear of disapproval by others, knowledge deficit). ("You seem to be unable to talk about your husband's illness. Is there anyone with whom you can talk about it?")
* Assess knowledge regarding patient's current health status and therapies. Provide information frequently, and allow sufficient time for questions. Reassess understanding at frequent intervals.
* Provide opportunities in a private setting to talk and share concerns with nurses or other health care providers. If appropriate, refer to psychiatric clinical nurse specialist for therapy.
* Offer realistic hope. Help family/significant others develop realistic expectations for the future and identify support systems that will assist them with planning for the future.
* Reduce anxiety by encouraging diversional activities (e.g., period of time outside of hospital) and interaction with outside support systems. ("I know you want to be near your son, but if you would like to go home to rest, I will call you if *any* changes occur.")

NIC Family Involvement Promotion; Family Mobilization; Family Support

Ineffective family coping: disabling, related to unexpressed feelings; ambivalent family relationships; disharmonious coping styles among family members/significant others

Desired outcomes: Before hospital discharge, family/significant others verbalize feelings, identify sources of support as well as ineffective coping behaviors that create ambivalence and disharmony, and do not demonstrate destructive behaviors.

* Establish open, honest communication and rapport. ("I am here to care for your mother and to help you, as well.")
* Identify ineffective coping behaviors (e.g., violence, depression, substance abuse, withdrawal). ("You seem to be angry. Would you like to talk to me about your feelings?") Refer to psychiatric clinical nurse specialist, clergy, or support group as appropriate.
* Identify perceived or actual conflicts. ("Are you able to talk freely among yourselves?" "Are your brothers and sisters able to help and support you during this time?")
* Encourage healthy functioning. For example, facilitate open communication and encourage behaviors that support cohesiveness. ("Your mother enjoyed your last visit. Would you like to see her now?")
* Assess knowledge about patient's current health status. Provide opportunities for questions; reassess understanding at frequent intervals.
* Assist with developing realistic goals, plans, and actions. Refer to clergy, case manager, psychiatric nurse, social services, financial counseling, and family therapy as appropriate.

- Encourage family/significant others to spend time outside of the hospital and to interact with support individuals. Respect the need for occasional withdrawal.
- Include the family/significant others in the patient's plan of care. Offer them opportunities to become involved in patient care, for example, ROM exercises, patient hygiene, and comfort measures (e.g., back rub).

NIC Family Support; Family Process Maintenance

Fear related to patient's life-threatening condition; knowledge deficit
Desired outcome: After intervention, family/significant others relate that fear has been lessened or is manageable.

- Assess fears and understanding related to the patient's clinical situation. Evaluate verbal and nonverbal responses.
- Acknowledge the fears. ("I understand these tubes must frighten you, but they are necessary to help nourish your son.")
- Assess history of coping behavior. ("How do you react to difficult situation?") Determine resources and significant others available for support. ("Who/what usually helps during stressful times?")
- Provide opportunities for expression of fears and concerns. Recognize that anger, denial, withdrawal, and demanding behavior may be adaptive coping responses during initial period of crisis.
- Provide information at frequent intervals about patient's status and the therapies and equipment used. Demonstrate a caring attitude.
- Encourage use of positive coping behaviors by identifying the fear(s), developing goals, identifying supportive resources, facilitating realistic perceptions, and promoting problem solving.
- Recognize anxiety, and encourage family/significant others to describe their feelings. ("You seem very uncomfortable tonight. Can you describe your feelings?")
- Be alert to maladaptive responses to fear: potential for violence, withdrawal, severe depression, hostility, and unrealistic expectations of staff or of patient's recovery. Provide referrals to psychiatric clinical nurse specialist or other as appropriate.
- Offer *realistic* hope, even if it is the hope for the patient's peaceful death.
- Explore desires for spiritual, religious, or psychologic counseling.
- Assess your own feelings about the patient's life-threatening illness. Acknowledge that your attitude and fear may be reflected to the family/significant others.
- For other interventions, see previous nursing diagnoses: **Altered family processes; Ineffective family coping: Compromised;** and **Ineffective family coping: Disabling.**

NIC Coping Enhancement; Security Enhancement; Support System Enhancement

Knowledge deficit: patient's current health status; therapies
Desired outcome: After intervention, family/significant others verbalize knowledge and understanding about the patient's current diet, disease process, health resources, medication, prescribed activity, treatment procedures, and treatment regimen.

- At frequent intervals, inform the family/significant others about the patient's current health status, therapies, and prognosis. Use individualized verbal, written, and audiovisual strategies to promote understanding.
- Evaluate family/significant others at frequent intervals for understanding of information that has been provided. Adjust teaching as appropriate. Some individuals in crisis need repeated explanations before comprehension can be assured. ("I have explained many things to you today. Would you mind summarizing what I've told you so that I can be sure you understand your husband's status and what we are doing to care for him?")
- Encourage family/significant others to relay correct information to the

patient. This also reinforces comprehension for family/significant others and patient.

- Ask if needs for information are being met. ("Do you have any questions about the care your mother is receiving or about her condition?")
- Help family/significant others use the information they receive to guide health care decisions (e.g., regarding patient's surgery, resuscitation, organ donation).
- Promote active participation in patient care when appropriate. Encourage family/significant others to seek information and express feelings, concerns, and questions.

NIC Learning Facilitation; Learning Readiness Enhancement

Ethical considerations in critical care

More controversy surrounds health care decisions made by and for critical care patients than in any other health care area. Issues surrounding these decisions have been debated vigorously in the literature. Although some of these issues have been settled, others continue to be argued. Here we will examine what is currently considered morally acceptable practice.

Health care providers must develop a clear understanding of ethical issues to ensure that the care they provide is morally and legally acceptable. Ethical reasoning enables the health care professional to examine the moral principles involved in decision making and determine what we ought to do. There are four predominant principles used in health care ethics: (1) respect for autonomy (recognizing that each patient has a right to make decisions for himself), (2) nonmaleficence (not harming a patient), (3) beneficence (helping a patient), and (4) justice (treating patients equally). Ethical dilemmas occur when one of these principles conflicts with another. When a patient refuses needed treatment, the principles of autonomy and beneficence are in conflict.

INFORMED CONSENT

Without adequate knowledge, patients and significant others cannot make good decisions. Part of a nurse's obligation is to inform patients and families, in a caring manner, what is to be expected regarding different treatments. Informed consent serves not only to protect the health care provider from liability; its primary purpose is to support the ethical principle of respect for autonomy. Informed consent is instrumental to a patient's right to accept, continue, or reject all or part of health care interventions of any sort. The elements of informed consent should be used as a guide but are not absolutely necessary for all nursing or medical interventions (Table 1-42).

If a patient is unsure, does not understand, or feels pressured about consenting to the treatment plan, nurses are responsible to advocate for the patient and communicate this to the physician and to the hospital administration if necessary.

ADVANCE DIRECTIVES

Advance directives refer to a patient's directions on how to provide care in the event that the patient becomes unable to make decisions. An advance directive can be written or verbal and can be in the form of a living will or a durable power of attorney for health care (DPAHC).

A living will specifies what treatment a patient wants or does not want in the event that the condition is terminal and the patient cannot make health care decisions. A DPAHC appoints a person to make decisions for a patient when the patient cannot make decisions.

A surrogate decision-maker is someone named in the DPAHC. When no DPAHC exists, the legal next of kin becomes the surrogate decision-maker for

TABLE 1-42   Elements of Informed Consent

Threshold elements (preconditions)
  1. Competence (to understand and decide)
  2. Voluntariness (in deciding)

Information elements
  3. Disclosure (of material information)
  4. Recommendation (of a plan)
  5. Understanding (of nos. 3 and 4)

Consent elements
  6. Decision (in favor of a plan)
  7. Authorization (of the chosen plan)

From Beauchamp TL, Childress JF. *Principles of biomedical ethics,* ed 4, pp. 145-146, New York, 1994, Oxford University Press.

the patient. If the patient does not have family or a DPAHC, a court-appointed guardian becomes the surrogate decision-maker. This person is obligated to make choices that the patient would make. If those choices are unknown, the surrogate decision-maker must try to determine, based on the patient's values, what the patient would want.

Advance directives appeal to the ethical principle of respect for autonomy. When no advance directive is available, we then turn to the ethical principle of beneficence by making decisions in the patient's best interest. Advance directives are supported by the Patient Self-Determination Act,which encourages their use as well as prompts health care providers and institutions to honor them. Interpretation of advance directives can be problematic. Although many patients express a desire for no "extraordinary measures," the meaning of this term can vary. For example, a ventilator can be considered "extraordinary," but it is also part of quite common temporary treatments regularly used in critical care.

CONFIDENTIALITY

Confidentiality in a relationship between a health care provider and a patient means that we do not identify or expose information that is not relevant to care. Also, we do not communicate information gained from a patient except with providers and decision-makers identified by the patient. Confidentiality appeals to the ethical principles of respect for autonomy, beneficence, and nonmaleficence. Almost all nursing and medical codes provide for keeping all information about a patient confidential. Any disclosure of patient information should be considered very carefully.

There are situations, however, in which we are legally obligated to breech patient confidentiality. These situations include public welfare risks, sexually transmitted diseases, gunshot wounds, and suspected abuse of children, elders, or developmentally disabled individuals. Whereas we are *legally* obligated to report such incidents, we are *morally* obligated to let the patient know that we have reported the incident.

QUALITY OF LIFE

Most quality-of-life dilemmas in health care appeal to the ethical principle of justice. A person's quality of life is based on physical, intellectual, emotional, and social components. Although improving quality of life is a primary focus of health care, assessing quality of life is difficult at best. Numerous studies have demonstrated that health care providers consistently rate patients' quality of life lower than the patients do themselves. In addition, studies have revealed that such judgments by health care providers do affect care. Nurses in critical care need to be aware that they are seeing only a minuscule part of a patient's entire life. They tend to base quality-of-life assessments on a patient's medical condition during this time. However, patients take into account things such as family, relationships, and finances when assessing their own quality of life.

It is important to be aware that a patient's assessment of quality of life is compromised when that patient becomes depressed or newly disabled (e.g., stroke, paraplegia, quadriplegia). Whereas critical care nurses care for many patients in such situations, it is usually the first time that this patient or family has faced such life-altering circumstances. The stress of the situation makes evaluation of quality of life difficult for them. It is important to provide the patient and family with support and time before making these critical decisions.

Besides judging quality of life based on a patient's medical condition, studies indicate that health care providers have social prejudices that also can affect care. These include prejudices against the elderly, persons with alternative life-styles, and patients with alcohol and substance abuse and criminal activity. Judgments about a patient may be passed on to other nurses during nursing reports. This serves only to promote prejudice rather than to promote good care. Our justice system, not our health care system, determines what behaviors to punish and how they should be punished.

WITHHOLDING AND WITHDRAWING TREATMENT

Withholding (not starting) and withdrawing (stopping) treatment are widely considered to have no moral or legal difference. However, health care providers and patients' family members are more comfortable withholding than with withdrawing treatment. This comfort is misguided. Once a treatment has been started and is determined to be of no benefit to the patient, any reasons that would have justified not initiating the treatment can be used to justify stopping it. The decision can be reinforced by the knowledge that it has not benefited the patient.

It has been noted that when decisions to withhold resuscitation (do not resuscitate [DNR]) have been made, it seems unclear what other care should be provided. DNR does not mean do not treat. Many patients with DNR orders receive critical care interventions, surgery, and other treatments and then survive to discharge. Once a decision has been made to withhold resuscitation, it is important to clearly define treatments to be withheld or provided.

ASSISTED SUICIDE

Assisted suicide occurs when someone provides a means for a patient to commit suicide (such as deliberately providing enough medicine for an overdose) but the patient actually performs the act that results in death. Although controversy surrounds assisted suicide, the American Nurses Association (ANA), the American Association of Critical Care Nurses (AACN), the American Medical Association (AMA), and the National Hospice Organization (NHO) explicitly oppose it. Most states have laws that make assisted suicide a criminal act. In 1994 Oregon became the first and only state to allow physician-assisted suicide for terminally ill patients. In the summer of 1997 the U.S. Supreme Court determined that there is no constitutional right to physician-assisted suicide.

EUTHANASIA

Euthanasia refers to one person killing another person without causing pain. Several studies reveal that a significant number of nurses believe that euthanasia is justifiable and should be legalized. This indicates a serious conflict of interest by health care providers. Euthanasia is illegal, is opposed by nursing and medical codes, and is morally unacceptable. Even if the intent of euthanasia is "compassion" and the patient requests it, if the health care provider kills a patient, that health care provider is morally and legally responsible for that patient's death.

COMFORT CARE

Patients who are chronically ill, debilitated, or dying are generally isolated from and by society as well as by health care providers. Health care providers are beginning to realize that they have been undertreating pain and depression not only in the routine care of patients, but specifically while caring for those who are chronically ill and dying. Concerns center around fears of causing dependence, unresponsiveness, and even death. When faced with a dying patient, it is unreasonable to worry about potential dependence on medicine. The benefits of analgesics far outweigh the risks of dependence. Health care providers should try to provide the maximal pain relief possible while preserving responsiveness. When that is not possible, most patients and families choose to accept a decreased responsiveness to ensure that adequate pain relief is provided for the dying patient.

Many health care providers voice concerns that giving potent opioids to a dying patient may actually kill the patient. This concern is magnified when decisions to withdraw and withhold treatments have been made simultaneously. Opioid analgesics afford a broad therapeutic index and a long history of safe use in medically frail patients. Patients with a history of opioid use can tolerate large doses without adverse respiratory or cardiovascular effects.

Even though it is very difficult to determine what amount of opioid will cause a person's death, such medicines can still be given by appealing to the principle of double effect. Simplified, this principle explains that giving narcotics to relieve pain is morally acceptable, even while knowing that it may also cause the patient to die sooner. When narcotics and sedatives are given to a patient at the end of life, the intent is to provide comfort until death; the health care provider does not intend to cause the patient to die. If the health care provider gives a medicine with the primary intent of killing a patient, the health care provider is euthanizing that patient and the action is immoral and illegal.

ETHICAL REASONING

When nurses find themselves in a situation in which they think something is "wrong," they should first consider the situation logically and systematically. By doing this, nurses can defend their position rationally and provide ethically as well as medically sound care.

The first thing to do when feeling uncomfortable with a situation is to identify the problem. Is the care provided inappropriate? Once the problem is identified, determine the relevant facts of the case. These facts include the patient's medical, mental, and emotional condition as well as the current plan of care. Then the nurse must consider his or her personal values and ethical position regarding the situation. Nurses should also consider the values and ethical position of all of the decision-makers involved. If the patient is incompetent, does he or she have an advance directive? Next explore every possible option for resolving the dilemma. Then consider the consequences of each option, and apply relevant ethical principles to the situation. For example, a question asked may be "Will continued aggressive treatment respect the patient's autonomy by following the advance directive?"

Once the ethical principles involved have been considered, rank the acceptable options in order of importance and develop and implement a plan. Often, the first step to resolving an ethical dilemma involves clarifying the expectations and wishes of those involved. Table 1-43 outlines steps used to begin clarifying our understanding of the situation and allow us to move forward from there. If direct communication with those involved does not resolve the issue, the bedside nurse should then involve the unit manager. The medical director's involvement may be beneficial also. If assistance is still needed in resolving the dilemma, the Joint Commission on Accreditation of Healthcare Organizations (JCAHO) requires that health care providers have access to institutional means for resolving ethical dilemmas (such as an ethics consultant or committee). If a nurse strongly believes that unethical care is

TABLE 1-43   Components of Ethical Reasoning

1. Identify the actual problem.
2. Determine the relevant facts of the case.
3. Consider the values and ethical positions of everyone involved.
4. Determine possible options for resolving the dilemma.
5. Consider consequences of each option identified.
6. Apply relevant ethical principles to each option identified.
7. Prioritize acceptable options.
8. Develop and implement a plan to resolve the dilemma.
9. Evaluate the resolution of the dilemma.

Modified from Rushton CH: Ethical decision-making in critical care. II. Strategies for nurse preparation, *Pediatr Nurs* 14(6):497-499, 502, 1988.

being provided and an acceptable resolution to the issue is not found, the nurse should withdraw from caring for that patient. Before withdrawing from that patient, however, the nurse must be replaced by another equally competent nurse who does not oppose the plan of care.

PREVENTIVE ETHICS

Just as it is easier to prevent heart disease than it is to cure it, it is easier to prevent an ethical conflict than it is to resolve one. When evaluating actions taken to resolve a dilemma, nurses should consider how those actions can provide help with future dilemmas. When the bedside nurse first sees signs of a problem, strategies used in previous similar situations should be employed to prevent this situation from developing into a conflict. Nurses should refrain from speculation or gossip and instead openly communicate with the patient, family, and other members of the care team about the plan of care. The nurse should promote discussions in advance of all possible outcomes. Last and most important, nurses should respect each patient as a person and treat that patient accordingly.

NURSING DIAGNOSES AND INTERVENTIONS

Knowledge deficit: medical/nursing interventions
Desired outcome: Before any medical or nursing intervention, patient/significant others will know, understand, and agree to or refuse the intervention.
• Determine appropriate decision-maker
• Assess decision-making capacity
• Assess decision-maker's understanding of intervention; provide information as indicated
• Determine voluntariness
• Accept patient's/significant others' permission for or refusal of the intervention
NIC Teaching: Procedure/Treatment; Teaching: Disease Process; Learning Facilitation
Knowledge deficit: end-of-life decisions
Desired outcome: Patient will know and understand options regarding living wills and DPAHC.
• Provide patient with information regarding living wills and DPAHC.
• Assess understanding of living wills/DPAHC; provide information as indicated.
NIC Health System Guidance; Patient Rights Protection
Anticipatory grieving related to withholding/withdrawal of treatment; anticipation of loss

Desired outcome: After interventions, patient and significant others communicate feelings and participate in decisions regarding death and dying.

- Assess patient's/significant others' understanding of medical prognosis and planned interventions.
- Provide specific information regarding what to expect, what care/interventions will be given, and what will be withheld/discontinued; answer questions openly.
- Allow for significant others to be with patient during the dying process.
- Provide all comfort measures possible for patient/significant others.

NIC Grief Work Facilitation; Support System Enhancement; Active Listening; Family Support; Environmental Management: Comfort; Spiritual Support

Bibliography

Acute Pain Management Guideline Panel: *Acute pain management: operative and medical procedures and trauma, clinical practice guideline,* AHCPR Pub No 92-0032, Agency for Health Care Policy and Research, Public Health Service, Rockville, Md, 1992, US Department of Health and Human Services.

Aimone LD: Neurochemistry and modulation of pain. In Sinatra RS et al, editors: *Acute pain: mechanisms and management,* St Louis, 1992, Mosby.

Anderson J: Management of four arterial blood gas problems in adult mechanical ventilation: decision-making algorithms and rationale for their use, *Crit Care Nurse* 16(3):62-73, 1996.

Asch DA, DeKay ML: Euthanasia among US critical care nurses: practices, attitudes, and social and professional correlates, *Med Care* 35:890-900, 1997.

Baranoski S: Wound dressings: challenging decisions, *Home Healthc Nurse* 17(1):19-25, 1999.

Beauchamp TL, Childress JF: *Principles of biomedical ethics,* ed 4, New York, 1994, Oxford University Press.

Benjamin M, Curtis J: *Ethics in nursing,* ed 3, New York, 1992, Oxford University Press.

Borg GV: Psychophysical basis of perceived exertion, *Med Sci Sports Exerc* 14:377-381, 1982.

Bos S: Coma stimulation. *Online J Knowledge Synthesis* 4(1), 1997.

Bozeman M: Cultural aspects of pain management. In Salerno E, Willens JS, editors: *Pain management handbook: an interdisciplinary approach,* St Louis, 1996, Mosby.

Byas-Smith M: Management of acute exacerbation of chronic pain syndromes. In Sinatra RS et al, editors: *Acute pain: mechanisms and management,* St Louis, 1992, Mosby.

Celesia G: Persistent vegetative state: clinical and ethical issues, *Theo Med* 18:221-236, 1997.

Conwell Y, Caine ED: Rational suicide and the right to die: reality and myth, *N Engl J Med* 325:1101-1102, 1991.

Davis A, Gimenez A: *Auditory sensory stimulation in comatose brain injured patients.* Manuscript in preparation, 1998.

Davis A, White J: Innovative sensory input for the comatose brain-injured patient, *Crit Care Nurs Clin North Am* 7(2):351-361, 1995.

Davis AJ et al: Nurses' attitudes toward active euthanasia, *Nurs Outlook* 43(4):174-179, 1995.

Duff D, Wells D: Postcomatose unawareness/vegetative state following severe brain injury: a content methodology, *J Neurosci Nurs* 29(5):305-317, 1997.

Fahey PJ, Tobin MJ: Weaning from ventilatory support. In Baum GL et al, editors: *Textbook of pulmonary diseases,* ed 6, Philadelphia, 1998, Lippincott-Raven.

Folstein M, Folstein S, McHugh P: Mini-mental state: a practical method for grading the cognitive state of patients for clinicians, *J Psychiatr Res* 12(5):189-198, 1975.

Giacino J: Disorders of consciousness: differential diagnosis and neuropathologic features, *Semin Neurol* 17(2):105-111, 1997.

Howard CA: Mechanical ventilation. In Keen JH, Swearingen PL, editors: *Mosby's critical care nursing consultant,* St Louis, 1997, Mosby.

Hunt TK, Hopf HW: Wound healing and wound infection: what surgeons and anesthesiologists can do, *Surg Clin North Am* 77(3):567-606, 1997.

Inaba-Roland K, Maricle R: Assessing delirium in the acute care setting, *Heart Lung* 21(2):48-55, 1992.

Inouye S et al: Clarifying confusion: the confusion assessment method. A new method for detection of delirium, *Ann Intern Med* 113(12):941-948, 1990.

Jonsen AR et al: *Clinical ethics,* ed 4, New York, 1998, McGraw-Hill.

Kim MJ, McFarland GK, McLane AM: *Pocket guide to nursing diagnoses,* ed 7, St Louis, 1997, Mosby.

Kirby RR, Taylor RW, Civetta JM: Ventilatory support modes. In Kirby RR, editor: *Handbook of critical care,* ed 2, Philadelphia, 1997, Lippincott-Raven.

Lode HM et al: Nosocomial pneumonia in the critical care unit, *Crit Care Clin* 14(1):119-133, 1998.

MacIntyre N: Mechanical ventilatory support. In Baum GL et al, editors: *Textbook of pulmonary diseases,* ed 6, Philadelphia, 1998, Lippincott-Raven.

Mackay L et al: Early intervention in severe head injury: long-term benefits of a formalized program, *Arch Phys Med Rehabil* 73:635-641, 1992.

Malkmus D, Booth B, Kodimer C: *Rehabilitation of the head-injured adult: comprehensive cognitive management,* Downey, Calif, 1980, Professional Staff Association of the Rancho Los Amigos Hospital.

McCaffery M: How to calculate a rescue dose, *Am J Nurs* 94(4):65-66, 1996.

McCloskey JC, Bulechek GM, editors: *Nursing interventions classifications (NIC),* ed 3, St Louis, 2000, Mosby.

Melltorp G, Nilstun T: The difference between withholding and withdrawing life-sustaining treatment, *Intensive Care Med* 23:1264-1267, 1997.

Milisen K et al: Delirium in the hospitalized elderly: nursing assessment and management, *Nurs Clin North Am* 33(3):417-436, 1998.

Olsen DP: When the patient causes the problem: the effect of patient responsibility on the nurse-patient relationship, *J Adv Nurs* 26:515-522, 1997.

Ozuna J: Persistent vegetative state: important considerations for the neuroscience nurse, *J Neurosci Nurs* 28(3):199-203, 1996.

Plum F, Posner J: *The diagnosis of stupor and coma,* ed 3, Philadelphia, 1980, Davis.

Portenoy RK: Morphine infusions at the end of life: the pitfalls in reasoning from anecdote, *J Palliat Care* 12:44-46, 1996.

Sanders KM, Stern TA: Management of delirium associated with use of the intra-aortic balloon pump, *Am J Crit Care* 2(5):371-377, 1993.

Schinner K et al: Effects of auditory stimuli on intracranial pressure and cerebral perfusion pressure in traumatic brain injury, *J Neurosci Nurs* 27(6):348-354, 1995.

Siegel MD, Matthay M: Sedatives, analgesics, and paralytic agents in the intensive care unit. In Bone R, editor: *Pulmonary and critical care medicine,* St Louis, 1997, Mosby.

Sosnowski C, Ustik M: Early intervention: coma stimulation in the intensive care unit, *J Neurosci Nurs* 26(6):336-341, 1994.

Stotts NA: Promoting wound healing. In MR Kinney et al, editors: *AACN's clinical reference for critical care nursing,* ed 4, St Louis, 1998, Mosby.

Stotts NA, Hunt TK: Managing bacterial colonization and infection, *Clin Geriatr Med* 13(3):565-574, 1997.

Teasdale G, Jennett B: Assessment of coma and impaired consciousness: a practical scale, *Lancet* 2:81, July 6, 1974.

Tess M: Acute confusional states in critically ill patients: a review, *J Neurosci Nurs* 23(6):398-402, 1991.

Tobin M: Mechanical ventilation: conventional modes and settings. In Fishman AP, editor: *Fishman's pulmonary diseases and disorders*, ed 3, New York, 1998, McGraw-Hill.

Wilson S et al: Vegetative state and responses to sensory stimulation: an analysis of 24 cases, *Brain Inj* 10(11):807-818, 1996.

Yagan MB: Hospital-acquired pneumonia and its management, *Crit Care Nurs Q* 20(3):43, 1997.

Multisystem Trauma

Major trauma

PATHOPHYSIOLOGY

Injuries are the leading cause of death in the United States for all persons younger than 40 years and result in more lost years of potential life than any other cause. Aggressive public education and other prevention measures are necessary to reduce the staggering burden posed by trauma: lost lives, lifetime disability, enormous health care costs, and lost wages. Approximately 60 million injuries occur annually in the United States, 30 million of those require medical care, and 3.6 million require hospitalization. According to the 1997 Advanced Trauma Life Support by the American College of Surgeons, trauma-related dollar costs exceed $400 billion annually. Immediate resuscitation and transport to a designated trauma center must occur to maximize the chance of survival and limit comorbidities and permanent disability associated with trauma.

Mechanisms of injury: Certain injuries can be predicted based on a knowledge of the object producing the injury (e.g., motor vehicle, handgun); type of energy released (e.g., kinetic, thermal, chemical); force of energy (e.g., velocity of vehicle or missile); and use of protective devices (e.g., seat belts, air bags, helmets).

Types of injury: *Blunt injuries* occur without interruption of skin integrity. The degree of injury is related to the transfer of energy causing tissue deformation and the responsiveness of the anatomic structure involved. For example, hollow organs (e.g., stomach, bladder), which tend to be compressible when force is applied, are less likely to rupture than solid organs (e.g., liver, spleen), which are less compressible. Common causes of blunt injury are vehicular collisions and falls.

Penetrating injuries are produced from the motion of foreign objects that penetrate tissue, causing direct damage. Indirect damage may occur because of tissue deformation associated with energy transference from the penetrating object into the surrounding tissues. As a missile penetrates tissue, the surrounding tissue is briefly displaced, creating a temporary cavity. This process is called *cavitation* and is responsible for the massive tissue damage caused by high-velocity missiles. Usually injury inflicted by stab wounds follows a more predictable pattern and involves less tissue destruction than does injury from gunshot wounds.

Oxygen delivery and consumption: Massive fluid shifts related to tissue damage and blood loss create a severe fluid volume deficit. Profound hypovolemic shock ensues unless replacement of estimated blood and fluid loss is initiated and euvolemia maintained until the bleeding is controlled. An oxygen debt is created by a profound imbalance between oxygen supply and demand that develops as a consequence of the hypovolemia and inadequate cellular tissue perfusion.

After initial restoration of circulating fluid volume, the body develops a hyperdynamic circulatory state, which can be associated with improved survival and fewer complications. The hyperdynamic circulatory state helps compensate for the oxygen debt incurred during the initial traumatic injury. This phase generally peaks at 48-72 h and diminishes within 7-10 days. The hyperdynamic state is evidenced by a higher than normal cardiac index (CI), oxygen delivery (Do_2), and oxygen consumption ($\dot{V}o_2$). Inability to achieve and maintain a hyperdynamic state is associated with higher mortality and shock-related organ failure.

Neuroendocrine stress response: To sustain functioning, the brain, blood, and bone marrow require glucose as an energy source. Immediately after major trauma, the central nervous system (CNS) triggers a series of reactions that promote compensation. Catecholamines such as epinephrine and norepinephrine are released. These hormones mobilize glycogen stores, increase available glucose, suppress pancreatic insulin secretion, and enhance peripheral use of glucose, resulting in a net increase in blood glucose. Glycogen stores are rapidly depleted (in <24 h), and energy is then generated from the breakdown of fat and protein. Breakdown of muscle tissue and viscera creates a negative nitrogen balance. Occasionally, subclinical adrenal insufficiency becomes clinically apparent after severe injury; exogenous steroids are administered if standard resuscitative measures fail to correct shock.

The centrally mediated release of antidiuretic hormone (ADH) promotes water absorption in the distal tubules, which increases intravascular volume and diminishes urinary output. The renin-angiotensin complex is stimulated, and aldosterone is released. The aldosterone promotes sodium and water reabsorption and contributes to intravascular volume.

Systemic inflammatory response syndrome: In patients who sustain major trauma, the inflammatory response is triggered by direct trauma as well as by the presence of foreign bodies such as road dirt, missiles, and catheters. In addition, an increase in circulating levels of catecholamines triggers the release and production of white blood cells. When widespread inflammation is present, the term *systemic inflammatory response syndrome (SIRS)* is used. Although the hemodynamic response and clinical findings associated with SIRS are similar to those with sepsis, the term *sepsis* should be used only when an infection is documented.

Multiple organ dysfunction syndrome: The overwhelming inflammation associated with SIRS ultimately can lead to multiple organ dysfunction syndrome (MODS). MODS is a major cause of late mortality in polytrauma patients and accounts for as many as 10% of all trauma deaths. Sepsis or direct organ injury, if present, adds to the likelihood of MODS. In addition, inadequate initial resuscitation or inability to achieve and maintain a compensatory hyperdynamic state contributes to the development of organ failure in trauma patients. The presence of endotoxin, tumor necrosis factor (TNF), interleukin-1, and other mediators of sepsis is associated with hypotension, acidosis, pulmonary compromise, and circulatory collapse, resulting in MODS. New therapies are directed against these mediators. Mediators for interleukin 1 and TNF are showing promise in MODS treatment.

Coagulopathy: Massive blood transfusion is associated with abnormal hemostasis caused by fluid resuscitation with stored blood, which is deficient in some coagulation factors and platelets. Replacement of clotting components with fresh-frozen plasma and platelet transfusions, as appropriate, helps prevent transfusion-related coagulopathies. Disseminated intravascular coagulopathy (DIC) is a severe acquired bleeding disorder that may be triggered by massive trauma and SIRS. Factors contributing to the development of DIC in the polytrauma patient include impaired tissue perfusion, capillary stasis, hypotension, hypoxemia, and acidemia.

Hypothermia: Multiple factors increase the likelihood of hypothermia in major trauma. Exposed body surface area or viscera may occur at the scene of injury or during the initial resuscitation. Cold blood and room-temperature resuscitation fluids lower the core body temperature. Prolonged exposure to cool temperatures in resuscitation or operative areas is an additional factor. When present, central thermoregulatory failure caused by CNS injury, intoxication, or hypoperfusion contributes to hypothermia. Mild hypothermia can help preserve the function and viability of major organs, particularly when tissue perfusion is diminished as a result of injury, shock, or surgical clamping of arteries. However, severe hypothermia creates significant physiologic alterations, including CNS depression, dysrhythmias, acidosis, and electrolyte imbalances.

Psychologic response: Victims of major trauma sustain life-threatening injuries. The patient often is aware of the situation and fears death. Even after the physical condition stabilizes, the patient may have a prolonged or severe reaction triggered by the trauma.

ASSESSMENT

Preservation of the patient's survival and optimization of the chance for life without disability depend on fast and accurate determination of the extent of all major injuries. It is essential to perform a complete and rapid assessment with the patient's clothing removed.

History and risk factors

Mechanism of injury: A knowledge of the events leading to the injury can predict certain patterns of injury. For example, an unrestrained driver in an automobile collision typically sustains injuries to the cranium, face, cervical vertebrae, torso, and lower extremities. High-velocity gunshot wounds typically result in large, ragged exit wounds with massive internal injury along the missile path.

Intoxicants: Acute alcohol intoxication is a common finding with blunt and penetrating trauma. The presence of alcohol and other intoxicants produces neurologic and pupillary changes that may be incorrectly attributed to CNS injury. In addition, acute alcohol or drug intoxication causes cardiovascular, hematologic, and ventilatory changes that compound injury-related alterations. Finally, intoxicants dull the pain response and may obscure important signs that are useful for accurate diagnosis of injuries.

Preexisting medical conditions: Chronic health conditions such as hypertension, diabetes, chronic obstructive pulmonary disease (COPD), cerebrovascular disorders, renal failure, and immune disorders produce physiologic alterations that increase the susceptibility for injury and impair physiologic responses to injury. Use of prescribed and illicit drugs should be determined. For example, beta- (β-) blocking medications inhibit sympathetic stimulation and limit the patient's ability to compensate for hypovolemia. Individuals with insulin-dependent diabetes may require additional insulin to respond to transient hyperglycemia. Chronic opiate use increases tolerance to opiates, and greater than usual amounts may be necessary for analgesia.

? - 1   Tetanus Prophylaxis in Routine Wound Management—United States, 1991

History of adsorbed tetanus toxoid (doses)	Clean, minor wounds		All other wounds*	
	Td†	TIG	Td†	TIG
Unknown or <3	Yes	No	Yes	Yes
≥3‡	No§	No	No‖	No

Modified from Centers for Disease Control: *MMWR* 40(RR10):1-28, 1991.

Td, Tetanus and diphtheria (toxoid); *TIG*, tetanus immunoglobulin.

*Such as, but not limited to, wounds resulting from missiles, crushing, burns, and frostbite.

†For children <7 yr: DPT (DT, if pertussis vaccine is contraindicated) is preferred to tetanus toxoid alone. For persons ≥7 yr, Td is preferred to tetanus toxoid alone.

‡If only three doses of *fluid* toxoid have been received, a fourth dose of toxoid, preferably an adsorbed toxoid, should be given.

§Yes, if >10 yr since last dose.

‖Yes, if >5 yr since last dose. (More frequent boosters are not needed and can accentuate side effects.)

Last meal: Information regarding time, quantity, and type of food or beverage ingested is necessary for planning care to prevent vomiting and reduce the risk of aspiration, especially if surgical intervention is imminent.

Tetanus immunization: Tetanus immunization history is necessary to determine the need for tetanus vaccine or immunoglobulin (Table 2-1).

Initial subjective presentation: Mild tenderness to severe pain may be present, with the pain either localized to the site of injury or diffuse. Pain may be referred, particularly if abdominal structures are involved. Dyspnea, shortness of breath (SOB), agitation, restlessness, and anxiety are associated with impaired tissue perfusion and oxygenation. Nausea and vomiting may occur, and the conscious patient who has sustained blood loss often complains of thirst, an early sign of hemorrhagic shock. Slurred speech and poor coordination are present with intoxication or CNS impairment caused by decreased cerebral O_2 delivery from blood loss.

Initial objective presentation: Should be assessed during the primary survey and resuscitation. Primary survey consists of the *A, B, C, D,* and *E's: A*—airway with cervical spine protection; *B*—breathing: oxygenation and ventilation; *C*—circulation with hemorrhage control; *D*—disability: brief neurologic examination (usually Glasgow coma scale [see Appendix 3]); *E*—exposure/environment.

Initial objective presentation my vary according to site of injury, blood loss, and involved structures. For posterior examination, ensure that spinal alignment is maintained while turning patient. General findings are listed below.

Inspection (secondary survey):   Abrasions and ecchymoses suggest mechanism of injury and involvement of underlying structures. Ecchymoses may take hours to days to develop, depending on rate of blood loss. Absence of external evidence of injury does not exclude the possibility of serious internal injury. Protrusion of bone fragments and viscera may be present. Entrance and exit wounds (if present) should be determined with penetrating injuries. Protruding instruments should not be removed because additional harm and renewed bleeding may occur.

Auscultation: Diminished or absent breath sounds, distant heart sounds, diminished or absent bowel sounds.

Palpation: Weak and irregular pulse, cool and clammy skin, subcutaneous emphysema over area of injury, swelling and point tenderness over injured area.

Percussion: Dullness over blood-filled areas or internal hematomas.

Vital signs and hemodynamics

Initial: Widely variable, according to catecholamine response, volume status, and drugs administered. Increased respiratory rate (RR) and compensatory tachycardia are typical. The absence of tachypnea suggests CNS injury or severe intoxication. Patients taking β-blocking medications may not experience tachycardia, and heart rate (HR) may remain within normal limits despite serious blood loss. Blood pressure (BP) may be normal, slightly elevated, or diminished, depending on volume of blood loss. In young adults, compensatory responses maintain a normal BP until major blood loss occurs. If left untreated, hypotension with mean arterial pressure (MAP) <70 mm Hg occurs, sometimes very rapidly. Decreased central venous pressure (CVP), positive airway pressure (PAP), and cardiac output/cardiac index (CO/CI) reflect hypovolemia and should be corrected to maintain euvolemia. Systemic vascular resistance (SVR) is elevated as a result of hypovolemia and catecholamine release.

Hyperdynamic phase: After fluid volume resuscitation, a hyperdynamic circulatory state compensates for the oxygen debt incurred during the initial traumatic injury. Increases in CO/CI are present. Do_2 is greatly increased because of hypermetabolism and other potential factors such as pain, agitation, infection, and tachycardia. $\dot{V}o_2$ may be double the normal of 250-300 ml/min. Svo_2 usually is >80%. SVR is <900 dynes/sec/cm^{-5} during this phase. If there is failure of compensatory mechanisms, MODS may ensue. In this case, CO/CI will be decreased and pulmonary artery wedge pressure (PAWP) will be increased. The patient may require pressor support to maintain MAP >70 mm Hg.

DIAGNOSTIC TESTS

Complete blood count (CBC): Serial determination of hematocrit/hemoglobin (Hct/Hgb) reflects the amount of blood lost. If drawn immediately after the injury, Hct/Hgb levels may be normal, but serial levels will reveal dramatic decreases during resuscitation and as extravascular fluid mobilizes during the recovery phase. Leukocytosis is expected with a moderate to high total white blood cell (WBC) count. Later, an increase in WBCs or a shift to the left reflects the anticipated inflammatory response or may signal infection.

Blood chemistries: Glucose is elevated initially because of catecholamine release and insulin resistance. Ionized calcium levels decline because of metabolic alterations associated with impaired tissue perfusion and binding with citrate from stored blood. Baseline levels of electrolytes, enzymes, and other chemistries are drawn for later comparison and to guide therapy. Venous lactate levels may be elevated if tissue perfusion is inadequate and anaerobic metabolism is present.

Arterial blood gas (ABG) analysis: May show pH <7.35 and HCO_3^- <22 mEq/L because of metabolic acidosis, which is present if inadequate tissue oxygen delivery leads to anaerobic metabolism and excess lactate production. Decreased Pao_2 is present if ventilation is compromised by pulmonary injury or altered level of consciousness (LOC).

Oximetry: Continuous pulse oximetry is used to assess oxygen saturation. Oxygen therapy should be titrated to maintain Spo_2 of ≥92%-94%, according to individual injuries and preexisting medical conditions.

Type and cross-match: To determine presence of antigens so that recipient and donor blood are compatible. If blood loss is very rapid, requiring immediate transfusion, O-negative (without major antigens) blood or type-specific blood is used until a full cross-match can be performed.

Blood alcohol, toxicology screen: To check for the presence of alcohol or other intoxicant, if suspected. Positive results are used to guide therapy and prevent acute withdrawal symptoms.

Urinalysis: Initially, to check for the presence of blood caused by urinary tract injury. Later, to check for presence of bacteria caused by urinary tract infection (UTI).

X-rays: To check for the presence of fractures, abnormal air or fluids, and foreign objects and to determine location of large organs. With polytrauma patients, cervical spine, chest, abdomen, pelvic, and extremity x-rays usually are necessary.

Computed tomography (CT): To detect magnitude of soft tissue injury, hematomas, and subtle fractures.

> *Caution:* Because of the risk of rapid deterioration, the patient should be accompanied by an experienced nurse during the CT. Appropriate monitoring and resuscitation equipment must be readily available.

COLLABORATIVE MANAGEMENT

Airway management: A patent airway must be secured when Glasgow coma scale (GCS) score #8 or potential for airway compromise is possible. Secure the airway by intubation or cricothyroidotomy, if necessary. If cervical spine injury is suspected, the cervical spine is stabilized during the procedure by maintaining constant in-line positioning with gentle traction. Nasal intubation is preferred to the oral route because there is less manipulation of the cervical spine. However, the success of a particular method depends on the individual patient and the experience of the clinician. Cricothyroidotomy is indicated when other means of intubation are not possible or are contraindicated.

Oxygen: All trauma patients require supplemental oxygen because of the reduced oxygen-carrying capacity of the blood that results from initial blood loss, and because of greatly increased tissue demand for oxygen during the hypermetabolic phase. High-flow oxygen by mask is indicated initially. Oxygen therapy can be titrated according to ABG and pulse oximetry values. Mechanical ventilation may be required.

Fluid management: Underresuscitation as well as overresuscitation of trauma patients during the initial 48-72 h may lead to shock, MODS, and death. The goal of resuscitation in any trauma patient should be to maintain euvolemia. Two or more large-bore (≥16-gauge) short catheters should be placed to maximize delivery of fluids and blood. Use of IV tubing with an exceptionally large internal diameter (trauma tubing), absence of stopcocks, and use of external pressure are techniques used to promote rapid fluid volume therapy when indicated. When rapid infusion of large amounts of fluid is required, all fluid should be warmed to body temperature to prevent hypothermia. Rapid warmer/infusor devices are available to facilitate rapid administration of blood products. A combination of crystalloids, colloids, and blood products is necessary for most major trauma patients. Patients with significant craniocerebral trauma have precise fluid requirements (see "Traumatic Brain Injury," p. 118).

Crystalloids: Balanced salt solutions such as 0.9% normal saline (NaCl) or lactated Ringer's (LR) are commonly used. These solutions are inexpensive and convenient to store, but intravascular retention is poor. Sustained use of normal saline (NS) can lead to hyperchloremic metabolic acidosis; therefore LR is generally preferred. NS is used when crystalloids are administered simultaneously through the same intravenous (IV) line as blood products. The ionized calcium in LR can interact with the citrate anticoagulant in banked blood, causing clot formation.

Colloids: These do not readily cross capillary walls and therefore do not pass between the tissue compartments as easily as crystalloids. The osmotic force generated by the large molecular weight (colloid) substances results in increased plasma osmotic pressure and promotes intravascular fluid retention. Albumin, dextran, and hetastarch are colloid substances in current use. Colloids are generally used as a supplement to crystalloid therapy.

Packed red blood cells (PRBCs): Some degree of blood loss is associated with most injuries, and massive transfusion is sometimes necessary. Massive transfusion is defined as replacement of one half of the patient's blood volume at one time or complete replacement of the patient's blood volume over 24 h. If blood loss is very rapid during the initial resuscitation, immediate transfusion with O-negative blood may be required. When bleeding continues, type-specific blood is used until a full cross-match can be performed. The patient must be properly and permanently identified with trauma alias or name, if known, to prevent transfusion errors. Complications of massive transfusion are numerous. Hypocalcemia caused by calcium binding with citrate in stored PRBCs results in depressed myocardial contractility, particularly in hypothermic patients or in those with impaired liver function. One ampule of 10% calcium chloride should be administered after every 4 units (U) of PRBCs. Abnormal hemostasis occurs, since stored PRBCs are deficient in some coagulation factors and platelets. Replacement of clotting components with fresh-frozen plasma and platelet transfusions, as appropriate, will help minimize transfusion-related coagulopathies.

Autotransfusion: Shed blood is filtered and reinfused into the patient. Shed blood is captured from chest tube drainage or the operative field and reinfused immediately. Various techniques are used to capture and reinfuse the blood. Advantages of autotransfusion include reduced risk of disease transmission, absence of incompatibility problems, and ready availability of blood. Disadvantages include risk of blood contamination and presence of naturally occurring factors that promote anticoagulation.

Gastric intubation: Permits gastric decompression, aids in removal of gastric contents, and is necessary to prevent vomiting and possible aspiration. Contraindicated in patients with basal skull fractures.

Urinary drainage: An indwelling catheter is inserted to obtain a specimen for urinalysis and to monitor hourly urine output. See "Renal and Lower Urinary Tract Trauma" p. 148, for precautions.

Pharmacotherapy

Antibiotics: Broad-spectrum antibiotics are used initially to prevent infections. More specific antimicrobial agents are used when results from culture and sensitivity tests are available.

Analgesics and anxiolytics: Relief of pain and relief of anxiety are important parts of the management of trauma patients. Effective therapy usually requires use of intravenous opiates and anxiolytics. All intravenous agents should be administered judiciously to enhance patient comfort and relieve anxiety while avoiding respiratory depression, masking injury, or disguising changes in physiologic parameters.

Tetanus prophylaxis: Tetanus immunoglobulin and tetanus toxoid are considered on the basis of Centers for Disease Control (CDC) recommendations (see Table 2-1).

Nutrition therapy: When present, infection and sepsis contribute to the negative nitrogen state and increased metabolic needs associated with injury. Prompt initiation of nutrition therapy is essential for rapid healing and prevention of complications. Parenteral nutrition may be necessary because of one or more of the following factors: postoperative status, ileus, and injury to the gastrointestinal (GI) tract. For more information, see "Nutritional Support," p. 1.

Surgery: Need for surgery depends on the type and extent of injuries. The surgical team is coordinated by the trauma surgeon. When several specialty surgeons are required because of injuries to various systems, the order of surgeries is coordinated carefully to preserve life and limit the potential for disability.

NURSING DIAGNOSES AND INTERVENTIONS

Fluid volume deficit related to active loss secondary to physical injury or inadequate resuscitation

Desired outcome: Within 12-24 h of this diagnosis, patient becomes euvolemic as evidenced by MAP ≥70 mm Hg; HR 60-100 beats per minute (bpm); normal sinus rhythm on electrocardiogram (ECG); CVP 2-6 mm Hg; PAWP 6-12 mm Hg; CI ≥2.5 L/min/m^2; systemic vascular resistance (SVR) 900-1200 dynes/sec/cm^{-5}; urinary output ≥0.5 ml/kg/h; specific gravity 1.010-1.0300; warm extremities; brisk capillary refill (<2 sec); and distal pulses >2+ on a 0-4+ scale.

- Monitor BP q15min, or more frequently in the presence of obvious bleeding or unstable VS. Be alert to changes in the MAP of >10 mm Hg. Even a small but sudden decrease in BP may be a signal to consult the physician, especially when the extent of injury is unknown.
- Monitor HR, ECG, and cardiovascular status q15min until volume is restored and vital signs (VS) are stable. Check ECG to note HR elevations and myocardial ischemic changes (i.e., ventricular dysrhythmias, ST-segment changes), which can occur because of dilutional anemia in susceptible individuals. Monitor intake and output hourly.
- In the patient with evidence of volume depletion or active blood loss, administer fluids through several large-caliber (≥16 gauge) catheters or central line. Use short, large-bore IV tubing (trauma tubing) to maximize flow rate. Avoid use of stopcocks, because they slow the infusion rate. Fluids should be warmed to prevent hypothermia.

Caution: Evaluate patency of IV catheters continuously during rapid-volume resuscitation. Hypocalcemia may develop in rapidly transfused patients as a result of stored citrate. Monitor for signs and symptoms such as hyperreflexia, positive Trousseau or Chvostek sign.

- Measure pulmonary artery (PA) pressures q1h or more frequently if blood loss is ongoing. Measure CO/CI and calculate SVR and pulmonary vascular resistance (PVR) q4-8h, or more often in unstable patients. Be alert to low or decreasing CVP and PAWP. An elevated HR, along with decreased PAWP, decreased CO/CI, and increased SVR, suggests inadequate fluid resuscitation. During the hyperdynamic phase, calculate Do_2 and $\dot{V}o_2$ and support higher-than-normal values by oxygen and fluid administration, conservation of energy, and other measures according to individual patient. Anticipate higher-than-normal CO/CI and lower-than-normal SVR.
- Measure urinary output q1h. Be alert to output <0.5 ml/kg/h for 2 consecutive hours. Low urine output usually reflects inadequate intravascular volume in the patient with abdominal trauma.
- Monitor for physical indicators of hypovolemia, including cool extremities, capillary refill >2 sec, and absent or decreased amplitude of distal pulses.
- Estimate ongoing blood loss. Measure all bloody drainage from tubes or catheters, noting drainage color (e.g., coffee-ground, burgundy, bright red [see Table 2-13]). Note the frequency of dressing changes as a result of saturation with blood to estimate amount of blood loss via wound site.
- Administer oxygen to maximize delivery of oxygen to tissues. Use continuous pulse oximetry to assess for adequate oxygenation. Evaluate arterial blood gas (ABG) values as available.

You may also wish to refer to the following interventions from the Nursing Interventions Classification (NIC):

NIC Electrolyte Management; Fluid Management; Fluid Monitoring; Hypovolemia Management; Bleeding Precautions

Pain related to physical injury secondary to external trauma or surgery

Desired outcome: Within 2 h of this diagnosis, patient's subjective or objective (in unconscious, sedated, or paralyzed) evaluation of discomfort improves. If patient can give subjective response, document by using pain scale.

- Evaluate patient for presence of preoperative and postoperative pain. Preoperative pain is anticipated and is a vital diagnostic aid. If able, use a pain scale with the patient to rate discomfort and effectiveness of strategies to relieve pain. Devise alternative methods to communicate with patients with endotracheal tubes or other barriers to communication.
- Administer opiates and other analgesics as prescribed. Avoid preoperative administration of large doses of opiate analgesics until the patient has been evaluated thoroughly by a trauma surgeon. Once analgesics are prescribed, inform patient of their availability. Postoperatively, administer prescribed analgesics promptly before the pain becomes severe. Analgesics are helpful in relieving pain, as well as in aiding in the recovery process by promoting greater ventilatory excursion. Be aware that substance abuse often is involved in traumatic events; victims therefore may be drug or alcohol users, with a higher-than-average tolerance to narcotics. These same persons may suffer symptoms of alcohol or narcotics withdrawal that need recognition and treatment. In addition, recognize that narcotic analgesics can decrease GI motility and may delay return to normal bowel functioning. Document the degree of pain relief obtained, using the pain scale or changes in assessment.
- Supplement analgesics with nonpharmacologic maneuvers (e.g., positioning, back rubs, distraction) to aid in pain reduction.
- See p. 61 for additional pain intervention.

NIC Analgesic Administration; Pain Management, Post Anesthesia Care; Positioning

Altered protection related to clotting factor alterations; decreased hemoglobin level

Desired outcomes: Patient is free of symptoms of bleeding as evidenced by absence of bleeding at venipuncture sites, mucous membranes, intravenous catheter insertion sites, incisions, and GI tract. Coagulation profiles return to normal by the time of transfer from ICU.

- Obtain blood for coagulation and related studies: prothrombin time (PT), thrombin time, partial thromboplastin time (PTT), Hct, Hgb, fibrinogen levels, and fibrinogen degradation products (FDPs).
- Observe for bleeding at venipuncture sites, mucous membranes, urinary catheter insertion sites, incisions, and GI tract. Test gastric drainage, emesis, and stool for the presence of occult blood.
- Administer misoprostol (Cytotec), omeprazole (Prilosec), histamine H_2-receptor antagonists, and/or sucralfate (Carafate) as prescribed to reduce gastric acid and prevent erosion of gastric mucosa. (Avoid cimetidine [Tagamet] because of reduction in hepatic blood flow.)
- Avoid intramuscular (IM) injections and multiple venipunctures. Use IV route for medication administration.
- If DIC is present, see "Disseminated Intravascular Coagulation," p. 579, for treatment.

NIC Infection Control, Infection Protection, Bleeding Precautions

Risk for infection related to inadequate primary defenses secondary to physical trauma or surgery; inadequate secondary defenses as a result of decreased hemoglobin or inadequate immune response; tissue destruction and environmental exposure; multiple invasive procedures

Desired outcome: Patient is free of infection as evidenced by core or rectal temperature <37.7° C (100° F); HR ≤100 bpm; orientation to time, place, and person; and absence of unusual redness, warmth, or drainage at surgical incisions and drain sites.

- Monitor vital signs (VS) for evidence of infection, noting temperature increases and associated increases in heart and respiratory rates. An elevated CO and a decreased SVR suggest sepsis. Consult surgeon if these are new findings. See Tables 10-1 and 10-2, pp. 597 and 598, for hemodynamic profiles of early and late septic shock. Also refer to "Septic Shock," p. 593.

Major trauma   **115**

- Evaluate orientation and level of consciousness (LOC) q2-4h.
- Ensure patency of all surgically placed tubes or drains. Irrigate or attach to low-pressure suction as prescribed. Promptly report unrelieved loss of tube patency.
- Evaluate incisions and wound sites for evidence of infection: unusual redness, warmth, delayed healing, and purulent or unusual drainage.
- Note color, character, and odor of all drainage. Consult physician and culture drainage if it is foul smelling or abnormal.
- Administer parenteral antibiotics in a timely fashion. Reschedule antibiotics if a dosage is delayed for more than 1 h. Recognize that failure to administer antibiotics on schedule may result in inadequate blood levels and treatment failure.
- Administer tetanus immunoglobulin and tetanus toxoid as prescribed (see Table 2-1). Ensure that patient receives documentation of tetanus immunization, if given.
- Change dressings as prescribed, using aseptic technique. Prevent cross-contamination from various wounds by changing one dressing at a time.

NIC Infection Control; Infection Protection; Incision Site Care; Vital Signs Monitoring; Tube Care

Impaired tissue integrity related to mechanical factors (including physical injury); related to altered circulation secondary to hemorrhage or direct vascular injury; related to nutritional deficit secondary to hypermetabolic state; and related to impaired physical mobility

Desired outcome: Patient has adequate tissue integrity as evidenced by wound healing within an acceptable time frame according to extent of injury.

- On admission, clean and irrigate all cutaneous injuries with 0.9% NaCl, or use some other procedure according to individual prescription or hospital protocol.
- Assess all wounds, fistulas, and drain sites q4-8h for signs of irritation, infection, and ischemia. Inspect for healing and presence of granulation tissue q8h.
- Identify infected and devitalized tissue. Aid in the removal of eschar by irrigation or wound packing, or prepare patient for surgical débridement.
- Turn patient q1-2h. Identify need for specialty bed in patients with multiple risk factors for impaired tissue integrity (use individual hospital protocol).
- Promptly change all dressings that become soiled with drainage or blood.
- Protect the skin surrounding tubes, drains, or fistulas, keeping the areas clean and free from drainage. If necessary, apply ointments, skin barriers, or drainage pouches to protect the surrounding skin. Consult wound specialist as necessary.
- Ensure adequate protein and calorie intake for tissue healing (see **Altered nutrition,** on next page).
- See "Wound and Skin Care," p. 55, for more information.

NIC Wound care; Incision Site care

Hypothermia related to exposure at the scene of injury; temporary loss of temperature regulatory mechanisms because of shock or CNS ischemia; surgical exposure of abdominal viscera; administration of large volumes of unwarmed fluid or blood

Desired outcomes: Patient's temperature remains or returns to normal within 24 h of this diagnosis. Complications of hypothermia are avoided as evidenced by normal sinus rhythm on ECG; patient oriented to time, place, and person; Pao_2 ≥80 mm Hg; and absence of prolonged bleeding from wounds, incisions, and venipuncture sites.

- Warm all fluids administered during the initial resuscitation phase and until the patient postoperatively approaches normothermia. Prewarm crystalloids so that they are ready for immediate use. Use rapid-volume infuser for rapid warming of large volumes of blood.

- Keep ambient room temperature as warm as possible in trauma receiving, surgical, and critical care areas. Keep patient dry, and cover head to reduce heat loss.
- Avoid unnecessary exposure of the patient. Keep patient covered with warmed blankets or warming blanket whenever possible.
- Monitor core temperature via rectal or esophageal probe, urinary catheter attachment, or PA catheter until normothermia is attained.
- Be aware that vasodilation during rewarming can result in an intravascular fluid volume deficit (see **Fluid volume deficit**, p. 112).
- Be aware that vasodilation during rewarming necessitates evaluation and frequent titration of vasoactive infusions.
- Monitor for and promptly report serious dysrhythmias (i.e., atrial fibrillation with rapid ventricular response, ventricular dysrhythmias, AV conduction block), which are associated with severe or prolonged hypothermia.
- Be aware that hypothermia compromises cortical functioning, and the patient may be confused, disoriented, or somnolent or may have other neurologic derangements. These symptoms may make it difficult to evaluate concurrent head injury.
- Monitor ABG values at frequent intervals for evidence of hypoxemia. Hypothermia causes a shift to the left in the oxyhemoglobin dissociation curve and may impair oxygen unloading to peripheral tissue.
- Because DIC may develop several days after a hypothermic episode, monitor for excessive bleeding from wounds, surgical incisions, and venipuncture sites and promptly report the presence of serious or progressive thrombocytopenia. (See "Disseminated Intravascular Coagulation," p. 579.)

NIC Hypothermia Treatment; Temperature Regulation; Vital Signs Monitoring

Altered nutrition: less than body requirements, related to increased need secondary to hypermetabolic posttrauma state; possible decreased intake secondary to direct injury or surgical disruption of GI tract or ileus

Desired outcome: Within 5 days of this diagnosis, patient has adequate nutrition as evidenced by maintenance of baseline body weight and state of nitrogen balance on nitrogen studies.

- Collaborate with physician, dietitian, and pharmacist to estimate patient's metabolic needs on the basis of type of injury, activity level, and nutritional status before injury.
- Consider patient's specific injuries and preexisting medical condition when planning nutrition.
- Monitor serum markers of nutritional status: prealbumin, transferrin, albumin.
- Start enteral feedings as soon as possible (i.e., bowel sounds are present, patient experiences hunger).
- Recognize that opiates decrease GI motility and may cause nausea and vomiting.
- Weigh patient daily to evaluate trend. Be alert to steady decreases in weight, and evaluate loss by assessing and comparing with volume status and fluid shifts.
- Collect 24-h urine specimen for urea nitrogen value, as prescribed, to evaluate nitrogen balance.
- For additional information, see "Nutritional Support," p. 1.

NIC Nutrition Management; Weight Gain Assistance

Fear related to potentially threatening situation (e.g., serious injuries, hospitalization) and supported by presence of pain, unfamiliarity, and noxious environmental stimuli present in critical care area; communication barrier (e.g., intubation); sensory impairment from direct injuries

Desired outcome: Within 24 h of this diagnosis, patient exhibits decreased symptoms of fear: apprehension, tension, nervousness, tachycardia, superficial vasoconstriction, aggressiveness, and withdrawal.

- Assess level of fear and understanding of present condition.
- Plan care to provide as restful an environment as possible.
- Provide information regarding nursing care, treatment plan, and progress. It is often necessary to repeat information because injury, stress, and fear can interfere with comprehension.
- Promote visits by family members and significant others.
- Offer to consult hospital chaplain or patient's clergy member as desired by patient.
- Assess and promote patient's usual coping strategies. It may be helpful to interview family members.
- Provide referral to support groups for trauma patients and family members.
- For more information, see this diagnosis in "Psychosocial Support," p. 83.

NIC Anxiety Reduction; Coping Enhancement; Security Enhancement; Support System Enhancement

Risk for injury related to potential for use of alcohol or illicit drugs; propensity for thrill-seeking behaviors

Desired outcomes: The potential for postdischarge use of alcohol or illicit drugs is identified by the time of hospital discharge. The potential for thrill-seeking behaviors is evaluated by the time of hospital discharge.

- Evaluate preinjury status regarding use of intoxicants.
- Assess for preinjury patterns of thrill-seeking behaviors.
- Initiate early referral to social services or discharge planner if need of rehabilitation is anticipated.
- Refer patient and family members or significant others to appropriate rehabilitation program or counseling as indicated. Immediately after serious injury, the patient and family members are very impressionable, making this period an ideal time to begin addressing behaviors that place that patient at risk for additional injury.
- Initiate injury prevention education. Provide instructions on proper seat belt application (across the pelvic girdle rather than across soft tissue of the lower abdomen), firearm safety, injury prevention for infants and children, and other factors suitable for the persons involved.

NIC Impulse Control Training; Risk Identification; Substance Use Prevention; Substance Use Treatment; Vehicle Safety Promotion

Posttrauma syndrome related to unanticipated serious physical injury or event resulting in physical trauma

Desired outcomes: By the time of hospital discharge, patient verbalizes that the psychosocial impact of the event has decreased; cooperates with treatment plan; and does not exhibit signs of severe stress reaction, such as display of inconsistent affect, suicidal or homicidal behavior, or extreme agitation or depression.

- Evaluate mental status at systematic intervals during the acute and recovery periods. Be alert to indicators of severe stress reaction such as display of affect inconsistent with statements or behavior, suicidal or homicidal statements or actions, extreme agitation or depression, and failure to cooperate with instructions related to care.
- Anticipate some re-experience of traumatic event. Reassure patient and significant others that this is common.
- Consult with specialist such as psychologist, psychiatric nurse clinician, or pastoral counselor if patient displays signs of severe stress reaction, as described in the first intervention.
- Consider organic causes that may contribute to posttraumatic stress response (e.g., severe pain, alcohol intoxication or withdrawal, electrolyte imbalance, metabolic encephalopathy, impaired cerebral perfusion).
- For other psychosocial interventions, see "Psychosocial Support," p. 83.

NIC Counseling; Support System Enhancement; Support Group

ADDITIONAL NURSING DIAGNOSES

Also see the following as appropriate: "Nutritional Support," p. 1; "Hemodynamic Monitoring," p. 28; "Sedating and Paralytic Agents," p. 38; "Alterations in Consciousness," p. 46; "Wound and Skin Care," p. 55; "Pain," p. 61; "Prolonged Immobility," p. 74; "Psychosocial Support," p. 83; "Psychosocial Support for the Patient's Family and Significant Others," p. 95; other trauma discussions in this chapter; and "SIRS and MODS," p. 604.

Traumatic brain injury

PATHOPHYSIOLOGY

Trauma to the head from blunt and penetrating forces can result in injury to the brain, support structures, blood vessels, and cranium in any combination. Blunt injuries to the head are caused by acceleration, deceleration, and rotational forces (e.g., vehicular collisions, falls, high-impact sports). Penetrating injuries occur from piercing forces that traverse the skull and, ultimately, damage underlying brain tissue and support structures.

Brain injury is a process that may lasts days to weeks but begins at the time of impact. The injury is a combination of neuronal damage, vascular insufficiency, and inflammatory effects. The neuronal component consists of both neurexcitation and deafferentation injuries. The neurexcitatory injury activates excitatory neurotransmitters (glutamate and aspartate), which in turn depolarize neurons. This neurotransmitter surge causes aberrant cell signaling, leading to long-lasting or permanent neuronal dysfunction. In the deafferentation injury, the neurofilament of the axon is destroyed, causing the axon to swell and retract. Permanent destruction of the neurons results. Ischemia, resulting in neuronal cell death, and infection are secondary brain injuries that often accompany the primary injuries. Injuries to the cerebral vasculature and skull are common associated injuries.

Outcome after traumatic brain injury is variable but can be predicted to some extent based on the type of lesion, severity of injury, and length of coma. However, age, preinjury medical status, mechanism of injury, intracranial pressure, and brainstem integrity are important factors influencing outcome.

Primary injuries

Primary brain injuries are classified as mild (Glasgow coma scale [GCS] score = 13-15), moderate (GCS score = 9-12), and severe (GCS score = $\leq$ 8).

Concussion: Mild neurexcitatory injury that may be accompanied by diffuse, axonal brain injuries classified as mild (no loss of consciousness, possible brief episodes of confusion or disorientation); moderate (brief loss of consciousness, transient focal neurologic deficits); or severe (prolonged loss of consciousness with sustained neurologic deficits lasting <24 h).

Contusion: Bruising of the brain tissue often associated with lacerations and capillary hemorrhages. Contusions can be described as *coup* if the brain injury is directly beneath the site of impact or *contrecoup* if the brain injury is opposite the site of impact.

Diffuse axonal injuries (DAI): Usually severe injury where diffuse areas of white matter have been torn or sheared; injury evolves over time, thus *initial* CT may not demonstrate a pathologic condition.

Secondary injuries

Ischemia: These secondary injuries are caused by decreased cerebral perfusion. Global ischemia occurs as a result of anoxia (obstructed airway or respiratory insufficiency) or hypoperfusion (hypotension or hypovolemia). Focal ischemia is a result of local disruption of blood supply possibly related to a cerebral vessel laceration, embolus, or thrombus.

Infection: Meningitis is typically bacterial in nature and occurs as a result of open wounds or tears in the dura (see "Meningitis," p. 460).

Associated injuries
Skull fractures: Occur as a result of blunt or penetrating impact force. Primary brain injuries are usually seen along with skull fractures.
Linear skull fractures: Nondisplaced, associated with low-velocity impact.
Basilar skull fractures: Linear, involving the base of the cranium's anterior, middle, and posterior fossae.
Depressed skull fractures: Characterized by depression of the skull over the point of impact; may be comminuted (usually closed without direct brain penetration), compressed, or compound (open).

Vascular injuries
Vascular injuries occur from impact force and result in bleeding of cerebral arteries or veins. These injuries usually accompany moderate and severe primary injuries.
Epidural hematomas: Commonly occur after a temporal linear skull fracture that lacerates the middle meningeal artery below it or from fractures of the sagittal and transverse sinuses. The hematoma develops rapidly in the space between the skull and dura.
Subdural hematomas: Bleeding from the veins between the dura and the arachnoid spaces; classified as acute, subacute, and chronic.
Subarachnoid hemorrhage: Seen over the convexities of the brain and in the basal cisterns; indicative of bleeding into the ventricular system.
Intracranial hematomas: Generally result from injury to the small arteries and veins within the subcortical white matter of the temporal and frontal lobes; usually associated with petechiae, contusions, and edema.

Neurologic complications
Herniation syndromes: Processes whereby a portion of the brain is displaced through openings within the intracranial cavity. Herniation occurs when there is a pressure difference between the supratentorial and infratentorial compartments. When herniation occurs, the vascular system is compressed, destroyed, or lacerated, resulting in ischemia, necrosis, and ultimately death. Several herniation syndromes may occur, and each has specific characteristics.
- *Cingulate herniation:* Occurs because of a unilateral hemispheric increase in intracranial pressure (ICP). It is best described as a shift to the side opposite the increased hemispheric pressure, as noted on CT. Cingulate herniation compresses the anterior cerebral artery and internal cerebral vein, contributing further to the development of cerebral edema, ischemia, and increased intracranial pressure (IICP). Associated neurologic deficits may include decreased LOC and unilateral or bilateral lower extremity weakness or paralysis.
- *Uncal herniation:* Life-threatening, emergent situation that occurs when an expanding lesion of the middle or temporal fossa forces the tip (uncus) of the temporal lobe toward the midline, causing it to protrude over the edge of the tentorium cerebelli and compress the oculomotor nerve (third cranial) and the posterior cerebral artery. During this process, the uncus may be lacerated and the midbrain is compressed and pushed against the tentorial edge. In addition to the fixed and dilated pupil on the side of herniation, there is deterioration of LOC and further elevation in ICP.
- *Transtentorial (central) herniation:* Occurs with expanding lesions of the frontal, parietal, or occipital lobes or with severe, generalized cerebral edema. Subcortical structures, including the basal ganglia and diencephalon (thalamus and hypothalamus), herniate through the tentorium cerebelli, causing compression of the midbrain and posterior cerebral arteries

bilaterally. Often, cingulate and uncal herniation precede this life-threatening process. Table 2-2 describes the clinical features of uncal and central herniation syndromes. It is important to note, however, that many of these manifestations may occur too rapidly to be observed and changes in respiratory patterns will not be seen in critically ill patients who are mechanically ventilated.

- **Transcranial (extracranial) herniation:** Occurs when intracranial contents under pressure are forced through an open wound, surgical site, or cranial vault fracture. Although the resultant loss of brain volume lowers ICP and may prevent intracranial herniation, this is an ominous sign and the patient is at risk for infection, further brain injury, and death.

Changes in intracranial pressure dynamics

Intracranial pressure dynamics (IPD) is based on the volume-pressure relationship within the cranium (Monro-Kellie hypothesis). Three volumes exist within the fixed, rigid cranial vault: the brain, blood, and cerebrospinal fluid (CSF). Under normal conditions these volumes exert a pressure that is <15 mm Hg. When any of these volumes increases, pressure increases and compensatory mechanisms (shunting of CSF into the intrathecal space or vasoconstriction to reduce blood volume) are activated to reduce the volume. In addition, the brain requires a constant blood supply to maintain normal function. With brain injury, the intrinsic compensatory mechanisms are damaged or overwhelmed and functions that serve to maintain cerebral perfusion are compromised. Extrinsic measures are necessary to maintain the normal pressure-volume relationship and preserve cerebral perfusion pressure (CPP). Table 6-3, p. 429, lists indicators of IICP. Treatment of derangements in IPD is based on the relationship between ICP and CPP and is stated simply:

$$CPP = MAP - ICP$$

MAP is calculated using the following equation:

$$MAP = \frac{Systolic\ BP + 2(Diastolic\ BP)}{3}$$

The goal of treatment is to maintain CPP >70 mm Hg and reduce ICP to <20 mm Hg.

ASSESSMENT

Baseline physical examination data should include assessment of mental status, cranial nerves, motor status, sensory status, and reflexes. Thereafter, continuous neurologic assessment should be based on the clinical status of the patient. Ideally, a complete neurologic assessment should be performed. However, many components of the examination require patients to follow commands. For patients unable to follow commands, the neurologic assessment should be tailored individually to the patient's abilities and redesigned as necessary. The Glasgow coma scale (Appendix 3) and the Rancho Los Amigos cognitive functioning scale (see Cognitive Rehabilitation Goals, Table 1-26) should be part of the neurologic assessment. Record specific patient responses to stimuli and the type of stimuli required to produce the response. The following are assessment findings related to specific injuries.

Epidural hematoma/linear skull fracture: Scalp lacerations, swelling, tenderness, and ecchymosis. Classic epidural signs are loss of consciousness, followed by a lucid interval and then rapid deterioration. Ipsilateral pupil dilation and contralateral weakness, followed by brainstem compression, occur if treatment is not initiated emergently.

TABLE 2-2   Assessment of Central and Uncal Herniations

| Criteria | Diencephalic | | Midbrain/upper pons | Lower pons/upper medulla |
	Early	Late		
Central herniation				
Respiratory pattern	Deep sighs, yawning	Cheyne-Stokes	Hyperventilation that is sustained and regular	Shallow, rapid, irregular
Pupils: size/reaction	Small; react to bright light; small range of contraction	Small; react to bright light; small range of contraction	Midpositioned; irregularly shaped; fixed reaction to light	Midpositioned; fixed
Oculocephalic/oculovestibular responses (doll's eyes phenomenon/ice water caloric)	Full conjugate or slightly roving eye movements; full conjugate lateral; ipsilateral response to ice water ear irrigation	Same as early; nystagmus absent	Impaired; may be dysconjugate	No response
Motor responses				
At rest	Contralateral paresis, which may worsen	Motionlessness	Abnormal extension posturing	Flaccidity
To stimulus	Bilateral Babinski	Abnormal flexion posturing	Rigidity	Bilateral Babinski

Continued

Modified from Plum F, Posner J: *Diagnosis of stupor and coma*, ed 3, Philadelphia, 1980, Davis.

TABLE 2-2   Assessment of Central and Uncal Herniations—cont'd

	Early third nerve	Late third nerve
Uncal herniation		
Respiratory pattern	Normal	Hyperventilation that is regular and sustained
Pupils: size/reaction	Moderate dilation; ipsilateral to primary lesion; sluggish constriction; brisk contralateral pupillary reaction	Widely dilated and fixed ipsilateral pupil
Oculocephalic/oculovestibular responses (doll's eyes phenomenon/ice water caloric)	Present or dysconjugate, full conjugate, slow ipsilateral eye movement or dysconjugate caused by contralateral eye not moving medially	Impaired or absent. Full lateral movement with contralateral eye; absence of medial movement with ipsilateral eye
Motor response to stimulus	Contralateral extensor plantar reflex	Ipsilateral hemiplegia; abnormal posturing; absence of all responses

Modified from Plum F, Posner J: *Diagnosis of stupor and coma*, ed 3, Philadelphia, 1980, Davis.

Basilar skull fracture: Dural tears resulting in rhinorrhea and otorrhea are common. Anterior fossa injuries are associated with periorbital ecchymosis (raccoon eyes), epistaxis, damage to cranial nerves I and II, and meningitis. Middle and posterior fossa injuries may damage cranial nerves VII and VIII and are associated with tinnitus, hemotympanum, and destruction of the cochlear vestibular apparatus. Ecchymosis of the mastoid process (Battle's sign) is common.

Compound depressed skull fracture: Neurologic changes are based on the extent of brain injury, but changes in LOC, pupillary changes, headache, cerebral edema, and IICP often accompany these injuries. Physical and diagnostic examination findings may include CSF leaks if the dura has been torn; tympanum rupture; and bruised, lacerated, or contused brain tissue.

Concussion: Headache, dizziness, vomiting, memory loss, and decreased attention and concentration skills. Moderate and severe injuries require close observation because cerebral edema and IICP can develop.

Contusion: Loss of consciousness common. Neurologic deficits may be generalized or focal, depending on the site and severity of injury. Cerebral edema and unstable intracranial pressure dynamics may often complicate the primary injury.

Diffuse axonal injury: May occur with other injuries and is characterized by an immediate loss of consciousness. Ischemia often a secondary complication. Edema and unstable intracranial pressure dynamics are common. Duration of coma varies depending on the severity of the injury, but often, coma is prolonged and recovery of function is minimal to moderate.

Subdural hematoma: With acute subdural hematoma, neurologic deterioration is seen within 24-72 h (or earlier) and is manifested by a changing LOC, ipsilateral dilated pupil, and contralateral extremity weakness. Subacute hematoma may present within 48 h to weeks after injury and manifests initially as a headache. Characteristically there is no clinical sign of improvement. LOC begins to deteriorate, and focal neurologic deficits ensue. Neurologic signs associated with a chronic subdural hematoma may occur weeks or months after injury. The progression of elusive, fluctuating deficits, such as personality changes, memory loss, headache, extremity weakness, and incontinence, may signal chronic subdural hematoma, especially in high-risk groups such as older adults or chronic alcohol users.

Subarachnoid hemorrhage (SAH): Highly associated with headache, changes in LOC, and meningeal signs such as nuchal rigidity, elevated temperature, and positive Kernig sign (loss of ability to extend leg when thigh is flexed on abdomen).

Intracranial hematoma: Neurologic deficits based on the site and severity of injury.

Other physical assessment data: Baseline cardiovascular, pulmonary, gastrointestinal, genitourinary, and integumentary data should be completed, with reassessment on an ongoing basis.

NON-NEUROLOGIC COMPLICATIONS

Cardiac dysrhythmias: Commonly seen in brain-injured patients and probably related to autonomic (sympathetic and parasympathetic) derangement or compression of midbrain and brainstem structures. ECG changes seen with elevated ICP are prominent U waves, ST-segment changes, notched T waves, and prolongation of the QT interval. Bradycardic, supraventricular, tachycardic, and ventricular dysrhythmias are seen, as well. Cushing syndrome, characterized by bradycardia, elevated systolic blood pressure (SBP), and a widening pulse pressure, is a late sign indicating mechanical compression or severe metabolic dysfunction of the brainstem.

Aspiration with resultant pneumonia: Prevalent complication after brain injury. Aspiration may occur at the time of injury or as an iatrogenic complication of intubation, enteral feedings, or prolonged use of artificial airways. Whatever the cause, early detection reduces associated morbidity and mortality. Early detection methods that should be incorporated into the plan of care include checking tracheobronchial secretions for glucose (a sign that tube feedings have been aspirated inasmuch as sputum is normally negative for glucose), initiating enteral feeding protocols, and performing swallowing assessments. See "Nutritional Support" for **Risk for aspiration,** p. 15, and Table 1-4, which discusses complications in the tube-fed patient.

Other complications: In addition, the patient with brain injury is predisposed to numerous complications that arise from injury to the central and autonomic nervous systems, concurrent injuries, hypoperfusion injury, and iatrogenic complications. These include adult respiratory distress syndrome (p. 229), pulmonary edema (p. 265), meningitis (p. 460), diabetes insipidus (p. 479), syndrome of inappropriate antidiuretic hormone (p. 428), gastrointestinal bleeding (p. 541), anemia (p. 558), and disseminated intravascular coagulation (p. 579).

DIAGNOSTIC TESTS

Skull x-ray: Detects structural deficits such as skull fractures and facial bone destruction, as well as air-fluid level in sinuses, abnormal intracranial calcification, pineal gland location (normally midline), and foreign bodies that are radiopaque.

Cervical spine x-ray: Demonstrates structural deficits of the spine and used to rule out associated cervical spine injuries, including fractures, dislocations, and subluxations. Cervical spine mobilization is mandatory in all trauma patients until the cervical spine (cervical 1 through thoracic 1 [C1-T1]) is visualized completely and fractures are ruled out.

Computed tomography (CT):   Gray and white matter, blood, and CSF are detectable because of their different radiologic densities. Because CT is capable of diagnosing cerebral hemorrhage, infarction, hydrocephalus, cerebral edema, and structural shifts, it continues to be the most important diagnostic tool for primary and secondary brain injury.

Magnetic resonance imaging (MRI):   Identifies type, location, and extent of injury. It provides spatial resolution, can follow metabolic processes, and detects structural changes.

Cerebral angiography: Invasive radiographic procedure that uses dye to examine the cerebral vasculature. It is used only as an adjunct study in diagnosing brain injury or if CT is unavailable.

Electroencephalography (EEG):   Measures spontaneous brain electrical activity via surface electrodes. It is useful in detecting areas of abnormal brain activity (irritability) associated with seizures and generalized brain activity related to drug overdose, coma, or suspected brain death. Drug therapy, especially anticonvulsants, alters brain activity, and therefore use of these drugs should be documented if the drug cannot be withheld 24-48 h before EEG.

Evoked responses: Evaluation of the electrical potentials (responses) of the brain to an external stimulus (i.e., auditory, visual, somatosensory), thereby providing information related to lesions of the cortex or ascending pathways of the spinal cord, brainstem, or thalamus. Evoked potentials can be useful in determining the extent of injury in uncooperative, confused, or comatose patients and should be used when planning rehabilitation.

CSF analysis: Useful in determining infection in the brain-injured patient. Analysis of CSF should include color, turbidity/cloudiness, RBC and WBC counts, protein, glucose, electrolytes, Gram stain, culture, and sensitivity. A promising new means of CSF analysis is via cerebral microdialysis, whereby levels of neurotransmitters and electrolytes are calculated, enabling treatment of abnormal levels.

Serum laboratory studies: To identify complications associated with injury. WBCs, Hgb, Hct, electrolytes, osmolality, albumin, and transferrin are monitored at least daily and more frequently during the acute phase.

COLLABORATIVE MANAGEMENT

Management focuses on treating the emergent pathologic condition, controlling ICP, preventing complications, and initiating rehabilitation.

Surgical intervention: Performed to evacuate mass lesions (epidural, subdural, and intracranial hematomas), place ICP monitoring system, elevate depressed skull fractures, débride open wounds and brain tissue, and repair dural tears or scalp lacerations. Frontal lobectomies may be necessary to control severe increases in ICP.

Management of intracranial pressure dynamics: ICP monitoring is accomplished using a variety of techniques (Table 2-3). All monitoring systems provide a digital display of ICP, but CPP must be calculated (see p. 434). The goal is to maintain CPP >70 mm Hg.

Reduction of ICP by CSF drainage: Accomplished only by using intraventricular or ventriculostomy systems. To prevent herniation when draining CSF, drainage collection bags must be maintained at the level of the tragus of the ear or higher, thereby preventing excessive CSF flow caused by a higher-to-lower pressure gradient.

Hyperventilation via mechanical ventilation: Hyperventilation is no longer recommended as a first-line treatment to reduce ICP. Evidence is sufficient to believe hyperventilation may cause neurologic dysfunction as a result of decreased cerebral perfusion. Maintaining $Paco_2$ at 35 ± 2 is now considered optimal ventilation.

Monitoring jugular venous oxygen saturation (Sjo_2):   Used to measure cerebral oxygenation by determining oxygen content of cerebral venous blood. Three types of blood flow can be discriminated: normal (Sjo_2 = 55%-70%), oligemic (Sjo_2 <55%), and hyperemia (Sjo_2 >70%). Treatment should be aimed at maintaining normal range.

Diuresis therapy: Reduces cerebral brain volume by extracting fluid from the brain's intracellular compartment. Mannitol 20%, an osmotic diuretic, and furosemide (Lasix), a loop diuretic, are used most commonly. Mannitol may be given in 25-50 g doses as needed to reduce ICP or may be given q4-6h. Furosemide may be given in conjunction with mannitol at doses between 20-40 mg. Dehydration is a major complication with continued use of diuretics, and therefore strict attention must be paid to serum electrolyte and osmolality values. In addition to maintenance fluid therapy (75-100 ml/h), replacement of urine losses may be prescribed. Replacement therapy is based on the volume of urine collected 1 h after administration of the diuretic and is given either ml for ml or 0.5 ml for ml over a 3- to 4-h period.

Maintenance of blood pressure within an acceptable range: Imperative because both hypotension and hypertension can contribute to cerebral edema. Hypotension can result in decreased oxygen delivery to brain cells, thereby decreasing pH, elevating $Paco_2$, and causing cerebral vessels to vasodilate. Hypotension also reduces MAP and thus CPP. Dopamine HCl (Intropin), used at doses between 3-5 µg/kg/min, can effectively increase MAP and raise CPP.

The effects of hypertension (elevated CPP and increased cerebral edema) have not been well studied, but increased capillary permeability and petechial hemorrhage are seen with hypertension. Antihypertensive medications, such as labetalol HCl (Normodyne) or nitroprusside sodium (Nipride), may be necessary.

Reduction of metabolic demand: Important strategy when treating ICP problems, because cerebral blood supply must match demand to maintain cerebral function.

- *Sedating agents:* Use of continuous drips of midazolam HCl (Versed), opiate analgesics, such as fentanyl citrate (Sublimaze) or morphine sulfate, and anesthetic agents, such as propofol (Diprivan), is common. In addition, nondepolarizing agents, such as vecuronium bromide (Norcuron) or atracurium, are used to reduce metabolic demand. Sedation,

TABLE 2-3 Types of Intracranial Monitoring

System	Type	Placement	Advantages/uses	Disadvantages
Fluid-filled or fiberoptic	Intraventricular cannula	Lateral ventricle in nondominant hemisphere through burr hole	CSF measurement CSF drainage Drug administration Volume-pressure response testing	Rapid CSF drainage can result in collapsed ventricles or subdural hematoma Cannula tip may catch on ventricular wall Risk of intracerebral bleeding and infection May become plugged with debris Possible difficult insertion because of shifting or collapse of ventricle
Fluid-filled	Subarachnoid screw	Subarachnoid space through twist drill hole	Pressure monitoring Less risk of infection than with cannula Useful with small ventricles Does not penetrate brain	Compliance testing may be unreliable No CSF drainage Some risk of infection Risk of hemorrhage or hematoma during insertion Brain may herniate into bolt, making recording unreliable
Electrical sensor	Epidural sensor	Epidural space Burr hole Fiberoptic sensor	Lowest risk of infection Easy to insert Dura not penetrated	No direct measurement of CSF No CSF drainage Inability to recalibrate to zero
Fiberoptic	Intraparenchymal	Intraparenchymal via twist drill Fiberoptic sensor	Easy to insert Direct pressure Compliance testing One-time zero and calibration before insertion	Cannot measure volume-pressure response Risk of intracerebral bleeding and infection No CSF drainage

CSF, Cerebrospinal fluid.

analgesia, and paralysis may be used as combination therapy or as individual therapies. See "Sedating and Paralytic Agents," p. 38.

- *Seizure control:* Seizure activity may occur, especially in the presence of focal injuries such as depressed, comminuted, or compound skull fractures; contusions; and lacerations. Because seizure activity increases the metabolic demand of the brain, seizure prophylaxis using an anticonvulsant agent is frequently used. Phenytoin sodium (Dilantin) is most commonly administered; however, phenobarbital can also be used. When using phenytoin, a loading dose consisting of 500-1000 mg IV is followed by a daily dose of 100 mg tid. Phenytoin must be administered slowly, 50 mg/min, and cannot be administered with a dextrose solution. Therapeutic levels should be maintained between 10-20 µg/ml; however, dosing should be patient specific (higher levels may be necessary to prevent breakthrough seizures, or lower levels if seizures are controlled).

- *Barbiturate coma:* Is a less often used method of reducing metabolic demand. High doses of barbiturates should never be used without continuous ICP and hemodynamic monitoring and controlled ventilation, because barbiturates induce profound cardiac and cerebral depression. Pentobarbital sodium (Nembutal) is the drug of choice. A loading dose between 5-10 mg/kg is given (discontinue if MAP falls <70 mm Hg), followed by a maintenance dose of 1-3 mg/kg/h to sustain a level of 3-5 mg/dl. Barbiturates are withdrawn gradually as the patient improves. Patients with barbiturate coma require intensive physical care and physiologic monitoring. When use of barbiturates does not improve the clinical condition, brain death criteria cannot be initiated until barbiturate levels return to zero.

- *Maintaining body temperature:* For every 1° C in temperature elevation, there is a 10%-13% increase in metabolic rate. Normal temperatures range from 35.8°-37.5° C (96.4°-99.5° F) with a diurnal variation of 1° C. Rectal temperatures are 0.2°-0.6° C higher than oral and can be 0.8° C higher than right atrial, esophageal, and oral temperatures during fever. With brain injury, evaluation of the etiology of fever is important because it will influence treatment choice. Fever can be attributed to brain injury (central fever), an infectious process (peripheral fever), or drugs (drug fever). Central fever reflects a derangement in the hypothalamic thermoregulatory mechanism and is characterized by lack of sweating, no diurnal variation, plateaulike elevation patterns, elevations up to 41° C (105.8° F), absence of tachycardia, persistence for days or weeks, and temperature reduction with external cooling rather than with antipyretic agents. Peripheral fever is associated with wound infections, meningitis, sepsis, pneumonia, and other bacterial invasion. Sweating, diurnal variation, response to antipyretic agents, and tachycardia are characteristic of peripheral fever. Shivering, associated with hypothermia therapy, is the body's mechanism to increase heat production. Shivering not only increases metabolic demand, it also may increase ICP. Wrapping distal extremities in bath towels before initiating hypothermia is an effective measure for controlling shivering. Chlorpromazine (Thorazine) also may be used to control shivering, but it should be used with caution because it may have a hypotensive effect. There is some support for use of hypothermia for the treatment of acute brain injury; however, the scientific evidence for this treatment is still evolving. If hypothermia is used, follow a strict treatment protocol.

Modifying nursing care activities that raise ICP: Brief and rapid elevations in ICP are commonly seen during position changes or performance of other nursing care and cannot always be avoided. However, these elevations are transient and generally the ICP returns to resting baseline within a few minutes. Sustained increases (>5 min) should be avoided. All nursing care activities that increase ICP should be spaced to enable a return of ICP to baseline and

---

TABLE 2-4   Guidelines for Suctioning Patients at Risk for Increased Intracranial Pressure

- Suction only if the clinical status of the patient warrants.
- Precede suctioning with preoxygenation using 100% oxygen.
- Limit each suctioning pass to ≤10 sec.
- Limit suction passes to 2.
- Follow each pass with 60 sec of hyperventilation using 100% oxygen.
- Use negative suction pressure <120 mm Hg.
- Keep patient's head in a neutral position.
- Use a suction catheter with an outer-to-inner diameter ratio of 2:1.

---

maximizing of CPP. Clustering nursing care such as bathing, turning, and suctioning creates a stair-step rise in ICP. Thus care activities should be performed to prevent sustained increases.

- *Suctioning:* Causes a significant rise in ICP. To minimize adverse effects associated with suctioning, implement the guidelines found in Table 2-4.
- *Neck positioning:* Flexion, extension, and lateral movements of the neck can significantly raise ICP. Maintaining the neck in a neutral position at all times is important. In patients with poor neck control, stabilize the neck with towel rolls or sandbags.
- *Elevating head of bed (HOB):* Although HOB elevation at 30 degrees is believed to improve venous drainage and contribute to ICP reduction, ICP may be improved at higher or lower elevations. Adjust HOB elevation to optimize the patient's CPP and minimize ICP.
- *Turning:* Turning the patient with IICP is not contraindicated but should be based on the patient's response to turning. Initially, turning from side to side will elevate pressure, but ICP should return to resting baseline after a few minutes. If the ICP does not return to resting baseline within 5 min, CPP may be compromised and the patient should be returned to a position that reduces ICP and maximizes CPP.
- *Bathing:* Although bathing itself has not been documented as raising ICP, rapid turning from side to side associated with linen changes raises ICP. These "turn procedures" are actually clustered activities because the length of the procedure does not allow sufficient time for the ICP to return to baseline. Evaluation of the patient's response may necessitate performing the linen change in stages or allowing adequate time for ICP to return to resting baseline.
- *Sensory stimulation:* A sensory stimulation program may be implemented safely in comatose patients early after injury when ICP is stable. This rehabilitative technique may be an important adjunct to traditional care. (See Table 2-5.)

Nutritional support: Enteral nutrition is most physiologically compatible with gut function and should be initiated as early as possible after injury. When transpyloric (duodenum or jejunum) feeding tubes are used, enteral feedings can be initiated before bowel sounds return to normal. In some cases, gastric tubes for gastric decompression are used simultaneously with the transpyloric tubes. See "Nutritional Support," p. 1, for documentation of proper placement and checking of residual volumes. If enteral feedings are contraindicated or not tolerated by the patient, parenteral feedings are started.

Rehabilitation: Brain injury is highly associated with physical (paralysis, spasticity, and contractures) and cognitive impairments. Initiate early consultations with physical, occupational, and speech therapists to minimize the deficits and prepare the patient for an active rehabilitative program. National Institutes of Health (NIH) Consensus Development Conference Recommendations on Rehabilitation of Persons with Brain Injury are available. Support also

T A B L E 2 - 5	**Management of Severe Brain Injury**	
Treatment	**Level of evidence***	**Recommendation**
Blood pressure and oxygenation	Guideline	Avoid early postinjury episodes of hypotension <90 mm Hg or hypoxia <60 mm Hg.
ICP treatment threshold	Guideline	Treatment to lower ICP should be initiated at 20-25 mm Hg.
CPP treatment	Option	CPP should be maintained at >70 mm Hg. Maintain MAP >90 mm Hg.
Hyperventilation	Guideline	Avoid prophylactic hyperventilation (<35 mm Hg) the first 24 hours postinjury. May use hyperventilation for refractory IICP.
Mannitol	Guideline	Use intermittent boluses of 0.25-1.00 mg/kg.
Barbiturates	Guideline	May be considered in hemodynamically stable patients refractory to other methods to reduce ICP.
Glucocorticoids	Standard	Use is not recommended.
Nutrition	Guideline	Replace 140% of resting metabolic expenditure in unparalyzed patients and 100% in paralyzed patients using parenteral or enteral methods. By day 7, feedings should contain at least 15% protein.
Seizure prophylaxis	Guideline	Anticonvulsants can be considered an option for high-risk patients early after injury.
	Standard	Not recommended for preventing late posttraumatic seizures.

Modified from Brain Trauma Foundation: Guidelines for the management of severe head injury, *J Neurotrauma* 13:639-734, 1996.
Standard = high level of certainty; *Guideline* = moderate clinical certainty; *Option* = unclear clinical certainty. Level of evidence is based on scientific literature where the highest degree of certainty is drawn from prospective randomized clinical trials.
*Level of evidence denotes the degree that the recommendation represents clinical certainty.

is available through the National Head Injury Foundation, 18A Vernon Street, Framingham, MA 01701; or the state chapter of the Head Injury Foundation.

NURSING DIAGNOSES AND INTERVENTIONS

Impaired gas exchange related to decreased oxygen supply and increased carbon dioxide production secondary to decreased ventilatory drive occurring with pressure on respiratory center, imposed inactivity, and possible neurologic pulmonary edema

Desired outcomes: $Paco_2$ values remain between 35 ± 2 mm Hg. By the time of discharge from ICU or transfer to rehabilitation unit, patient has adequate gas exchange as evidenced by orientation to time, place, and person; Pao$_2$ ≥80 mm Hg; RR 12-20 breaths/min with normal depth and pattern (eupnea); and absence of adventitious breath sounds.

- Assess patient's respiratory rate, depth, and rhythm. Auscultate lung fields for breath sounds q1-2h and prn. Monitor for respiratory patterns described in Table 2-2. Be alert to IICP (see Table 6-3, p. 429).
- Assess patient for signs of hypoxia, including confusion, agitation, restlessness, and irritability. Remember that cyanosis is a late indicator of hypoxia.
- Ensure a patent airway via proper positioning of neck and frequent assessment of the need for suctioning. Ensure hyperoxygenation of patient before and after each suction attempt to prevent dangerous, suction-induced hypoxia.
- Monitor ABG values; consult physician for significant findings or changes. Be alert to levels indicative of hypoxemia (Pao$_2$ <80 mm Hg) and to Paco$_2$ ≥35 ± 2 mm Hg, inasmuch as levels higher than this range may increase cerebral blood flow and thus ICP.
- Ensure that oxygen is delivered within prescribed limits.
- Assist with turning q2h, within limits of patient's injury, to promote lung drainage and expansion and alveolar perfusion. Unless contraindicated, raise HOB 30 degrees to enhance gas exchange.
- Encourage deep breathing at frequent intervals to promote oxygenation. Avoid coughing exercises for patients at risk for IICP.
- Evaluate the need for an artificial airway in patients unable to maintain airway patency or adequate ventilatory effort.

NIC Airway Management; Oxygen Therapy; Respiratory Monitoring

Risk for infection: CNS, related to inadequate primary defenses secondary to direct access to the brain in the presence of skull fracture, penetrating wounds, craniotomy, intracranial monitoring, or bacterial invasion caused by pneumonia or iatrogenic causes

Desired outcome: Patient is free of infection as evidenced by normothermia; WBC count ≤11,000/µl; negative culture results; HR ≤100 bpm; BP within patient's normal range; and absence of agitation, purulent drainage, and other clinical indicators of infection.

- Assess VS at frequent intervals for indicators of CNS infection. Be alert to elevated temperature and increased HR and BP.
- Monitor patient for signs of systemic infection, including discomfort, malaise, agitation, and restlessness.
- Inspect cranial wounds for the presence of erythema, tenderness, swelling, and purulent drainage. Obtain prescription for culture as indicated.
- Apply a loose sterile dressing (sling) to collect CSF drainage. Do not pack. Record amount, color, and character of drainage.
- Caution patient against coughing, sneezing, nose blowing, or other Valsalva-type maneuvers, because these activities can damage the dura further. Use orogastric tubes if basilar skull fractures or severe frontal sinus fractures are present.
- Ensure timely administration of prescribed antibiotics.
- Apply basic principles for care of invasive device used with ICP monitoring:
  ☐ Use good hand-washing technique before caring for patient.
  ☐ If patient is not comatose, encourage him or her not to touch device; apply restraints *only* if necessary to keep patient from harm. Restraints can increase ICP by causing straining.
  ☐ Maintain aseptic technique during care of device, following agency protocol.

NIC Infection Control; Infection Protection

Decreased adaptive capacity: intracranial, related to decreased cerebral perfusion pressure or infections that can occur with secondary head injury

Desired outcomes: Within 12-24 h of treatment/interventions, patient has adequate intracranial adaptive capacity as evidenced by equal and normoreactive pupils; RR 12-20 breaths/min with normal depth and pattern (eupnea); HR 60-100 bpm; ICP 0-15 mm Hg; CPP 60-80 mm Hg; and absence of headache, vomiting, and other clinical indicators of IICP. Optimally, by the time of discharge from ICU or transfer to rehabilitation unit, patient is oriented to time, place, and person and has bilaterally equal strength and tone in the extremities.

- Assess neurologic status at least hourly. Monitor pupils, LOC, and motor activity; also perform cranial nerve assessments (see Appendix 4). A decrease in LOC is an early indicator of IICP and impending herniation. Changes in the size and reaction of the pupils, a decrease in motor function (e.g., hemiplegia, abnormal flexion posturing), and cranial nerve palsies all indicate impending herniation.
- Monitor VS at frequent intervals. Be alert to changes in respiratory pattern, fluctuations in BP and pulse, widening pulse pressure, and slow HR.
- Monitor patient for indicators of IICP (see Table 6-3, p. 429).
- Monitor hemodynamic status to evaluate CPP and ensure that it is 60-80 mm Hg. Be alert to decrease in mean systolic arterial blood pressure (<80 mm Hg) or increase in MAP. Perform ongoing assessment of ICP and CPP, recording pressures at least hourly until stable. Consult physician if pressure changes significantly (e.g., >15 mm Hg or other preestablished range). Perform ongoing calibration and zeroing of transducer to ensure accuracy of readings.
- Maintain a patent airway, and ensure precise delivery of oxygen to promote optimal cerebral perfusion.
- Facilitate cerebral venous drainage by maintaining neck in neutral position.
- To help prevent fluid volume excess, which could add to cerebral edema, ensure precise delivery of IV fluids at consistent rates.
- Ensure timely administration of medications that are prescribed for the prevention of sudden increase or decrease in BP, HR, RR.
- Treat elevations in ICP immediately (Table 2-6).

NIC Cerebral Edema Management; Cerebral Perfusion Management; Intracranial Pressure (ICP) Monitoring; Neurologic Monitoring

Ineffective thermoregulation related to trauma associated with injury to or pressure on the hypothalamus

Desired outcome: Patient becomes normothermic within 24 h of this diagnosis.

- Monitor for signs of hyperthermia: temperature >38.3° C (101° F), pallor, absence of perspiration, torso that is warm to the touch.
- As prescribed, obtain specimens for blood, urine, and sputum cultures to rule out underlying infection.

TABLE 2-6   Nursing Interventions for Patients With Increased Intracranial Pressure

- Maintain HOB elevation at level that keeps ICP <20 mm Hg and CPP >70 mm Hg.
- Loosen constrictive objects around neck to facilitate venous blood flow from the head.
- With position changes, ensure ICP and CPP return to baseline or stay within acceptable parameters within 5 minutes of turn.
- Maintain head in neutral position.
- Correct factors that may increase ICP such as hypoxia, pain, anxiety, fear, and abdominal or bladder distention.
- Evaluate activities that increase ICP (e.g., suctioning, bathing, dressing changes) and reorganize care to minimize elevations.

ICP, Intracranial pressure; *CPP,* cerebral perfusion pressure.

- Be alert to signs of meningitis: fever, chills, nuchal rigidity, Kernig sign, Brudzinski sign (see "Meningitis," p. 460).
- Assess wounds for evidence of infection, including erythema, tenderness, purulent drainage.
- If patient has hyperthermia, remove excess clothing and administer tepid baths, hypothermic blanket, or ice bags to axilla or groin.
- As prescribed, administer antipyretics such as acetaminophen.
- As prescribed, administer chlorpromazine to treat or prevent shivering, which can cause further increases in ICP.
- Keep environmental temperature at optimal range.
- Assess for possible drug fever reaction, which can occur with antimicrobial therapy.

NIC Temperature Regulation, Fever Treatment

Risk for disuse syndrome related to immobilization and prolonged inactivity secondary to brain injury, spasticity, or altered LOC

Desired outcome: Patient has baseline/optimal ROM without verbal or nonverbal indicators of pain.

- Begin performing passive range-of-motion (ROM) exercises q4h on all extremities as soon as patient's acute condition stabilizes. Monitor ICP during exercise, being alert to dangerous elevations outside of the established parameters. Consult with physical therapist accordingly.
- Teach passive ROM exercises to significant others. Encourage their participation in patient exercise as often as they are able.
- Reposition patient q2h within restrictions of the head and other injuries, using log-rolling technique as indicated.
- Ensure proper anatomic position and alignment. Support alignment with pillows, trochanter rolls, wrapped sandbags.
- For patient with spasticity, use foot cradles to keep linen off the feet. To maintain dorsiflexion, provide patient with shoes that are cut off at the toes, with the shoes ending just proximal to the head of the patient's metatarsal joints. Because there is no contact of the balls of the feet with a hard surface, the risk of spasticity will be minimized. Consult occupational therapist for use of splints or other supportive device.
- For patient without spasticity, use foot supports to prevent plantarflexion and external hip rotation.
- To maintain anatomic position of the hands, provide spastic patient with a splint or cone that is secured with an elastic band. Either device will limit spasticity by pressing on the muscles, while the elastic band will stimulate the extensor muscles, thereby promoting finger extension.

NIC Exercise Therapy: Joint Mobility; Positioning

Impaired corneal tissue integrity (or risk for same) related to irritation associated with corneal drying and reduced lacrimal production secondary to altered consciousness or cranial nerve damage

Desired outcome: Patient's corneas are moist and intact.

- Assess for indicators of corneal irritation: red and itching eyes, ocular pain, sensation of a foreign object in the eye, scleral edema, and blurred vision. Avoid exposing patient's eyes to irritants such as baby powder or talc.
- Lubricate patient's eyes q2h with isotonic eye drops or ointment.
- Facilitate an ophthalmic consultation as indicated.

NIC Medication Administration: Eye

ADDITIONAL NURSING DIAGNOSES

Also see "Cerebral Aneurysm and Subarachnoid Hemorrhage" for **Decreased adaptive capacity: intracranial,** p. 434. As appropriate, see nursing diagnoses and interventions under "Alterations in Consciousness," p 46; "Care of the Patient After Intracranial Surgery," p. 437; and "Meningitis," p. 466. See "Status Epilepticus" for **Risk for trauma,** p. 441. Also see nursing diagnoses and interventions under "Nutritional Support" (particularly **Risk for aspiration,** p. 15); "Mechanical Ventilation," p. 17; "Hemodynamic Monitoring," p. 28; "Prolonged Immobility," p. 74; "Psychosocial Support," p. 83; and "Psychosocial Support for the Patient's Family and Significant Others," p. 95. The patient with craniocerebral trauma is at risk for diabetes insipidus and syndrome of inappropriate antidiuretic hormone. See "Diabetes Insipidus" for **Fluid volume deficit,** p. 479; and "Syndrome of Inappropriate Antidiuretic Hormone" for **Risk for injury,** p. 484.

Chest trauma

PATHOPHYSIOLOGY
Chest trauma is a complex and multidimensional problem. It is usually categorized by cause.
Blunt injury: Occurs as a result of a direct, forceful blow to the chest. Usually the injury is "closed" in that there is no communication of the chest cavity with outside atmospheric pressure. A typical occurrence is a vehicular collision, during which there is impact of the thorax with the steering wheel, but blunt injury also can occur as a result of a fall, beating, or crushing injury.
Penetrating injury: Occurs as a result of stab or missile wounds to the thorax. This is an open chest injury because there is communication between the chest cavity and outside atmospheric pressure. Gunshots are the most common missile-type penetrating injuries, whereas knife wounds represent the most common stabbing chest injuries.

• • •

Both blunt and penetrating chest wounds can lead to pneumothorax. In addition, thoracic injury can be severe enough to cause pulmonary or cardiac contusion, airway rupture, or tracheobronchial injury or can lead to interference with the mechanical functions of the heart and lungs. Therefore in-depth physical assessment is critical after the patient's injury.

ASSESSMENT
Subtle signs and symptoms and changes in the patient's condition can be clues to serious problems. Treat the patient as though a spinal cord injury has occurred until diagnostic tests have ruled it out. Be aware that subtle changes in mental status can signal a central nervous system insult as well as hypoxemia.
Blunt injury: Dyspnea, SOB, agitation, restlessness, anxiety, and severe chest pain during respirations that the patient can localize.
Potential complications: Pneumothorax, flail chest, hemothorax, pulmonary contusion, myocardial contusion, cardiac tamponade.
Inspection: RR >20 breaths/min; hyperpnea; ventilatory distress; use of accessory muscles of respiration; nasal flaring; decreased tidal volume; hemoptysis; asymmetric chest wall motion; paradoxic chest wall motion; inability to clear tracheobronchial secretions; splinting; jugular venous distention; cyanosis or pallor of the skin, lips, and nail beds; and ecchymosis, which can signal injury to underlying organs.
Palpation: Tracheal deviation; subcutaneous emphysema of the neck and upper portion of the chest; tenderness at fracture points; flail chest segment; weak pulse; cool, clammy skin; protrusion of bony fragments.
Percussion: Dullness over lung fields, which can signal hemothorax or atelectasis; hyperresonance over lung fields, signaling pneumothorax.
Auscultation: Diminished or absent breath sounds, respiratory stridor, bony crepitus over fracture sites, muffled heart tones, decreased BP, pericardial

friction rub, paradoxic pulse, apical tachycardia. In addition, bowel sounds may be heard in the thorax as a result of rupture or tear of the diaphragm, allowing herniation of abdominal contents into the thorax.

Penetrating injury: Dyspnea, SOB, moderate chest pain, restlessness, anxiety.

> **Note:** It is essential to perform a complete and rapid assessment with the patient's clothing removed. Entry sites may be deceptive, as the skin has an elastic quality and tends to close behind the penetrating object, thereby masking the size and extent of injury. Log roll the patient to visualize the exit wound, if present.

Potential complications: Hemothorax, pneumothorax, tension pneumothorax, hemorrhage, shock, and infection.

Inspection: RR >20 breaths/min; hyperpnea; respiratory distress; use of accessory muscles of respiration; nasal flaring; decreased tidal volume; asymmetric chest wall movement; inability to clear tracheobronchial secretions; splinting; and cyanosis or pallor of the skin, lips, and nail beds. During inspection, estimate blood loss on clothing and locate both entry and exit sites. Be alert to presence or severity of other wounds and to presence of ecchymosis, which can signal injury to underlying internal organs. Also note presence or absence of pulsations of the penetrating object, which may be imbedded in a major organ or blood vessel. Do not remove any penetrating object, because the object may have caused a sealing effect and removing it could result in uncontrollable bleeding of the organ or vessel.

Palpation: Tracheal deviation, subcutaneous emphysema, weak or irregular pulse, cool and clammy skin.

Percussion: Dullness over lung fields as a result of hemothorax or atelectasis; hyperresonance over lung fields as a result of pneumothorax.

Auscultation: Sucking sound over point of entry during inspiratory phase; diminished breath sounds; respiratory stridor; muffled heart tones; apical tachycardia or bradycardia, depending on stage of shock; bowel sounds in thorax.

Flail chest: A severe complication of blunt chest trauma that occurs when three or more adjacent ribs fracture in two or more places (or the sternum is fractured, along with ribs adjacent to the sternum fracture). The fracture segment is free of the bony thorax and moves independently in response to intrathoracic pressure. Paradoxic chest wall motion is the hallmark symptom in diagnosing flail chest. Normally the chest expands on inspiration, creating a negative intrathoracic pressure; on expiration the chest wall retracts in response to positive pressure inside the chest. Because a flail chest segment is no longer attached to the bony thorax, it follows the pressure and retracts on inspiration (negative pressure is a pulling pressure) and bulges on expiration (positive pressure is a pushing pressure).

DIAGNOSTIC TESTS

Chest x-ray: Confirms presence of air or fluid in the pleural space; assists in determining extent of hemothorax or pneumothorax; and confirms presence or absence of fractures of the bony thorax, as well as mediastinal shift.

ABG analysis: Evaluates adequacy of oxygenation and presence or absence of acid-base abnormalities. Typical results will reflect hypoxemia (Pao_2 <80 mm Hg) and hypercapnia ($Paco_2$ >45 mm Hg) with concomitant respiratory acidosis (pH <7.35). Pulse oximetry may be used for continuous monitoring of oxygen saturation (see discussion, p. 213).

ECG: Reveals presence or absence of life-threatening dysrhythmias and provides a more thorough analysis of the heart's electrical activity. Although dysrhythmias are a common complication after chest trauma, this important test often is overlooked.

Hgb/Hct values: Levels determine the need for blood transfusion or fluid volume replacement.

WBC count: Baseline indicator of an infectious process.

COLLABORATIVE MANAGEMENT

Interventions are directed toward managing acute respiratory compromise while correcting the underlying pathophysiology or injuries that complicate or aggravate the patient's condition.

Oxygen therapy: Delivered by mask or cannula, depending on extent of hypoxemia.

Intubation: Maintains patent airway, decreases airway resistance and respiratory effort, provides route for easy removal of airway secretions, and allows for manual or mechanical ventilation, as necessary.

Mechanical ventilation: For cases of extreme respiratory distress or ventilatory collapse (see p. 17).

Blood replacement: A high priority in the trauma victim. Generally, blood loss is replaced with packed RBCs or whole fresh blood, when available. Blood replacement via a commercially prepared autotransfusion system is a widely accepted therapy. Use of colloid versus crystalloid fluids for volume replacement remains controversial. Volume usually is replaced with crystalloid fluids (e.g., normal saline, lactated Ringer's solution) rather than colloidal IV fluids (e.g., plasma, albumin) because colloids increase the risk of developing acute respiratory distress syndrome (ARDS) and renal failure. In addition, colloids are more expensive and research has failed to demonstrate a significant benefit.

Chest tube insertion: To remove accumulation of fluid or air from the chest cavity. A large-bore (26-30 Fr) thoracic catheter is inserted into the chest cavity through the second intercostal space, midclavicular line, or fifth lateral intercostal space, midaxillary line. Placement depends on the location and extent of the hemothorax or pneumothorax and on principles of gravity drainage. The catheter then is connected to a one-way flutter valve or to a closed chest-drainage system.

Analgesia: Manages pain, which can interfere with work of breathing. Generally, opioid analgesics are avoided or used cautiously because of respiratory depressive side effects. Intercostal nerve block may be performed to provide local pain relief.

Thoracentesis: Relieves life-threatening tension pneumothorax. A 14-gauge needle is inserted into the second intercostal space at the midclavicular line to ventilate the pressurized chest cavity or, in an emergency situation, to remove a massive hemothorax.

Stabilization and fixation of flail chest: Most flail chest injuries stabilize within 10-14 days without surgical intervention. Internal fixation involves the use of a volume-cycled ventilator to stabilize the fracture(s). In some cases the flail segment is fixated externally during a surgical procedure by wiring or otherwise attaching the segment to the intact bony structures.

Thoracotomy: Generally avoided unless complications develop after stabilization. Indications for thoracotomy include massive air leak in a functioning drainage system, continued or increased bleeding through a chest tube, refractory hypotension, acute deterioration, and cardiac tamponade.

NURSING DIAGNOSES AND INTERVENTIONS

Risk for fluid volume deficit related to active loss secondary to excessive bleeding occurring with chest trauma

Desired outcome: Patient is normovolemic as evidenced by BP and HR within patient's normal limits; stable weight; urine output ≥0.5 ml/kg/h; chest drainage ≤100 ml/h; and RR ≤20 breaths/min with normal depth and pattern (eupnea).

- Note condition of dressings at frequent intervals. Be sure to check sheets underneath patient. Report excessive drainage or bleeding (e.g., if dressings are saturated more frequently than q4h during the first 24-48 h). After the first 48 h, bleeding should subside and the dressing should not require changing more often than bid. At that time drainage should be serosanguineous or serous; however, any bright red bleeding should be reported promptly.

- Monitor drainage in closed chest-drainage system. Report significant increase in bright red blood or excessive drainage. Amounts >100 ml/h usually are considered excessive.
- Monitor functioning of autotransfusion equipment. Collaborate with physician for additional transfusion/fluid requirements based on the amount and rate of bleeding. Record accurate I&O status.
- Assess VS at frequent intervals. Be alert to decreased BP and to increased HR and RR, which can signal an impending shock state.
- Assess patient's hydration status by monitoring daily weight, as well as amounts of fluid intake and urinary output.
- Monitor patient's Hgb as an indicator of hemostasis. Be alert to a decrease in Hgb, which can occur with blood loss. Normal Hgb is ≥12 g/dl (female) or ≥14 g/dl (male).

NIC Airway Management; Analgesic Administration; Bleeding Reduction; Blood Products Administration; Fluid/Electrolyte Management; Fluid Management; Fluid Monitoring; Hypovolemia Management; Oxygen Therapy; Pain Management; Respiratory Monitoring; Shock Management; Shock Management: Volume

ADDITIONAL NURSING DIAGNOSES

Also see "Major Trauma" for **Posttrauma response,** p. 106. See "Pneumothorax" for **Impaired gas exchange,** p. 242, and **Pain,** p. 243. For other nursing diagnoses and interventions, see "Psychosocial Support," p. 83, and "Psychosocial Support for the Patient's Family and Significant Others," p. 95.

Near drowning

PATHOPHYSIOLOGY

Near drowning can be defined as survival longer than 24 h after asphyxia related to submersion in a fluid medium. Many adult drownings or near drownings are preceded by alcohol or drug ingestion, diving injuries, or medical catastrophes such as seizures or myocardial infarctions. Hypoxia, hypotension, pulmonary edema, and respiratory and metabolic acidosis are the most common problems after near drowning. Potential complications include neurologic deficits from cerebral anoxia, acute renal failure secondary to acute tubular necrosis, and disseminated intravascular coagulation (DIC). Near drowning can be categorized in two ways.

Near drowning with aspiration (wet): Occurs in 85%-90% of victims of near drowning. The aspirant is either the submersion fluid or gastric contents. Hypoxia results from a variety of mechanisms, including laryngospasm, bronchospasm, airway obstruction from aspirated contaminants, or pulmonary edema. Freshwater (hypotonic) aspiration results in loss of surfactant, which is caused by the presence of hypotonic solution in the lungs. This can lead to atelectasis because surface tension of the lung tissue increases, causing alveoli to collapse. A decrease in lung compliance also occurs. In turn, the atelectasis and pulmonary edema lead to a ventilation-perfusion mismatch, which adds to the hypoxia and acidosis. Saltwater (hypertonic) aspiration results in a rapid shift of water and plasma proteins from the circulation into the alveoli. These fluid-filled alveoli are not ventilated, and the continued perfusion leads to ventilation-perfusion mismatch and hypoxia. Because the aspirated volume of either freshwater or saltwater is usually small, there is little effect on total blood volume. The intravascular depletion frequently seen is caused by increased capillary permeability (from anoxia) and loss of protein in the pulmonary edema fluid. Any contaminants that are aspirated (e.g., algae, chemicals, sand) can cause or contribute to obstruction and lead to asphyxiation. Bacterial pneumonia can develop, depending on the type of contaminant in the aspirant, and chemical pneumonitis can occur if gastric contents were aspirated.

Near drowning without aspiration (dry):   Represents 10%-15% of cases of near drowning. Death, if it occurs, results from asphyxiation secondary to laryngospasm. Laryngospasm usually results from irritation of the trachea by minimal aspiration of fluid, although it can be triggered by fear or pain.

Many deaths that have been attributed to near drowning may, in fact, be the result of one of two separate phenomena that can lead to aspiration: (1) immersion syndrome, which occurs with sudden immersion in cold water, resulting in hyperventilation; this increases the risk of swallowing or inhaling large amounts of cold water, which can lead to vagally stimulated bradycardia that results in loss of consciousness and can progress to asystolic cardiac arrest; and (2) hyperventilation syndrome, which occurs when divers hyperventilate to increase the duration time of breath-holding underwater. The normal impetus to breathe (increased $Paco_2$) is not present, and with exercise, oxygen stores continue to be used. Because breath-holding may not be terminated before oxygen supplies have reached dangerously low levels, dysrhythmias, seizure, or death from hypoxia can occur.

Hypothermia also is significant in near drowning. It is defined as a drop in core temperature to 33° C (91.4° F) or below. Its progression can cause muscle activity and vital functions to cease and ventricular fibrillation to occur (this happens at 28° C [82.4° F]). In some instances hypothermia protects the brain from permanent damage, depending on the victim's age and the degree of hypothermia, because of the decrease in cerebral metabolism that occurs when core body temperature reaches 25° C (77° F). This decrease in cerebral metabolism helps protect the brain from the effects of anoxia. Resuscitation should be continued until the victim is rewarmed to at least 32° C (89.6° F), because the heart may start beating at that temperature. Resuscitation is possible, even after 30 min of submersion. Resuscitation efforts frequently need to be continued for at least 1 h.

ASSESSMENT

The following criteria are based on postresuscitation findings.

Clinical presentation: Depending on the severity and duration of the hypoxia, may include unconsciousness, seizures, nonspecific alterations in mental status (e.g., confusion, irritability, lethargy), neurologic deficits (motor, speech, visual), mild coughing, pink and frothy sputum, vomiting, substernal chest pain, mottled and cold skin, cyanosis, fixed and dilated pupils, and abdominal distention.

Physical assessment: In the presence of pulmonary edema, there may be resonance over lung fields and normal tactile fremitus. Auscultation of lung fields may reveal apnea, tachypnea (RR >20 breaths/min), shallow or gasping respirations, crackles, rhonchi, wheezes, supraventricular dysrhythmias, bradycardia (HR <60 bpm), tachycardia (HR >100 bpm), and ventricular fibrillation.

DIAGNOSTIC TESTS

ABG values: Initially may reflect hypoxemia (Pao_2 <80 mm Hg), hypercapnia ($Paco_2$ >45 mm Hg), and metabolic and respiratory acidosis (pH <7.35, serum bicarbonate <22 mEq/L). Often the $Paco_2$ will return to normal but the hypoxemia will persist. Pulse oximetry may be initiated for continuous monitoring of oxygen saturation (see p. 213).

Note: Initial ABG values may be within acceptable range, but because respiratory status can deteriorate quickly, serial monitoring is essential.

CBC: To determine baseline hematologic status and presence of infection.
Serum electrolyte levels: Life-threatening changes in electrolyte levels are unusual after near drowning. Electrolyte disturbances are related to the quantity and tonicity of the water aspirated.
BUN and creatinine levels: To determine effects of hypoxia on renal tubular function. Creatinine is the most sensitive indicator of renal dysfunction. Acute tubular necrosis is a potential complication of near drowning.
Chest x-ray: Serial x-rays are necessary to determine presence or development of infiltrates, atelectasis, and pulmonary edema. The alveolar filling pattern, which is evaluated with pulmonary edema, is evidenced on x-ray by a soft, fluffy appearance with poorly demarcated lesions, often referred to as a *ground-glass* appearance.
Skull and spine x-rays: If CNS trauma has not been ruled out as a precipitating event, obtaining these x-rays is crucial. Until x-ray results are known, the patient's neck and spine must be immobilized.

COLLABORATIVE MANAGEMENT

Oxygen therapy: Oxygen (100%) is initiated immediately to treat hypoxia. High concentrations of oxygen are continued, even in alert patients with spontaneous ventilation, because of the risk of hypoxia and acidosis. Warmed oxygen 40°-43° C (104°-109.4° F) may be used as part of the rewarming process for patients with hypothermia.
Endotracheal intubation and mechanical ventilation: Used in respiratory failure when lung compliance is decreased or when the patient is unable to maintain effective respiratory effort. Intubation also assists in the maintenance of patent airways in patients who are unable to manage secretions independently. Patients with freshwater aspiration require 1½-2 times normal tidal volume at slower rates to allow optimal lung expansion and ventilation of alveoli. If neurologic involvement is present, decreased levels of $Paco_2$ can be achieved via mechanical hyperventilation.
Positive end-expiratory pressure (PEEP):   Required when pulmonary edema or hypoxia is present and unresponsive to increasing levels of oxygen (Fio_2 ≥0.50 to maintain a Pao_2 ≥60 mm Hg). PEEP improves oxygenation by preventing the collapse of alveoli during expiration, and it is especially useful after freshwater aspiration because the pressure keeps alveoli open in the absence of adequate surfactant. PEEP should be removed cautiously, because levels of surfactant can remain low for 48-72 h after freshwater aspiration.
Bronchoscopy: To remove aspirated contaminants, if necessary.
Rewarming for hypothermia: Warm, moist oxygen 40°-43° C (104°-109.4° F) may be used to elevate core temperature. Peritoneal lavage also is used for rewarming. Fluid for lavage is warmed to 37° C (98.6° F). The goal is quick rewarming to achieve a normal core temperature.
Pharmacotherapy: Profound metabolic acidosis is treated with sodium bicarbonate and careful monitoring of arterial pH. If bronchospasm is present, aerosolized bronchodilators such as epinephrine or isoproterenol HCL may be used.

Note: Use of steroids and prophylactic antibiotics is controversial. Temperature elevation up to 38° C (100.4° F) during the first 24 h can be a normal response to injury. Antibiotics may be prescribed if fever ≥38° C (100.4° F) persists for longer than 24 h after the submersion.

Fluid and electrolyte management: Although uncommon, fluid and electrolyte abnormalities may occur. Usually no specific therapy is required for minor disturbances. Fluid volume may be replaced with crystalloid solutions (Ringer's lactate or normal saline).

Neurologic support: Depends on the severity of the neurologic impairment. Severe impairment may necessitate intracranial pressure monitoring, steroids, hyperosmolar diuretics (e.g., mannitol), mechanical ventilation to maintain $Paco_2$ <30 mm Hg or a barbiturate coma (see "Traumatic Brain Injury," p. 118), and deep hypothermia (core temperature <30° C [86° F]).

Management of event that precipitated the near drowning: Conditions such as alcohol or drug ingestion, seizure, myocardial infarction, or cervical spine fracture.

NURSING DIAGNOSES AND INTERVENTIONS

Impaired gas exchange related to alveolar-capillary membrane changes secondary to fluid accumulation in the lung or loss of surfactant

Desired outcomes: Within 12 h of initiation of treatment, patient has adequate gas exchange as evidenced by the following ABG values: Pao_2 ≥60 mm Hg and $Paco_2$ ≤45 mm Hg. Within 3 days of treatment, RR is ≤20 breaths/min with normal depth and pattern (eupnea); breath sounds are clear and bilaterally equal; and patient is oriented to time, place, and person (depending on degree of permanent neurologic impairment).

- Assess patient for indicators of increased respiratory effort: complaints of SOB, tachypnea (RR >20 breaths/min), change in the use of accessory muscles of respiration, nasal flaring, grunting, restlessness, and anxiety.
- Auscultate lung fields at frequent intervals. Note the type and extent of adventitious breath sounds (e.g., crackles, rhonchi, friction rubs); document findings. Consult physician if acute changes occur.
- Assess patient's need for suctioning at frequent intervals. Document color, consistency, amount of sputum; frequency of suctioning to maintain clear airway; and patient's response to the procedure.
- Monitor ABG values and/or oxygen saturation via pulse oximetry. Hypoxemia is common. Progressive hypoxemia may require increased concentrations of oxygen or mechanical ventilation. Alert physician accordingly.
- Place patient in semi-Fowler's position to optimize lung expansion and decrease work of breathing.
- If patient is receiving PEEP therapy, be aware that alveoli collapse when PEEP is removed. Oxygenation levels achieved before suctioning will not be attained immediately after PEEP is reinstituted because the effect PEEP exerts on alveoli is not instantaneous. To prevent dramatic decreases in Pao_2 with suctioning, use of a PEEP adapter or manual resuscitator is recommended for patients receiving high levels of PEEP. (See "Mechanical Ventilation," p. 17, for details.) An in-line suction device may prevent hypoxia associated with suctioning.
- Provide rest periods between activities to decrease oxygen demands.
- Explain all procedures to patient, and provide emotional support to decrease anxiety, which can contribute to oxygen consumption.

Hypothermia related to prolonged exposure to cold water during submersion

Desired outcomes: Within 24 h of initiating therapy, patient's core temperature increases to 35°-37° C (95°-98.6° F). BP, RR, and HR are within patient's normal limits.

- Use temperature probe or PA catheter to continuously measure patient's core temperature. The temperature of inspired gases may affect the accuracy of PA catheter measurements. Other methods for measuring core temperature include bladder thermometry, rectal probe, or esophageal temperature probe, which is positioned in the lower third of the esophagus.
- Monitor patient's response to rewarming. Assess temperature and humidity level of inspired oxygen. Monitor temperature of instilled peritoneal lavage fluid. Do not attempt surface or external warming until core temperature is within acceptable limits (i.e., 35°-37° C [95°-98.6° F]). Premature surface rewarming can lead to the return of cold blood to the heart and precipitate an "after-drop" in core temperature.

- After core temperature has reached acceptable limits, monitor patient's response to active rewarming of body surface. Rewarming can be achieved by warm baths, heating pads, or lights. Cover patient's head to prevent heat loss from this exposed area. Use of blankets alone is an inadequate method of rewarming surface areas except in cases of mild hypothermia.
- Be aware of the likelihood of decreased drug metabolism during patient's hypothermic period.

Risk for infection related to increased environmental exposure secondary to aspiration of water and contaminants present in water

Desired outcome: Patient is free of infection as evidenced by body temperature ≤37.5° C (99.5° F) after the first 24 h; WBC count within normal limits for patient; clear sputum; and negative culture results.

- Monitor temperature q2h. Increases in temperature up to 38° C (100.4° F) are common during the first 24 h. After 24 h, an increased temperature may be indicative of infection.
- Monitor WBC count, being alert to increases from baseline values.
- Inspect sputum for changes in color, consistency, and amount.
- Use meticulous aseptic technique when suctioning patient's secretions.
- Collect sputum specimen for Gram stain and culture and sensitivity as prescribed. These tests will identify the pathogen if infection is present.

NIC Acid Base Management; Acid Base Monitoring; Airway Management; Bedside Laboratory Testing; Laboratory Data Interpretation; Oxygen Therapy; Respiratory Monitoring; Temperature Regulation; Vital Signs Monitoring

ADDITIONAL NURSING DIAGNOSES

Also see "Major Trauma" for **Posttrauma response,** p. 106. See other nursing diagnoses and interventions in "Psychosocial Support," p. 83; and "Psychosocial Support for the Patient's Family and Significant Others," p. 95.

Cardiac trauma

PATHOPHYSIOLOGY

Cardiac trauma may be caused by blunt or penetrating injuries to the heart. *Blunt cardiac trauma* commonly is caused by acceleration-deceleration injuries during a vehicular collision if the driver slams forward against the steering wheel. When this occurs, the heart muscle is injured by one or more of four mechanisms: compression of the heart between the sternum and vertebrae, bruising of heart tissue by bony structures, rupture or compression of coronary arteries by the blow, or cardiac rupture caused by intrathoracic or intraabdominal pressure. Other causes of blunt cardiac trauma are direct blows to the chest, falls from great heights, sporting and industrial injuries, and kicks by animals.

Blunt cardiac trauma can be classified as cardiac concussion or cardiac contusion. With cardiac concussion, the less severe injury, the patient will demonstrate many of the clinical signs and symptoms of cardiac trauma, without any evidence of cellular injury. Cardiac concussion leads to a transient myocardial dysfunction and some tissue edema but not to cellular damage or increase in serum creatine kinase–myocardial band isoenzyme (CK-MB). The tissue damage, however, may lead to temporary cardiac dysrhythmias. In comparison, cardiac contusion involves demonstrable cellular damage. The patient has varying degrees of cellular injury and necrosis, ranging from small areas of bruising to full-thickness cellular necrosis and permanent myocardial scarring. The patient may exhibit signs and symptoms similar to those manifested by individuals with myocardial infarction. The walls of the right ventricle are those most often injured because they are located directly behind the sternum. Blunt trauma also may damage cardiac valves, particularly the aortic and mitral valves, the ventricular septum, and the papillary muscle attachment. Rupture of the left ventricle from blunt forces generally leads to

> **Research Brief 2-1** Investigators at a level I trauma center found that, over a 10-year span, of 70 patients with blunt cardiac trauma, only 12 required inotropes for management of cardiac pump problems and only 3 patients died from causes directly attributable to the cardiac injury. Most frequently the myocardial contusion was of little importance clinically and did not affect the patient's outcome after injury.

From Wijngaarden MH et al: Blunt cardiac injury: a 10-year institutional review, *Injury* 28(1):51-55, 1997.

death in a few minutes, whereas rupture of the right ventricle sometimes can be successfully managed. Ventricular rupture also may occur up to 2 wk after injury if the contused area of the heart fails to heal and instead softens and weakens.

Penetrating cardiac trauma is caused by gunshot wounds, stab wounds, or foreign bodies in the heart. The right ventricle, because of its anterior location, is the most common chamber involved in this type of injury. Penetrating injuries are the most common cause of intrapericardial hemorrhage (see "Acute Cardiac Tamponade," p. 144).

ASSESSMENT
History and risk factors: Motor vehicle collision, assault, sporting injuries, car-pedestrian collision.
Clinical presentation
Blunt injury: Precordial chest pain (difficult to distinguish from angina), bradycardia or tachycardia, SOB, guarded breathing.
Penetrating injury: Tachycardia, SOB, weakness, diaphoresis, acute anxiety, cool and clammy skin.
Physical assessment
Blunt injury: Contusion marks on chest (may outline shape of steering wheel), flail chest (loss of continuity of bony thorax because of rib fracture) with resulting paradoxic respiratory movement of the chest wall, murmurs indicating valvular injury, atrial or ventricular gallops (if cardiac injury has decreased ventricular contractility). Note that upper body cyanosis associated with the symptoms of cardiac tamponade may indicate cardiac rupture after blunt trauma to the heart.
Penetrating injury: Protrusion of penetrating instrument (e.g., knife, ice pick), external puncture wound, signs of cardiac tamponade (see "Acute Cardiac Tamponade," p. 144).
ECG and hemodynamic measurements
Cardiac monitor: Sinus tachycardia, sinus bradycardia, ventricular tachycardia, ventricular fibrillation, asystole, and ST-segment and T-wave changes.
Arterial blood pressure: Decreased.

DIAGNOSTIC TESTS
There is no clear agreement on the diagnostic criteria for the medical diagnosis of cardiac contusion. Elevations of the CK-MB fraction, troponin I, and troponin t, as well as the results of echocardiography, ECG, and myocardial scanning are considered useful aids in making the diagnosis, but no single test is widely accepted as the definitive diagnostic tool. In addition, these diagnostic methods lack sensitive and specific indicators of myocardial damage. The following diagnostic tests may demonstrate abnormal results with cardiac contusion.
Chest x-ray: Although heart muscle damage will not appear on routine chest x-ray, findings may reveal damage to bony structures of the chest.
Cardiac enzyme levels: CK and the MB subfraction may increase in the first 3-4 h after injury to levels >7%-8% of the total CK. In the patient with multiple

trauma, however, the myocardium may not be the only source of CK-MB release. Injury to the liver, skeletal muscles, stomach, pancreas, and bowel also may lead to CK-MB elevations.

Troponin: Cardiac markers, troponins I and t, are recently used as diagnostic tools to indicate cardiac injury. Troponins I, C, and t form a complex that regulates calcium interaction with striated muscle fibers. Cardiac troponins I (cTnI) and t (cTnt) are not present in adult skeletal muscles. Initial research indicates that cTnI in particular, as well as cTnt, may be the most specific markers to indicate cardiac injury after blunt injury if specimens are obtained 24 h after injury.

ECG: Cardiac injury may cause alterations in depolarization, repolarization, and muscle perfusion. The following abnormalities may occur: ST-segment changes, T-wave changes, prolongation of the QT interval, sinus tachycardia, heart block, and ventricular dysrhythmias. The ability of the ECG to determine myocardial contusion currently is being questioned. ECG changes are detected in <40% of all contusions, possibly because the right ventricle is the heart's most anterior structure and thus the area most likely to be damaged. The majority of ECG changes reflect changes in the large muscle mass of the left ventricle rather than the right.

Multiple-gated acquisition (MUGA) scan: In the presence of a contusion, detects decreased ability of the heart to pump efficiently.

Echocardiography: Detects abnormalities in wall motion and valvular function and presence of intracavity thrombi or pericardial effusion.

Transesophageal echocardiography (TEE):   A useful diagnostic tool when hemodynamic compromise occurs after chest trauma. It is particularly helpful in differentiating severe right ventricular contusion from acute cardiac tamponade. High-frequency sound waves are emitted from a transducer fitted to the end of a standard gastroscope approximately 9 mm in diameter. When the gastroscope is introduced into the esophagus, the transducer produces clear posterior images of the heart.

Technetium pyrophosphate myocardial scan: Identifies localized area(s) of radioisotope uptake by damaged myocardial cells, revealed as "hot spot(s)" on the scan.

COLLABORATIVE MANAGEMENT
For blunt injuries

Treatment of dysrhythmias: Antidysrhythmic agents (e.g., lidocaine for ventricular dysrhythmias; digitalis for pump failure or tachycardia) or temporary pacemakers for heart block. If rhythm disturbances do not appear in the first 5 days after trauma, they rarely occur later.

Relief of acute pain: Usually with IV morphine sulfate in small increments unless hypotension occurs.

Restriction of activity and institution of continuous observation

Immediate corrective surgical repair: For ruptured valve, torn papillary muscle, or torn intraventricular septum accompanied by hemodynamic instability.

Research Brief 2-2   In a prospective study over 1 year, 60 patients with penetrating cardiac injuries were evaluated to determine the characteristics of survivors. More patients with stab wounds (68%) survived than did patients with gunshot wounds (14%). The presence of cardiac tamponade and the anatomic site of injury did not predict survival, but the mechanism of injury (stab versus gun shot wound) and the presence of sinus rhythm when the pericardium was penetrated were predictors of survival.

From Asensio JA et al: Penetrating cardiac injuries: a prospective study of variables predicting outcomes, *J Am Coll Surg* 186:24-34, 1998.

Treatment of shock: With fluid resuscitation, pressor agents.
Treatment of myocardial failure: Oxygen, diuretics, positive inotropic agents, and monitoring with a pulmonary artery catheter for right- and left-sided heart pressures.

For penetrating injuries
Surgical intervention: Foreign bodies of reasonable size are localized by fluoroscopic examination and removed surgically.

> *Caution:* Because of the potential for hemorrhage or pneumothorax, never remove a penetrating object until a surgeon is present.

Antimicrobial agents: To control infections that occur secondary to contamination by the penetrating instrument.

NURSING DIAGNOSES AND INTERVENTIONS

Altered tissue perfusion: peripheral, cardiopulmonary, renal, and cerebral, related to interruption of arterial and venous flow secondary to decreased cardiac contractility
Desired outcome: Within 12 h after injury, patient has adequate perfusion as evidenced by systolic BP ≥90 mm Hg (or within patient's normal range); HR ≤100 bpm; RR 12-20 breaths/min with normal depth and pattern (eupnea); ease of respiration; clear lung fields; urine output ≥0.5 ml/kg/h; brisk capillary refill (<2 sec); peripheral pulses >2+ on a 0-4+ scale; normal sinus rhythm; absence of neck vein distention with the HOB elevated to 30 degrees; and orientation to time, place, and person.
- Perform a complete cardiac assessment q4h, noting peripheral pulses, heart sounds, and capillary refill; assess heart rate and rhythm and BP hourly. For more assessment information, see **Decreased cardiac output,** p. 146, in "Acute Cardiac Tamponade" and **Impaired gas exchange,** p. 139, in "Pneumothorax."
- Perform a complete pulmonary assessment q4h, noting respiratory rate, depth, and effort. Auscultate lung fields q4h and as needed to evaluate for pulmonary congestion.
- Consult physician for changes in mental status, systolic BP <90 mm Hg or a drop of >20 mm Hg from trend, delayed capillary refill, or absent or thready peripheral pulses.
- Administer fluids as prescribed to maintain systolic BP at ≥90 mm Hg and urine output at ≥0.5 ml/kg/h.
- Maintain continuous cardiac monitoring for the first 3-4 days after cardiac trauma.
- If dysrhythmias occur, prepare to administer antidysrhythmic agents or assist with insertion of a transvenous temporary pacemaker.
- If hemodynamic instability occurs, place patient in supine position, if injuries allow, and prepare for initiation of pulmonary artery pressure monitoring.

NIC Cardiac Care: Acute; Circulatory Precautions; Emergency Care; Invasive Hemodynamic Monitoring; Dysrhythmia Management; Respiratory Monitoring; Shock Management; Vital Signs Monitoring; Oxygen Therapy; Fluid/Electrolyte Management

Pain (acute precordial chest pain) related to biophysical injury secondary to myocardial damage and chest wall injury
Desired outcomes: Within 2 h after initiation of analgesic therapy, patient's subjective evaluation of discomfort improves, as documented by a pain scale. Nonverbal indicators, such as grimacing or diaphoresis, are absent or reduced.
- Assess and document location, type, severity, and duration of patient's discomfort. Devise a pain scale with patient, rating discomfort from 0 (no pain) to 10. Administer IV morphine or other analgesic agent as prescribed, and record its effectiveness, using the pain scale. Pain may begin

immediately after injury or after approximately 8 h. Usually, it is not affected by coronary vasodilators.

- Place patient in a position of comfort. Patients often prefer the HOB elevated at 30-45 degrees.
- If bony structures are damaged and pain limits coughing and deep breathing, assist patient with chest splinting during chest physiotherapy. For some patients, intercostal nerve blocks may be necessary.
- Teach patient to recognize signs of posttraumatic pericarditis (i.e., fever, diaphoresis, precordial chest pain) and to notify physician promptly if they occur.

NIC Analgesic Administration; Pain Management; Positioning; Presence

ADDITIONAL NURSING DIAGNOSES

For other nursing diagnoses and interventions, see also "Major Trauma," p. 106; "Acute Cardiac Tamponade," p. 144; "Psychosocial Support," p. 83; and "Psychosocial Support of the Patient's Family and Significant Others," p. 95.

Acute cardiac tamponade

PATHOPHYSIOLOGY

Acute cardiac tamponade is the sudden accumulation of blood, fluid, clots, pus, and/or gas in the pericardial space, resulting in compression of the heart muscle and interference with cardiac filling during diastole and cardiac ejection during systole. Tamponade may occur as a result of blunt or penetrating cardiac trauma or as a complication after cardiac catheterization, anticoagulant therapy, myocardial infarction, or acute pericarditis. Pericardial disease with the potential for cardiac tamponade occurs in approximately 20% of patients with HIV infections as a result of opportunistic infections, tumors, and metabolic or hemodynamic abnormalities. Those HIV-positive patients who become symptomatic generally have infections or a neoplasm.

The primary effect of sudden cardiac tamponade is hemodynamic compromise, with inadequate cardiac output and decreased tissue perfusion. Normally the pericardial sac contains 10-20 ml of fluid that protects the myocardium. Because the pericardial sac has minimal stretching ability, the sudden addition of as little as 50-100 ml of fluid can increase intrapericardial pressure markedly. On the other hand, in a slowly accumulating tamponade as much as 1 liter of fluid can collect without life-threatening cardiac compromise.

As intrapericardial pressure increases and exceeds central venous pressure, the atria, ventricles, and coronary arteries become compressed. The compressed heart chambers, which no longer can hold their usual volume, cause a reduction in end-diastolic volume and end-diastolic fiber stretch and a decrease in stroke volume. Ultimately, decreased cardiac output and poor tissue perfusion occur.

ASSESSMENT

Clinical presentation: Tachycardia, decreased BP, shock, pallor, confusion, restlessness, cold and clammy skin, dyspnea, oliguria, thready pulse, unwillingness to lie supine because of difficulty breathing.

Classic signs: Beck's triad (distended neck veins, hypotension, muffled heart tones). Distended neck veins usually are not present in acute traumatic tamponade (as compared with constrictive pericarditis) because of hypovolemia and an acceleration of blood into the right atrium during inspiration. Beck's triad occurs in <10%-33% of patients with acute cardiac tamponade. Muffled heart tones may not be present if the patient is sitting upright because gravity pulls the blood toward the bottom of the pericardial sac.

Physical assessment: See Table 2-7.

TABLE 2-7 Physical Signs of Acute Cardiac Tamponade

Physical sign	Explanation for findings
Muffled heart sounds	Accumulation of fluid surrounding the heart diminishes sounds of valve closure
CVP elevated to >12 mm Hg	Mean right atrial pressure is elevated because diastolic filling is impeded by atrial compression
Decreased BP	Compression by tamponade reduces ventricular filling, decreasing CO and BP
Jugular venous distention	As atria and ventricles become compressed, there is less space for diastolic filling, causing impairment of venous return
Pulsus paradoxus: a fall of ≥10 mm Hg in systolic BP during inspiration	Two possible explanations: (1) during each inspiration, blood pools in pulmonary veins, reducing left ventricular filling and output; (2) with inspiration, intraventricular septum shifts toward left ventricle, causing more volume to be drawn to right side rather than to left side of heart
Absence of Kussmaul sign: Kussmaul sign is a rise, rather than fall, in venous pressure during inspiration	On inspiration, blood is accelerated toward the right atrium because of septal shift toward left ventricle

CVP, Central venous pressure; *BP*, blood pressure; *CO*, cardiac output.

Note: In severe hypovolemic states, physical signs may be masked.

ECG and hemodynamic measurements
Cardiac monitor: May show evidence of sinus tachycardia or electrical alternans (see "ECG," below).
Pulmonary artery pressure: Elevation of right atrial pressure (early sign if severe hypotension does not occur); elevation of left ventricular end-diastolic pressure (late sign).

DIAGNOSTIC TESTS

ECG: May reveal ST-segment elevation, nonspecific ST and T-wave changes (representing myocardial ischemia), and electrical alternans (alternation of the QRS axis from beat to beat) caused by the heart's movement like a pendulum within the pericardial effusion. The underlying mechanism for this movement is not understood.
Chest x-ray: May reveal normal cardiac silhouette, clear lung fields, dilation of the superior vena cava, and an enlarged mediastinum.
Echocardiography: May show echo-free space anterior to the right ventricular wall and posterior to the left ventricular wall, with a decrease in right

ventricular chamber size. There will be right-to-left intraventricular septal shift during inspiration.

TEE: See discussion with "Cardiac Trauma," p. 140.

COLLABORATIVE MANAGEMENT

Pericardiocentesis: Needle aspiration of the pericardium by the subxiphoid or left parasternal approach to drain the pericardial space of the excess fluid. Often the blood removed from the pericardium will not clot because of breaking down of clotting factors (defibrination) within the pericardial sac by heart action. Evidence exists that pericardiocentesis alone does not manage acute pericardial tamponade; surgical exploration is recommended after this procedure because of the high incidence of recurrent bleeding if surgery is not performed.

Surgical procedures: Subxiphoid pericardiostomy involves a resection of the xiphoid process to drain the pericardial sac; it can be performed with the patient under either local or general anesthesia. In addition, other more extensive surgical procedures such as a pericardiectomy can be used to decompress a pericardial tamponade. If the patient suddenly has signs of bradycardia (HR <50 bpm), severe hypotension (systolic BP <70 mm Hg), or cardiac arrest, an immediate thoracotomy is performed in the emergency department or ICU to allow for pericardial sac evacuation, hemorrhage control, and internal cardiac massage if needed.

Fluid resuscitation: To increase filling pressures during diastole, resulting in increased cardiac output and BP. Blood products, colloids, or crystalloids may be used.

Inotropic agents: To increase myocardial contractility and support cardiac output. Examples include dopamine, norepinephrine, phenylephrine, isoproterenol, and amrinone. For more information, see Appendix 7.

Oxygen, intubation, mechanical ventilation: Usually oxygen is administered via face mask; more aggressive therapy is used, as necessary, to correct hypoxia.

NURSING DIAGNOSES AND INTERVENTIONS

Decreased cardiac output related to decreased preload secondary to compression of ventricles by fluid in the pericardial sac

Desired outcome: Within 4-6 h after management with fluids or evacuation of tamponade, patient has adequate cardiac output as evidenced by mean right atrial pressure (RAP) 4-6 mm Hg; mean PAWP 6-12 mm Hg; pulmonary artery pressure (PAP) 20-30/8-15 mm Hg; cardiac output (CO) 4-7 L/min; systolic BP ≥90 mm Hg (or within patient's normal range); HR 60-100 bpm; normal sinus rhythm on ECG; and absence of new murmurs or gallops, distended neck veins, and pulsus paradoxus.

- Assess cardiovascular function by evaluating heart sounds and neck veins hourly. Consult physician for muffled heart sounds, new murmurs, new gallops, irregularities in rate and rhythm, and distended neck veins.
- Monitor all patients with blunt or penetrating trauma to the chest and abdomen for physical signs of acute cardiac tamponade (see Table 2-6), persistent hemodynamic instability, and shock out of proportion to the apparent blood loss.
- Evaluate patient for pulsus paradoxus: an abnormal decrease in arterial systolic BP during inspiration compared with that with expiration. See Table 2-8.
- Measure and record hemodynamic parameters. Consult physician for abnormalities or changes in trend. Early signs of tamponade include elevated RAP with normal BP. Later signs include elevated PAP in the presence of hypotension.
- Evaluate ECG for ST-segment changes, T-wave changes, rate, and rhythm.

T A B L E   2 - 8   Measuring Paradoxic Pulse

- After placing BP cuff on patient, inflate it above the known systolic BP. Instruct patient to breathe normally.
- While slowly deflating the cuff, auscultate BP.
- Listen for the first Korotkoff sound, which will occur during expiration with cardiac tamponade.
- Note the manometer reading when the first sound occurs, and continue to deflate the cuff slowly until Korotkoff sounds are audible throughout inspiration and expiration.
- Record the difference in millimeters of mercury between the first and second sounds. This is the pulsus paradoxus.

The optimal is sinus rhythm or sinus tachycardia. Maintain continuous cardiac monitoring.
- Administer blood products, colloids, or crystalloids as prescribed. For trauma patients, use large-bore IV lines in the periphery, if possible. Use pressure infusers and rapid volume/warmer infusers for patients who require massive fluid resuscitation. Be prepared to administer pressor agents if fluid resuscitation does not support patient's BP.
- Have emergency equipment available for immediate pulmonary artery catheterization, central line insertion, pericardiocentesis, or thoracotomy.

NIC Cardiac Care; Cardiac Care: Acute; Emergency Care; Hemodynamic Regulation; Invasive Hemodynamic Monitoring; Fluid Monitoring; Fluid Management; Blood Product Administration; Medication Administration; Oxygen Therapy; Resuscitation; Shock Management: Cardiac; Vital Sign Monitoring; Dysrhythmia Management

Altered tissue perfusion: cardiopulmonary, peripheral, cerebral, and renal, related to interruption of arterial and venous flow secondary to compression of the myocardium by the collection of blood

Desired outcome: Within 4-6 h after management with fluids or evacuation of tamponade, patient has adequate perfusion as evidenced by orientation to time, place, and person; systolic BP ≥90 mm Hg (or within patient's normal range); RR 12-20 breaths/min with normal depth and pattern (eupnea) and ease of respirations; Sao_2 >95%; peripheral pulses >2+ on a 0-4+ scale; equal and normoreactive pupils; warm and dry skin; brisk capillary refill (<2 sec); and urine output ≥0.5 ml/kg/h.

- Assess tissue perfusion by evaluating the following at least hourly: LOC, BP, pulses, pupillary response, skin temperature, and capillary refill.
- Evaluate urine output hourly to ensure that it is at least 0.5 ml/kg/h. Assess urine specific gravity q4h; elevations (>1.030) may signal hypovolemia and inadequate renal perfusion.
- Maintain tissue perfusion by delivering prescribed blood products, colloids, or crystalloids.
- If hypotension occurs, be prepared to administer medication to maintain BP. Be familiar with dosage, side effects, and calculations necessary for administration. At frequent intervals, assess peripheral IV lines for evidence of infiltration. Pressor agents, which infiltrate subcutaneous tissues, jeopardize future tissue perfusion.

Note: When it is feasible, all pressor agents (e.g., norepinephrine, dopamine) should be infused through a central line.

- Have emergency equipment available for delivery of humidified oxygen, intubation, and mechanical ventilation.

NIC Cardiac Care: Acute; Circulatory Care; Emergency Care; Invasive Hemodynamic Monitoring; Respiratory Monitoring; Shock Management; Vital Signs Monitoring; Cerebral Perfusion Promotion; Neurologic Monitoring; Medication Administration; Medication Management; Oxygen Therapy; Intravenous Therapy; Fluid/Electrolyte Management

ADDITIONAL NURSING DIAGNOSES

For other nursing diagnoses and interventions see also "Major Trauma," p. 106; "Cardiac Trauma," p. 140; "Hemodynamic Monitoring," p. 28; "Psychosocial Support," p. 83; and "Psychosocial Support for the Patient's Family and Significant Others," p. 95.

Renal and lower urinary tract trauma

PATHOPHYSIOLOGY

Injuries to the kidneys and lower urinary tract (LUT), which includes the ureters, urinary bladder, and urethra, occur in <1% of all trauma patients but have the potential for lifelong complications or even death. These injuries often are overlooked in the initial trauma assessment because they frequently accompany life-threatening injuries that require aggressive and immediate management.

Blunt injuries are responsible for most renal and LUT trauma and are caused by vehicular collisions, falls, sports-related injuries, and assaults. Renal and LUT trauma also can occur after penetrating injuries, such as stab and gunshot wounds. The specific pathophysiology for each type of renal and LUT trauma is discussed in Table 2-9.

Urethral injury presents males with a particular set of long-term complications that my interfere with quality of life. Sexual and voiding dysfunction may occur. Sexual dysfunction may be the result of damage of neural and vascular structures, whereas incontinence may be caused by damage to the sphincters themselves or the nerves that innervate them. In patients with complete urethral disruption, approximately 20% have voiding dysfunction and 25% have sexual dysfunction.

ASSESSMENT

Renal trauma
Clinical presentation: Abdominal or flank pain, back tenderness, colicky pain with passage of blood clots, hemorrhage (pallor, diaphoresis, hypotension, tachycardia, restlessness, confusion), gross or microscopic hematuria.

Note: Gross hematuria is present in slightly more than half of patients with renal trauma and is considered an unreliable diagnostic sign.

Physical assessment: Hematoma over the flank of the eleventh or twelfth ribs; obvious wounds, contusions, or abrasions in the flank or abdomen; abdominal distention; Grey Turner sign (bruising over the lower portion of the back and the flank caused by a retroperitoneal hemorrhage); pain at the costovertebral angle; flank or abdominal mass.

Note: Physical signs may be masked because of the protection of the kidneys by abdominal organs, back muscles, and bony structures.

Ureteral trauma
Clinical presentation: May be few early signs. Microscopic or gross hematuria may be present. If the ureter is completely transected, normal urine

TABLE 2-9   Pathophysiology for Renal and Lower Urinary Tract Trauma

Type of injury	Anatomic considerations	Pathophysiology and mechanism of injury	Result of injury
Renal trauma	Kidneys are well protected from injury posteriorly by muscles of the back, anteriorly by organs of the GI tract, and by a tough outer capsule and adipose tissue Kidneys are fixed in retroperitoneal space only by renal pedicle (vascular stem in renal hilum) and ureters Blunt renal injury is often caused by compression of kidney by the twelfth rib, which rotates kidney inwardly and squeezes kidney into lumbar spine	Renal trauma can be divided into three classifications: **Minor trauma: Incidence 85%** Bruising of renal parenchyma; superficial lacerations of renal cortex without rupture of renal capsule **Major trauma: Incidence 10%-15%** Major lacerations through cortex and medulla; continuation of laceration through renal capsule **Critical trauma: Incidence <5%** Renal vascular trauma in which kidney is shattered and renal pedicle is injured; fragmentation (renal fracture)	**Minor trauma:** Hematuria and flank tenderness that will usually result in a full recovery with rest and observation **Major trauma:** Hematuria, flank pain, and possible hypotension that may require surgical intervention **Critical injury:** Severe blood loss and shock requiring immediate surgical intervention
Ureteral trauma	Injury to upper part of ureter is uncommon because of its location deep in retroperitoneum Ureteral lacerations are most common at ureteropelvic junction, where upper ureter joins renal pelvis	Ureteral injury is most commonly associated with iatrogenic injuries during gynecologic, colonic, and vascular surgery Blunt injury may occur when ureter becomes crushed against spinal column	Extravasation of urine or blood may lead to infection, abscess formation, hemorrhage, or shock; late complications include prolonged voiding time, ureteral strictures, and fistula formation

Continued

TABLE 2-9 Pathophysiology for Renal and Lower Urinary Tract Trauma—cont'd

Type of injury	Anatomic considerations	Pathophysiology and mechanism of injury	Result of injury
Ureteral trauma—cont'd		When ureteral injury is not associated with iatrogenic injury, it usually occurs in the setting of severe abdominal compression or significant penetrating abdominal injury	
Bladder trauma	When bladder is distended, it extends above umbilicus and has less protection from trauma; the bladder ruptures at its point of least resistance (the dome), and blood and urine extravasate into the peritoneal cavity (intraperitoneal rupture)	Motor vehicle crashes are the most common cause of bladder rupture; bladder contusion often results from a direct blow or the cavitational effect of missiles (outward tissue acceleration away from the tract of the bullet); bladder rupture does not require extensive force, which may be a blunt blow to the lower abdomen	Bladder lacerations or rupture can lead to blood or urine extravasation outside of the peritoneal cavity (80%) and into the peritoneal cavity (20%); infection or hemorrhage can follow
	Extraperitoneal rupture occurs most often in conjunction with pelvic fractures; sharp bone fragments perforate bladder at its base, leading to extravasation of blood and urine into space surrounding bladder base		
Urethral trauma	Urethral injury is more common in males than females because the male urethra is 5 times longer; the male urethra is also rigidly fixed at the urogenital diaphragm (bulbous urethra), whereas the female urethra is short and mobile	Perineal trauma, straddle injuries, and pelvic fractures are often the causes of urethral injury; vehicular collisions with deceleration and shearing may also lead to injury of the posterior urethra	Urethral injury may lead to extravasation of blood and/or urine within penis; if disruption to Buck's fascia occurs, extravasation into upper thighs and peritoneum follows; hemorrhage or infection may also occur

from the unaffected kidney may be voided. *Late signs* may include fever and flank or abdominal discomfort.

Physical assessment: Urine at the entrance or exit sites of penetrating wound, enlarging retroperitoneal mass.

Bladder trauma

Clinical presentation: Suprapubic tenderness, inability to void spontaneously, gross hematuria (present in approximately 95% of patients). *Late signs* may include fever and abdominal discomfort.

Physical assessment: Perineal or scrotal edema and hematoma, abnormal position of prostate, abdominal distention, palpable suprapubic mass, palpable and overdistended bladder.

Urethral trauma

Clinical presentation: Inability to void spontaneously, urethral bleeding, prostate tenderness, microscopic or gross hematuria, pain and tenderness of genitalia.

Physical assessment: Blood at urethral meatus, tracking of urine into tissues of the thighs or abdominal wall, bruised to discolored genitalia.

DIAGNOSTIC TESTS

Retrograde urethrogram: A small urinary catheter is inserted and the balloon inflated to 2 ml in the distal anterior urethra, 2 cm from the urinary meatus. Contrast material, 5-10 ml, is injected and a single x-ray is taken to outline the inner size and shape of the urethra. In urethral rupture, extravasation of the contrast material occurs, usually near the membranous urethra.

Cystogram: If no urethral tear is found on retrograde urethrogram, a catheter is inserted into the bladder. The bladder is filled with 300 ml of contrast material. After x-rays are obtained to determine if intraperitoneal or extraperitoneal extravasation of contrast material occurs, the bladder is drained and repeat x-rays are taken to check for small posterior ruptures.

Excretory urogram/intravenous pyelogram (IVP): Contrast material is administered intravenously and is filtered by the kidneys before excretion through the urinary tract. X-rays provide visualization of the normal or injured structures of the kidneys, ureters, or bladder.

> *Caution:* Check patient for a history of allergy to iodine, iodine-containing foods, or contrast material. Adequate hydration and sometimes diuretics are needed to rid the body of contrast material after this test.

Renal ultrasound: A transducer transmits high-frequency sound waves through the urinary tract. The resultant echoes are amplified and converted into electrical impulses that are displayed on an oscilloscope. The sound waves demonstrate the presence or absence of fluid accumulation, blood clots, and LUT structural damage.

Radionuclide imaging: After IV injection of a radionuclide, a radioactivity-detecting device scans and records the radioactive uptake to evaluate for injured LUT structures and alterations in renal blood flow. It takes 6-24 h for the substance to be excreted from the patient's body.

Blood urea nitrogen values: Measurement of the nitrogen fraction of urea, the end product of protein metabolism. Renal dysfunction causes insufficient excretion of urea, elevating nitrogenous wastes in the blood. In renal trauma, blood urea nitrogen (BUN) level also may increase because of body catabolism or dehydration. Normal value is 10-20 mg/dl.

Serum creatinine levels: Measurement of a nonprotein end product of creatinine metabolism. Creatinine level measures renal damage more accurately than does the BUN level because renal impairment is virtually the only cause of elevated serum creatinine. Creatinine production is fairly constant day to day

Research Brief 2-3 Although ureteral injuries are rare, delay in diagnosis can lead to the loss of renal function. This study was performed to determine the effectiveness of preoperative testing after suspected ureteral injury. In 20 patients, a total of 10 diagnostic studies were performed but only 2 were diagnostic for ureteral injury (one IVP and one CT). The rest of the injuries were discovered during surgery by primary visualization. The authors concluded that direct visualization is the best and most accurate diagnostic modality in ureteral injury.

From Medina D et al: Ureteral trauma: preoperative studies neither predict injury nor prevent missed injuries, *J Am Coll Surg* 186:641-644, 1998.

because production is proportional to muscle mass. Creatinine is freely filtered at the glomerulus and minimally reabsorbed, causing creatinine excretion to be roughly proportional to glomerular filtration rate. Normal value is 0.7-1.5 mg/dl.

Note: If an intraperitoneal bladder rupture has occurred, hyperkalemia, hypernatremia, uremia, and acidosis may occur as a result of resorption of urine from the peritoneal cavity.

Clearance tests: Clearance is the volume of plasma that can be cleared of a specific substance during a specified period of time. Clearance tests evaluate the extent of injury by assessing renal filtration, reabsorption, secretion, and renal plasma flow. Creatinine, inulin (a plant starch), and urea are the substances usually tested.

Kidney-ureter-bladder (KUB) radiography: Evaluates position, size, structure, and defects of kidney and LUT structures. Abnormal findings include retroperitoneal hematoma, fracture of the lower ribs or pelvis, foreign bodies, organ displacement, or fluid accumulation.

CT: Imaging of the kidneys via a series of cross-sectional slices that are then interpreted by computer. CT after renal trauma may reveal hematomas, renal lacerations, renal infarcts, or extravasation of urine. Contrast-enhanced CT detects kidney laceration and shows arterial occlusion. CT is the method of choice to assess patients with severe renal trauma.

Renal angiography: Arterial injection of a contrast medium, permitting identification on x-ray of renal vasculature and functional tissue. After renal trauma, angiography permits identification of renal pedicle injury, renal infarct, intrarenal hematoma, lacerations, and shattered kidney.

Note: Assess patient for allergy to contrast medium, and maintain adequate hydration during and after the procedure.

MRI: Clarifies the surgical approach necessary for trauma such as traumatic posterior urethral injury and enables estimation of the length of injury.

COLLABORATIVE MANAGEMENT

Pharmacotherapy

Antibiotics: For positive urine culture results, penetrating injuries, or peritonitis.

Analgesics: IV morphine sulfate usually relieves the pain and can be readily reversed with naloxone if complications, such as hypotension or bradypnea, occur.

Management of complications

Hemorrhage shock: Volume resuscitation with crystalloids, colloids, or blood products as indicated.

T A B L E   2 - 1 0   Surgical Procedures for Renal and Lower Urinary Tract Trauma

Type of injury	Surgical indications/surgical management
Minor renal trauma	None needed. Rest and observation with careful follow-up to prevent progressive deformity and to evaluate BP.
Major renal trauma	Surgical intervention if hypotension and hemodynamic instability occur.
Critical renal trauma	Immediate surgical exploration; low rates of renal salvage.
Proximal ureteral injury	Primary ureterostomy with end-to-end anastomosis.
Distal ureteral injury	Ureteral stenting or percutaneous nephrostomy, depending on location and extent of injury.
Bladder injury	Use of suprapubic drainage versus indwelling urethral catheter drainage is controversial. Use of suprapubic catheter avoids complications of prolonged urethral catheterization, particularly in males who are prone to the development of urethral strictures.
Urethral injury	Suprapubic cystotomy and drainage for temporary urinary evacuation. Urethral splinting and surgical reconstruction usually are delayed for 3-6 mo to allow reduction in bruising and swelling, which could delay healing of urinary structures.

Infections: Blood and urine cultures, antibiotics.

Renal dysfunction: Evaluation of need for fluid restriction; dietary restrictions of protein, sodium, phosphorus, and potassium; peritoneal dialysis; continuous arteriovenous hemofiltration (CAVH); continuous venovenous hemofiltration (CVVH); or hemodialysis. See "Renal Replacement Therapies," p. 395, for more information.

Catheterization: If patient is unable to void. Catheter should be passed only as far as it will progress without undue force. If any resistance is met during catheterization, a urethrogram is indicated. If blood is present at the urethral meatus, the patient should not be catheterized until a urethrogram is obtained inasmuch as the blood may signal urethral injury. In the presence of urethral injury, an improperly placed catheter can cause subsequent incontinence, impotence, and urethral strictures. In renal trauma, diversion of urine may be required by nephrostomy tube, depending on location of injury or in cases of coexisting pancreatic and duodenal injury. A suprapubic catheter may be used to manage severe urethral lacerations and urethral disruption. Internal ureteral catheters (ureteral stents) may be indicated for ureteral trauma, particularly for gunshot wounds, to maintain ureteral alignment, ensure urinary drainage, and provide support during anastomosis.

Surgical correction: Indicated for transected ureter, partial ureteral tears of more than a third of the circumference of the ureter, bladder perforation with associated abdominal injuries or intraperitoneal rupture, and injuries accompanied by rapidly expanding, pulsating hematomas. See Table 2-10 for examples of procedures for the various types of renal and LUT injuries.

NURSING DIAGNOSES AND INTERVENTIONS

Altered urinary elimination related to mechanical trauma secondary to injury to the kidney and LUT structures

Desired outcome: Within 6 h after immediate trauma management, patient has a urinary output of ≥0.5 ml/kg/h with no evidence of bladder distention.

- Ensure adequate urinary outflow by encouraging patient to void. If patient is unable to void, assess the need for urinary catheterization or suprapubic drainage by palpating gently for a full bladder. As indicated, discuss the need for a urinary catheter with physician. Monitor for the following signs of kidney or LUT trauma:
  - ☐ Urge but inability to void spontaneously in spite of adequate volume replacement
  - ☐ Blood at the urethral meatus
  - ☐ Difficult or unsuccessful urinary catheterization
  - ☐ Anuria after urinary catheterization
  - ☐ Hematuria
- Do not catheterize patient if there is blood at the urethral meatus unless a urethrogram has indicated that catheterization can be performed safely. Do not force a catheter if resistance is felt. Call physician for consultation if urethral injury is suspected.
- Monitor serum BUN and creatinine. Elevations reflect ineffective removal of waste products. Normal values are as follows: serum BUN ≤20 mg/dl; serum creatinine ≤1.5 mg/dl.
- Document I&O hourly. Assess patency of urinary collection system hourly to determine if clots are occluding the system. If indicated, obtain prescription for catheter irrigation or call physician to irrigate catheter, according to agency policy.
- Sudden cessation of urine flow through the collection system (particularly if past output was >50 ml/h) indicates possible catheter obstruction. If catheter irrigation does not resume urine drainage, consider changing the urinary catheter after discussion with physician.
- Ensure that the nephrostomy tube is not occluded by patient's weight or external pressure. Irrigate the nephrostomy tube *only* if prescribed, and with ≤5 ml of fluid, because the renal pelvis can hold no more than 10 ml of fluid.
- Assess entrance site of the nephrostomy tube for bleeding or leakage of urine. Catheter blockage with clots or catheter dislodging can cause a sudden decrease in urine output. Consult physician if urine output is <0.5 ml/kg/h.
- Assess urine for color and presence or absence or clots. Expect hematuria for the first 24-48 h after nephrostomy tube insertion. Consult physician if gross bleeding (with or without clots) occurs.
- Ensure adequate hydration to allow for clearing of contrast material from patient's system after diagnostic testing.

NIC Urinary Elimination Management; Urinary Catheterization; Fluid Management; Fluid Monitoring; Tube Care: Urinary

Risk for infection related to inadequate primary defenses and tissue destruction secondary to bacterial contamination of the urinary tract system occurring with penetrating trauma, rupture of the bladder into the perineum, or instrumentation

Desired outcome: Patient is free of infection as evidenced by normothermia; WBC count ≤11,000/mm^3; and negative results of urine and wound drainage testing for infective organisms.

- Use aseptic technique when caring for urinary drainage systems. Maintain catheters and collection container at a level lower than the bladder to prevent reflux; ensure that drainage tubing is not kinked.
- Record the color, odor, and specific gravity of urine each shift. Culture urine specimen when infection is suspected.
- Monitor patient's WBC count daily and temperature q4h for elevations.
- Assess patient each shift for signs of peritonitis: abdominal pain, abdominal distention with rigidity, nausea, vomiting, fever, malaise, and weakness.

- Assess catheter exit site each shift for the presence of erythema, swelling, or drainage.
- Assess thigh, groin, and lower portion of abdomen for indicators of urinary extravasation: swelling, pain, mass(es), erythema, tracking of urine along fascial planes.
- Assess surgical incision for approximation of suture line and evidence of wound healing, noting presence of erythema, swelling, and drainage. Note and record color, odor, and consistency of wound drainage. As prescribed, culture any drainage that appears purulent or is foul smelling; notify physician of results.
- At least q8h assess skin at all catheter entrance sites for indicators of irritation: erythema, drainage, and swelling.
- Cleanse insertion site q8h with antimicrobial solution. Apply sterile gauze pad(s) over suprapubic catheter exit site, and tape securely with paper tape. Change dressings q24h or as soon as they become wet. If erythema and swelling occur as a result of maceration from contact with urine, consider use of a pectin wafer skin barrier for extra protection.

NIC Incision Site Care; Infection Protection; Wound Care; Infection Control; Surveillance; Tube Care: Urinary

Pain (acute tenderness in lower abdomen) related to physical injury associated with LUT structural injury, procedures for urinary diversion, or surgical incisions

Desired outcomes: Within 2 h after giving analgesic agent, patient's subjective evaluation of discomfort improves, as documented by a pain scale. Nonverbal indicators of discomfort, such as grimacing, are absent.

- Assess patient for pain at least q4h. Devise a pain scale with patient, rating discomfort from 0 (no pain) to 10. Be alert to shallow breathing in the presence of abdominal pain, which can cause inadequate pulmonary excursion. Medicate promptly, and document patient's response to analgesic agent, using the pain scale. IV narcotics may be indicated if the injury is severe.
- Explain the cause of the pain to the patient.
- Assist patient into a position of comfort. Often knee flexion will relax lower abdominal muscles and help reduce discomfort.
- Implement nonpharmacologic measures for coping with pain: diversion, touch, conversation. Also see discussion of pain, p. 61.

NIC Analgesic Administration; Pain Management; Positioning; Presence

Pelvic fractures

PATHOPHYSIOLOGY

The pelvis is composed of three bones: two innominate bones and the sacrum. The innominate bones are each composed of three bones (ilium, pubis, and ischium) that fuse after childhood. The two innominate bones are joined by the symphysis pubis, a fibrous cartilage joint that connects the two pubic bones anteriorly, and attached posteriorly to a third bone, the sacrum, by a system of ligaments termed the *posterior osseous ligamentous structures.*

Motor vehicle collisions and auto-pedestrian trauma cause approximately two thirds of all pelvic fractures, which have mortality up to 50% in some studies. For a pelvic fracture to occur, a large force is needed because these bones are stabilized by a strong network of ligaments. Pelvic fractures have been classified by several systems, but perhaps the most helpful are the systems that classify fractures by their stability and mechanism of injury (Table 2-11). Pelvic fractures are considered stable fractures when the posterior osseous ligamentous structures are intact. An unstable pelvic fracture occurs when the osseous ligamentous structures are disrupted posteriorly and portions of the pelvis can move in any direction.

TABLE 2-11   Classification of Pelvic Fractures

Classification of injury	Mechanism of injury	Description
Anteroposterior compression	External rotation is caused by a crushing force on the posterior superior iliac spines.	"Open book injury"; the force causes the symphysis pubis to spring open. Rupture of anterior sacroiliac and sacrospinous ligaments occurs, but posterior ligaments are intact. Stable vertically but can rotate externally. May be associated with ruptured bladder (intraperitoneal) if injury occurs when bladder is full.
Lateral compression	Internal rotation from a high-energy injury that causes direct pressure to crush anterior sacrum. Pressure on the greater trochanter causes the femoral head to displace the anterior pubic rami.	Most common type of injury. Often does not affect posterior ligamentous complex. Partially unstable fracture that is rotationally unstable but vertically stable. May have extensive soft tissue injury. May be associated with ruptured bladder (extraperitoneal).
Vertical shear (Malgaigne fracture)	Excessive force from trauma such as falls and crush injuries in a vertical plane leads to unstable disruption of the anterior and posterior ring.	Most severe injury with the highest mortality rates. Very unstable. Complete disruption of the posterior osseous ligamentous system. Often accompanied by injuries of the skin and subcutaneous tissues or injuries to the gastrointestinal, genitourinary, vascular, and neurologic systems.
Complex fracture	Excessive and powerful forces from many directions.	Pelvic ring disruptions resulting in bizarre fractures or dislocations in a combination of injury patterns. Usually very unstable.

Research Brief 2-4   After pelvic fractures, 255 women were interviewed to determine the effect of trauma on their genitourinary, sexual, and reproductive function. Urinary complaints occurred more frequently in women with residual pelvic fracture displacement of 5 mm or more as compared with those without displacement and more frequently in women with residual lateral and vertical displacement as compared with those with medial displacement. Women with a fractured pelvis also reported more cesarean sections than controls but there was no difference in the incidence of miscarriage or infertility. Pain during sex was most common in women with fractures displaced 5 mm or more.

From Copeland CE et al: Effect of trauma and pelvic fracture on female genitourinary, sexual, and reproductive function, *J Orthop Trauma* 11(2):73-81, 1997.

The most serious complications from a pelvic fracture are hemorrhage and exsanguination, which cause up to 60% of the deaths from pelvic injuries. The pelvis receives a rich supply of blood from a complex system of interconnected collateral arteries and the venous plexus of the iliac system, often called the *vascular sink*. The aorta and internal iliac artery have proximity to the pelvis as well. This complex vascular network easily can be damaged or disrupted by the same forces that injure the pelvis, or pelvic fragments can damage vascular structures. Because the retroperitoneal space can hold as much as 4 liters (L) of blood before spontaneous tamponade occurs, acute blood loss is difficult to identify until systemic symptoms, such as those with shock, appear. In addition, damage to the sciatic and sacral nerves may occur with sacral and sacroiliac disruption.

Pelvic fractures in older adults, which most often occur from falls as compared with motor vehicle crashes in younger people, present a particular constellation of problems because of the likelihood of other serious conditions. Despite a less severe mechanism of injury, rates of sepsis and death are higher in older adults than in those trauma patients younger than 65 years with similar injuries. One reason for an increased mortality is preexisting cardiovascular disease, which causes insufficient compensatory function to manage the stress of injury.

ASSESSMENT

History and risk factors: Motor vehicle or motorcycle crash, auto-pedestrian collision, fall, industrial accident, crush injury, sports injury.

Clinical presentation: Suprapubic tenderness; pain over the iliac spines; signs and symptoms of hemorrhagic shock (tachycardia, delayed capillary refill, decreased urinary output, decreased extremity temperature, pallor, hypotension); signs and symptoms of urinary injuries (as many as 15% of trauma victims with a pelvic fracture have associated renal and lower urinary tract injuries; see p. 148).

Note: Initial evaluation of a patient with multiple trauma and a pelvic fracture may reveal no obvious evidence of pelvic injury.

Note: Of patients with both pelvic fractures and urologic injuries, 50% have accompanying abdominal injuries.

Accompanying injuries: in victims <65 years, common accompanying injuries include upper and lower extremity fractures and head injuries; in victims >65 years, abdominal and chest trauma are more common accompanying injuries.

Physical assessment: Groin, genitalia, and suprapubic swelling, ecchymosis, or lacerations; swelling, ecchymosis, or lacerations of medial thigh or lumbosacral area; increased diameter of the root of the thigh; pelvic instability (asymmetry or abnormal movement on downward pressure of the iliac crests); crepitus; lower extremity shortening; abnormal lower extremity internal rotation; "frog-leg positioning" of the lower extremities; hematuria or urethral bleeding; vaginal bleeding; blood in the rectum; high-riding prostate; lower extremity paresis or hypoesthesia (in particular at the L5 and S1 levels); absence of plantar flexion and ankle jerk reflexes; unequal or weak peripheral pulses.

> **Note:**   Lacerations of the perineum, groin, or buttocks are assumed to be caused by compound open pelvic fractures until proven otherwise.

DIAGNOSTIC TESTS
Pelvic x-ray
Anteroposterior view: Differentiates between a stable and unstable fracture; shows overall alignment, hip assessment, and location of fractures.
Inlet view: Determines rotational displacement, posterior displacement, sacral fractures.
Outlet view: Demonstrates superior rotation, vertical migration, sacral fractures.
CT: Ascertains pattern of pelvic injury. This is the most reliable method for determining injury to the posterior portion of the pelvis and is particularly successful in identifying sacral and sacroiliac joint injury.
Angiography: Identifies the site of bleeding, which often occurs at multiple points in the pelvic circulation. Two groups of patients have angiograms: those who undergo full laparotomy and are discovered to have an expanding pelvic retroperitoneal hematoma, and those with a pure pelvic injury who bleed internally.
Hematocrit: A value that fails to stabilize, falls, or fails to rise with transfusion is an indication of ongoing bleeding. A falling Hct is a late sign of hemorrhage and occurs only after significant blood loss.
Excretory urography (intravenous pyelogram [IVP]), cystography, and urography: Used to determine associated injuries (see "Renal and Lower Urinary Tract Trauma," p. 148).

COLLABORATIVE MANAGEMENT
Pelvic stabilization
External immobilization: Defined as any device that is applied to immobilize the pelvis either externally or percutaneously through the skin into the bone. External fixation can be accomplished at the scene of injury to preserve function and prevent further orthopedic and neurovascular injury. If abnormal shortening or rotation has occurred with the injury, the lower extremities should be supported and stabilized in the position in which they were found with a wooden backboard and supported by pillows, towels, or blankets taped in place with cloth tape. Most patients are managed with bed rest, spica cast, or sling traction. Emergency external fixation devices, consisting of one pin in each iliac wing connected by a bar, can be inserted to provide pelvic stability. If an emergency laparotomy is performed, more complex fixation devices may be applied.

> **Note:**   Use of an external fixation device is not sufficient for maintaining reduction in the posterior pelvis or for stabilizing the pelvic posterior elements. As long as the patient is on bed rest or in traction, it will, however, sufficiently manage the patient's fracture in the acute phase.

Internal immobilization: Surgical open reduction and immobilization of unstable pelvic ring disruptions with plates, screws, or other devices that are surgically implanted internally. Permanent fixation requires close anatomic reduction because it will be the final form of pelvic stabilization.

Surgical exploration: May occur along with ligation or vessel repair when the patient is hemorrhaging. The surgeon can limit blood inflow to the pelvic circulation by ligation of the internal iliac artery to control pelvic bleeding. Because many collateral vessels exist in the pelvic circulation, infarction is unusual after this procedure. Surgical exploration, however, is not always recommended. When the peritoneal space is entered, the tamponade is released and bleeding can increase. In addition, the extensive vascular sink makes identification of bleeding vessels difficult. Instead of surgical exploration, some patients undergo angiography and selective embolization of bleeding points with either an autologous blood clot or particulate gel foam.

Massive fluid resuscitation: Rapid fluid replacement with blood, colloids, or crystalloids. If >2 L of blood are required in the 8 h after the initial resuscitation, additional measures to manage bleeding are indicated. Current thinking in many institutions is to withhold aggressive fluid resuscitation until after operative repair, since an increase in MAP will increase intravascular hydrostatic pressure and may promote blood loss from torn vessels.

Pharmacotherapy

Antibiotics: Initially for prophylaxis with open fractures (controversial) and later if positive cultures of wounds, blood, or urine.

Analgesics: IV morphine sulfate usually relieves pain and can be readily reversed with naloxone if complications, such as hypotension or bradypnea, occur.

Vasopressors: For hypotension *only* after sufficient volume replacement has occurred (see Appendix 7).

Tetanus immunization: Booster is given if history is unknown or if a booster is needed (see Table 2-1).

NURSING DIAGNOSES AND INTERVENTIONS

Fluid volume deficit related to active blood loss secondary to injury to the pelvis and pelvic sink

Desired outcomes: Within 12 h after injury, patient's fluid status is adequate as evidenced by regular HR ≤100 bpm; bilaterally strong and equal peripheral pulses; warm and dry extremities; brisk (<2 sec) capillary refill; systolic BP ≥90 mm Hg (or within 10% of patient's normal range); and urine output ≥0.5 ml/kg/h. If hemodynamic monitoring is present, PAWP is ≥6 mm Hg and CI is ≥2.5 L/min/m². Patient is awake, alert, and oriented to time, place, and person without restlessness or confusion.

- Perform a complete assessment of fluid balance qh until patient is stable, noting all cardiac, hemodynamic, urinary, and CNS parameters. Consult physician for early signs of hemorrhage: decreased urinary output, delayed capillary refill, tachycardia, and changes in mental status.
- Prepare to move the patient to the operating room rapidly if necessary for repair of pelvic vasculature.
- Administer blood products, colloids, or crystalloids as prescribed through a large-bore peripheral IV or trauma catheter. Unless peripheral access is unavailable, avoid using standard central lines or triple-lumen catheters for fluid resuscitation inasmuch as their length and narrow gauge increase resistance to flow and slow fluid administration. Note that in many situations fluid resuscitation may occur only after surgical repair to reduce preoperative fluid loss from torn vessels.
- Use pressure infusers and rapid warmer/infusers for patients who require massive fluid/blood resuscitation. Be prepared to administer pressor agents only after fluid replacement is in progress. Vasopressors never should be

used to maintain BP in the patient without adequate fluid volume replacement.

- Place the patient flat until fluid volume status is stabilized if other injuries do not preclude position and if the patient has adequate airway and breathing in that position. Avoid Trendelenburg position because of the risk of aspiration, negative hemodynamic consequences, and decreased pulmonary excursion.

NIC Bleeding Reduction; Blood Products Administration; Shock Management: Volume; Fluid Management; Fluid/Electrolyte Management; Fluid Monitoring; Fluid Resuscitation; Electrolyte Monitoring; Hypothermia Treatment

Risk for infection related to inadequate primary defenses secondary to open pelvic fractures, percutaneous external fixation devices, or surgical procedure
Desired outcomes: Within 24 h after injury, soft tissues begin to heal without purulent drainage or erythema; WBC count is $\leq11,000/mm^3$; cultures of blood and wounds are negative; pin insertion site is free of erythema, edema, or purulent drainage; and surgical wounds are well approximated and without erythema, edema, or purulent drainage.

- For initial wound care, remove any gross contamination from the wound and cover any exposed soft tissue and bone with wet sterile dressings. Avoid dressings soaked in povidone-iodine to minimize iodine absorption and local tissue irritation. Prevent reentry of a portion of dirty bone or soft tissue into a wound. See "Infection Prevention and Control," Appendix 8, for indications for use of sterile gloves, mask, and eye protection when managing large wounds.
- Perform pin care as prescribed (e.g., q4-6h). Pin care is controversial and may include removing dried exudate to allow the pin holes to drain freely. In contrast, some experts believe that exudate is a part of the normal healing process and provides a tight interface between the skin and pin, thereby limiting bacterial invasion into the wounds. Unless contraindicated, wrap a loose, open-gauze dressing around the insertion site of the pin.
- Monitor all wounds, incisions, and pin insertion sites on external fixation devices q4h for presence of warmth, erythema, drainage, edema, or purulence. Monitor patient for temperature $\geq38.3°$ C ($101°$ F) and increased WBC count.

NIC Incision Site Care; Infection Protection; Wound Care; Traction/Immobilization Care; Infection Control; Surveillance

Impaired physical mobility related to pelvic immobilization secondary to pelvic ring instability
Desired outcomes: Immediately after pelvic immobilization, patient maintains appropriate body alignment; external fixation devices and traction remain in place. At the time of hospital discharge, patient exhibits full ROM in uninjured extremities.

- Position patient in proper body alignment.
- Apply compression boots if appropriate to limit the effects of venous stasis. Remove boots at least every shift to provide skin care. Consider using compression boots on upper extremities if appropriate to aid in venous return.
- Provide active and passive ROM to uninjured extremities every shift as appropriate.
- Maintain traction by keeping it free hanging. Do not remove weights even when repositioning.
- Use caution when turning and positioning to maintain body alignment. If patient has an unstable fracture that has not yet been reduced, consult orthopedic surgeon before moving patient. Some patients can be turned from side to side until internal fixation is accomplished. Also consult physician regarding the appropriate HOB elevation, and put this information on the patient's individual plan of care.
- Do not turn patient by holding on to the external fixation.
- Provide pain relief appropriate to level of activity.

NIC Exercise Therapy: Joint Mobility; Positioning; Traction/Immobilization Care; Bed Rest Care; Body Mechanics Promotion; Pain Management; Pressure Management

Impaired skin integrity related to initial injury, physical immobility, and placement of external fixation or pneumatic antishock garment (PASG) secondary to pelvic injury

Desired outcomes: Within 12 h of injury and throughout hospitalization, patient has timely wound healing. Patient does not develop pressure ulcers or experience tissue injury from the external fixation device.

- Cover the ends of all wires on the external fixation device with cork or gauze to protect the patient from injury.
- Apply padding to any traction slings.
- Apply alternating air mattress or other specialty mattress.
- If patient can be positioned laterally, pad the external fixation device to prevent damage to the patient's skin. Provide padding over bony prominences and any body area that comes in contact with a rigid surface.
- Keep all skin areas clean and dry to minimize the risk of pressure ulcers.
- If cast is used, inspect cast for signs of drainage or odor from wounds under cast; pad rough cast edges.

NIC Incision Site Care; Positioning; Pressure Management; Pressure Ulcer Prevention; Skin Surveillance; Traction/Immobilization Care; Wound Care; Cast Care: Maintenance

- See "Wound and Skin Care," p. 55, for more interventions.

> **Note:** Also see "Pain," p. 61, for management of discomfort.

Compartment syndrome (ischemic myositis)

PATHOPHYSIOLOGY

Compartment syndrome is defined as increased pressure within an anatomic compartment that compromises the circulation, viability, and function of tissues within the compartment. Failure to diagnose compartment syndrome is a frequent cause of litigation against the medical profession in North America. It is a surgical emergency that requires rapid intervention to prevent permanent cosmetic or functional deformity or loss of limb. Although compartment syndrome most commonly follows fractures, especially those of the tibia and fibula, it can occur from a variety of conditions (Table 2-12). Although compartment syndrome may be acute or chronic (exercise-related forms), this discussion focuses on acute forms.

As compartmental tissue pressure increases, it compromises capillary blood flow. Unremitting pressure results in tissue injury, which causes the release of histamine, producing vasodilation and increased capillary permeability. Dilated blood vessels and loss of fluids and proteins through the more permeable capillaries contribute to higher tissue pressures. These higher pressures eventually exceed capillary pressure and, ultimately, venous pressure, which in turn promotes further tissue ischemia. Tissue ischemia results in the release of additional histamine, which further exacerbates the problem. As a result of impaired venous return, anaerobic metabolism creates more lactic acid, which stimulates vasodilation, increases BP, and elevates tissue pressure even further. Finally, as compartmental pressure continues to increase, arteriolar spasm occurs from vascular compression, further contributing to lower capillary hydrostatic pressure. As this cycle continues, ischemic tissue begins to necrose, resulting in permanent tissue changes.

Sustained hypotension and shock have been associated with a greater incidence of compartment syndrome. As systemic BP decreases, the likelihood of tissue ischemia increases, because it then takes less compartmental pressure

TABLE 2-12 Causes of Compartment Syndrome			
Localized compartmental trauma	Tissue reaction/edema formation	Coagulation defects	Other
Fractures	Prolonged use of operative tourniquets	Hemophilia	Compression during obtundation (anesthesia, drug overdose)
Surgery		Anticoagulant therapy	
Hematoma			
Venomous bites (snake, spider)	Arterial or venous obstruction		Infiltrated IV therapy
Vascular injury	Limb reimplantation		Muscle hypertrophy (e.g., shin splints)
Postischemic swelling	Burns (especially when circumferential)		Constrictive dressings, inflatable splints or casts
Crush injuries	Excessive exercise (e.g., march gangrene)		Closure of fascial defects
Electrical injuries	Nephrotic syndrome		Hypothermia or hyperthermia
			Clostridium perfringens infections
			Rocky Mountain spotted fever
			Use of pneumatic antishock garment (PASG)

Modified from Callahan J: *Orthop Nurs* 4(4):11-15, 1985.

to result in arteriolar spasm. Therefore periods of hypotension may result in increased tissue injury at lower compartmental pressure, and persons in shock are more susceptible to compartment syndromes.

The average interval between the initial injury to the compartment and the beginning symptoms of compartment syndrome is 2 h. Compartmental tissue ischemia that lasts longer than 6 h results in tissue necrosis and irreversible tissue changes. Neurologic injury begins within 30 min of inadequate blood supply and may become functionally irreversible after 4 to 6 h.

Late-onset compartment syndrome can occur in patients who are comatose or confused and thus unable to identify symptoms such as pain. Late-onset compartment syndrome has also been associated with worsening compartment syndrome, even after treatment with fasciotomy. Late-onset compartment syndrome can occur in compartments that have already been treated with fasciotomy, since deceptively healthy granulation tissue may overlie necrotic muscle within incompletely opened compartments. With sufficient muscle tissue injury, for example, especially after crush injuries, rhabdomyolysis can develop and result in secondary myoglobinemia that leads to acute tubular necrosis (ATN), which may progress to acute renal failure (ARF).

ASSESSMENT

History and risk factors: Any patient with a peripheral injury listed in Table 2-11 is at risk. Patients admitted for acute renal failure after treatment for crush injuries or compartment syndrome should be suspected of having late-onset or continuing compartment syndrome.

Clinical presentation

Early indicators: Pain out of proportion to the injury is the cardinal symptom. Passive motion of the involved muscle group (via passive extension of the digits) significantly increases the pain. Palpation of the compartment reveals a tense compartment and slowed capillary refill. Tissue pressures vary with the method of measurement; in general, normal tissue pressures vary from 0-10 mm Hg and sustained pressures >30 mm Hg result in tissue necrosis. Pressures >16 mm Hg are sufficient to collapse thin-walled lower extremity veins, further contributing to the pathogenesis.

Late indicators: With late-onset compartment syndrome, persistent peripheral edema or continued elevation of tissue pressures may be present, even after fasciotomy.

If compartment syndrome is left untreated, the necrosed muscle becomes fibrosed and contracted, resulting in a functionally useless compartment (e.g., Volkmann ischemic contracture), which drastically impairs function of the involved limb. The importance of early recognition and treatment of compartment syndrome is reinforced by the fact that decompression fasciotomy seldom restores lost myoneural function.

Physical assessment

Muscle involvement: Inability to control pain with usual amounts of opiates in any patient at risk for compartment syndrome requires closer evaluation. Pain on passive extension or flexion of the digits is an early finding indicative of muscle tissue involvement.

Neurovascular involvement: Increasing extremity circumference, decrease in or loss of two-point discrimination, sluggish capillary refill, and tautness and tenderness over tissue compartments are signs of early neurovascular involvement. Eventually, all neurovascular structures traversing the involved compartment will show deficit. *Late findings* include the *six P's: p*ain (increased with pressure applied over the compartment and passive movement of the digits), *p*allor, *p*olar (coolness), *p*ulselessness, *p*aresthesia, and *p*aralysis.

DIAGNOSTIC TESTS

Blood chemistries: Creatine phosphokinase (CPK) is released by injured muscle tissue and elevates with muscle necrosis; continued elevation in the presence of treatment may indicate late-onset compartment syndrome. Extensive muscle necrosis may lead to myoglobinemia and myoglobinuria. BUN and creatinine levels will be elevated if acute renal failure ensues.

Intracompartmental pressure monitoring: Although simple needle manometers may be used to measure compartment tissue pressures, they are subject to obstruction from muscle tissue and are inappropriate for continuous monitoring. Wick or slit catheters allow continuous pressure monitoring via fluid-filled catheters and pressure monitors. Pressures that indicate the need for fasciotomy vary with clinical indicators, the patient's systemic condition, and the measurement technique. Methods of measuring compartment pressure and associated critical values include *needle* (pressure within 10-30 mm Hg of diastolic BP), *continuous infusion* (pressure >45 mm Hg), and *wick* or *slit catheter* (>30-35 mm Hg). In the presence of factors favorable to the development of compartment syndrome (see Table 2-11) and low systemic BP, the delta pressure should be determined (delta pressure equals mean arterial pressure minus compartmental pressure). Delta pressures of ≤30 mm Hg for 6 h or ≤40 for 8 h require prompt consultation with the physician.

Research Brief 2-5 Recent research by McQueen and Court-Brown suggests that a delta pressure of 30 mm Hg should be used as the definitive assessment of the need for fasciotomy. The authors conclude that the absolute tissue pressures, e.g. the pressure within the compartment alone, is not sufficient to predict the need for fasciotomy.

From McQueen MM, Court-Brown CM: Compartment monitoring in tibial fractures, *J Bone Joint Surg Br* 78-B(1):99-104, 1996.

Arteriograms and venograms: Radiologic examination of blood vessels may be performed when embolus, thrombus, or other vascular injury is suspected.

Transcutaneous Doppler venous flow and/or duplex imaging: Enable noninvasive determination of impaired venous flow as an adjunct to the clinical signs for diagnosing compartment syndrome.

MRI spectroscopy: May be used to determine presence of muscle ischemia.

Pulse oximetry: May be used to assess perfusion of distal tissues. Readings should be compared with readings from a contralateral, uninvolved extremity.

COLLABORATIVE MANAGEMENT

Release of external pressure: Loosening or removing circumferential casts and padding or dressings; escharotomy for circumferential burns or frostbite.

Analgesia: Parenteral opiates often with sedative adjuncts (e.g., hydroxyzine HCl, promethazine HCl).

Ice and extremity elevation: Recommended with fractures to promote vasoconstriction when there is no evidence of impaired microcirculation (i.e., decreased capillary refill, pallor, pulselessness, or coolness of the extremity). Once microcirculation has been impaired, however, use of ice and extremity elevation is *contraindicated* inasmuch as further impairment of circulation is likely to result.

Intravenous hypertonic mannitol: May be used as a preliminary measure. It reduces compartmental pressure via systemic diuresis.

Fasciotomy of myofascial compartment: Imperative for strongly suspected compartment syndrome to permit unrestricted swelling. After a few days, the fasciotomy is closed primarily; skin grafting may be needed to ensure complete coverage of the exposed compartments. The compartment with identified increased tissue pressure may be opened singularly or, more commonly, adjacent or all tissue compartments in the area are incised prophylactically. Persistent peripheral edema and elevated CPK or the presence of ARF may justify reexploration and wide excision of all necrotic muscle in involved and adjacent compartments.

After 7-10 days, the fasciotomy wound may be closed primarily; skin grafting is commonly needed to ensure complete coverage of the exposed compartments. In an attempt to reduce the need for another surgery, some surgeons advocate alternative wound closure methods. Delayed wound closure may involve use of several buttons sutured on either side of the wound and held together under tension with rubber bands to slowly pull wound edges together. Another method involves use of adhesive strips on either side of the wound as a base to place adhesive strips applied with tension across the wound (similar to the butterfly dressing used in first aid) as a means of drawing the wound edges together over time.

Complications of fasciotomy include wound infection, the potential for osteomyelitis, and large scars.

Compartment syndrome caused by vascular injury: Requires exploration of the involved vessel to facilitate application of papaverine (i.e., a smooth muscle relaxant that causes local vasodilation), injection of a bolus of fluid to regain normal internal artery dynamics, and repair of lacerations or resection of involved vessels.

NURSING DIAGNOSES AND INTERVENTIONS

Altered tissue perfusion (or risk for same): peripheral (compartment), related to interruption of capillary blood flow secondary to increased pressure within the anatomic compartment

Desired outcomes: Throughout duration of the hospitalization, patient has adequate perfusion to compartment tissues as evidenced by brisk (<2 sec) capillary refill; peripheral pulses >2+ on a 0-4+ scale; normal tissue pressures (0-10 mm Hg); and absence of edema, tautness, and the six P's for the involved compartment. Within 2 h of admission, patient verbalizes understanding of the importance of reporting symptoms indicative of impaired neurovascular status.

- Monitor neurovascular status of injured extremity with each VS check (at least q2h). Assess for increased pain on passive extension or flexion of the digits. Monitor for sluggish capillary refill, decrease in or loss of two-point discrimination, increasing limb edema, and tautness over individual compartments. Use pulse oximetry to assess distal tissue perfusion, and report significant differences from oximetry readings taken from the uninvolved contralateral extremity. Also assess for the six P's: *p*ain (especially on passive digital movement and with pressure over the compartment), *p*allor, *p*olar (coolness), *p*ulselessness, *p*aresthesia, and *p*aralysis.
- Report deficits in neurovascular status promptly. Loosen circumferential dressings as indicated. Apply ice when appropriate (see p. 164).
- Teach patient the symptoms that necessitate prompt reporting: increasing pain, paresthesia (diminished sensation, hyperesthesia, or anesthesia), paralysis, coolness, sluggish capillary refill, or pulselessness.
- Monitor tissue pressures on a continuous basis if an intracompartmental pressure device is present. Consult physician if pressures exceed normal or preestablished levels. Be aware that pressures >10 mm Hg may be significantly elevated above normal.
- Be alert to increased susceptibility to tissue injury with slightly increased compartmental tissue pressures in hypotensive states.

NIC Cast care: Maintenance; Circulatory Precautions; Heat/Cold Application; Peripheral Sensation Management; Shock Management; Skin Surveillance; Teaching: Disease Process

Pain related to physical factors (tissue ischemia) secondary to compartment syndrome

Desired outcomes: Throughout duration of the hospitalization, patient's subjective evaluation of discomfort improves as documented by a pain scale. Nonverbal indicators of discomfort, such as grimacing, are absent or diminished. Within 2 h of admission, patient verbalizes understanding of the need to report uncontrolled or increasing pain.

- Assess the patient's complaints of pain for onset, duration, progression, and intensity. Devise a pain scale with patient, rating discomfort "0" for no pain to "10" for unbearable. Patients with impaired ability to communicate may require a visual scale.
- Determine if passive stretching of digits and pressure over limb compartments increase the pain, inasmuch as both are likely to occur with compartment syndrome.
- Adjust the medication regimen to the patient's needs; document medication effectiveness. Promptly report uncontrolled pain.
- Prevent pressure on involved compartment and neurovascular structures.
- If patient has had a fasciotomy, be aware that if the pain does not subside after this procedure, it could indicate an incomplete fasciotomy. Pain that increases several days after a fasciotomy may signal compartmental infection.

- Continue to monitor neurovascular function with each VS check to assess for recurring compartment syndrome or infection.

█NIC Analgesic Administration; Anxiety Reduction; Coping Enhancement; Pain Management; Progressive Muscle Relaxation; Simple Guided Imagery

Risk for infection related to inadequate primary defenses secondary to necrotic tissue, wide compartmental fasciotomy, and open wound

Desired outcomes: Throughout duration of the hospitalization, patient is free of infection as evidenced by normothermia; WBC count ≤11,000/mm^3; erythrocyte sedimentation rate (ESR) ≤20 mm/h (women) or ≤15 mm/h (men); and absence of wound erythema and other clinical indicators of infection. Within 24 h of admission, patient verbalizes understanding of the need to report promptly any indicators of infection.

- Monitor patient for fever, increasing pain, and laboratory data indicative of infection (e.g., increased WBC count, increased ESR).
- Assess exposed wounds and dressings for erythema, increasing wound drainage, purulent wound drainage, increasing wound circumference, edema, and localized tenderness.
- Assess neurovascular structures for deficit, which can signal infection or pressure from adjacent inflamed tissues.
- After primary closure or grafting of wound, continue to assess wound for signs of infection.
- Be aware of and assess for chronic infection and osteomyelitis as potential complications after compartment syndrome.
- Caution patient about the need to report the following indicators of infection: fever, localized warmth, increasing pain, increasing wound drainage (especially if purulent), swelling, and redness.
- Consult with physician promptly regarding significant findings.

█NIC Environmental Management; Infection Protection; Medication Management; Surveillance; Vital Signs Monitoring; Wound Care; Wound Care: Closed Drainage

Body image disturbance related to physical changes secondary to large, irregular fasciotomy wound and skin-grafted scar; loss of function and cosmesis of an extremity; amputation

Desired outcomes: Within the 24-h period before discharge from ICU, patient acknowledges body changes and demonstrates movement toward incorporating changes into self-concept. Patient does not exhibit maladaptive response (e.g., severe depression) to wound or functional loss.

- Encourage questions about compartment syndrome, therapeutic interventions, and long-term effects.
- Provide time for verbalization of feelings regarding change in appearance and function. Encourage discussion of these feelings with patient's significant others.
- Identify and emphasize patient's strengths to facilitate adaptation to cosmetic and functional loss. Help patient set realistic goals for recovery.
- Facilitate patient's progression through the grieving process, as appropriate.
- Recognize individuality in adjustment; enable patient to determine when to view or discuss the injury.
- If the extremity will be amputated (and it is feasible within the time frame), collaborate with physician regarding visit by an amputee who has successfully adapted and who can serve as patient's role model.
- Begin to encourage maximal self-care. Provide necessary adjunctive aids (e.g., built-up utensils, button hooks, orthotics) to facilitate independence.
- For patients with functional loss or amputation, introduce the ability for compensation via use of orthotics and adjunctive devices to facilitate self-care.

█NIC Active Listening; Amputation Care; Anxiety Reduction; Body Image Enhancement; Coping Enhancement; Emotional Support; Self-Care Assistance; Wound Care

Acute spinal cord injury

PATHOPHYSIOLOGY

A spinal cord injury (SCI) results from concussion, contusion, laceration, transection, hemorrhage, or impairment of blood supply to the spinal cord. This trauma to the spinal cord may be secondarily increased by the ischemia and subsequent edema. Most often (47%), SCI is caused by a vehicular collision, a fall, an act of violence, or a sports-related incident. Of those affected, 75%-82% are males between the ages of 15 and 35 years. Approximately 10,000 new SCIs occur per year; half of these are complete injuries of the spinal cord with loss of voluntary motor and sensory function below the level of the lesion. Approximately two thirds of these have injuries to the cervical area of the spinal cord. Although life expectancy is good after injury, morbidity and mortality most often are the result of infection. Pulmonary complications (atelectasis, pneumonia), renal complications (infection, calculi, urosepsis), and pulmonary disease account for 30%-40% of all deaths. A higher incidence of left lower lobe pneumonia and atelectasis is associated with high-level injuries, possibly because of changes in respiratory patterns, ineffective cough, positioning problems, and the anatomy of the left mainstem bronchus, which branches at an oblique angle, making it more difficult to access for suctioning.

SCI is classified in several ways according to: *type and cause,* such as open (gunshot, stab wound) or closed (motor vehicle collision, fall, sports-related incident); *site* (level of the spinal cord involved); *mechanism,* such as flexion (e.g., occurring as a result of sudden deceleration in a head-on collision, backward fall down a flight of stairs, diving into a swimming pool) or extension (e.g., whiplash or fall involving hyperextension of the neck); *stability* (integrity of the supporting structures such as ligaments or bony facets); and whether the injury is *complete* or *incomplete* ("complete" meaning the absence of all voluntary motor, sensory, and vasomotor function below the level of injury, and "incomplete" meaning the presence of some percentage of voluntary motor or sensory function below the level of injury).

Fractures involving the vertebral bodies: These fractures may or may not cause SCI. Conversely, severe SCI can occur without evidence of damage to the vertebrae. With more severe fractures, such as the "burst" fracture (fragmentation of a vertebral body with penetration of the spinal cord), paralysis almost always occurs. Penetration of the spinal cord with bony fragments may cause hemorrhage, infection, and leakage of CSF.

Spinal shock: Immediately after SCI, most patients experience a period of spinal shock, which is the loss of all reflex activity below the level of injury. It may last minutes or be prolonged for days or weeks. Generally, the duration is 1-6 wk, although periods of 6 mo to 1 yr have been reported. Generally, the more quickly the individual shows signs of return to function, the better the prognosis.

Neurogenic shock: Patients with injuries to the upper thoracic and cervical regions may experience cardiovascular instability because of interruption of the descending sympathetic pathways. This interruption results in loss of vasomotor tone and sympathetic innervation to the heart. The loss of sympathetic innervation causes venous pooling in the extremities and splanchnic vasculature, which decreases venous return to the heart, resulting in low cardiac output and low tissue perfusion pressure. This causes bradycardia and hypotension.

ASSESSMENT

Clinical presentation

Spinal shock: Flaccid paralysis of all skeletal muscles; absence of deep tendon reflexes (DTRs), cutaneous sensation, proprioception (position sense), visceral and somatic sensation, and penile reflex; urinary and fecal retention; anhidrosis (absence of sweating).

Neurogenic shock: Vasodilation, bradycardia, hypotension.

> **Note:** Although spinal shock is seen in SCIs at *any* level, the loss of central control of peripheral vascular tone (neurogenic shock) occurs most dramatically in high cervical spine injuries, with interruption of the sympathetic nervous system. Profound bradycardia and hypotension are possible. With spinal cord injuries lower than the midthoracic area, the patient will experience a phase of neurogenic shock, with loss of sympathetic innervation to vasculature below the level of the lesion; however, the effects of that loss are not as dramatic.

Recovery phase of spinal shock: As spinal shock subsides, the patient may experience the following: (1) flexor spasms evoked by cutaneous stimulation, (2) reflex emptying of the bowel and bladder, (3) extensor or flexor rigidity, (4) hyperreflexic DTRs, and (5) reflex priapism or ejaculation in the male, evoked by cutaneous stimulation.

Levels of cord injury

C4 AND ABOVE: Loss of all muscle function, including muscles of respiration. With complete cord transection the patient will die, probably at the scene of the injury, unless immediate ventilation is initiated.

C4-C5: Same as preceding but with possible sparing of the phrenic nerve. This means that the patient probably will require assisted ventilation because of weak or absent intercostal muscle function. Patient will be tetraplegic/quadriplegic.

C6-C8: Quadriplegia will occur, but patient will retain function of diaphragm and accessory muscles of respiration and may have some movement of neck, shoulders, chest, and upper portion of arms.

T1-T3: Will have neck, shoulder, chest, arm, hand, and respiratory function; will experience difficulty maintaining a sitting position.

T4-T10: Same as preceding but with more stability of trunk muscles. The lower the lesion, the greater the independence. The patient will be paraplegic.

> **Note:** Of persons with lesions at or above T6 (tetraplegics/quadriplegics/high paraplegics), 80% will have episodes of autonomic dysreflexia (AD). See discussion that follows.

T11-L2: Will have use of upper extremities, neck, and shoulders. Chest and trunk muscles will provide stability, and patient will have some muscle function of upper portion of thigh. At this level there may be loss of voluntary bowel and bladder control, but the patient will have reflex emptying of the bowel. Men may experience difficulty achieving and maintaining an erection and may have decreased seminal emission.

L3-S1: Will have muscle function of all muscle groups in the upper portion of the body and most of the muscle function in the lower extremities. Voluntary bowel and bladder function will be lost, with reflex emptying. Men may experience decreased ability or lack of ability to have an erection, with decreased seminal emission.

S2-S4: Will have function of all muscle groups but may have some lower extremity weakness. There may be flaccidity of bowel and bladder, as well as loss of the ability to have a reflex erection.

Cord syndromes

Anterior cord syndrome: This syndrome involves injury to the anterior portion of the spinal cord supplied by the anterior spinal artery and may be associated with acute traumatic herniation of an intervertebral disk. High-dose methylprednisolone is used in the acute phase, with surgical decompression as necessary. The prognosis varies with each patient and depends on the degree of structural damage and edema.

- *Clinical presentation:* Varying degrees of paralysis occur below the level of the injury, along with diminution of pain and temperature sensations. Patient will retain senses of touch, position, and vibration.

Central cord syndrome: Generally seen with hyperextension injuries or interruption of blood supply to the cervical spinal cord. Usually it is seen in older adults, with some evidence of vertebral injury noted on radiography. In this syndrome, motor and sensory deficits are less severe in the lower extremities than in the upper extremities because of the central arrangement of cervical fibers in the spinal cord. Incomplete injuries carry a relatively good prognosis. Steroids are used to decrease edema. Many patients can ambulate with an assistive device and may regain bowel and bladder function. Regaining useful function in the hands carries a less favorable prognosis.

  • *Clinical presentation:* Motor and sensory deficits usually are severe in the upper extremities and profound in the hands and fingers. With sparing of sacral and some lumbar fibers there will be some motor and sensory function in the perineum, genitalia, and lower extremities.

Lateral cord (Brown-Séquard) syndrome: Results from a horizontal hemisection of the spinal cord (e.g., from a gunshot or stab wound). Patients usually have bilateral motor and sensory impairment, with a relative difference in function from one side to the other. High-dose methylprednisolone is used for the acute phase, with treatment of fracture-dislocation as needed. Prognosis usually is good for recovery of upper and lower extremity function.

  • *Clinical presentation:* Ipsilateral weakness and decrease in light touch, vibratory, and position senses, with contralateral hypalgesia. Usually there are bilateral motor and sensory deficits, but motor activity will be better on one side and sensory activity will be better on the other.

Autonomic dysreflexia (AD): Life-threatening response of the autonomic nervous system to a stimulus, creating an exaggerated sympathetic nervous system response. This response can occur during the acute phase of SCI, or it may not appear until several years after injury. It affects individuals with lesions at or above T6. If AD is not identified promptly, treated, and reversed, the potential consequences include seizures, subarachnoid hemorrhage, fatal cerebrovascular accident, and myocardial infarction.

  • *Causes:* Stimuli to the *bladder* (most common), such as distention, infection, calculi, cystoscopy; *bowel,* such as fecal impaction, rectal examination, suppository insertion; or *skin,* such as tight clothing or sheets, temperature extremes, sores, or areas of broken skin.

  • *Clinical presentation:* Classic triad includes a throbbing headache, cutaneous vasodilation, and sweating, which occur above the level of the lesion. The patient also may exhibit the following: hypertension (BP >250-300/150 mm Hg), nasal congestion, flushed skin (above the level of the lesion), blurred vision, nausea, bradycardia, and chest pain. Below the level of the lesion there will be pilomotor erection (goose bumps), pallor, chills, and vasoconstriction.

DIAGNOSTIC TESTS

Spinal x-rays: AP and lateral films are obtained to detect fractures or dislocations of vertebral bodies, narrowing of the spinal canal, and hematomas. Additional views (odontoid [open-mouth], bilateral oblique, flexion-extension) or tomograms may be necessary to view some levels of the spinal cord, particularly in obese and heavily muscled patients.

> *Caution:* This stage in the evaluation of the patient with a possible SCI is extremely dangerous, because any sudden or incorrect movement of the injured area could cause further trauma to the spinal cord.

COLLABORATIVE MANAGEMENT

Immobilization of the injured site: With or without surgical intervention.
Cervical spine injury: Cervical traction to immobilize and reduce the fracture or dislocation is most often achieved through the use of a halo system. Traction

may also be achieved via Vinke, Gardner-Wells, or Crutchfield tongs, which are inserted through the outer table of the skull. These tongs are attached to ropes and pulleys with weights to achieve bony reduction and proper alignment. The patient may be placed on a special frame or bed (e.g., RotoRest® kinetic treatment table). The use of the halo device and a plaster or fiberglass jacket for skeletal fixation of the head and neck allows for earlier mobilization and rehabilitation.

Surgical intervention during the immediate postinjury phase is controversial. Surgery may be performed if (1) the neurologic deficit is progressing, (2) there are compound fractures, (3) the injury involves a penetrating wound of the spine, (4) there are bone fragments in the spinal canal, or (5) there is acute anterior spinal cord trauma. Surgeries may include decompression laminectomy, closed or open reduction of the fracture, or spinal fusion for stabilization.
Thoracic and lumbar spine injuries: May require surgical stabilization with laminectomy with or without fusion and insertion of Harrington or Cotrel-Dubousset (CD) rods. If the injury is stable, it may be treated with closed reduction. Some patients with lumbar spine injury may be immobilized with a halo device with femoral distraction. This device may be connected to traction with weights for reduction and stabilization before surgery.
Respiratory management: The need for assisted ventilation is based on level of injury, ABG values, and the results of pulmonary function tests, pulmonary fluoroscopy, and physical assessment data. In addition, the need for ventilatory assistance is considered likely with injuries at C4 and above, patients older than 40 yr, smokers, associated chest trauma, and immersion injuries. Initially, the patient may require intubation, and later, tracheotomy. Persons with high cervical injury who survive the initial injury but have paralysis of the muscles of respiration may require permanent tracheostomy with mechanical ventilation.
Aggressive pulmonary care: To prevent, detect, and treat atelectasis, pulmonary infection, and respiratory failure inasmuch as pulmonary problems are a major source of morbidity and mortality in the patient with SCI. Chest physiotherapy, intubation, and ventilation are instituted as indicated.
Fluid management: In patients with neurogenic shock, blood volume is normal but the vascular space is enlarged, causing peripheral pooling, decreased venous return, and decreased cardiac output. Careful fluid repletion, usually with crystalloids, is indicated. Pressor therapy is initiated for patients unresponsive to fluid volume replacement (see discussion under "Pharmacotherapy," below). For fluid management in patients with multisystem trauma, see "Major Trauma," p. 106.
Gastric tube placement: To decompress the stomach, prevent aspiration of gastric contents, and decrease the risk of paralytic ileus (often seen within 72 h of injury in patients with lesions higher than T6).
Urinary catheterization: Insertion of an indwelling or intermittent catheter to decompress an atonic bladder in the immediate postinjury phase (spinal shock). With the return of the reflex arc after spinal shock subsides, a reflex neurogenic bladder that fills and empties automatically will develop in patients with lesions above T12. Patients with lesions at or below T12 generally will have an atonic, areflexic neurogenic bladder that overfills, distending the bladder and causing overflow incontinence. Intermittent catheterization may be necessary.
Pharmacotherapy
Methylprednisolone: Because neuromembranes are 40% fat (compared with 5%-10% fat for other body cell membranes), administration of this adrenal steroid within 8 h of injury inhibits lipid peroxidation, which in turn protects the neuromembrane from further destruction. In addition, it improves blood flow to the injury site, facilitating tissue repair. A loading dose (30 mg/kg) is administered by IV bolus over a 15-min period. After a 45-min wait, 5.4 mg/kg/h is then administered in a continuous IV infusion over a 23-h period

and then stopped. If the infusion is interrupted for any reason, it must be recalibrated so that the entire dose can be completed within the original 23 h.

Antacids (e.g., Maalox):   To prevent gastric ulceration, which may occur post-SCI because of hyperacidity of gastric secretions and increased production of gastric acid. The risk of ulceration with hemorrhage is further increased if steroids are used. Maintain gastric pH >5.0 by using Maalox 30 ml q3h.

Histamine H₂-receptor antagonists (e.g., cimetidine, ranitidine):   To suppress secretion of gastric acid and to prevent or treat ulcers in the patient with increased production of gastric acid and an increased susceptibility to gastric ulceration and perforation.

Stool softeners (e.g., docusate sodium):   To begin bowel retraining program and prevent fecal impaction with distention of the bowel, which could stimulate an episode of AD.

Hyperosmolar laxatives (e.g., glycerin suppository):   To prevent fecal impaction and facilitate movement of the bowels on a regular basis (part of a bowel program).

Irritant or stimulant laxatives (e.g., bisacodyl):   To stimulate bowel movements as part of a bowel training program.

Analgesics (e.g., acetaminophen or acetaminophen with codeine):   To decrease pain associated with the injury or surgery.

Sedatives: To decrease anxiety caused by the injury, hospitalization, or fear of the prognosis.

Antihypertensives (e.g., hydralazine hydrochloride, methyldopa, nitroprusside sodium):   To treat the severe hypertension that occurs in AD.

Vasopressors (e.g., epinephrine):   To treat the hypotension that may occur in the immediate postinjury stage because of loss of vasomotor control below the level of injury, with resultant vasodilation and a relative hypovolemia (see Appendix 7).

> **Note:**   Orthostatic hypotension may become a permanent problem, especially in patients with cervical and high thoracic injuries. Caregivers must be taught to move the patient slowly into the upright position to avoid a sudden drop in BP, which can cause cerebral hypoxia and loss of consciousness. Abdominal binders and Ace bandages or thigh-high antiembolic stockings also may aid in preventing orthostatic hypotension.

Bronchodilators (theophylline):   To dilate bronchioles and facilitate removal of secretions. Early use of theophylline is recommended in patients with a history of COPD, smoking, and evidence of difficulty moving secretions. Some research indicates that theophylline may increase diaphragmatic contractility and reduce respiratory fatigue.

Mucolytic agents (guaifenesin, acetylcysteine):   To reduce tenacity and viscosity of purulent and nonpurulent secretions.

Antibiotics: To prevent or treat respiratory infection or UTI.

Anticoagulants (heparin or low-molecular-weight heparins such as enoxaparin [Lovenox]):   To prevent thrombophlebitis, deep vein thrombosis, and pulmonary emboli.

> **Note:**   Patients with SCI are at high risk for development of vascular complications because they are immobilized, have lost vasoconstrictive capabilities below the level of injury, and cannot constrict the muscles in the lower extremities to facilitate venous flow. Patients who are not candidates for anticoagulation may have an inferior vena cava umbrella or Greenfield filter inserted to trap emboli traveling from the lower extremities to the lungs.

NURSING DIAGNOSES AND INTERVENTIONS

Impaired gas exchange related to altered oxygen supply associated with hypoventilation secondary to paresis or paralysis of the muscles of respiration (diaphragm, intercostals) occurring with high cervical spine injury or ascending cord edema

Desired outcomes: Within 24 h of this diagnosis and throughout remaining hospitalization, patient has adequate gas exchange as evidenced by orientation to time, place, and person; Pao_2 ≥80 mm Hg; and $Paco_2$ ≤45 mm Hg. RR is 12-20 breaths/min with normal depth and pattern (eupnea), HR is 60-100 bpm, BP is stable and within patient's normal range, and vital capacity is ≥1 L. Motor and sensory losses remain at the same spinal cord level as the initial findings.

> **Note:**   Patients with cervical injuries usually arrive in the ICU already intubated. However, with some high thoracic or low cervical lesions, patients who ventilate independently in the emergency department may arrive in the ICU without assisted ventilation. Such a patient is at risk for an increasingly higher level of cord damage because of hemorrhage and edema, which can result in a higher level of dysfunction and a change in respiratory status that requires assisted ventilation.

- Assess for signs of respiratory dysfunction: shallow, slow, or rapid respirations; vital capacity <1 L; changes in sensorium; anxiety; restlessness; tachycardia; pallor; and inability to move secretions.
- Monitor ABG studies; report abnormalities. Be particularly alert to Pao_2 <60 mm Hg, $Paco_2$ >50 mm Hg, and decreasing pH, inasmuch as these findings indicate the need for assisted ventilation, possibly caused by atelectasis, pneumonia, or respiratory fatigue.
- Monitor vital capacity at least q8h. If it is <1 L, Pao_2/PAo_2 ratio is ≤0.75, or copious secretions are present, intubation is recommended.
- Monitor chest x-rays, and consult physician for abnormalities.
- Monitor patient for evidence of ascending cord edema: increasing difficulty with swallowing secretions or coughing, presence of respiratory stridor with retraction of accessory muscles of respiration, bradycardia, fluctuating BP, and increased motor and sensory loss at a higher level than the initial findings.
- Before attempting oral intubation with neck flexion, ensure that cervical x-rays have confirmed the absence of cervical involvement. If patient exhibits evidence of respiratory distress and cervical involvement has not been ruled out, do not hyperextend the neck for resuscitation; instead, use either nasal intubation or orotracheal intubation with manual cervical spine immobilization.
- If patient has undergone immobilization via placement of cranial tongs or traction with a halo apparatus, monitor patient's respiratory status q1-2h for the first 24-48 h and then q4h if patient's condition is stable. Be alert to absent or adventitious breath sounds, and inspect chest movement to ensure that the plaster or fiberglass vest is not restricting diaphragmatic movement.
- If intubation via endotracheal (ET) tube or tracheostomy becomes necessary, explain the procedure to patient and significant others.
- See "Mechanical Ventilation," p. 17, for interventions related to mechanical ventilation.

NIC Airway Management; Oxygen Therapy; Respiratory Monitoring; Mechanical Ventilation

Ineffective airway clearance (or risk for same) related to decreased or absent cough reflex secondary to cervical or high thoracic spine injury

Desired outcome: Within 24-48 h of this diagnosis, patient has a clear airway as evidenced by absence of adventitious breath sounds.

- Monitor patient's respiratory status, and be alert to the following indicators of ineffective airway clearance: adventitious breath sounds (i.e., crackles, rhonchi), decreased or absent breath sounds (bronchial, bronchovesicular, vesicular), increased HR (>100 bpm) and BP (>10 mm Hg over patient's normal), decreased tidal volume (<75%-85% of predicted value) or vital capacity (<1 L), shallow or rapid respirations (>20 breaths/min), pallor, cyanosis, increased restlessness, and anxiety.

- Monitor and report abnormal ABG values (i.e., decreased Pao_2 or increased $Paco_2$) and chest x-ray results.
- Suction secretions as needed, according to auscultation findings. Always hyperoxygenate before suctioning.

Note: Be alert for bradycardia associated with tracheal suctioning. Some authorities suggest giving atropine before suctioning.

- If indicated by the assessment findings, prepare patient for intubation or tracheostomy with mechanical ventilation. See "Mechanical Ventilation," p. 17, for more information.
- If patient does not require intubation with mechanical ventilation, implement the following measures to improve airway clearance:
  ☐ Place patient in semi-Fowler's position unless it is contraindicated (e.g., patient is in cervical tongs with traction).
  ☐ Turn patient from side to side at least q2h to help mobilize secretions.
  ☐ Keep room humidified to help loosen secretions.
  ☐ Unless contraindicated, keep patient hydrated with at least 2-3 L fluid/day.
  ☐ If patient has respiratory muscle control, teach coughing and deep-breathing exercises, which should be performed at least q2h.
  ☐ If patient's cough is ineffective, implement the following method, known as *quad coughing:* Place palm of hand under patient's diaphragm, and push up on the abdominal muscles as patient exhales.

Note: Be aware that using the *quad cough* maneuver in patients with intracaval filters to prevent pulmonary emboli has been reported to have significant complications, including bowel perforation and filter migration and deformation.

NIC Airway Management; Cough Enhancement; Respiratory Monitoring
Dysreflexia (AD) (or risk for same) related to abnormal response of the autonomic nervous system to a stimulus
Desired outcomes: Patient has no symptoms of AD as evidenced by dry skin above the level of injury; BP within patient's normal range; HR ≥60 bpm; and absence of headache and other clinical indicators of AD. ECG demonstrates normal sinus rhythm.

- Assess for the classic triad of AD: throbbing headache, cutaneous vasodilation, and sweating above the level of injury. In addition, extremely elevated BP (e.g., ≥250-300/150 mm Hg), nasal stuffiness, flushed skin (above the level of the injury), blurred vision, nausea, bradycardia, and chest pain can occur. Be alert to the following signs of AD that occur below the level of injury: pilomotor erection, pallor, chills, and vasoconstriction.
- Assess for cardiac dysrhythmias, optimally via cardiac monitor during initial postinjury stage (2 wk).
- Be aware of and implement measures to prevent factors that may precipitate AD: *bladder stimuli* (i.e., distention, calculi, infection, cystoscopy); *bowel stimuli* (i.e., fecal impaction, rectal examination, suppository insertion); *skin stimuli* (i.e., pressure from tight clothing or sheets, temperature extremes, sores, areas of broken skin).
- If indicators of AD are present, implement the following measures:
  ☐ Elevate HOB, or place patient in a sitting position. This will decrease BP by promoting cerebral venous return.
  ☐ Monitor BP and HR q3-5min until patient stabilizes.

☐ Determine and remove offending stimulus. If, for example, the patient's bladder is distended, catheterize cautiously, using a sufficient amount of a lubricant that contains a local anesthetic. If patient has an indwelling urinary catheter, check for obstruction, such as granulation in catheter or kinking of tubing; as indicated, irrigate catheter, using no more than 30 ml normal saline. If UTI is suspected, obtain a urine specimen for culture and sensitivity once the crisis stage has passed. Check for fecal impaction; perform the rectal examination gently, using an ointment containing a local anesthetic (e.g., Nupercainal). Check for sensory stimuli, and loosen clothing, bed covers, or other constricting fabric as indicated.

- Consult physician for severe or prolonged hypertension or other symptoms that do not abate. Severe or prolonged elevations of BP may result in life-threatening consequences: seizures, subarachnoid or intracerebral hemorrhage, fatal cerebrovascular accident.
- As prescribed, administer antihypertensive agent and monitor its effectiveness.
- Remain calm and supportive of patient and significant others during these episodes.
- Upon resolution of the immediate crisis, answer patient's and significant others' questions regarding cause of the AD. Provide patient and family teaching regarding signs and symptoms and methods of treatment of AD. This is particularly critical for the patient with SCI who has sustained injury above T6, because these patients are at risk for AD for life.

NIC Dysreflexia Management

Decreased cardiac output related to relative hypovolemia secondary to enlarged vascular space occurring with neurogenic shock

Desired outcome: Within 24 h of this diagnosis, patient has adequate cardiac output as evidenced by orientation to time, place, and person; systolic BP ≥90 mm Hg (or within patient's normal range); HR 60-100 bpm; RAP 4-6 mm Hg; PAP 20-30/8-15 mm Hg; PAWP 6-12 mm Hg; SVR 900-1200 dynes/sec/cm^{-5}; normal amplitude of peripheral pulses (>2+ on a 0-4+ scale); urinary output ≥0.5 ml/kg/h; and normal sinus rhythm on ECG.

- Monitor patient for indicators of decreased cardiac output: drop in systolic BP >20 mm Hg, systolic BP <90 mm Hg, or a continuous drop of 5-10 mm Hg with each assessment; HR >100 bpm, irregular HR, lightheadedness, fainting, confusion, dizziness, flushed skin; diminished amplitude of peripheral pulses; change in BP, HR, mental status, and color associated with a change in position. Monitor I&O, and be alert to urine output <0.5 ml/kg/h for 2 consecutive hours. Also assess hemodynamic measurements. In the presence of neurogenic shock, anticipate decreased RAP, PAP, PAWP, and SVR. (See Table 1-13, pp. 30-31.)
- Continuously assess cardiac rate and rhythm per cardiac monitor; report changes in rate and rhythm.
- Implement measures to prevent episodes of decreased cardiac output caused by orthostatic hypotension:
  ☐ Change patient's position slowly.
  ☐ Perform ROM exercises q2h to prevent venous pooling.
  ☐ Apply elastic antiembolic hose as prescribed to promote venous return.
  ☐ Avoid placing pillows under patient's knees, "gatching" the bed, or allowing patient to cross the legs or sit with legs in a dependent position.
  ☐ Collaborate with physical therapy personnel in progressing patient from a supine to upright position, using a tilt table.
- As prescribed, administer fluids to control *mild* hypotension.
- Administer and monitor for therapeutic effects of vasopressors (see Appendix 7).
- Ensure adequate volume repletion before or concurrent with pressor therapy.

NIC Cardiac Care; Hemodynamic Regulation; Fluid Management

Risk for injury related to risk of development of gastric ulcer (Cushing) or gastritis secondary to increased gastric acid production
Desired outcome: Result of patient's gastric pH test is >5, and patient has no symptoms of gastric ulcer as evidenced by gastric aspirate and stool culture that are negative for blood; BP within patient's normal range; HR ≤100 bpm; and absence of midepigastric or referred shoulder pain.

> **Note:** Patients sustaining major trauma are at high risk for development of gastritis/gastric ulcers caused by increased production of gastric acid. Although ulceration can occur at any time in the patient with SCI, it is most likely to occur within 3 wk of the injury.

- Assess for indicators of GI ulceration or hemorrhage: midepigastric pain (dull, gnawing, burning ache) if patient has sensation; and hematemesis, melena, constipation, anemia, pallor, decreased BP, increased HR, and complaints of shoulder pain.
- Test gastric aspirate and stools for blood q8h. Promptly consult physician if blood is present.
- Monitor CBC for signs of anemia: decreases in Hct, Hgb, and RBCs. Normal values are as follows: Hct 40%-54% (male) or 37%-47% (female); Hgb 14-18 g/dl (male) or 12-16 g/dl (female); and RBCs 45-60 million/mm^3 (male) or 40-55 million/mm^3 (female).
- As prescribed, implement measures to treat or prevent ulceration and hemorrhage:
  - ☐ Monitor gastric pH q2h; administer antacids q2-4h or as prescribed to maintain gastric pH >5.
  - ☐ Administer histamine H_2-receptor antagonists to suppress secretion of gastric acids, decrease irritating effects of gastric secretions, and facilitate healing.
  - ☐ Insert gastric tube and attach to low, intermittent suction to remove gastric contents.
  - ☐ Prepare patient for surgery as indicated.
- For the patient with GI ulceration and hemorrhage, bowel perforation is an added risk. Be alert to the following indicators: pallor, shock state, abdominal distention, vomiting of material that resembles coffee grounds, absent bowel sounds, elevated WBC count (>11,000/mm^3), and presence of air on abdominal x-ray. In some cases the only indicators are tachycardia and shoulder pain. Bowel perforation is an emergency situation, requiring immediate surgical intervention.

NIC Surveillance; Medication Administration; Bleeding Precautions; Risk Identification

Altered tissue perfusion (or risk for same): peripheral and cardiopulmonary, related to interruption of blood flow associated with thrombophlebitis, deep vein thrombosis (DVT), and pulmonary emboli (PE) secondary to venous stasis, vascular intimal injury, and hypercoagulability occurring as a result of decreased vasomotor tone and immobility
Desired outcome: Patient is free of symptoms of thrombophlebitis, DVT, and PE within 48 h of initiation of therapy as evidenced by absence of heat, swelling, discomfort, and erythema in the calves and thighs; HR ≤100 bpm; RR ≤20 breaths/min with normal pattern and depth (eupnea); BP within patient's normal range; Pao$_2$ ≥80 mm Hg; and absence of chest or shoulder pain.
- The high-risk interval for this diagnosis is the 6-12 wk period after injury. Assess for indicators of thrombophlebitis and DVT: unusual heat and erythema of calf or thigh, increased circumference of calf or thigh, tenderness or pain in extremity (depending on patient's level of injury and whether injury is complete or incomplete), pain in the calf area with dorsiflexion (positive reaction for Homans sign).

- Assess for indicators of pulmonary emboli: sudden chest or shoulder pain, tachycardia, dyspnea, tachypnea, hypotension, pallor, cyanosis, cough with hemoptysis, restlessness, increasing anxiety, low Pao_2.
- Implement measures to prevent development of thrombophlebitis, DVT, and PE:
  - ☐ Change patient's position at least q2h to prevent venous pooling.
  - ☐ Perform ROM exercises on all extremities q1-2h to promote venous return and prevent venous stasis.
  - ☐ Avoid use of knee gatch or pillows under the knees, which can compromise circulation.
  - ☐ If patient is out of bed and in a chair, do not allow patient to cross legs at the knee or sit with legs dependent for longer than ½-1 h. For the patient experiencing some return of spinal reflex arcs below the level of the injury with spasticity of lower extremities, caution patient to alert nurse should legs become crossed.
  - ☐ Apply sequential compression devices or antiembolic hose as prescribed.
  - ☐ Maintain adequate hydration of at least 2-3 L/day, unless contraindicated, to prevent dehydration and concomitant increase in blood viscosity, which can promote thrombus formation.
  - ☐ Administer prophylactic low-dose, low-molecular-weight heparin as prescribed.
- If the patient exhibits signs of thrombophlebitis or DVT:
  - ☐ Consult physician.
  - ☐ Maintain bed rest unless otherwise directed.
  - ☐ Maintain rest of affected extremity, keeping extremity in a neutral or elevated position, as prescribed.
  - ☐ Administer anticoagulants and antiplatelet aggregating agents as prescribed.

Note: Patients with SCI who are not candidates for anticoagulation may require surgical intervention (intracaval filter) to prevent pulmonary emboli as a result of thrombophlebitis or DVT.

  - ☐ Apply warm, moist heat as prescribed. Use of heat is controversial, however, because of concern that heat causes vasodilation, which may mobilize a thrombus.
- If patient exhibits evidence of PE, perform the following, in addition to the aforementioned interventions for thrombophlebitis and DVT:
  - ☐ Elevate HOB if not contraindicated.
  - ☐ Administer oxygen.
  - ☐ As prescribed, administer vasopressors (for hypotension) and analgesics (for pain).
  - ☐ Prepare patient for diagnostic procedure (i.e., perfusion lung scan) or surgical intervention (e.g., insertion of intracaval filter).
  - ☐ Remain calm, and provide support and reassurance to patient and significant others.
- See "Pulmonary Emboli," p. 232, for more information.

NIC Circulatory Care: Arterial Insufficiency; Circulatory Care: Venous Insufficiency; Peripheral Sensation Management; Cardiac Care: Acute; Respiratory Monitoring; Shock Management: Cardiac

Risk for impaired skin integrity related to prolonged immobility secondary to immobilization device or paralysis

Desired outcome: Patient's skin remains intact during hospital course.
- Perform a complete skin assessment at least q8h. Pay close attention to skin that is particularly susceptible to breakdown (i.e., skin over bony promi-

nences and around halo vest edges). Be alert to erythema, warmth, open or macerated tissue, and foul odors (indicative of infection with tissue necrosis).

- Turn and reposition patient and massage susceptible skin at least q2h. Post a turning schedule, and include patient in the planning and initiating of this schedule.

> *Caution:* Do not turn patient without a written prescription until the injured area of the spinal cord has been stabilized. If turning is allowed before immobilization with tongs, halo, or surgery, use log-rolling technique only, using at least three people to turn patient: *one to support the head and neck and keep them in alignment during the procedure, and two to turn the patient.*

- Keep skin clean and dry.
- Pad halo jacket edges (e.g., with sheepskin) to minimize irritation and friction.
- Provide pressure-relief mattress most appropriate for patient's injury.
- For more information related to the maintenance of skin and tissue integrity, see "Wound and Skin Care," p. 55.

NIC Pressure Management; Pressure Ulcer Prevention; Skin Surveillance

Altered nutrition: less than body requirements, related to decreased oral intake secondary to anorexia, difficulty eating in prone position, fear of choking and aspiration, and inability to feed self because of paralysis of upper extremities; decreased GI motility secondary to autonomic nervous system dysfunction

Desired outcome: Within 24-72 h of this diagnosis, patient has adequate nutrition as evidenced by balanced nitrogen state per nitrogen balance studies; serum albumin 3.5-5.5 g/dl; thyroxine-binding prealbumin 20-30 mg/dl; and retinol-binding protein 4-5 mg/dl.

- Perform a complete baseline assessment of patient's nutritional status. See "Nutritional Support," p. 1.
- Assess patient's readiness for oral intake: presence of bowel sounds, passing of flatus, or bowel movement.

> **Note:**   Next to fecal impaction, paralytic ileus is the second most common GI disorder of patients with SCI. It usually occurs within 72 h of the injury and is associated with gastric distention. (See **Constipation**, p. 180.)

- When the patient begins an oral diet, progress slowly from liquids to solids as tolerated.
- Monitor and record percentage of each meal eaten by patient.
- Implement measures to maintain or improve patient's intake.
  - ☐ Obtain dietary consultation to provide patient with his or her favorite foods, as well as those that are highly nutritious.
  - ☐ Make mealtime pleasant: provide oral hygiene before and after meals, and decrease external stimuli (which also will help patient concentrate on chewing and swallowing and thus minimize the risk of aspiration).
  - ☐ Provide small, frequent feedings, inasmuch as they may be more readily digested; less likely to cause abdominal distention, which may compromise respiratory movement; and less fatiguing.
  - ☐ If patient is on a Stryker wedge frame or Foster frame, feed in a prone position to minimize the risk of aspiration. If patient is in a halo device or has been stabilized, feed in high Fowler's position.
  - ☐ Feed patient slowly, providing small, bite-size pieces, which facilitate digestion and help prevent choking.
  - ☐ Provide straws for liquids; teach patient to sip slowly.
- Once patient's condition has been stabilized, consult with occupational

therapy personnel for selection of assistive devices that will enable patient to feed self.

NIC Fluid/Electrolyte Management; Nutrition Management; Swallowing Therapy; Self-Care Assistance: Feeding

Urinary retention related to inhibition of the spinal reflex arc secondary to spinal shock after SCI

Desired outcome: Within 24 h of this diagnosis, patient has urinary output ≥0.5 ml/kg/h with output comparable to intake.

> **Caution:** Urinary retention with stretching of the bladder muscle may trigger AD. Therefore it is critical to assess for retention and to treat it promptly.

- Assess for indicators of urinary retention: suprapubic distention and intake greater than output.
- Catheterize patient on admission as prescribed. Patients usually have an indwelling catheter for the first 48-96 h after injury, followed by intermittent catheterization in an attempt to retrain the bladder.
- Ensure continuous patency of the drainage system to prevent reflux of urine into the bladder or blockage of flow, which could cause urinary retention or UTI, which may precipitate AD.
- Maintain a fluid intake of at least 2.5-3 L/day to prevent early stone formation caused by mobilization of calcium.
- Tape the catheter over the pubis in both the male and female patient to prevent traction on the catheter, which can lead to ulcer formation in the urethra and erosion of the urethral meatus.
- If an episode of AD is triggered by a distended bladder, obstructed catheter, kinked tubing, or UTI, implement the following:
  ☐ Have someone notify physician.
  ☐ If patient is not already catheterized, catheterize patient, using an anesthetic jelly.
  ☐ If the catheter is obstructed, gently instill no more than 30 ml normal saline in an attempt to open the catheter.
  ☐ If the catheter remains obstructed, remove it and insert another, using an anesthetic lubricating agent.
  ☐ If a UTI is the suspected triggering factor, obtain a specimen of urine for culture and sensitivity testing.
  ☐ For other treatment interventions, see **Dysreflexia**, p. 173.

NIC Urinary Catheterization; Urinary Retention Care

Reflex incontinence related to uninhibited activity of the spinal reflex arc secondary to recovery phase from spinal shock in patients with cord lesions above T12

Desired outcome: Patient does not experience urinary incontinence.

- As prescribed, catheterize patient on a regularly scheduled basis (e.g., q3-4h).
- If episodes of urinary incontinence occur, catheterize more frequently. If >400 ml of urine is obtained, catheterize more often and reduce fluid intake.
- Measure the amount of residual urine, and attempt to increase the length of time between catheterizations as indicated by decreased amounts (e.g., <50-100 ml urine).

> **Note:** Recent studies recommend continuing 3- to 4-h intermittent catheterizations to prevent >300-400 ml of urine from accumulating in the bladder. Amounts of urine >400 ml are associated with a significant increase in the rate of infection.

- Monitor and record I&O. Encourage a consistent intake of fluids, evenly distributed throughout the day, to prevent overdistention, which can cause incontinence and increase the risk for AD.

- Decrease fluid intake before bedtime to prevent nighttime incontinence.
- Discourage intake of caffeine-containing beverages and foods (e.g., colas, chocolate, coffee, tea) because they have a diuretic effect and may stimulate increased urine production, bladder spasms, and reflex incontinence.
- Teach patient and significant others the procedure for intermittent catheterization. Alert them to the indicators of UTI (restlessness, incontinence, malaise, anorexia, fever, cloudy or foul-smelling urine) and the importance of adequate fluid intake, regular urine cultures, good hand-washing technique, and cleansing of the urinary catheter before catheterization. (The patient with a lesion above T12 whose bladder indicates a neurogenic reflex eventually may be able to empty the bladder automatically and may not require catheterization.)

Caution: UTI is one of the leading causes of morbidity and mortality in the patient with SCI. This patient may not be aware of the presence of UTI until he or she is severely ill as a result of pyelonephritis.

Urinary retention (with overflow incontinence) related to loss of reflex activity for micturition and bladder flaccidity secondary to cord lesion at or below T12
Desired outcome: Patient has urinary output without incontinence.
- As prescribed, either insert an indwelling urinary catheter or catheterize patient intermittently on a regularly scheduled basis (e.g., q3-4h).
- If intermittent catheterization is used and episodes of urinary incontinence occur, catheterize more frequently. If >400 ml of urine is obtained, catheterize more often and reduce fluid intake.
- Measure the amount of residual urine, and attempt to increase the length of time between catheterizations, as indicated by decreased amounts (i.e., <50-100 ml urine).
- Monitor and record I&O. Distribute fluids evenly throughout the day to prevent overdistention, which can cause incontinence and increase the risk for AD.
- Decrease fluid intake before bedtime to prevent nighttime incontinence.
- Discourage intake of caffeine-containing beverages and foods (e.g., colas, chocolate, coffee, tea) because they have a diuretic effect and may stimulate increased urine production.
- When patient or significant other is ready, teach bladder-emptying techniques such as straining or Credé method.

Note: Even with these techniques, patients may experience dribbling of urine, which will necessitate catheterization or incontinence undergarments.

- Teach patient and significant others the procedure for intermittent catheterization. Alert them to the indicators of UTI (restlessness, incontinence, malaise, anorexia, fever, cloudy or foul-smelling urine) and the importance of adequate fluid intake, regular urine cultures, good hand-washing technique, and cleansing of the urinary catheter before catheterization.

Caution: UTI is one of the leading causes of morbidity and mortality in the patient with SCI. This patient may not be aware of the presence of UTI until he or she is severely ill as a result of pyelonephritis (calculi, infection, septicemia).

Ineffective thermoregulation related to inability of the body to adapt to environmental temperature changes secondary to poikilothermic reaction occurring with SCI
Desired outcome: Within 2-4 h of this diagnosis, patient becomes normothermic.

Note: With SCI the patient may become poikilothermic, meaning that the patient adapts his or her own body temperature to that of the environment and cannot control core body temperature via vasodilation to lose heat or vasoconstriction to conserve heat.

- Monitor patient's temperature at least q4h, and assess patient for signs of ineffective thermoregulation: complaints of being too warm, excessive diaphoresis, warmth of skin above level of injury, complaints of being too cold, pilomotor erection (goose bumps), or cool skin above the level of injury.
- Implement measures to attain normothermia:
  ☐ Regulate room temperature.
  ☐ Provide extra blankets to prevent chills.
  ☐ Protect patient from drafts.
  ☐ Provide warm food and drink if patient is chilled; provide cool drinks if patient is warm.
  ☐ Use fans or air conditioners to prevent overheating.
  ☐ Remove excess bedding to facilitate heat loss.
  ☐ Provide a tepid bath or cooling blanket to facilitate cooling.

NIC Temperature Regulation; Environmental Management

Risk for injury related to potential of paralytic ileus with concomitant risk of AD secondary to SCI

Desired outcomes: Patient remains free of symptoms of paralytic ileus, as evidenced by auscultation of normal bowel sounds, and free of symptoms of AD, as evidenced by BP within patient's normal range; vision normal for patient; dry skin above the level of injury; HR ≥60 bpm; and absence of headache, nasal congestion, flushed skin above the level of injury, and nausea; as well as absence of the following findings below the level of injury: pilomotor erection (goose bumps), pallor, chills.

Note: Paralytic ileus occurs most often in patients with SCI at T6 and above and usually within the first 72 h after the injury.

- Assess for indicators of paralytic ileus: decreased or absent bowel sounds, abdominal distention, anorexia, vomiting, and altered respirations as a result of pressure on the diaphragm. Report significant findings promptly.
- Observe closely for signs of AD, which can be triggered by distention of the abdomen (for assessment and treatment of AD, see interventions with **Dysreflexia,** p. 173).
- If indicators of paralytic ileus appear, implement the following, as prescribed:
  ☐ Restrict oral or enteral intake.
  ☐ Insert gastric tube to decompress the stomach; attach to suction.
  ☐ Insert a rectal tube if prescribed.

Caution: Stimulation of the rectum by a rectal tube may precipitate an episode of AD; therefore application of anesthetic ointment before insertion is recommended.

- If patient has a rectal tube in place, he or she may not have sensation in the rectal area. Therefore special care is necessary to prevent damage to the rectal mucosa and anal sphincter. Remove the tube as soon as possible.

NIC Surveillance: Safety; Dysreflexia Management; Tube Care

Constipation or fecal impaction related to neuromuscular impairment secondary to spinal shock

Desired outcome: Within 24-48 h of this diagnosis and subsequently q2-3 days (or within patient's preinjury pattern), patient has bowel elimination of soft and formed stools.

- Monitor patient for indicators of constipation (nausea, abdominal distention, malaise) and fecal impaction (nausea, vomiting, increasing abdominal distention, palpable colonic mass, or presence of hard fecal mass on digital examination).
- Until bowel sounds are present and paralytic ileus has resolved, maintain patient on nothing by mouth (NPO) status, with gastric suction.
- Perform a gentle digital examination to determine presence of fecal impaction and check for rectal reflexes.
- Before the return of rectal reflex arc, it may be necessary to remove feces from the rectum manually. If a fecal impaction is present in an atonic bowel, a small-volume enema may be necessary.

> *Caution:* Be aware that overdistention of the bowel or stimulation of the anal sphincter caused by impaction, rectal examination, or enema may precipitate AD. Use generous amounts of anesthetic lubricant when performing rectal examination or administering an enema.

Constipation related to lack of voluntary control of the anal sphincter and lack of sensation of a fecal mass after return of reflex arc associated with neuromuscular impairment
Desired outcome: Within 24-48 h of this diagnosis and subsequently q2-3 days (or within patient's preinjury pattern), patient has bowel elimination of soft and formed stools.
- Obtain history of patient's preinjury bowel elimination pattern.
- Assist patient with selection of menu items that are high in fiber.
- Unless contraindicated, maintain a minimum fluid intake of 2-3 L/day.
- Administer stool softeners (e.g., docusate sodium) daily.
- If possible, avoid enemas for long-term bowel management, because the patient with SCI cannot retain the enema solution. If, however, impaction occurs, a gentle, small-volume cleansing enema, followed by manual removal of fecal material, may be necessary.
- Assess patient's readiness for bowel retraining program, including neurologic status and current bowel patterns, noting frequency, amount, and consistency. Usually bowel retraining is initiated when the patient is neurologically stable and can resume a sitting position.
- Because use of a bedpan may impair the patient's ability to evacuate the bowel, provide a bedside commode, if allowed.
  - ☐ Provide ample time each day for bowel elimination. One-half hour after mealtime coincides with the gastrocolic reflex.
  - ☐ Ensure patient's privacy.
  - ☐ Stimulate the rectal sphincter with digital stimulation or insert suppository (i.e., bisacodyl) to initiate reflex peristalsis with reflex evacuation.

> *Caution:*   See precautions with **Dysreflexia**, p. 173.

  - ☐ If patient has upper extremity function, teach him or her how to perform digital rectal stimulation, insert suppository, and massage abdomen to facilitate bowel movement.
NIC Constipation/Impaction Management
Risk for infection related to inadequate primary defenses (broken skin) secondary to presence of invasive immobilization devices
Desired outcome: Patient is free of infection at insertion site for tongs or halo device as evidenced by normothermia; negative culture results; and absence of erythema, swelling, warmth, purulent drainage, or tenderness at insertion site.
- Assess insertion sites q8h for indicators of infection: erythema, swelling, warmth, purulent drainage, and increased or new tenderness. Also be alert to pin migration. If the pin appears to be loose, consult physician and instruct patient to remain still until the pin can be secured.

- Perform pin care as prescribed. One regimen involves cleansing the site with povidone-iodine or half-strength normal saline and hydrogen peroxide, leaving any superficial crust intact, followed by application of an antibiotic ointment. An alternative regimen involves cleansing with povidone-iodine or hydrogen peroxide and no antibiotic ointment. Sterile dressings may be applied around the pins, or the area may be left open to air according to physician or agency policy. Collaborate with physician to develop an effective pin care regimen for the patient. Use sterile applicators, and follow aseptic technique during all pin care procedures.

NIC Infection Control; Infection Protection; Skin Surveillance

Sensory/perceptual alterations: visual, related to presence of immobilization device; use of therapeutic bed

Desired outcome: After intervention(s), patient expresses satisfaction with visual capabilities.

- Assess for factors that limit the patient's visual capabilities: presence of tongs, cervical traction, halo device; and use of Stryker wedge frame or Foster frame or RotoRest® kinetic treatment table.
- Provide for increased visualization of patient's surroundings:
  - ☐ Obtain prism glasses for patient who must remain supine or cannot turn his or her head because of halo traction device. If prism glasses are unavailable, provide a hand mirror for patient with upper extremity function.
  - ☐ Position mirrors to increase the amount of area that can be visualized from patient's position.
  - ☐ Approach patient and converse within patient's visual field.
  - ☐ Keep clocks, calendars, and other personal objects within patient's visual field.

NIC Environmental Management; Positioning

Sexual dysfunction or altered sexuality patterns related to trauma associated with SCI

Desired outcome: Patient verbalizes sexual concerns before discharge from ICU.

- Assess patient's level of sexual function or loss from a neurologic and psychologic perspective. The general rule for men is that the higher the lesion, the greater the chance of maintaining the ability to have an erection, but with less chance for ejaculation. For women, ovulation may stop for several months because of stress after the injury. Ovulation usually returns, however, and the woman can become pregnant and have a normal pregnancy. Both men and women with high lesions may experience feelings of excitement similar to a preinjury orgasm.
- Evaluate your own feelings about sexuality. If you are uncomfortable discussing this subject with the patient, arrange for a knowledgeable staff member to speak with patient about his or her concerns.
- Elicit patient's knowledge, concerns, and questions about his or her sexual function after the SCI.
- It is normal for men to experience a reflex erection upon resolution of the spinal shock, particularly for individuals with lesions in the cervical and thoracic areas. Reassure patient that this is normal and therefore nothing to be embarrassed about.
- Expect acting-out behavior related to the patient's sexuality. This is a normal response to the patient's concern regarding his or her sexual prognosis.
- Provide accurate information regarding expected sexual function in an open, interested manner, based on your assessment of the patient's readiness for information.
- Facilitate communication between the patient and his or her partner.
- Refer patient and his or her partner to a sex therapist or other knowledgeable rehabilitation professional upon resolution of the critical stages of SCI.

- Also provide patient with the following addresses and phone numbers:
  - ☐ National Spinal Cord Injury Association, 1-800-962-9629; e-mail: www.spinalcord.org.
  - ☐ Spinal Cord Injury Network International, 3911 Princeton Drive, Santa Rosa, CA 95405-7013; 1-800-548-CORD (2673), 1-707-577-8796; fax:1-707-577-0605; URL: http://www.sonic.net/~spinal/; e-mail: spinal @sonic.net

NIC Sexual Counseling; Anxiety Reduction; Body Image

ADDITIONAL NURSING DIAGNOSES

Also see nursing diagnoses and interventions as appropriate under "Nutritional Support," p. 1; "Mechanical Ventilation," p. 17; "Prolonged Immobility," p. 74; "Psychosocial Support," p. 83; and "Psychosocial Support for the Patient's Family and Significant Others," p. 95.

Abdominal trauma

PATHOPHYSIOLOGY

The degree of injury to abdominal contents is related to the nature of the force applied and the consistency of the affected structures. Forces involved may be blunt or penetrating, and organs are categorized as solid (e.g., liver, spleen, pancreas) or hollow (e.g., stomach, intestine). Penetrating abdominal trauma typically results in injury to organs in the direct path of the instrument or missile, but high-velocity weapons (e.g., rifles) cause injury not only to tissue in the direct path of the missile but to adjacent organs as well because of energy shock waves that surround the missile path. Injury inflicted by stab wounds follows a predictable pattern and involves less tissue destruction than does injury from gunshot wounds, although stab wounds to major vascular structures (e.g., aorta) and organs (e.g., liver) can be fatal. Blunt abdominal trauma typically results in injury to solid viscera because hollow viscera tend to be more compressible. Hollow organs, however, may rupture, especially when full, if there is a sudden increase in intraluminal pressure. The rate of complications and death increases greatly if injury to multiple abdominal organs is sustained.

The three distinct but overlapping areas of the abdomen are the peritoneal cavity, the retroperitoneal space, and the pelvis. The upper region of the abdomen is covered by the bony thorax and the peritoneal cavity. It includes the diaphragm, liver, spleen, stomach, and transverse colon. The two most commonly injured *solid* abdominal organs are the spleen (blunt trauma) and the liver (penetrating trauma), and the small bowel is the most commonly injured *hollow* abdominal organ.

The retroperitoneum contains the aorta, vena cava, pancreas, kidneys, adrenal glands, ureters, and some of the duodenum and colon.

The pelvis contains the rectum, bladder, iliac vessels, and, in women, the genitalia.

Abdominal trauma results in direct injury to organs, blood vessels, and supporting structures. Other pathophysiologic changes associated with abdominal trauma include (1) massive fluid shifts related to tissue damage, blood loss, and shock; (2) systemic inflammation and metabolic changes associated with stress and catecholamine release; (3) coagulation problems associated with massive hemorrhage and multiple transfusions; (4) inflammation, infection, and abscess formation caused by release of GI secretions and bacteria into the peritoneum; and (5) nutritional and electrolyte alterations that develop as a consequence of disruption of GI tract integrity. Prolonged hypovolemia and shock result in organ ischemia and ultimately failure (see "Major Trauma," "Acute Respiratory Distress Syndrome," "Cardiogenic Shock," "Acute Renal

Failure," "Hepatic Failure," and "Disseminated Intravascular Coagulation"). The following brief overview summarizes common injuries.

Diaphragm: Commonly after blunt trauma, the diaphragm may be injured at the left posterior portion. The tear will be visualized best by chest x-ray (CXR), which will show an elevation of the left hemidiaphragm and a bubble of air in the chest.

Spleen: The organ most frequently injured after blunt trauma and the most common cause of major abdominal injury. Damage to the spleen may occur with the most trivial of injuries, so index of suspicion must be high. Massive hemorrhage from splenic injury is common. Splenic injury often is associated with hepatic or pancreatic injury. All efforts are made to repair the spleen, because total splenectomy increases the long-term risk of infection, especially in children and young adults.

Liver: Because of its large size and location, it is the organ most frequently involved in penetrating trauma (80%) and often is affected by blunt injury (20%) as well. Control of bleeding and bile drainage are major concerns with hepatic injury. Mortality from liver injuries is about 10%. In most patients, bleeding from a liver injury can be controlled with conventional techniques. About 5% of injuries require packing for bleeds. The biliary tree also may be injured and should always be suspected with concomitant liver injury. The patient may have few or no symptoms.

Lower portion of esophagus and stomach: Occasionally, the lower portion of the esophagus is involved in penetrating trauma. Because the stomach is flexible and readily displaced, it usually is not injured with blunt trauma, but it may be injured by direct penetration. Injury to either one results in the escape of irritating gastric fluids (gastric perforation) and the release of free air below the level of the diaphragm. Esophageal injuries often are associated with thoracic injuries.

Pancreas and duodenum: Although traumatic pancreatic or duodenal injury occurs relatively infrequently, it is associated with high morbidity and mortality because of the difficulty of detecting these injuries, the likelihood of massive injury to nearby organs, and the spillage of fluid, activated enzymes, and bile, contributing to a significant inflammatory response. Because these organs are retroperitoneal, clinical indicators of injury often are not obvious for several hours.

Small intestine and mesentery: The three most common injuries associated with penetrating abdominal trauma are small bowel, liver, and colon, whereas with blunt trauma they are liver, spleen, and kidney. Compromised intestinal blood flow with eventual infarction is the consequence of undetected mesenteric damage. Perforations or contusions can result in release of bacteria and intestinal contents into the abdominal cavity, causing serious infection.

Colon: Injury most frequently caused by penetrating forces, although lap belts, direct blows, and other blunt forces cause a small percentage of colonic injuries. Because of the high bacterial content, infection is even more a concern than it is with small bowel injury. Most patients with significant colon injuries require temporary colostomy.

Pelvis: See "Renal and Lower Urinary Tract Trauma," p. 148.

Major vessels: Injuries to the abdominal aorta and inferior vena cava most often are caused by penetrating trauma, but they also occur with deceleration injury. Hepatic vein injuries frequently are associated with juxtahepatic vena caval injury and result in rapid hemorrhage. Blood loss after major vascular injury is massive, and survival depends on rapid transport to a trauma center and immediate surgical intervention.

Retroperitoneal vessels: Tears in retroperitoneal vessels associated with pelvic fractures or damage to retroperitoneal organs (pancreas, duodenum, kidney) can cause bleeding into the retroperitoneum. Even though the retroperitoneal space can accommodate up to 4 L of blood, detection of retroperitoneal hematomas is difficult and sophisticated diagnostic techniques may be required.

Abdominal compartment syndrome (ACS);   Intraabdominal hypertension is common with abdominal injuries because of the inflammatory response and volume resuscitation. The clinical effects of abdominal hypertension are well documented, but only recently have large clinical studies confirmed the adverse effects and outcomes from intraabdominal pressure (IAP). The hypertensive effects are known to decrease lung compliance and assumed to create a type of obstructive renal failure. These clinical problems are relieved if abdominal decompression occurs. Key features of IAP/ACS include (1) elevated ventilatory pressures, (2) elevated CVP, (3) decreased urine output, (4) massive abdominal distention, and (5) reversal of these derangements with abdominal decompression.

ASSESSMENT

History: Details regarding circumstances of the accident and mechanism of injury are invaluable in detecting the presence of specific injuries. In addition, the time of the patient's last meal, previous abdominal surgeries, and use of safety restraints (if appropriate) should be ascertained. Hollow viscous injury should always be suspected with a visible contusion on the abdomen and is often missed. If possible, information concerning current medications and allergies, particularly to contrast material, antibiotics, and tetanus toxoid, should be obtained. The history may be difficult to obtain because of alcohol or drug intoxication, head injury, breathing difficulties, or impaired cerebral perfusion. In such cases, family members and emergency personnel may be valuable sources of information.

Clinical presentation: A wide variation can occur. Mild tenderness to severe abdominal pain may be present, with the pain either localized to the site of injury or diffuse. Blood or fluid collection within the peritoneum causes irritation that results in involuntary guarding, rigidity, and rebound tenderness. Fluid or air under the diaphragm may cause referred shoulder pain. Kehr sign (left shoulder pain caused by splenic bleeding) also may be noted, especially when the patient is recumbent. Nausea and vomiting may occur, and the conscious patient who has sustained blood loss often complains of thirst—an early sign of hemorrhagic shock. Symptoms of abdominal injury may be minimal or absent in the patient who is intoxicated or has sustained head or spinal cord injury.

> **Note:**   The absence of signs and symptoms does not exclude the presence of major abdominal injury. Blood in the peritoneum does not produce peritoneal signs. According to Beachly and Farrar (1993), outward signs of injury are absent in as many as 36% of patients with abdominal trauma.

Physical assessment: Abdominal assessment is highly subjective, and serial evaluations by the same examiner are strongly recommended to detect subtle changes. Abdominal assessment after blunt injury is often unreliable.

Inspection: Abrasions and ecchymoses may indicate underlying injury. Ecchymosis over the left upper quadrant (LUQ) suggests splenic rupture, and erythema and ecchymosis across the lower portion of the abdomen suggest intestinal injury caused by lap belts. *Grey Turner sign,* a bluish discoloration of the flank, may indicate retroperitoneal bleeding from the pancreas, duodenum, vena cava, aorta, or kidneys. *Cullen sign,* a bluish discoloration around the umbilicus, may be present with intraperitoneal bleeding from the liver or spleen. Ecchymoses may take hours to days to develop, depending on the rate of blood loss. The absence of ecchymosis does not exclude major abdominal

---

TABLE 2-13   Signs and Symptoms That Suggest Peritoneal Irritation

- Generalized abdominal pain and tenderness
- Involuntary guarding of the abdomen
- Abdominal wall rigidity
- Rebound tenderness
- Abdominal pain with movement or coughing
- Decreased or absent bowel sounds

---

trauma and massive internal bleeding. In the event of gunshot wounds, entrance and exit (if present) wounds should be identified. Careful evaluation of the patient including log roll, counting the bullet wounds, and exploration of the body creases and perineum is essential.

Auscultation: It is important to auscultate before palpation and percussion, because these maneuvers can stimulate the bowel and confound assessment findings. Bowel sounds are likely to be decreased or absent with abdominal organ injury or intraperitoneal bleeding. The presence of bowel sounds, however, does not exclude significant abdominal injury. Immediately after injury, bowel sounds may be present, even with major organ injury. Bowel sounds should be auscultated in each quadrant q1-2h in patients with suspected abdominal injury. Absence of bowel sounds is expected immediately after surgery. Failure to auscultate bowel sounds within 24-48 h after surgery suggests ileus, possibly caused by continued bleeding, peritonitis, or bowel infarction.

Palpation: Tenderness to light palpation suggests pain from superficial or abdominal wall lesions, such as that occurring with seat-belt contusions. Deep palpation may reveal a mass in the area of hematoma. Internal injury with bleeding or release of GI contents into the peritoneum results in peritoneal irritation and certain assessment findings. Table 2-13 describes signs and symptoms that suggest peritoneal irritation. Subcutaneous emphysema of the abdominal wall usually is caused by thoracic injury but also may be produced by bowel rupture. Measurements of abdominal girth may be helpful in identifying increases in girth attributable to gas, blood, or fluid. Visual evaluation of abdominal distention is a late and unreliable sign of bleeding.

Percussion: Unusually large areas of dullness may be percussed over ruptured blood-filled organs. For example, a fixed area of dullness in the LUQ suggests a ruptured spleen. An absence (or decrease in the size) of liver dullness may be caused by free air below the diaphragm, a consequence of hollow viscus perforation, or, in unusual cases, displacement of the liver through a ruptured diaphragm. The presence of tympany suggests gas; dullness suggests that the enlargement is caused by blood or fluid.

Vital signs and hemodynamic measurements: Ventilatory excursion often is diminished because of pain, thoracic injury, or diaphragmatic elevation caused by abdominal distention. With initial compensatory tachycardia and vasoconstriction caused by blood loss, a normal BP usually is maintained until blood loss becomes major. At that point BP deteriorates to a MAP <70 mm Hg. Vascular resistance remains high. A diminished CVP and PAP reflect hypovolemic shock; CO decreases because of hypovolemia but will normalize with correction. Initial hypothermia is common. See "Major Trauma," p. 106, for hemodynamic findings associated with hyperdynamic responses to injury.

DIAGNOSTIC TESTS

Hct level: Serial levels reflect the amount of blood lost. If measured immediately after the injury, the Hct level may be normal, but serial levels will reveal dramatic decreases during resuscitation and as extravascular fluid mobilizes during the recovery phase. Major blood loss is common with intraabdominal injury.

WBC count: Leukocytosis is expected immediately after injury. Splenic injuries in particular result in the rapid development of a moderate to high WBC count. A later increase in WBCs or a shift to the left reflects an increase in the number of neutrophils, which signals an inflammatory response and possible intraabdominal infection. In the patient with abdominal trauma, ruptured abdominal viscera must be considered as a potential source of infection.

Platelet count: Mild thrombocytosis occurs immediately after traumatic injury. Spontaneous bleeding and a very low platelet count (<20,000-30,000/mm^3) signal the need for platelet transfusion.

Glucose levels: Initially elevated because of catecholamine release and insulin resistance associated with major trauma. Glucose metabolism is abnormal after major hepatic resection, and patients with significant hepatic injury should be monitored at frequent intervals to prevent severe hypoglycemic episodes.

Electrolytes: Sodium, potassium, and chloride levels may drop because of gastric suctioning or vomiting.

BUN: Elevations are associated with shock, dehydration, GI bleeding, infection, and impaired kidney function.

Amylase levels: Elevated serum levels are associated with pancreatic or upper small bowel injury, but values may be normal even with severe injury to these organs. Delayed elevation suggests traumatic pancreatitis.

Liver enzymes: Elevations of aspartate aminotransferase (AST), alanine aminotransferase (ALT), and alkaline phosphatase (ALP) reflect hepatic dysfunction as a result of liver ischemia during prolonged hypotensive episodes or direct traumatic damage. Fluctuations in these enzyme levels during the postoperative period can be used to detect evidence of liver necrosis.

Bilirubin: Elevated direct (conjugated) indicates the liver's inability to excrete bilirubin. Elevated indirect (unconjugated) indicates rapid destruction of RBCs or possible retroperitoneal hematoma.

X-rays: Flat and upright chest x-rays exclude chest injuries (frequently associated with abdominal trauma) and establish a baseline, inasmuch as surgery is likely. In addition, chest, abdominal, and pelvic x-rays may reveal fractures, missiles, free intraperitoneal air, hematoma, or hemorrhage.

Occult blood: Gastric contents and stool should be tested for blood in the initial and recovery periods because GI bleeding can occur as a result of both direct injury and later complications, including gastric erosion.

Abdominal ultrasound: Indications for abdominal ultrasound are similar to those for diagnostic peritoneal lavage (DPL). Accuracy of the ultrasound depends on the experience of the operator. However, the test is quick and noninvasive.

DPL: Involves insertion of a peritoneal dialysis catheter into the peritoneum to check for intraabdominal bleeding. DPL is indicated for confirmed or suspected blunt abdominal trauma for the following patients: (1) those in whom signs and symptoms of abdominal injury are obscured by intoxication, head or spinal cord trauma, opiate administration, or unconsciousness; (2) those about to undergo general anesthesia for repair of other injuries (e.g., orthopedic, facial); and (3) any patient with equivocal assessment findings. DPL is unnecessary for patients with obvious intraabdominal bleeding or other indications for immediate laparotomy (see "Surgical Considerations," p. 189, in the following section).

If gross blood is recovered when the catheter is inserted, immediate laparotomy is indicated. If blood is not recovered, 1 L of normal saline or Ringer's lactate is infused rapidly through the catheter and then drained into a sterile bedside drainage device. If possible, the patient is moved from side to side after fluid instillation to distribute the lavage fluid evenly. If the drained lavage is grossly bloody, intraperitoneal bleeding is confirmed. Other indicators of positive lavage results are >100,000 RBC/μl; >500 WBC/μl; amylase >175 U/dl; presence of bile or bacteria; or obvious intestinal contents in the drainage.

> **Note:**   An indwelling urinary catheter is inserted before DPL to prevent inadvertent puncture of a full bladder. The stomach is decompressed with a gastric tube to check for bleeding and avoid pressure on a full stomach, vomiting, and aspiration.

CT: Can detect intraperitoneal and retroperitoneal bleeding and free air (associated with rupture of hollow viscera). It is most useful in assessing injury to solid abdominal organs.

Angiography: Performed selectively to evaluate injury to spleen, liver, pancreas, duodenum, and retroperitoneal vessels when other diagnostic findings are equivocal.

> *Caution:*   Because of the large amount of contrast material used during this procedure, monitor urine output closely for several hours for a decrease and ensure adequate hydration.

ADDITIONAL DIAGNOSTIC TESTS

Abdominal injuries often are associated with multisystem trauma. Also see diagnostic test discussions in "Major Trauma," p. 106, "Traumatic Brian Injury," p. 118, "Chest Trauma," p. 133, "Cardiac Trauma," p. 140, "Renal and Lower Urinary Tract Trauma," p. 148, and "Acute Spinal Cord Injury," p. 167.

COLLABORATIVE MANAGEMENT

Oxygen: Abdominal injury may result in poor ventilatory efforts caused by pain or compression of thoracic structures. High-flow supplemental oxygen is indicated initially and then titrated according to ABG values.

Fluid management: Because massive blood loss is associated with most abdominal injuries, immediate volume resuscitation is critical. Initially, Ringer's lactate or a similar balanced salt solution is given. Colloid solutions may be helpful in the postoperative period if there are low filling pressures and evidence of decreased plasma oncotic pressure. Typed and cross-matched fresh blood is the optimal fluid for replacement of large blood losses. However, inasmuch as fresh whole blood is rarely available, a combination of packed cells and fresh frozen plasma often is used. Overaggressive use of colloids and PRBC may increase third spacing and systemic inflammatory response syndrome (SIRS). See "Major Trauma," p. 106, for more information.

Gastric intubation: Gastric tube permits gastric decompression, aids in removal of gastric contents, and prevents accumulation of gas or air in the GI tract. Aspirated contents can be checked for blood to aid in the diagnosis of lower esophageal, gastric, or duodenal injury. The tube usually remains in place until bowel function returns.

Pharmacotherapy

Antibiotics: Abdominal trauma is associated with a high incidence of intraabdominal abscess, sepsis, and wound infection, particularly with injury to the terminal ileum and colon. Persons with penetrating or blunt trauma and suspected intestinal injury are started on parenteral antibiotic therapy immediately. Broad-spectrum antibiotics are continued postoperatively and stopped after approximately 72 hours unless there is evidence of infection.

Analgesics: Because opiates alter the sensorium, making evaluation of the patient's condition difficult, they seldom are used in the early stages of trauma. Analgesics are used in the immediate postoperative period to relieve pain and promote ventilatory excursion.

Tetanus prophylaxis: Tetanus immunoglobulin and tetanus toxoid are considered on the basis of Center for Disease Control (CDC) recommendations (see Table 2-1).

Nutrition: Patients with abdominal trauma have complex nutritional needs because of the hypermetabolic state associated with major trauma and traumatic or surgical disruption of normal GI function. Often infection and sepsis contribute to a negative nitrogen state and increased metabolic needs. Prompt initiation of parenteral feedings in patients unable to accept enteric feedings and the administration of supplemental calories, proteins, vitamins, and minerals are essential for healing. For additional information, see "Nutritional Support," p. 1.

Surgical considerations for penetrating abdominal injuries: Removing penetrating objects can result in additional injury; thus attempts at removal should be made only under controlled situations with a surgeon and operating room immediately available. The issue of mandatory surgical exploration versus observation and selective surgery, especially with stab wounds, remains controversial. There is a trend toward observation of patients without obvious injury or peritoneal signs. Indications for laparotomy include one or more of the following: (1) penetrating injury suspected of invading the peritoneum; (2) positive peritoneal signs (e.g., tenderness, rebound tenderness, involuntary guarding); (3) shock; (4) GI hemorrhage; (5) free air in the peritoneal cavity as seen on x-ray; (6) evisceration; (7) massive hematuria; and (8) positive findings on diagnostic peritoneal lavage.

Note: The patient should be evaluated for peritoneal signs at least hourly by the same examiner. Consult surgeon immediately if the patient shows peritoneal signs, evidence of shock, gastric or rectal bleeding, or gross hematuria.

Surgical considerations for nonpenetrating abdominal injuries: Physical examination usually is reliable in determining the necessity for surgery in alert, cooperative, unintoxicated patients. Additional diagnostic tests such as abdominal ultrasound, DPL, or CT are necessary to evaluate the need for surgery in the patient who is intoxicated or unconscious or who has sustained head or spinal cord trauma. Immediate laparotomy for blunt abdominal trauma is indicated under the following circumstances: (1) clear signs of peritoneal irritation (see Table 6-16); (2) free air in the peritoneum; (3) hypotension caused by suspected abdominal injury or persistent and unexplained hypotension; (4) positive DPL findings; (5) GI aspirate or rectal smear positive for blood; (6) other positive findings in diagnostic tests such as CT or arteriogram; (7) abdominal gunshot wound; and/or (8) abdominal stab wound with evisceration, hypotension, or peritonitis. Carefully evaluated, stable patients with blunt abdominal trauma may be admitted to a critical care unit for observation. These patients should be evaluated in the same manner as that described in "Surgical Considerations for Penetrating Abdominal Injuries," above. It is important to note that damage to retroperitoneal organs such as the pancreas and duodenum may not cause significant signs and symptoms for 6-12 h or longer. Relatively slow bleeding from abdominal viscera may not be clinically apparent for 12 h or longer after the initial injury. In addition, the nurse should be aware that complications such as bowel obstruction caused by adhesions or narrowing of the bowel wall from localized ischemia, inflammation, or hematoma may develop days or weeks after the traumatic event. The need for vigilant observation in the care of these patients cannot be overemphasized.

NURSING DIAGNOSES AND INTERVENTIONS

Fluid volume deficit related to active loss secondary to physical injury
Desired outcome: Within 12 h of this diagnosis, patient becomes normo-

volemic as evidenced by MAP ≥70 mm Hg; HR 60-100 bpm; normal sinus rhythm on ECG; CVP 2-6 mm Hg; PAWP 6-12 mm Hg; CI ≥2.5 L/min/m²; SVR 900-1200 dynes/sec/cm⁻⁵; urinary output ≥0.5 ml/kg/h; warm extremities; brisk capillary refill (<2 sec); and distal pulses >2+ on a 0-4+ scale. Although hemodynamic parameters are helpful to determine adequacy of resuscitation, serum lactate and base deficit are essential to evaluate cellular perfusion.

- Monitor BP q15min, or more frequently in the presence of obvious bleeding or unstable VS. Be alert to changes in MAP of >10 mm Hg. Even a small but sudden decrease in BP signals the need to consult the physician, especially with the trauma patient in whom the extent of injury is unknown.
- Monitor HR, ECG, and cardiovascular status q15min until volume is restored and VS are stable. Check ECG to note HR elevations and myocardial ischemic changes (i.e., ventricular dysrhythmias, ST-segment changes), which can occur because of dilutional anemia in susceptible individuals.
- In the patient with evidence of volume depletion or active blood loss, administer pressurized fluids rapidly through several large-caliber (16-gauge or larger) catheters. Use short, large-bore IV tubing (trauma tubing) to maximize flow rate. Avoid use of stopcocks, because they slow the infusion rate. Fluids should be warmed to prevent hypothermia.

> *Caution:* Evaluate patency of IV catheters continuously during rapid-volume resuscitation.

- Measure central pressures and thermodilution CO q1-2h or more frequently if blood loss is ongoing. Calculate SVR and PVR q4-8h or more often in unstable patients. Be alert to low or decreasing CVP and PAWP. An elevated HR, along with decreased PAWP, decreased CO/CI, and increased SVR, suggests hypovolemia (see Table 4-22, p. 345, for hemodynamic profile of hypovolemic shock). Anticipate slightly elevated HR and CO caused by hyperdynamic cardiovascular state in some patients who have undergone volume resuscitation, particularly during the preoperative phase. Also anticipate mild to moderate pulmonary hypertension, especially in patients with concurrent thoracic injury, such as pulmonary contusion, smoke inhalation, or early ARDS. ARDS is a concern in patients who have sustained major abdominal injury, inasmuch as there are many potential sources of infection and sepsis that make the development of ARDS more likely (see "Acute Respiratory Distress Syndrome," p. 243).
- Measure urinary output q1-2h. Be alert to output <0.5 ml/kg/h for 2 consecutive hours. Low urine output usually reflects inadequate intravascular volume in the patient with abdominal trauma.
- Monitor for physical indicators of arterial hypovolemia, which may include cool extremities, capillary refill >2 sec, absent or decreased amplitude of distal pulses, elevated serum lactate, and base deficit (see p. 110).
- Estimate ongoing blood loss. Measure all bloody drainage from tubes or catheters, noting drainage color (e.g., coffee ground, burgundy, bright red [Table 2-14]). Note the frequency of dressing changes as a result of saturation with blood to estimate amount of blood loss via wound site.

NIC Electrolyte Management; Fluid Management; Fluid Monitoring; Hypovolemia Management

Pain related to physical injury secondary to external trauma or surgery

Desired outcomes: Within 2 h of this diagnosis, patient's subjective evaluation of discomfort improves, as documented by a pain scale. Nonverbal indicators of discomfort, such as grimacing, are absent.

- Evaluate patient using a pain scale for presence of preoperative and postoperative pain. Preoperative pain is anticipated and is a vital diagnostic aid. The nature of postoperative pain also can be important. Incisional and some visceral pain can be anticipated, but intense pain or prolonged pain,

TABLE 2-14 Characteristics of Gastrointestinal Drainage	
Source	**Composition and usual character**
Mouth and oropharynx	Saliva; thin, clear, watery; pH 7
Stomach	Hydrochloric acid, gastrin, pepsin, mucus; thin, brown to green, acidic
Pancreas	Enzymes and bicarbonate; thin, watery, yellowish brown; alkaline
Biliary tract	Bile, including bile salts and electrolytes; bright yellow to brownish green
Duodenum	Digestive enzymes, mucus, products of digestion; thin, bright yellow to light brown, may be green, alkaline
Jejunum	Enzymes, mucus, products of digestion; brown, watery with particles
Ileum	Enzymes, mucus, digestive products, greater amounts of bacteria; brown, liquid, feculent
Colon	Digestive products, mucus, large amounts of bacteria; brown to dark brown, semiformed to firm stool
Postoperative (GI surgery)	Initially, drainage expected to contain small amounts of fresh blood appearing bright to dark; later, drainage mixed with old blood appearing dark brown (coffee-ground); and then approaches normal composition
Infection present	Drainage cloudy, may be thicker than usual; strong or unusual odor, drain site often erythematous and warm

especially when accompanied by other peritoneal signs, can signal bleeding, bowel infarction, infection, or other complications.

- Recognize that opiate analgesics can decrease GI motility, causing nausea, vomiting, and delay of bowel activity. These factors are especially significant if the patient has had a recent laparotomy.
- See this diagnosis in "Major Trauma," p. 113, and in Chapter 1, p. 61, for additional pain interventions.

NIC Pain Management; Bowel Management

Risk for infection related to inadequate primary defenses secondary to physical trauma or surgery; inadequate secondary defenses caused by decreased hemoglobin or inadequate immune response; tissue destruction and environmental exposure (especially to intestinal contents); multiple invasive procedures

Desired outcome: Patient is free of infection as evidenced by core or rectal temperature <37.7° C (100° F); HR ≤100 bpm; CI ≤4 L/min/m^2; SVR ≥900 dynes/sec/cm^{-5}; orientation to time, place, and person; and absence of unusual redness, warmth, or drainage at surgical incisions and drain sites.

- Note color, character, and odor of all drainage. Report the presence of foul-smelling or abnormal drainage. See Table 2-13 for a description of the *usual* character of GI drainage.
- As prescribed, administer pneumococcal vaccine to patients with total splenectomy to minimize the risk of postsplenectomy sepsis.

- If evisceration occurs initially or develops later, do not reinsert tissue or organs. Place a saline-soaked gauze over the evisceration, and cover with a sterile towel until the evisceration can be evaluated by the surgeon.
- For more interventions, see this diagnosis in "Major Trauma," p. 114.

NIC Infection Control; Infection Protection

Altered tissue perfusion: gastrointestinal, related to interruption of arterial or venous blood flow or hypovolemia secondary to physical injury

Desired outcome: By the time of hospital discharge, patient has adequate GI tract tissue perfusion as evidenced by normoactive bowel sounds; soft, nondistended abdomen; and return of bowel elimination.

- Auscultate for bowel sounds hourly during the acute phase of abdominal trauma and q4-8h during the recovery phase. Report prolonged or sudden absence of bowel sounds during the postoperative period, because these signs may signal bowel ischemia or mesenteric infarction.
- Evaluate patient for peritoneal signs (see Table 2-12), which may occur initially as a result of injury or may not develop until days or weeks later if complications caused by slow bleeding or other mechanisms occur.
- Ensure adequate intravascular volume (see **Fluid volume deficit,** p. 112).
- Evaluate laboratory data for evidence of bleeding (e.g., serial Hct) or organ ischemia (e.g., AST, ALT, lactic dehydrogenase [LDH]). Desired values are as follows: Hct >28%-30%, AST 5-40 IU/L, ALT 5-35 IU/L, and LDH 90-200 U/L.
- Document amount and character of GI secretions, drainage, and excretions. Note changes that suggest bleeding (presence of frank or occult blood), infection (e.g., increased or purulent drainage), or obstruction (e.g., failure to eliminate flatus or stool within 3-4 days after surgery).
- Stress the importance of seeking medical attention if indicators of infection or bowel obstruction occur (e.g., fever, severe or unusual abdominal pain, nausea and vomiting, unusual drainage from wounds or incisions, change in bowel habits).

NIC Circulatory Care

Impaired tissue integrity related to mechanical factors (including physical injury); increased metabolic needs secondary to trauma/stress response; altered circulation secondary to hemorrhage or direct vascular injury; exposure to irritants (gastric secretions)

Desired outcome: Patient has adequate tissue integrity by the time of hospital discharge as evidenced by wound healing within an acceptable time frame (according to extent of injury) and absence of skin breakdown caused by GI drainage.

- Protect the skin surrounding tubes, drains, or fistulas, keeping the areas clean and free from drainage. Gastric and intestinal secretions and drainage are highly irritating and can lead to skin excoriation. If necessary, apply ointments, skin barriers, or drainage pouches to protect the surrounding skin. If available, consult ostomy nurse for complex or involved cases.
- For other interventions, see this diagnosis in "Major Trauma," p. 115.

NIC Wound Care; Skin Surveillance; Tube Care

Altered nutrition: less than body requirements, related to decreased intake secondary to disruption of GI tract integrity (traumatic or surgical); increased need secondary to hypermetabolic posttrauma state

Desired outcome: Within 5 days of this diagnosis, patient has adequate nutrition as evidenced by maintenance of baseline body weight and state of nitrogen balance on nitrogen studies.

- Collaborate with physician, dietitian, and pharmacist to estimate patient's metabolic needs on the basis of type of injury, activity level, and nutritional status before injury.
- Consider patient's specific injuries when planning nutrition. For example, expect patients with hepatic or pancreatic injury to have difficulty with blood sugar regulation. Patients with trauma to the upper GI tract may be fed

enterally, but feeding tube must be placed distal to the injury. Disruption of the GI tract may require a feeding gastrostomy or jejunostomy. Patients with major hepatic trauma may have difficulty with protein tolerance.
- Ensure patency of gastric or intestinal tubes to maintain decompression and encourage healing and return of bowel function. Avoid occlusion of the vent side of sump suction tubes, because this may result in vacuum occlusion of the tube. Use caution when irrigating gastric or other tubes that have been placed in or near recently sutured organs.
- For additional information, see this diagnosis in "Major Trauma," p. 116.

NIC Electrolyte Management; Feeding; Nutrition Management; Nutrition Therapy; Tube Feeding

Body image disturbance related to creation of stoma (often without the patient's prior knowledge); mutilating physical injury

Desired outcomes: By the time of hospital discharge, patient acknowledges body changes, views and touches affected body part, and demonstrates movement toward incorporating changes into self-concept.
- Evaluate the patient's reaction to the stoma or missing/mutilated body part by observing and noting evidence of body image disturbance (see Table 1-40, p. 92).
- Anticipate feelings of shock and disbelief initially. Be aware that trauma patients usually do not receive the emotional preparation for ostomy, amputation, and other disfiguring surgery that the patient undergoing elective surgery receives.
- Anticipate and acknowledge normalcy of feelings of rejection and isolation (and uncleanliness in the case of fecal diversion).
- Offer patient opportunity to view stoma/altered body part. Use mirrors if necessary.
- Encourage patient and significant others to verbalize feelings regarding altered/missing body part.
- Offer patient the opportunity to participate in care of ostomy, wound, or incision.
- Confer with surgeon regarding advisability of a visit by an ostomate or a patient with similar alteration in body part.
- Be aware that most colostomies are temporary in persons with colonic trauma. This fact can be reassuring to the patient, but it is important to verify the type of colostomy with the surgeon before explaining this to the patient.

NIC Body Image Enhancement; Ostomy Care

ADDITIONAL NURSING DIAGNOSES

Also see "Major Trauma" for **Hypothermia,** p. 115, and **Posttrauma response,** p. 117. For additional information, see other diagnoses under "Major Trauma," as well as nursing diagnoses and interventions in the following sections, as appropriate: "Hemodynamic Monitoring," p. 28; "Prolonged Immobility," p. 74; "Psychosocial Support," p. 83; "Psychosocial Support for the Patient's Family and Significant Others," p. 95; "Peritonitis," p. 536; "Enterocutaneous Fistula," p. 549; "Septic Shock," p. 593; and "Arterial Blood Gas Monitoring," p. 671.

Burns

PATHOPHYSIOLOGY

Burns usually involve damage to the skin, but other major organ systems (e.g., cardiac—caused by electrical burn; pulmonary—caused by smoke inhalation) may be involved as well. The causative agent in burn injury may be thermal, electrical, chemical, or radiation. The burn agent, intensity and duration of exposure, location and depth of burn, percentage of body exposure, and the patient's age are factors in determining outcome.

TABLE 2-15 ABA Classification System

| Magnitude of burn injury | Partial thickness | | Full thickness adults and children (%BSA) | Special location* | Complications (poor risk, fractures, other trauma) |
	Adult (%BSA)	Children (%BSA)			
Major	>25%	>20%	>10%	+	+
Moderate	15%-25%	10%-20%	<10%	—	—
Minor	<15%	<10%	<2%	—	—

ABA, American Burn Association; *TBSA*, total body surface area.
*Hands, face, eyes, ears, feet, and/or genitalia.

Burns are categorized based on depth or magnitude. The longer and more intense the exposure to the burn agent, the greater the severity of burn depth and magnitude. A burn injury may be described as superficial, partial thickness, or full thickness, relative to the layer(s) of skin and tissues involved. Partial-thickness injuries are further differentiated into superficial and deep partial-thickness categories. *Superficial injury,* commonly referred to as "first-degree" burn (e.g., sunburn), damages the epidermis. These burns usually heal within 3-5 days. *Deep partial-thickness injury,* called a "second-degree" burn, involves varying levels of the dermis, which contain structures essential to skin function (e.g., sweat and sebaceous glands, hair follicles, sensory and motor nerves, capillary network). These burns heal within 14-21 days or longer, depending on depth. *Full-thickness injury,* a "third-degree" burn, exposes the poorly vascularized fat layer, which contains adipose tissue, roots of sweat glands, and hair follicles; these burns destroy all epidermal elements. Burn wounds may heal by granulation and migration of healthy epithelium from wound margins; if wound requires more than 2 weeks to heal, surgical excision may be required to improve functional and cosmetic outcomes; larger wounds are closed via skin grafting.

Electrical burn injuries often reveal only superficial injury on initial inspection, but extensive damage may occur to deep and underlying tissues, nerves, blood vessels, and muscles along the conduction path and at the electrical current exit site. Careful assessment is needed to determine the full extent of these injuries.

The American Burn Association (ABA) has developed an injury severity grading system that categorizes burns as minor, moderate, and major (Table 2-15). The ABA advocates that patients with major burns be treated in a burn center or facility with expertise in burn care. Moderate burns usually require hospitalization, although not necessarily in a burn unit, and minor burns often are treated on an outpatient basis.

Care for the patient with burn injury is provided in three stages, based on the pathologic changes that occur. The resuscitative period lasts from the time of injury to 48 h postburn. The second stage, the acute phase, begins with resolution of the fluid shift and continues until all wounds are closed or, in some agencies, until open wound areas are <10% of the total body surface area (TBSA). This stage can last from 3 days to a month or longer. The last stage, the rehabilitative stage, can continue for many years and seldom is a focus for critical care nurses, although early rehabilitative efforts such as patient and family teaching begin in critical care.

ASSESSMENT

History and risk factors: History of having been burned in a confined area predisposes to smoke inhalation injury. Preexisting cardiac or respiratory

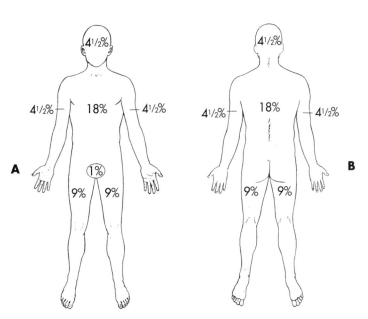

Figure 2-1: Estimation of adult burn injury: rule of nines. **A,** Anterior view. **B,** Posterior view.
From Thompson JM et al: *Mosby's clinical nursing,* ed 4, St Louis, 1997, Mosby.

condition and history of smoking increase susceptibility to respiratory complications. Patients with renal disease, diabetes, or preexisting cardiac, vascular, or respiratory conditions may have complications associated with fluid resuscitation therapy. History of compromised renal function, chronic cardio-vascular disease, diabetes mellitus, and collagen-vascular disease predispose to renal complications. Conditions such as immunosuppression, diabetes mellitus, invasive procedures, history of cardiopulmonary or vascular disease, and delayed antimicrobial therapy contribute to the likelihood of infection and may prolong healing.

General clinical presentation: The primary survey should include the basic *ABCDEFs*: *a*irway, *b*reathing, *c*irculation, *d*isability or neurologic deficit, *e*xposure and *e*valuation, and *f*luid resuscitation. The secondary survey includes a detailed head-to-toe assessment, exploration of the circumstances of the injury, and the patient's medical history. Evaluate severity according to percentage of body surface area burned, burn depth and location, potential for inhalation injury, and patient's age and past medical history.

The extent of the burn wound in adults is estimated quickly by means of the Berkow formula, commonly known as the *rule of nines* (Figure 2-1). For odd-shaped burns the surface area of the patient's palm usually equals 1% of the TBSA. A more accurate assessment tool is the Lund and Browder chart (Figure 2-2), which is more detailed and accounts for the changes in body parts according to age.

Respiratory system: Check for airway obstruction as a result of swelling caused by heat, smoke, or chemical injury to nasopharyngeal mucosa or by constriction around the neck or chest caused by eschar formation. Assess for singed nasal hairs, perioral burns, change in voice, or coughing, especially if

Relative percentages of areas affected by growth
(age in years)

	0	1	5	10	15	Adult
A: Half of head	9½	8½	6½	5½	4½	3½
B: Half of thigh	2¾	3¼	4	4¼	4½	4¾
C: Half of leg	2½	2½	2¾	3	3¼	3½

Second degree_____and
Third degree_____ =
Total percent burned___

Figure 2-2: Estimation of burn injury: Lund and Browder chart. Areas designated by letters *(A, B,* and *C)* represent percentages of body surface area that vary according to age. The accompanying table indicates the relative percentages of these areas in various stages of life.
From Sabiston DC, Jr, editor: *Textbook of surgery: the biological basis of modern surgical practice,* ed 11, Philadelphia, 1977, Saunders.

productive for soot. The lower respiratory tract can be damaged by contact with products of combustion and inhalation of vaporized caustic substances, such as sulfur, nitrogen, aldehydes, and hydrochloric acid. Damage may not appear immediately. Epithelial sloughing with bronchitis and respiratory distress occur 6-72 h postburn. Carbon monoxide (CO), a by-product of combustion, displaces oxygen from hemoglobin, resulting in hypoxia.
Clinical indicators: Include crackles, rhonchi, stridor, severe hoarseness, hacking cough, labored breathing, dyspnea, tachypnea, and possible altered LOC caused by hypoxia. Cherry-red skin coloring, headache, decreased visual acuity, tinnitus, vertigo, and convulsions may be signs of CO poisoning.

Note: Physical evidence of respiratory compromise may be absent initially, despite pulmonary injury. Progression to airway obstruction and acute respiratory distress can occur rapidly.

Cardiovascular system: Circulatory compromise secondary to burn injury results from fluid shifts, direct damage to the heart or blood vessels, obstruction of microcirculation, compression of blood vessels, and hemorrhage caused by clotting disorders. Increased capillary permeability caused by the inflammatory response results in a shift of intravascular fluid into the interstitial spaces. This causes a decrease in circulating volume and increased blood viscosity. Other systemic responses include increases in catecholamine, cortisol, renin-angiotensin, antidiuretic hormone (ADH), and aldosterone production as the body struggles to retain sodium and water to replenish intravascular fluid. Rapid fluid shifts can result in hemoconcentration and thrombus formation.

Clinical indicators: Signs of shock, such as thirst, pallor, dry mucous membranes, decreased LOC, and cool skin temperature; tachycardia, hypotension, and decreased filling pressures (CVP, PAP, PAWP); decreased or absent peripheral pulses and delayed capillary refill; impaired peripheral perfusion with possible obstruction caused by vascular compression with circumferential burns or thrombus formation; cardiac dysrhythmias caused by direct cardiac damage (electrical burns) and electrolyte imbalance (e.g., hyperkalemia caused by cellular hemolysis); and peripheral edema as a result of fluid shifts and hypoproteinemia. Muscle weakness caused by elevated fat mobilization from fatty acids and triglycerides, as well as by electrolyte imbalances, may occur with major burns.

Gastrointestinal system: Blood flow is shunted away from the GI tract, and peristalsis is slowed or stopped completely, causing paralytic ileus (usually resolves within 72 h after burn injury). Life-threatening stomach and intestinal ulceration and hemorrhage (associated with a gastric pH of ≤5) may occur. This condition is referred to as *Curling ulcer.*

Clinical indicators: Diminished or absent bowel sounds; presence of nausea and vomiting, possibly with hematemesis; abdominal distention caused by accumulated flatus.

Renal system: Hemoconcentration and reduced circulatory volumes result in decreased renal blood flow and low urinary output. A high myoglobin or hemoglobin load may be reflected by dark, concentrated urine. Continued poor renal perfusion can result in acute tubular necrosis and renal failure with buildup of metabolic waste products and electrolyte imbalances (see "Acute Renal Failure," p. 371).

Clinical indicators: Urine output <30 ml/h in adults and ≤0.5 ml/kg/h in children; dark, amber, "thick" urine.

Integumentary system: Loss of skin integrity results in fluid loss through evaporation, hypothermia, and increased risk of infection. Hypertrophic scar formation can result in contractures with limitations in extremity ROM. Keloids, an overgrowth of scar tissue most commonly found in individuals of dark pigmentation, may present a challenge to normal healing and require special treatment. Circumferential burns can cause constriction of underlying tissue, blood vessels, and muscles (see "Compartment Syndrome," p. 161) with circulatory compromise to underlying muscle.

Clinical indicators: Deep partial-thickness and full-thickness burn wounds of varied magnitude (Tables 2-16 and 2-17).

Invasive wound infection: Ongoing evaluation for wound sepsis is imperative, because sepsis is a serious and frequent complication. The larger the wound, the greater the risk for infection.

Clinical indicators: Rapid eschar separation, increased exudate, and pockets of purulent material. Disappearance of well-defined burn margins and presence of edema, discoloration, and superficial ulceration of burned skin at wound

TABLE 2-16   Burn Wound Classification

Degree of burn	Cause of injury	Depth of injury	Wound characteristics	Treatment course
First-degree burn	Prolonged ultraviolet light exposure; brief exposure to hot liquids	Limited damage to epithelium; skin intact	Erythematous, hypersensitive, no blister formation	Complete healing within 3 to 5 days without scarring
Superficial partial-thickness burn (second degree)	Brief exposure to flash, flame, or hot liquids	Epidermis destroyed; minimal damage to superficial layers of dermis; epidermal appendages intact	Moist and weepy, pink or red, blisters, blanching, hypersensitive	Complete healing within 21 days with minimal or no scarring
Deep partial-thickness burn (second degree)	Intense radiant energy; scalding liquids, semi-liquids (e.g., tar) or solids; flame	Epidermis destroyed; underlying dermis damaged; some epidermal appendages remain intact	Pale; decreased moistness; blanching absent or prolonged; intact sensation to deep pressure but not to pinprick	Prolonged healing (often longer than 21 days); may require skin grafting to achieve complete healing with better functional outcome
Full-thickness burn (third degree)	Prolonged contact with flame, scalding liquids; steam; hot objects; chemicals; electrical current	Epidermis, dermis, and epidermal appendages destroyed; injury through dermis	Dry, leatherlike; pale, mottled brown, or red; thrombosed vessels visible; insensate	Requires skin grafting
Full-thickness burn (fourth degree)	Electrical current; prolonged contact with flame (e.g. unconscious victim)	Epidermis, dermis, and epidermal appendages destroyed; injury involves connective tissue, muscle, and possibly bone	Dry; charred, mottled brown, white, or red; no sensation; limited or no movement of involved extremities or digits	Requires skin grafting; amputation of involved extremities or digits likely

From Carrougher GJ: Burn wound assessment and topical treatment. In Carrougher GJ: *Burn care and therapy*, St Louis, 1998, Mosby.

TABLE 2 - 17 Factors Determining Burn Severity

Criterion	Factors
Extent	Severity depends on intensity and duration of exposure
Depth	Severity depends on intensity and duration of exposure
Age	Patients <2 yr and >60 yr
Medical history	Preexisting conditions such as heart disease, chronic renal failure
Body part	Special burn areas: hands, face, eyes, ears, feet, and genitalia
Complications	Burns with concomitant trauma (e.g., fractures)

margin/skin interface are other indicators. Granulation tissue may become pale and boggy. Focal black, dark brown, or violet areas of discoloration may appear in the wound. Partial-thickness burn may advance to full-thickness. Vesicular lesions may appear in healing partial-thickness injury, and erythematous, nodular lesions may be present in unburned skin. In addition, there may be hemorrhagic discoloration of subeschar fat, cellulitis of unburned skin (common with gram-positive invasion); turquoise, sweet-smelling exudate (with *Pseudomonas* infection).

Signs of systemic/septic shock: Include tachycardia, tachypnea, decreased BP with low SVR, labile temperature, changes in LOC (confusion, disorientation, agitation), hyperglycemia, gastric distention, and paralytic ileus. (See "Septic Shock," p. 593.)

DIAGNOSTIC TESTS

Arterial blood gases: Early ABGs may be normal. Later studies show hypoxemia and metabolic acidosis.

Carboxyhemoglobin level: Determines presence of carbon monoxide in the blood secondary to smoke inhalation.

Pulse oximetry: For continuous monitoring of oxygenation. Probe placed on uninjured area. Not reliable in patients who are profoundly hypovolemic or in shock.

Serial chest x-rays: Usually normal on patient's admission; 24-48 h after injury may show atelectasis or increased lung water, reflecting fluid shifts, ARDS, or pulmonary edema in susceptible individuals.

Laryngoscopy and bronchoscopy: Not routine, but may help determine presence of extramucosal carbonaceous material and the state of the mucosa (e.g., edema, denudation, erythema, blistering) in inhalation injuries.

Culture and sensitivity studies: To evaluate sputum, blood, urine, and wound tissue for evidence of infection. Burn wound infection is defined as microorganisms 10^5/g of burn wound tissue with active invasion of adjacent, viable, unburned skin. Typical gram-negative organisms include *Pseudomonas aeruginosa, Klebsiella, Serratia, Escherichia coli,* and *Enterobacter cloacae.* Less frequently, gram-positive organisms *(Staphylococcus* and *Streptococcus)* and fungal pathogens *(Candida* and *Aspergillus)* may be present.

> **Note:** If a burn wound culture is positive for group A *Streptococcus* sp., this may signal the need for an epidemiologic investigation. Contact your facility's infection control department for assistance, especially if more than one patient is involved.

Urine specimen: Culture and sensitivities (C&S) performed for early detection of UTI. Urinalysis and 24-h urine collection for total nitrogen, urea nitrogen, creatinine, and amino acid nitrogen values may indicate return of capillary integrity (3-5 days postburn) and mobilization of third-space fluids, the degree of catabolism present, and the onset or resolution of acute renal failure. Myoglobinuria may be present as a result of muscle injury.

Hematology: Hct increased because of hemoconcentration. Hgb decreased secondary to hemolysis. WBC elevated because of systemic inflammatory response or sepsis.

Electrolytes: Sodium decreased secondary to massive fluid shifts into interstitial spaces. Potassium elevated because of cell lysis and fluid shifts. BUN elevated because of hypovolemic state, increased protein catabolism, or possible acute renal failure. Persistent elevation of BUN and creatinine signals inadequate fluid intake or acute renal failure. Total protein, albumin decreased secondary to leakage of plasma proteins into interstitial spaces. Creatine kinase (CK) is index of muscle damage; thus it is particularly important in electrical injuries. High CK levels indicate extensive muscle damage.

ECG: Myocardial damage secondary to electrical burn injury may be evident.

COLLABORATIVE MANAGEMENT

Humidified oxygen therapy: Treats hypoxemia and prevents drying and sloughing of the mucosal lining of the tracheobronchial tree. If patient is awake, oxygen by mask may be sufficient; intubation may be required if the patient is stuporous.

Intubation and mechanical ventilation: Indicated for respiratory distress or to maintain airway patency. Because laryngeal edema resolves in 3-5 days, tracheostomy is avoided for upper airway distress unless there is acute obstruction.

Bronchodilators and mucolytic agents: Aid in the removal of secretions.

Escharotomy and fasciotomy: Relieves respiratory distress secondary to circumferential, full-thickness burns of neck and trunk, or in extremities to lessen pressure from underlying edema and to restore adequate perfusion. It may be performed at the bedside or in the emergency room. Indications for escharotomy include cyanosis of distal unburned skin, delayed capillary filling, progressive neurologic changes (may mimic compartment syndrome), burns of thorax that restrict respiratory motion, and weak or absent peripheral pulses. See "Compartment Syndrome," p. 161, for more information.

Fluid resuscitation: Fluid replacement protocols are based on body weight and percentage of body surface area burned. Various formulas are used to estimate fluid requirements for burn patients during the acute phase of injury (Table 2-18). Colloids generally are avoided during the first 24 h after burn injury because increased capillary permeability causes leakage of protein into the interstitial tissues. In general, crystalloid fluids are used in the first 24 h, with small amounts of colloid fluids added during the second 24 h postinjury. The Parkland formula, which is most commonly used, recommends administration of 4 ml fluid/kg body weight/percentage body area burned. The first half of the calculated volume is infused over the first 8 h when fluid shifts are greatest. For example, if the patient was injured 2 h before arrival at the hospital and initial infusion of fluid, the first half of the calculated 24-h fluid need is infused over the next 6 h. The second half is then infused over the following 16 h.

> **Note:**   Calculate fluid infusion time from the time of injury, not the time of hospital admission. Fluid formulas should be modified, based on individual patient responses and needs. Patients with electrical injuries may have greater fluid needs than suggested by cutaneous injury. The presence of inhalation injury, ethanol intoxication, or crushing injuries also affects acute fluid requirements.

Indwelling urinary catheter: Essential for accurate measurement of urine output and evaluation of renal status.

TABLE 2-18 Adult Burn Resuscitation Formulas

Formula name	Recommended solutions	Formula for estimating fluid needs
Initial 24 h after injury		
Evans*	0.9% Normal saline plus	1 ml/kg/% TBSA burn
	colloid solution	1 ml/kg/% TBSA burn
Brooke*	Lactated Ringer's solution plus	1.5 ml/kg/% TBSA burn
	colloid solution	0.5 ml/kg/% TBSA burn
Hypertonic saline (Monafo)	Na^+ 250 mEq/liter	Volume to maintain urine output at 30 ml/hr
Modified Brooke*	Lactated Ringer's solution	2 ml/kg/% TBSA burn
Parkland*	Lactated Ringer's solution	4 ml/kg/% TBSA burn
Second 24 h after injury		
Evans	0.9% Normal saline plus	50% of first 24-h requirement
	5% dextrose in water	2000 ml
Brooke	Lactated Ringer's solution plus	50% to 75% of first 24-h fluid requirements
	5% dextrose in water	2000 ml
Hypertonic saline	33% Isotonic salt solution	0.6 ml/kg/% TBSA burn plus replacement of insensible losses
Modified Brooke	Colloid solution (diluted to physiologic concentration) plus	0.3-0.5 ml/kg/% TBSA burn (0.3 ml/kg/% TBSA burn for injuries of 30% to 50%; up to 0.5 ml/kg/% TBSA burn for injuries >50% TBSA)
	5% dextrose in water	Volume to maintain desired urine output
Parkland	25% Albumin plus	20% to 60% of calculated plasma volume
	5% dextrose in water	Volume to maintain desired urine output

From Gordon MD, Winfree JH: Fluid resuscitation after a major burn. In Carrougher GJ: *Burn care and therapy,* St Louis, 1998, Mosby.
TBSA, Total body surface area.
*The total estimated volume is calculated with one-half administered over the initial 8 hours after injury and the remaining half over the subsequent 16 hours.

Gastric suction: Allows aspiration of gastric contents, a necessary procedure because of the potential for paralytic ileus in patients with a ≥30% BSA burn or concomitant alcohol intoxication.
Tetanus-toxoid prophylaxis: Given intramuscularly to prevent tetanus. See Table 2-1.
IV morphine sulfate: Choice agent for pain management. It usually is

initiated as a large dose and then given in small increments as needed for comfort.

> **Note:** All medications, except tetanus toxoid, are administered intravenously to avoid sequestration of medication, which then would "flood" the vascular system with the return of capillary integrity and the diuresis of third-spaced fluids.

Antacids/histamine H_2-receptor antagonists: Maintain gastric pH >5, and prevent development of Curling ulcer. Early initiation of gastric tube feedings also helps to prevent Curling ulcer.

Dietary regimen: High metabolic activity and increased protein catabolism related to burn injury result in dramatic increases in energy requirements and nutritional needs. Energy requirements are estimated using one of several formulas based on body size and extent of burn with adjustment for age. Additional injury or poor preburn nutritional status may increase nutritional needs. The appropriate mix of protein, fat, and carbohydrates is controversial, but a positive nitrogen state has been achieved with patients who are administered high-protein, high-carbohydrate diets. Use of high-fat, low-carbohydrate diets has been suggested to facilitate weaning of patients from the ventilator, since increased CO_2 production results from high-carbohydrate loads. Oral, enteral, or central methods of delivery are used, based on patient tolerance. Enteral feedings are an inexpensive method of delivery that, if tolerated, may decrease GI acidity and ulcer formation. Central parenteral nutrition may be initiated for the patient with paralytic ileus or inability to tolerate an adequate amount of enteral feedings.

Multivitamin and mineral supplements: Vitamins A and C and zinc are especially important for promoting wound healing.

IV antibiotics: As indicated according to culture and sensitivity findings.

Wound care: Wound cleansing is accomplished with antibacterial surgical scrubs (e.g., chlorhexidine). Burns are débrided using manual, enzymatic, or surgical techniques. Topical antimicrobial agents such as silver sulfadiazine (Silvadene), mafenide (Sulfamylon), and silver nitrate control bacterial proliferation and promote tissue granulation.

Wound coverage and closure:

- Cutaneous autograft—include split-thickness skin graft (STSG) and cultured epithelial grafts
- Cutaneous allograft—fresh donor and cadaver
- Cutaneous xenograft—temporary closure usually porcine
- Amniotic graft
- Synthetic closure

NURSING DIAGNOSES AND INTERVENTIONS

Impaired gas exchange (or risk for same) related to smoke inhalation with tracheobronchial swelling and carbonaceous debris; competition of carbon monoxide (CO) with O_2 for hemoglobin; hypoventilation associated with circumferential burns to neck and thorax

Desired outcome: Within 1 h of treatment/intervention, patient exhibits adequate gas exchange as evidenced by Pao_2 ≥80 mm Hg; oxygen saturation ≥95%; RR 12-20 breaths/min with a normal pattern and depth (eupnea); absence of adventitious breath sounds and other clinical indicators of respiratory dysfunction; and orientation to time, place, and person.

- Assess and document respiratory status hourly, noting rate and depth, breath sounds, and LOC. Be alert to a declining respiratory status as evidenced by indicators of upper airway distress (e.g., severe hoarseness, stridor, dyspnea) and lower airway distress (e.g., crackles, rhonchi, hacking cough, labored or rapid breathing). Consult physician promptly for all significant findings.

- Administer humidified oxygen therapy, mechanical ventilation, or broncho-dilator treatment (i.e., theophylline, sympathomimetics) as prescribed.
- Monitor serial ABG values for decreasing Pao_2 and oxygen saturation and increasing $Paco_2$ as evidence of worsening hypoxemia. Also be alert to gradually declining values in vital capacity, tidal volume, and inspiratory force (see Table 3-1, p. 214).
- Place patient in high Fowler's position to enhance respiratory excursion.
- Teach patient the necessity of coughing and deep-breathing exercises q2h, including incentive spirometry.

NIC Airway Management; Respiratory Monitoring; Oxygen Therapy; Bedside Laboratory Testing; Cough Enhancement; Laboratory Data Interpretation

Ineffective airway clearance (or risk for same) related to increased secretions and inflammation and swelling of nasopharyngeal mucous membranes secondary to smoke irritation and impaired cough; compression of neck and chest cavity and decreased expansion of alveoli secondary to circumferential burns

Desired outcome: Patient has a clear airway within 10-30 min of treatment/intervention as evidenced by auscultation of normal breath sounds over the lung fields; a state of eupnea; and orientation to time, place, and person.

- Assess and document respiratory status hourly, noting breath sounds, rate and depth of respirations, and LOC. Be alert to a declining respiratory status as evidenced by crackles, rhonchi, stridor, labored breathing, dyspnea, tachypnea, restlessness, and decreasing LOC. Consult physician promptly for all significant findings.
- Assess and document character and amount of secretions after each coughing and deep-breathing exercise.
- Reposition patient from side to side q1-2h to help mobilize secretions; specialized rotation bed may be used.
- As prescribed, administer percussion and postural drainage to facilitate airway clearance (this is contraindicated with fresh skin grafts). Perform oropharyngeal or ET suctioning as indicated by the presence of adventitious breath sounds and the patient's inability to clear the airway effectively by coughing.

NIC Airway Management; Airway Suctioning; Artificial Airway Management; Aspiration Precautions; Cough Enhancement; Mechanical Ventilation

Fluid volume deficit related to active loss through the burn wound and leakage of fluid, plasma proteins, and other cellular elements into the interstitial space

Desired outcome: Within 24-48 h of this diagnosis, patient becomes normovolemic as evidenced by BP 110-120/70-80 mm Hg (or within patient's normal range); peripheral pulses >2+ on a 0-4+ scale; balanced I&O; urine output ≥0.5 ml/kg/h; and urine specific gravity 1.010-1.030.

- Monitor patient for evidence of fluid volume deficit, including tachycardia, decreased BP, decreased amplitude of peripheral pulses, urine output <0.5 ml/kg/h, thirst, and dry mucous membranes.
- Monitor I&O; administer fluid therapy using formula or as prescribed. Adjust infusion to maintain urine output at a minimum of 30-50 ml/h. Avoid colloids during first 24 h of burn injury.
- Monitor weight daily; report significant gains or losses. Recognize that weight loss also may be caused by catabolism and an increased metabolic rate as the body attempts to heal itself.
- Monitor urine specific gravity. An elevated value occurs with hypovolemia and reflects the need for additional volume.
- Monitor serial Hct, Hgb, serum sodium, and serum potassium values. As the circulating volume is restored, hemoconcentration is no longer present and Hct returns to within normal limits (WNL). Be aware that Hgb values may decrease secondary to hemolysis within the first 1-2 h after burn injury. Usually potassium is elevated during the first 24-36 h postburn because of hemolysis and other cellular lysis. After 72-96 h, hypokalemia may occur as cell membranes regain their integrity and the patient experiences diuresis. At

Research Brief 2-6   The effect of therapeutic touch on pain and anxiety in burn patients was explored. The McGill Pain Questionnaire, Visual Analogue Scales for Pain, Anxiety and Satisfaction With Therapy, and an Effectiveness of Therapy Form were used to determine if patients who were provided therapeutic touch and patients provided a sham form of therapeutic touch would report a difference in pain experienced or demonstrate a difference in pain medication usage or alteration in plasma T-lymphocyte concentration. Subjects receiving therapeutic touch reported a significantly greater reduction in pain on the McGill questionnaire and greater reduction in anxiety on the visual analogue scale for anxiety than those patients receiving sham therapeutic touch. A decreasing total $CD8^+$ lymphocyte concentration was noted for 11 subjects in the therapeutic touch group. There was no significant difference between groups on medication usage.

From Turner JG et al: *J Adv Nurs* 28(1):10-20, 1998.

this point it may be necessary to add potassium to the IV solutions. Consult physician for significant anemia or electrolyte imbalance.

- Monitor patient for evidence of fluid volume excess secondary to rapid fluid resuscitation, especially in patients with preexisting respiratory or cardiac disease. Be alert to crackles, SOB, tachypnea, and excessive urine output. Central hemodynamic monitoring is recommended for patients who have preexisting heart or lung disease.
- Confer with physician regarding use of mannitol to promote osmotic diuresis and prevent renal tubular sludging caused by myoglobinuria. Other diuretics are avoided because they further deplete an already compromised intravascular volume.
- With the onset of spontaneous diuresis, decrease infusion rates by 25% for 1 h as prescribed if the urine output is 30-50 ml/h for 2 consecutive hours. Continue to reduce rates gradually according to intake/output ratio and clinical status.

NIC Fluid/Electrolyte Management; Fluid Monitoring; Hypovolemia Management; Shock Prevention; Venous Access Devices Maintenance

Pain related to burn injury

Desired outcomes: Within 1 h of treatment/intervention, patient's subjective evaluation of discomfort improves as documented by a pain scale. Nonverbal indicators of discomfort are absent or diminished.

- Assess patient's level of discomfort at frequent intervals. Use a pain scale, asking patient to rate discomfort from 0 (no pain) to 10 (the most pain he or she could have). Patients with partial-thickness burns may experience severe pain because of exposure of sensory nerve endings. Pain tolerance decreases with prolonged hospitalization and sleep deprivation.
- Monitor patient for clinical indicators of pain: increased BP, tachypnea, dilated pupils (opiates may also dilate pupils), shivering, rigid muscle tone, or guarded position.
- Administer opioid analgesia and anxiolytics as prescribed. Time dosage for optimal effectiveness before painful procedures.
- Provide a full explanation of procedures and honest feedback, using a calm, organized, and firm manner.
- Employ nonpharmacologic interventions as indicated: relaxation breathing, guided imagery, therapeutic touch, soft music.
- Ensure that patient receives periods of uninterrupted sleep (optimally 90 min at a time) by grouping care procedures when possible and limiting visitors.
- See "Pain," p. 61, for additional information about pain management.

NIC Analgesic Administration; Anxiety Reduction; Environmental Management: Comfort; Pain Management

Impaired tissue integrity/Altered tissue perfusion: peripheral, related to thermal injury; circumferential burns; edema; hypovolemia

Desired outcomes: Patient's wound exhibits evidence of granulation and healing by primary intention or split-thickness skin grafting within an acceptable time frame. Tissue healing occurs without hypertrophic scarring.

> **Note:** Healing time varies with the extent of injury. Tissue perfusion in burned extremities is adequate as evidenced by peripheral pulses >2+ on a scale of 0-4+, brisk capillary refill (<2 sec), and skin temperature warm to the touch.

- Assess and document time and circumstances of burn injury, as well as extent and depth of burn wound (see Tables 2-15 and 2-16).
- In burned extremities, evaluate tissue perfusion by hourly monitoring of capillary refill, temperature, and peripheral pulses. Be alert to signs of decreased peripheral perfusion, including coolness of the extremity, weak or absent peripheral pulses, and delayed capillary refill. Immediately consult physician for evidence of impaired tissue perfusion, which could result in ischemia.
- Cleanse and débride wound as prescribed. Control ambient temperature carefully to prevent hypothermia.
- Apply topical antimicrobial treatments as prescribed, using aseptic technique.
- Elevate burned or recently grafted extremities at or above heart level to promote venous return and to prevent excessive dependent edema formation.
- To prevent pooling of fluid or seroma formation, which contributes to graft loss, express fluid between graft and recipient bed as prescribed by using a rolling motion with sterile applicators. Always roll the applicator in the same direction over the graft to prevent disruption of graft "take." If prescribed, aspirate hematomas or seromas with a tuberculin syringe and a 26-gauge needle.
- Monitor type and amount of drainage from wounds. Promptly report the presence of bright red bleeding, which would inhibit graft "take," and purulent exudate, which indicates infection.
- Maintain immobility of grafted site for 3 days or as prescribed. This is achieved with a combination of positioning, splinting, or light pressure and sedation. In some instances, restraints, stents, bulky dressings, or occlusive dressings may be required to maintain immobilization and promote hemostasis of graft.
- Apply elastic wraps to legs that have grafts to promote venous return.
- Use bed cradle to prevent bedding from coming in contact with burned or grafted area.
- Provide donor site care as prescribed, and be alert to signs of donor site infection (see **Risk for infection,** p. 207.)
- Apply compression netting to graft and incision sites. Teach patient about need for extended compression to prevent hypertrophic scarring.

NIC Infection Protection; Positioning; Wound Care

Altered tissue perfusion: gastrointestinal, related to hypovolemia and interruption in blood flow associated with splanchnic vasoconstriction secondary to fluid shifts and catecholamine release

Desired outcome: Patient has adequate GI tissue perfusion as evidenced by auscultation of 5-34 bowel sounds/min within 48-72 h after burn injury; bowel elimination and appetite within patient's normal pattern; and absence of nausea and vomiting.

> **Note:** Be aware that prolonged impaired perfusion to GI organs increases the likelihood of such complications as impaired gastric motility, adynamic ileus, gastritis, and Curling ulcer.

- Assess bowel function q2-4h. Be alert to abdominal distention and decreasing or absent bowel sounds, which occur with adynamic ileus.
- During period of absent bowel sounds, maintain gastric tube to intermittent low suction as prescribed. Check at intervals to ensure patency and position of the tube. Before removing tube, clamp for several hours to be certain patient has sufficient GI motility. Abdominal distention, nausea, vomiting, or return of a large volume of gastric contents when tube is reconnected indicates insufficient motility to tolerate tube removal.
- Maintain NPO status until return of bowel sounds. Provide mouth care for comfort and hygiene.
- Administer histamine H_2-receptor antagonists, antacids, and other agents prescribed to reduce formation of gastric acids. If prescribed, start enteral feedings to protect the patient's gastric mucosa from irritation.
- Test gastric aspirate for occult blood q8h. Promptly report presence of blood to physician.

NIC Gastrointestinal Intubation; Hemodynamic Regulation; Nutritional Management; Tube Care: Gastrointestinal

Altered nutrition: less than body requirements of protein, vitamins, and calories, related to hypermetabolic state secondary to burn wound healing

Desired outcome:　By the time of discharge from the critical care unit, patient has adequate nutrition as evidenced by stable weight; balanced nitrogen state per nitrogen studies; serum albumin ≥3.5 g/dl; thyroxine-binding prealbumin 20-30 mg/dl; retinol-binding protein 4-5 mg/dl; and evidence of burn wound healing and graft "take" within an acceptable time frame.

- Record all intake for daily calorie counts. Measure weight daily, and evaluate on the basis of patient's preburn weight.
- Monitor serum albumin, thyroxine-binding prealbumin, retinol-binding protein, and urine nitrogen measurements. Long periods of catabolism cause serum values to decrease. Be alert to measures of protein deficiencies, weight loss, and poor graft "take," all of which are signals that nutritional needs are not being met.
- Provide high-protein, high-calorie diet as prescribed. When patient can take foods orally, promote supplemental feedings of snacks such as milkshakes and ice cream between meals.
- Patients with burns >10% BSA, preinjury illness, or associated injuries have greatly increased calorie requirements and are likely to require nutritional supplements. Patients with ileus that persists for more than 4 days or those unable to meet caloric needs enterally will require TPN.
- Assess individual food preferences, and encourage those high in protein and carbohydrates. As appropriate, encourage family members to provide desired foods.
- For additional information, see "Nutritional Support," p. 1.

NIC Nutrition Management; Nutrition Therapy; Nutritional Monitoring; Weight Gain Assistance

Sensory/perceptual alterations: tactile and visual, related to altered reception secondary to medications, sleep pattern disturbance, pain, and altered dermal status

Desired outcomes:　Within 24-48 h of this diagnosis, patient verbalizes orientation to time, place, and person and describes rationale for necessary treatments.

- Assess patient's orientation to time, place, and person.
- Answer patient's questions simply and succinctly, providing information regarding immediate surroundings, procedures, and treatments. During the emergent phase of the burn injury, anticipate the necessity of having to repeat information at frequent intervals.
- For patient with full-thickness injury, explain why tactile sensation is decreased or absent and explain that it will return with eschar separation and débridement.

- If patient's eyelids are swollen shut because of facial edema, reassure patient that he or she is not blind and that swelling will resolve within 3-5 days.
- Touch patient often on unburned skin to provide nonpainful tactile stimulation.
- For additional information, see this nursing diagnosis in "Psychosocial Support," p. 83.

NIC Peripheral Sensation Management; Surveillance: Safety; Communication Enhancement: Visual Deficit; Environmental Management

Body image disturbance related to biophysical changes secondary to burn injury

Desired outcomes: Within 72 h of this diagnosis, patient begins to acknowledge body changes and demonstrates movement toward incorporating changes into self-concept. Patient does not exhibit maladaptive responses such as severe depression.

- Assess patient's perceptions and feelings about the burn injury and changes in life-style and relationships, especially those with significant others.
- Involve significant others in as much care as possible to maintain bond with patient.
- Respect patient's need to express anger over body changes.
- Provide information about cosmetic aids and use of clothing to help conceal burns.
- Praise patient's attempts to enhance appearance. Praise and encourage patient's expressed desires regarding public excursions after hospital discharge.
- Provide names and telephone numbers of support groups for burn patients.
- The American Burn Association, National Headquarters Office, 625 N. Michigan Avenue, Suite 1530, Chicago, IL 60611; URL: www.ameriburn. org; Phone: (800) 548-2876.

NIC Anxiety Reduction; Body Image Enhancement; Coping Enhancement; Grief Work Facilitation; Self-Esteem Enhancement; Support System Enhancement; Wound Care

- For additional information, see this nursing diagnosis, p. 92, and Table 1-40, p. 92.

Risk for disuse syndrome related to immobilization from pain, splints, or scar formation

Desired outcome: Patient displays complete ROM without verbal or nonverbal indicators of discomfort.

- Provide ROM exercises q4h while awake. When possible, combine with hydrotherapy.
- Apply splints as prescribed to maintain body parts in functional positions and to prevent contracture formation.
- For patient with graft, institute ROM exercises and ambulation on fifth postgraft day, or as prescribed. Premedicate with analgesic to aid mobility.

NIC Exercise Therapy: Ambulation; Exercise Therapy: Joint Mobility; Exercise Promotion; Nutrition Management; Positioning; Surveillance

Risk for infection related to inadequate primary and secondary defenses secondary to traumatized tissue, bacterial proliferation in burn wounds, presence of invasive lines or urinary catheter, and immunocompromised status

Desired outcome: Patient is free of infection as evidenced by normothermia; WBC count $\leq 11,000/mm^3$; negative culture results; well-defined burn wound margin; and absence of purulent matter and other clinical indicators of burn wound infection.

- Except for eyebrows, shave all hair within 5 cm of wound margin to prevent contamination of wound.
- Monitor temperature q2h. Report temperatures >38.8° C (102° F).
- Assess burn wound daily for status of eschar separation and granulation tissue formation, color, vascularity, sensation, and odor. Be alert to signs of infection, including fever, elevated WBC count, rapid eschar separation,

increased amount of exudate, pockets that contain purulent material, disappearance of a well-defined burn margin with edema formation, wound discoloration (e.g., black, dark brown), change in color of partial-thickness burn from pink or mottled red to full-thickness necrosis, superficial ulceration of burned skin at wound margins, pale and boggy granulation tissue, hemorrhagic discoloration of subeschar fat, and spongy and poorly demarcated eschar. Consult physician for significant changes.

- Assess appearance of grafted site, including adherence to recipient bed, appearance, and color. Be alert to erythema, hyperthermia, increasing tenderness, purulent drainage, and swelling around the grafted site.
- Observe for clinical indicators of sepsis: tachypnea, hypothermia, hyperthermia, ileus, subtle disorientation, unexplained metabolic acidosis, and glucose intolerance (see "Septic shock," p. 593). If sepsis is suspected, obtain wound, blood, sputum, and urine culture specimens.
- Administer antipyretic and antimicrobial agents as prescribed. Ensure aseptic technique when administering care to burned areas and performing invasive techniques. Rotate intravenous access sites at regular intervals.
- Practice Standard Precautions to reduce the risk of transmission of microorganisms. Consult the hospital's infection control professional to assist with placement of patients with infections if private rooms are not available.
- For patients with skin grafts, monitor donor site for evidence of infection, including purulent drainage, poorly defined borders, and foul odor.

NIC Environmental Management; Infection Control; Infection Protection; Surveillance; Wound Care; Shock Management

Knowledge deficit: self-care during the rehabilitative stage

Desired outcome: Within the 24-h period before discharge from the critical care unit, patient and significant others verbalize knowledge about prescribed medications and demonstrate and verbalize knowledge about techniques that facilitate continued wound healing and limb mobility.

- Review the splinting and exercise program for contracture prevention, as directed by physical therapist. Teach patient and significant others to monitor for pain or pressure caused by improperly applied splint and to assess splinted extremity for coolness, pallor, cyanosis, decreased pulses, and impaired function.
- Discuss skin care, emphasizing the following:
  - ☐ Explain that a lubricating cream without alcohol (e.g., Nivea) should be applied several times a day and after bathing to promote soft and pliant skin and assist with control of pruritus.
  - ☐ Explain that dressings or padding should be applied to areas that may be traumatized by pressure.
  - ☐ Teach patient to avoid exposure to sun, because healed skin is highly sensitive to ultraviolet rays for up to 1 year.
  - ☐ Explain to a darker-skinned patient that permanent pigmentation changes are likely to occur because of destruction of melanocytes and that burned areas usually will stay pink.
  - ☐ Review wound care. Provide simplified dressing change procedure; explain indicators of infection and importance of notifying physician should they appear.
  - ☐ Teach patient the importance of wearing pressure garment as prescribed to prevent excessive or hypertrophic scarring.
- Review nutrition needs: explain the importance of maintaining an adequate intake of protein and calories for optimal wound healing.
- Provide a list of medications, including drug name, purpose, dosage, schedule, precautions, and potential side effects.
- Discuss home care and the importance of counseling to provide support for adjustment to life outside the hospital environment after disfiguring injury.

- Provide addresses and telephone numbers of local support groups for burn patients.
- Stress the importance of follow-up care; confirm date and time of first appointment if it has been established.

NIC Learning Facilitation; Learning Readiness Enhancement; Teaching: Individual

ADDITIONAL NURSING DIAGNOSES

For other nursing diagnoses and interventions, see the following, as appropriate: "Nutritional Support," p. 1; "Mechanical Ventilation," p. 17; "Wound and Skin Care," p. 55; "Pain," p. 61; "Prolonged Immobility," p. 74; "Psychosocial Support," p. 83; "Psychosocial Support for the Patient's Family and Significant Others," p. 95; and "Infection Prevention and Control," Appendix 8.

Bibliography

Adams JE: Utility of cardiac troponins in patients with suspected cardiac trauma or after cardiac surgery, *Clin Lab Med* 17(4):613-623, 1997.

Alost T, Waldrop RD: Profile of geriatric pelvic fractures presenting to the Emergency Department, *Am J Emerg Med* 15(6):576-578, 1997.

American College of Surgeons: *Advanced trauma life support for doctors—first impression,* Chicago, 1997, ACS.

Ball JB, Morrison WL: Cardiac tamponade, *Postgrad Med J* 73:141-145, 1997.

Banning AP, Pillai R: Non-penetrating cardiac and aortic trauma, *Heart* 78:226-229, 1997.

Beachly M, Farrar J; Abdominal trauma: putting the pieces together, *Am J Nurs* 93(11):26-34, 1993.

Better OS, Rubinstein I: Management of shock and acute renal failure in casualties suffering from crush syndrome, *Ren Fail* 19(5):647-653, 1997.

Brain Trauma Foundation: Guidelines for cerebral perfusion pressure, *J Neurotrauma* 13(11):693-698, 1996.

Brain Trauma Foundation: Intracranial pressure threshold, *J Neurotrauma* 13(11):681-684, 1996.

Brain Trauma Foundation: Nutritional support of brain-injured patients, *J Neurotrauma* 13(11):721-730, 1996.

Brain Trauma Foundation: Resuscitation of blood pressure and oxygenation, *J Neurotrauma* 13(11):661-666, 1996.

Brain Trauma Foundation: The role of antiseizure prophylaxis following head injury, *J Neurotrauma* 13(11):731-734, 1996.

Brain Trauma Foundation: The role of glucocorticoids in the treatment of severe head injury, *J Neurotrauma,* 13(11):715-718, 1996.

Brain Trauma Foundation: The use of barbiturates in the control of intracranial hypertension, *J Neurotrauma* 13(11):711-714, 1996.

Brain Trauma Foundation: The use of hyperventilation in the acute management of severe traumatic brain injury, *J Neurotrauma* 13(11):699-704, 1996.

Brain Trauma Foundation: The use of mannitol in severe head injury, *J Neurotrauma* 13(11):705-710, 1996.

Crosby L, Parsons C: Cerebrovascular response of closed head-injured patients to a standardized endotracheal tube suctioning and manual hyperventilation procedure, *J Neurosci Nurs* 24(1):40-49, 1992.

Davis A, Briones T: Intracranial disorders. In Kinney M et al: *AACN Clinical Reference,* 685-709, St Louis, 1998, Mosby.

Davis A, Briones T: Neurological clinical physiology. In Kinney M et al: *AACN Clinical Reference,* 637-662, St Louis, 1998, Mosby.

Davis A, Hinkle J: *Constructing cerebral dynamic profiles.* (Manuscript in preparation, 2000.)

DeBoer S: Neurologic outcomes after near drowning, *Crit Care Nurse* 17(4):19-25, 1997.

Dillard TA, Grathwohl KW: Near drowning and diving accidents. In Baum GL et al, editors: *Textbook of pulmonary diseases,* ed 6, Philadelphia, 1998, Lippincott-Raven.

Estok L, Wallach F: Cardiac tamponade in a patient with AIDS: a review of pericardial disease in patients with HIV infection, *Mt Sinai J Med* 65(1):33-39, 1998.

Evans-Murray A: Adult respiratory distress syndrome after near drowning, *Crit Care Nurse* 17(2):41-44, 1997.

Fratianne RB, Brandt CP: Improved survival of adults with extensive burns, *J Burn Care Rehabil* 18:347-351, 1997.

Gennarelli T: The pathobiology of brain injury, *Neuroscientist* 3:73-80, 1997.

Goff CD, Collin GR: Management of renal trauma at a rural, level I trauma center, *Am Surg* 64(3):226-230, 1998.

Goldman SM et al: Blunt urethral trauma: a unified, anatomical mechanical classification, *J Urol* 157:85-89, 1997.

Gordon M, Goodwin CW: Initial assessment, management, and stabilization, *Nurs Clin North Am* 32(2):237-249, 1997.

Heath FR, Blum F, Rockwell S: Physical examination as a screening test for pelvic fractures in blunt trauma patients, *W V Med J* 93(5):267-269, 1997.

Hinkle J, Davis A: *Positioning effects on intracranial and cerebral perfusion pressures: an integrated review.* (Manuscript in preparation, 2000.)

Howard CA: Chest trauma. In Keen JH, Swearingen PL, editors: *Mosby's critical care nursing consultant,* St Louis, 1997, Mosby.

Howard CA: Flail chest. In Keen JH, Swearingen PL, editors: *Mosby's critical care nursing consultant,* St Louis, 1997, Mosby.

Howard CA: Near drowning. In Keen JH, Swearingen P, editors: *Mosby's critical care nursing consultant,* St Louis, 1997, Mosby.

Iowa Outcomes Project. Johnson M, Maas M, editors: *Nursing outcomes classification (NOC),* St Louis, 1997, Mosby.

Jordan BS, Harrington DT: Management of the burn wound, *Nurs Clin North Am* 32(2):251-271, 1997.

Kaiser L, DiPierro F: Thoracic trauma. In Fishman AP: *Fishman's pulmonary diseases and disorders,* New York, 1998, McGraw-Hill.

Kerr M, Lovasik D: Evaluating cerebral oxygenation using jugular venous oximetry in head injuries, *AACN Clin Issues Nurs* 6:11-20, 1995.

Kim MJ, McFarland GK, McLane AM: *Pocket guide to nursing diagnoses,* ed 6, St Louis, 1995, Mosby.

Kirby RR, Taylor RW, Civetta JM: Primary triage of the trauma patient. In Kirby RR, Taylor RW, Civetta JM: *Handbook of critical care,* ed 2, Philadelphia, 1997, Lippincott-Raven.

Kotkin L, Koch MO: Impotence and incontinence after immediate realignment of posterior urethral trauma: result of injury or management? *J Urol* 155:1600-1603, 1996.

MacLeod M, Powell JN: Evaluation of pelvic fractures: clinical and radiologic, *Orthop Clin North Am* 28(3):331-344, 1997.

Mbubaegbu CE, Stallard MC: A method of fasciotomy wound closure, *Injury* 27(9):613-615, 1996.

McCance KL, Huether SE: *Pathophysiology: the biologic basis for disease in adults and children,* ed 3, St Louis, 1998, Mosby.

McCloskey JC, Bulechek GM: *Nursing interventions classification (NIC),* ed 2, St Louis, 1996, Mosby.

McQueen MM, Court-Brown CM: Compartment monitoring in tibial fractures, *J Bone Joint Surg Br* 78-B(1):99-104, 1996.

Montgomery KD et al: Thromboembolic complications in patients with pelvic trauma, *Clin Orthop* 329:68-87, August, 1996.

Naranja RL Jr et al: Treatment considerations in patients with compartment syndrome and inherited bleeding disorder, *Orthopedics* 20(8):706-709, 1997.

Porter JM, Ivatury RR: Unwillingness to lie supine? A sign of pericardial tamponade, *Am Surg* 63:365-366, April, 1997.

Rogers FB, Leavitt BJ: Upper torso cyanosis: a marker for blunt cardiac rupture, *Am J Emerg Med* 15:275-276, 1997.

Saffle JR: Predicting outcomes of burns, *N Engl J Med* 338(6):387-389, 1998.

Shaw CJ, Spencer JD: Late management of compartment syndromes, *Injury* 26(9):633-635, 1995.

Spodick DH: Pathophysiology of cardiac tamponade, *Chest* 113:1372-1378, 1998.

St. John RE: Near drowning. In Alspach JG, editor: *American Association of Critical Care Nurses core curriculum for critical care nurses,* ed 5, Philadelphia, 1998, Saunders.

Swaanenburg JC et al: Troponin I, troponin T, CKMB-activity and CKMB-mass as markers for the detection of myocardial contusion in patients who experienced blunt trauma, *Clinica Chimica Acta* 272:171-181, 1998.

Taffet R: Management of pelvic fractures with concomitant urologic injuries, *Orthop Clin North Am* 28(3):389-396, 1997.

Turner JG et al: The effect of the therapeutic touch on pain and anxiety in burn patients, *J Adv Nurs* 28(1):10-20, 1998.

Williams A, Coyne S: Effects of neck position on intracranial pressure, *Am J Crit Care* 2(1):68-71, 1993.

Winfree, J, Barillo, DJ: Nonthermal injuries, *Nurs Clin North Am* 32(2):275-287, 1997.

CHAPTER 3

Respiratory Dysfunctions

Status asthmaticus

PATHOPHYSIOLOGY

Status asthmaticus (SA) is a severe, life-threatening bronchospasm that critically diminishes the diameter of the patient's airway. The hyperreactive bronchial airways respond to a variety of irritants with diffuse narrowing as a result of bronchospasm and bronchial inflammation, causing mucosal edema, increased mucus production, and plugging. When an episode of bronchospasm is not reversed after 24 h of maximal doses of traditional beta- (β-) agonist and theophylline therapy, the patient is diagnosed with SA. Precipitating factors include allergens (airborne or ingested), respiratory infection, chemical irritants (e.g., smoke, air pollution), physical irritants (e.g., cold air, exercise), and, in some individuals, emotional stress. Although the attack can happen suddenly, onset is usually more gradual, with symptoms of increased sputum production, coughing, wheezing, and dyspnea occurring over several days. The patient experiences increased work of breathing, which increases insensible water loss through exhaled water vapor and diaphoresis. Oral intake may be decreased, which contributes further to the hypovolemia. Mucus becomes thick and begins to plug the airways. Terminal bronchioles become occluded completely from mucosal edema and tenacious secretions. Ventilation-perfusion mismatch occurs as poorly ventilated alveoli continue to be perfused. Shunting of blood from nonventilated alveoli to other alveoli cannot compensate for the diminished ventilation, and hypoxia occurs. Tachypnea and tachycardia evolve as compensatory mechanisms. As a result, oxygen requirements and work of breathing increase. If the patient is not treated promptly, respiratory collapse can occur and death by asphyxiation is possible.

ASSESSMENT

Clinical presentation: Coughing, chest tightness, increased sputum production, increased respiration rate (RR) (>20 breaths/min), labored breathing, dyspnea, fatigue, insomnia, anorexia, restlessness, and confusion.

Physical assessment: Agitation, use of accessory muscles of respiration, chest retractions, nasal flaring, diaphoresis, decreased tactile fremitus and hyperresonance over lung areas in which there is air trapping, and dullness over

Research Brief 3-1 The purpose of this study was to compare arterial oxygen saturation as measured by pulse oximetry with standard arterial blood gas analysis. A meta-analysis of 74 studies from 1976 to 1994 was conducted. Results of the analysis supported that pulse oximeters are accurate within 2%-5% and that finger probes give more accurate readings than ear probes.

From Jensen LA, Onyskiw JE, Prasad NGN: Meta-analysis of arterial oxygen saturation monitoring by pulse oximetry in adults, *Heart Lung* 27(6):387-408,1998.

areas of atelectasis. Expiratory wheezing, prolonged expiratory phase, and coarse rhonchi may be auscultated. In addition, the patient may have hypotension, pulsus paradoxus >10 mm Hg, and apical tachycardia (HR >100 beats per minute [bpm]). Cyanosis of the lips and nail beds is a late sign of respiratory compromise.

Note: An absence of wheezing in the presence of other signs and symptoms of respiratory distress may be a result of severe bronchial constriction, which dangerously narrows airways during both inspiratory and expiratory phases. The volume of air moved through the airways is so minimal that it does not cause a sound. If this occurs, respiratory collapse may be imminent.

DIAGNOSTIC TESTS

Arterial blood gas (ABG) analysis: Evaluates status of oxygenation and acid-base balance. Initially, Pao_2 is normal and then decreases as the ventilation-perfusion mismatch becomes more severe. Usually, $Paco_2$ is decreased in early stages of SA because of hyperventilation. When $Paco_2$ is normal or greater than normal, respiratory failure may be imminent because of relative hypoventilation.

Pulse oximetry (Spo_2): Noninvasive technology that measures the oxygen saturation of arterial blood, which then can be displayed continuously. Pulse oximetry uses red and infrared wavelengths of light to calculate arterial saturation based on the difference between light transmitted and light absorbed by the red blood cells (RBCs). Correlation of peripheral oxygen saturation values measured by oximetry with arterial saturation (Sao_2) is within 2% when Sao_2 is >50%. Factors that may affect the oxyhemoglobin dissociation curve (temperature, pH, $Paco_2$, anemia, hemodynamic status) may adversely affect the accuracy of pulse oximetry measurements. Also, the presence of other forms of Hgb in the blood (carboxyhemoglobin, a byproduct of smoking and smoke, or methemoglobin, which is formed by the use of drugs such as lidocaine and nitroglycerin) can produce falsely high readings. Normal reading is ≥90%. When initiating pulse oximetry, it is helpful to obtain ABG values to compare Pao_2 and evaluate $Paco_2$ and pH.

Pulmonary function testing: Forced expiratory volume (FEV) is decreased during acute episodes because severely narrowed airways prevent forceful exhalation of inspired volume (Table 3-1).

Chest x-ray: Useful in ruling out other causes of respiratory failure (e.g., foreign body aspiration, pulmonary edema, pulmonary embolism, pneumonia). The x-ray usually shows lung hyperinflation caused by air trapping and a flat diaphragm related to increased intrathoracic volume.

Sputum: Gross examination may show increased viscosity or actual mucous plugs. Culture and sensitivity may show microorganisms if infection is the precipitating event.

Complete blood cell count (CBC): Differential will show increased eosinophils in patients not receiving corticosteroids, which is indicative of inflammatory response. The hematocrit (Hct) may be increased because of hypovolemia and hemoconcentration.

TABLE 3-1   Pulmonary Function Tests in Status Asthmaticus

Test	Description	Normal values	Parameters in SA
FVC	Total amount of gas exhaled as forcefully and rapidly as possible after maximal inspiration	≥80% of predicted normal	Normal or slightly decreased because of air trapping
FEV_1	Volume of gas exhaled over first second of FVC	≥75% of predicted normal	Decreased because of obstruction; may return to normal after inhalation of aerosolized bronchodilator
FEF	Average rate of flow during middle half of FEV; an accurate estimate of airway resistance	≥80% of predicted normal	Decreased because of small airways obstruction; may return to normal after inhalation of aerosolized bronchodilator

SA, Status asthmaticus; *FVC*, forced vital capacity; *FEV₁*, forced expiratory volume in 1 sec; *FEF*, forced expiratory flow.

Serum theophylline level: Important baseline indicator for patients who are on this therapy regimen. Acceptable therapeutic range is 10-20 µg/ml The therapeutic level is close to the toxic level, and the patient must be monitored for side effects (e.g., nausea, nervousness, dysrhythmias). Serial levels are drawn at frequent intervals.

Electrocardiogram (ECG):   Presence of sinus tachycardia is an important baseline indicator, because the use of some bronchodilators (e.g., metaproterenol) may produce cardiac stimulant effects and dysrhythmias.

COLLABORATIVE MANAGEMENT

Respiratory failure in SA is relative to the increased work of breathing and increased minute ventilation requirements. Primarily, management is directed toward decreasing bronchospasm and increasing pulmonary ventilation. Other interventions are directed toward treatment of sequelae.

Oxygen therapy: Generally, patients with SA have profound hypoxia and can tolerate high doses of oxygen (4-8 L/min). However, if the patient has chronic carbon dioxide (CO_2) retention, he or she may not tolerate >2-3 L/min oxygen, since higher doses might impair the drive to breathe, which in patients with chronic obstructive pulmonary disease (COPD) is a hypoxic drive. Oxygen therapy is begun immediately to correct hypoxemia, and the Pao_2 is kept above normal to compensate for the increased oxygen demands imposed by the increased work of breathing. The oxygen is humidified to help liquefy secretions. The degree of hypoxemia and patient response determine the method of oxygen delivery. The patient may prefer a nasal cannula, but a high-flow system delivers more precise and higher Fio_2. Comfort, however, is important, especially if the patient will not wear a mask because of feelings of suffocation.

Intubation and mechanical ventilation: Elected if $Paco_2$ continues to rise, if Pao_2 falls to <60 mm Hg, or if patient experiences intolerable respiratory distress. Therapy ensures adequate alveolar ventilation and provides a pathway for clearing airway secretions via suctioning. See discussion, p. 17.

Pharmacotherapy: Vigorous therapy is initiated to improve bronchospasm. Treatment is continued until wheezing is eliminated and pulmonary function tests return to baseline.

Bronchodilators: Dilate smooth muscles of the airways (Table 3-2).

Corticosteroids: Given intravenously during the acute phase of SA to decrease the inflammatory response. Dosage varies according to severity of episode and whether patient currently is taking steroids.

> **Note:** Acute adrenal insufficiency can develop in patients who take steroids routinely at home if these drugs are not given to the patient during hospitalization.

Anticholinergics: Atropine may have some bronchodilator effect in patients with mild to moderate asthma, but it is not as effective as a β-adrenergic bronchodilator. Atropine and quaternary ammonium compounds are available for administration by nebulizer and do show additive effects when used in combination with β-adrenergic agonists.

Sedatives and tranquilizers: Generally avoided unless patient is extremely agitated and unable to cooperate with therapy, inasmuch as these agents depress the central nervous system (CNS) response to hypoxia and hypercapnia.

Buffers: Metabolic acidosis may develop as a compensatory mechanism for early respiratory alkalosis during which patient is hyperventilating and exhaling greater-than-normal amounts of CO_2. Sodium bicarbonate may be given to correct severe metabolic acidosis. The physiologic response to bronchodilators improves with correction of metabolic acidosis.

Antibiotics: Given if infectious pulmonary process is suspected, as evidenced by fever, purulent sputum, or leukocytosis.

Fluid replacement: To liquefy secretions and replace insensible losses. Generally, crystalloid fluids (e.g., D_5W, D_5NS) are used.

Chest physiotherapy: Generally contraindicated in acute phases of SA because of acute respiratory decompensation and hyperreactive airways. Once the crisis is over, the patient may benefit from percussion and postural drainage q2-4h to help mobilize secretions.

NURSING DIAGNOSES AND INTERVENTIONS

Impaired gas exchange related to altered oxygen supply secondary to decreased alveolar ventilation present with narrowed airways

Desired outcomes: Within 2-4 h of initiation of treatment, patient has adequate gas exchange as evidenced by Pao_2 >60 mm Hg; $Paco_2$ 35-45 mm Hg; and pH 7.35-7.45 (or ABG values within 10% of patient's baseline). Within 24-48 h of initiation of treatment, RR is 12-20 breaths/min with normal depth and pattern (eupnea) and breath sounds are clear and bilaterally equal.

- Observe for signs and symptoms of hypoxia (e.g., restlessness, agitation, changes in level of consciousness [LOC]). Remember that cyanosis of the lips and nail beds is a late indicator of hypoxia.
- Auscultate breath sounds at frequent intervals. Monitor for decreased or adventitious sounds (e.g., wheezes, rhonchi).
- Position patient for comfort and to promote optimal gas exchange. Usually this is accomplished by high Fowler's position, with the patient leaning forward and elbows propped on the over-the-bed table to promote maximal chest excursion. Record patient's response to positioning.

T A B L E   3 - 2   Bronchodilators Used in Status Asthmaticus

Medication	Usual dosage	Action	Side effects
Epinephrine	0.2-0.5 ml of 1:1000 solution given SC q15-30min	Immediate adrenergic effects; activates adrenergic sympathomimetic receptors; acts on alpha-, $beta_1$-, and $beta_2$-receptors; relieves bronchospasm	Cardiac stimulation, palpitations, anxiety
Terbutaline (Brethine)	0.2-0.3 ml given SC q30min × 3 doses	Selective beta-adrenergic; relaxes bronchial smooth muscle	Fewer than with epinephrine and usually transient; increased HR (>120 bpm), nervousness, tremor, palpitations, nausea, vomiting, headache
Methylxanthines (theophylline, aminophylline)	*Loading dosage:* 6 mg/kg given as IV bolus. **Note:** Loading dose may be omitted if the patient is already taking oral methylxanthine and serum level is therapeutic *Maintenance dosage:* 0.1-0.5 µg/kg/h given via continuous IV infusion	Short-acting nonadrenergic; directly relaxes smooth muscle of bronchial airways and pulmonary vasculature	Nausea, vomiting, GI bleeding, gastric distress, HR >120 bpm, decreased BP, restlessness. **Note:** Toxic levels are close to therapeutic levels; serum levels should be monitored closely; theophylline toxicity may cause dysrhythmias

Note: Isoproterenol and isoetharine are two inhalants usually avoided during acute status asthmaticus because the patient's gas flow may be too minimal to provide adequate distribution of medication. Aerosolized drugs (e.g., albuterol, Proventil) may be used once other routes achieve bronchodilation.

SC, Subcutaneous; *IV,* intravenous; *HR,* heart rate; *bpm,* beats per minute; *GI,* gastrointestinal; *BP,* blood pressure.

- Encourage patient to breathe slowly and deeply. Teach pursed-lip breathing technique to assist patient with controlling his or her respirations:
  1. Inhale through the nose.
  2. Form lips in an "O" shape as if whistling.
  3. Exhale slowly through pursed lips.
- Record patient's response to breathing technique. Educate significant others in coaching.
- Deliver oxygen as prescribed; monitor Fio_2 to ensure that oxygen is within prescribed concentrations.
- Monitor ABG and pulse oximetry values. Be alert to decreasing Pao_2 and increasing $Paco_2$ or decreasing O_2 saturation levels, which are signals of respiratory failure.

Ineffective airway clearance related to presence of increased tracheobronchial secretions; decreased ability to expectorate secondary to fatigue
Desired outcome: Within 24-48 h of initiating treatment, patient's airway is free of excess secretions as evidenced by eupnea and absence of adventitious breath sounds and excessive coughing.

- At frequent intervals, assess patient's ability to clear tracheobronchial secretions. Keep emergency suction equipment at the bedside.
- Encourage oral fluid intake within patient's prescribed limits to help decrease viscosity of the secretions.
- Encourage patient to cough effectively at frequent intervals to clear secretions:
  1. Instruct patient to take several deep breaths. Instruct significant others in coaching this technique.
  2. After the last inhalation, teach patient to perform a succession of coughs (usually three to four) on the same exhalation until most of the air has been expelled.
  3. Explain that patient may need to repeat this technique several times before the cough becomes productive.
- After crisis phase of SA has been resolved, ensure that patient receives chest physiotherapy as prescribed; document patient's response to treatment. If appropriate, teach significant others to perform chest physiotherapy.
- Ensure that oxygen is humidified to aid in liquefying tracheobronchial secretions.

Activity intolerance related to imbalance between oxygen supply and demand secondary to decreased alveolar oxygen supply and greater metabolic oxygen demands caused by increased work of breathing
Desired outcome: Within 24-48 h of initiation of treatment, patient verbalizes a decrease in fatigue and associated symptoms.

- Organize and group assessment procedures and activities to provide patient with frequent rest periods (optimally, at least 90-120 min).
- Teach patient progressive muscle relaxation technique (see **Health-seeking behavior,** p. 302). Teach significant others how to coach patient in using relaxation techniques.
- Decrease metabolic demands for oxygen by limiting or pacing patient's activities and procedures.
- If patient is restless, which increases oxygen demand, ascertain the cause of the restlessness (e.g., if restlessness is related to anxiety, help reduce anxiety by providing reassurance, enabling family members to stay with patient, and offering distractions such as soft music or television). Be aware that restlessness may be an early sign of hypoxemia.
- Explain all procedures and offer support to minimize fear and anxiety, which can increase oxygen demands.
- Schedule rest times after meals to avoid competition for oxygen supply during digestion.
- Monitor Spo_2 by pulse oximetry during activity to evaluate limits of activity and recommend optimal positions for oxygenation.

Research Brief 3-2   The investigators assessed the impact of an evidence-based multidisciplinary asthma pathway on patient outcomes and expenses. Data were collected over a 6-month period and included demographics about the patients, as well as health-related information such as peak expiratory flow rates, pulse oximetry measurements, and length of stay (LOS). Nineteen patients were placed into the study group and were placed on the pathway. Twenty-three patients were not treated according to the pathway, and thirty-eight patients were in the historical control group. The results showed that, although there was not a significant reduction in LOS, use of the pathways was associated with a significant increase in conversion from nebulizer treatments to metered-dose inhaler use, resulting in a substantial cost savings.

From Bailey R et al: Impact of clinical pathways and practice guidelines on the management of acute exacerbations of bronchial asthma, *Chest* 113(1):28-33, 1998.

- Assess temperature q2-4h. Consult physician for increases, and provide treatment as prescribed to decrease temperature and thus oxygen demands.

You may also wish to refer to the following interventions from the Nursing Interventions Classification (NIC):

 Acid-Base Management; Acid-Base Monitoring; Airway Management; Anxiety Reduction; Bedside Laboratory Testing; Cough Enhancement; Emotional Support; Energy Management; Fluid Management; Fluid Monitoring; Laboratory Data Interpretation; Oxygen Therapy; Positioning; Respiratory Monitoring; Vital Signs Monitoring

ADDITIONAL NURSING DIAGNOSES

Also see "Acute Pneumonia" for **Risk for infection** (nosocomial pneumonia), p. 218. For other nursing diagnoses and interventions, see "Psychosocial Support," p. 83, and "Psychosocial Support for the Patient's Family and Significant Others," p. 95.

Acute pneumonia

PATHOPHYSIOLOGY

Pneumonia is an acute infection that causes inflammation of the parenchyma (alveolar spaces and interstitial tissue) of the lung. As a result of the inflammation, the involved lung tissue becomes swollen and the air spaces fill with liquid. Pneumonias can be classified into two groups: community acquired and hospital associated (nosocomial). Pneumonias that occur in the immunocompromised host can be acquired in the community or can be associated with hospitalization. The infecting organisms are often distinctive in this population and will be described separately. (See Table 3-3 for a detailed discussion by pneumonia type.)

Community acquired: Persons with this type of pneumonia seldom require hospitalization and are generally seen in intensive care areas only when an underlying medical condition such as COPD, cardiac disease, diabetes mellitus, or an immunocompromised state necessitates special care.

Hospital associated (nosocomial):   These pneumonias often occur after aspiration of oropharyngeal flora in an individual whose resistance is altered or whose coughing mechanisms are impaired (e.g., artificial airway, thoracoabdominal surgery). Bacteria invade the lower respiratory tract via four routes: aspiration of oropharyngeal organisms (most common route); inhalation of aerosols that contain bacteria; contamination of caregiver's hands or respiratory equipment; or hematogenous spread to the lung from another site of infection (rare). Alteration of oropharyngeal flora frequently occurs in

Text continued on p. 223

TABLE 3 - 3 Assessment Guidelines by Pneumonia Type

Type/pathogen	Risk groups	Onset	Defining characteristics	Complications/comments
Community acquired				
Pneumococcal (*Pneumococcus pneumoniae*, *Streptococcus pneumoniae*)	Persons >40 yr, especially males. Risk increases with alcoholism and debilitating diseases (e.g., COPD, heart failure, multiple myeloma, sickle cell disease). Viral upper respiratory tract infections often precede this pneumonia.	Abrupt	Single shaking chill, fever, pleuritic chest pain, severe cough, SOB, rust-colored sputum, and diaphoresis. Many patients also have herpes labialis, abdominal pain and distention, and paralytic ileus.	Pleural effusions, empyema, impaired liver function, bacteremia, and meningitis. Incidence of pneumococcal pneumonia peaks in winter and early spring. Mortality rate increases if more than one lobe is involved.
Mycoplasma (*Mycoplasma pneumoniae*)	School-age children to young adult (5-30 yr). Intrafamilial spread is common.	Gradual	Cough, sore throat, fever, headache, chills, malaise, anorexia, nausea, vomiting, diarrhea. In children, arthralgia involving the large joints is common.	Rare. Persistent cough and sinusitis are possible. Pulse-temperature dissociation is common.
Legionnaires (*Legionella pneumophila*)	Middle-age, elderly (males at increased risk) populations; smokers; individuals with malignancy, immunosuppression, or chronic renal failure; exposure to contaminated construction site.	Abrupt	Malaise, headache within 24 h, fever with normal HR, shaking chills, progressive dyspnea, cough that may become productive; GI symptoms, including anorexia, vomiting, diarrhea; arthralgia, myalgia.	Respiratory failure, hypotension, shock, acute renal failure.

COPD, Chronic obstructive pulmonary disease; *SOB*, shortness of breath; *HR*, heart rate; *GI*, gastrointestinal.

Continued

TABLE 3-3   Assessment Guidelines by Pneumonia Type—cont'd

Type/pathogen	Risk groups	Onset	Defining characteristics	Complications/comments
Community acquired—cont'd				
Viral influenza A	Elderly persons with chronic diseases (e.g., COPD, diabetes mellitus, heart failure); pregnancy.	1 wk after onset of influenza symptoms	Severe dyspnea, cyanosis, scant sputum occasionally with blood, fever, persistent and dry cough.	Rapid course leading frequently to acute respiratory failure; secondary bacterial pneumonia.
Haemophilus influenzae	Adults (especially ≥50 yr of age) with chronic diseases (e.g., diabetes mellitus, COPD, chronic alcohol ingestion).	2-6 wk after URI	Fever, chills, dyspnea, cough, nausea, vomiting, pain.	Fever may be minimal or absent; HR and RR may be normal.
Nosocomial				
Klebsiella (*Klebsiella pneumoniae*) (also may be acquired in the community), *Enterobacter, Serratia*	Males >40 yr of age, chronic disease (e.g., diabetes mellitus, COPD, chronic alcohol ingestion, heart disease); those previously treated with antibiotics or ET intubation.	Abrupt	Chills, fever, productive cough (copious, purulent, green or "currant jelly" sputum). Severe pleuritic chest pain, dyspnea, cyanosis, jaundice, vomiting, and diarrhea.	Lung abscess and empyema, necrotizing pneumonitis with cavitation, acute respiratory failure. High mortality rate (up to 50%). Aspiration of oropharyngeal flora believed responsible for many nosocomial and community-acquired cases.

Organism	Risk factors	Onset	Signs and symptoms	Comments
Pseudomonas (also may be acquired in the community)	Patients neutropenic from chemotherapy or immunosuppressed secondary to cortisone therapy or other illnesses.	Gradual	Fever, chills, confusion, delirium, bradycardia, purulent sputum (green, foul smelling).	Rarely occurs in previously healthy adults; high mortality rate.
Proteus	Older adults with debilitating underlying diseases.	Abrupt	High fever, chills, pleuritic chest pain.	Rare. Localizes to areas that already are damaged. Occurs as a mixed infection; has four pathogenic species with differing antibiotic susceptibilities.
Staphylococcus aureus, methicillin-resistant *Staphylococcus aureus* (MRSA)	Patients with debilitating diseases (e.g., diabetes mellitus, renal failure, liver disease, COPD); prior viral influenza infection; IV drug abusers.	Abrupt with community acquired; insidious with hospital associated.	Cough, chills, high fever, pleuritic pain, progressive dyspnea, cyanosis, bloody sputum.	Pulmonary abscesses, empyema, pleural effusions; slow response to antibiotics.
Aspiration of gastric contents	Patients with impaired gag/cough reflexes; general anesthesia; presence of NG/ET tube.	Gradual: latent period between aspiration and onset of symptoms.	Fever, wheezes, crackles (rales), rhonchi, dyspnea, cyanosis.	Physiologic response depends on pH of material aspirated: ≥2.5, little necrosis occurs; <2.5, atelectasis, pulmonary edema, hemorrhage, and necrosis can occur.

Continued

URI, Upper respiratory infection; *RR,* respiratory rate; *ET,* endotracheal; *IV,* intravenous; *NG,* nasogastric.

TABLE 3 - 3   Assessment Guidelines by Pneumonia Type—cont'd

Type/pathogen	Risk groups	Onset	Defining characteristics	Complications/comments
Immunocompromised patient				
Pneumocystis (*Pneumocystis carinii*)	Patients with AIDS or organ transplants.	Insidious	Several weeks of fever, nonproductive cough, night sweats, dyspnea; hypoxemia with few auscultatory signs.	Bronchoscopy with transbronchial biopsy usually required for diagnosis.
Aspergillosis (*Aspergillus*)	Patients with AIDS, COPD, and transplants (especially autologous bone marrow transplant); also those receiving cytotoxic agents or steroids.	Abrupt with immunosuppression; insidious with COPD.	High fever; fungal ball within lung cyst or cavity; nonproductive cough; pleuritic chest pain.	Cavitation frequently occurs; hematogenous spread common in immunocompromised patients.

AIDS, Acquired immunodeficiency syndrome.

debilitated hospitalized patients, especially those receiving antibiotics. Gram-negative pneumonias are associated with a high mortality, even with appropriate antibiotic therapy. *Aspiration pneumonia* is a nonbacterial cause of hospital-associated pneumonia that occurs when gastric contents are aspirated. If the alveolar-capillary membrane is affected, acute respiratory distress syndrome (ARDS) may develop.

Immunocompromised patient: Immunosuppression and neutropenia are predisposing factors in the development of nosocomial and community-acquired pneumonias, from both common and unusual pathogens. Usually, patients with neutropenia resulting from acute leukemia or cytotoxic agents have gram-negative bacilli as the source of pneumonia. Severely immunocompromised patients are affected not only by bacteria but also by fungi (*Candida, Aspergillus*), viruses (*Cytomegalovirus*), and protozoa (*Pneumocystis carinii*). Most commonly, *P. carinii* is seen in patients with HIV disease or in those who have received organ transplants.

ASSESSMENT

Findings are influenced by the patient's age, extent of the disease process, underlying medical condition, and pathogen involved.

Risk factors: In addition to the risk factors listed in Table 3-3, any factor that alters the integrity of the lower airways, thereby inhibiting ciliary activity, increases the likelihood of pneumonia. These factors may include hypoventilation, hyperoxia (increased Fio_2), hypoxia, airway irritants such as smoke, and the presence of an artificial airway.

Clinical presentation: Cough (productive and nonproductive), sputum (rust colored, purulent, bloody, or mucoid), fever, pleuritic chest pain (more common in community-acquired bacterial pneumonias), dyspnea, chills, headache, myalgia. The older adult may be confused or disoriented and run low-grade fevers but initially may have few other signs and symptoms.

Physical assessment: Presence of nasal flaring and expiratory grunt, use of accessory muscles of respiration, restricted chest expansion caused by pleuritic pain, dullness to percussion, tachypnea (respiratory rate [RR] >20 breaths/min), tachycardia (heart rate [HR] >100 bpm), decreased or bronchial breath sounds (absent if severe), high-pitched and inspiratory crackles (increased by or heard only after coughing), and low-pitched inspiratory crackles caused by airway secretions.

DIAGNOSTIC TESTS

ABG analysis: Hypoxemia (Pao_2 <80 mm Hg) and hypocapnia ($Paco_2$ <35 mm Hg), with a resultant respiratory alkalosis (pH >7.45), will be seen in the absence of an underlying pulmonary disease. In severe cases the $Paco_2$ can be <35 mm Hg because CO_2 elimination may be affected.

Pulse oximetry (Spo_2): O_2 saturation will be diminished. See description, p. 213.

CBC: White blood cell (WBC) count will be increased (>11,000/mm^3) in the presence of bacterial pneumonias. Normal or low WBC count will be seen with viral or mycoplasma pneumonias.

Sputum for Gram stain and culture and sensitivity tests: Sputum culture should be obtained from the lower respiratory tract before initiation of antimicrobial therapy. The most reliable specimens are obtained via transtracheal aspiration, bronchoscopy, or open-lung biopsy. Expectorated sputum specimens may not originate from the lower airways and are therefore unreliable. Pleural effusion fluid may also be cultured.

Blood culture and sensitivity: Secondary bacteremia is a frequent finding, and blood cultures help aid in identification of the causative organism.

Diagnostic fiberoptic bronchoscopy: Performed to obtain specimen for the purpose of diagnosing microorganism responsible for infection. Two diagnostic techniques (protected specimen brush [PSB] and bronchoalveolar lavage

[BAL]) make it possible to obtain specimens during simple bronchoscopy without contaminating the aspirate.

Serologic studies: Acute and convalescent titers are drawn to diagnose viral pneumonia. Rises in antibody titers are a positive sign for viral infection.

Acid-fast stain: To rule out mycobacterial infection (e.g. tuberculosis).

Chest x-ray: To identify anatomic involvement, extent of disease, and presence of consolidation, pleural effusions, and cavitation:
- ☐ *Lobar:* Entire lobe involved
- ☐ *Segmental (lobular):* Only parts of a lobe involved
- ☐ *Bronchopneumonia:* Affects alveoli contiguous to the involved bronchi

COLLABORATIVE MANAGEMENT

Oxygen therapy: Administered when ABG values demonstrate presence of hypoxemia. Special care must be taken not to abolish the drive to breathe if patient has a chronic lung disorder and is known to retain CO_2. Initially, in patients with chronic CO_2 retention, oxygen is delivered in low concentrations while closely monitoring ABG levels. If Pao_2 does not rise to acceptable levels (e.g., >60 mm Hg), Fio_2 is increased in small increments, with concomitant ABG checks or monitoring via pulse oximetry.

Intubation and mechanical ventilation: Intubation may be necessary if patient is unable to maintain a patent airway because of tenacious or copious secretions, ineffective cough, or fatigue. Mechanical ventilation is required if patient is unable to maintain adequate ABG values (Pao_2 >60 mm Hg) with supplemental oxygen. High concentrations of oxygen and positive end-expiratory pressure (PEEP) may be necessary in severe cases of pneumonia that lead to acute respiratory failure.

Pharmacotherapy

Antibiotics: Prescribed empirically on the basis of presenting signs and symptoms, clinical findings, and chest x-ray results until sputum or blood culture results are available. Erythromycin is the most commonly used antibiotic in community-acquired pneumonia. Antimicrobial therapy in critically ill patients usually is parenteral and guided by sensitivity of the causative organism. Many of the organisms responsible for nosocomial pneumonias are resistant to multiple antibiotics. Proper identification of the organism, determination of antibiotic sensitivity, and attainment of therapeutic drug levels are critical for effective therapy.

Antipyretics and analgesics: To reduce temperature and provide relief for pleuritic pain. Patients with pneumonia may have significant pleuritic pain that requires administration of opioid analgesics for relief. When opiates (e.g., codeine, morphine sulfate, meperidine) are given, varying degrees of respiratory depression occur. Careful and frequent monitoring of the patient's respiratory rate and depth, as well as oxygen saturation, via pulse oximetry is necessary.

Hydration: Intravenous (IV) fluids may be necessary to replace fluids lost from insensible sources (e.g., tachypnea, diaphoresis with fever).

Isolation: Some patients with pneumonia may require isolation and Transmission-Based Precautions (see "Infection Prevention and Control," Appendix 8).

Percussion and postural drainage: Indicated if deep breathing, coughing, and moving about in bed or ambulation are ineffective in raising and expectorating sputum.

NURSING DIAGNOSES AND INTERVENTIONS

Risk for infection (nosocomial pneumonia) related to inadequate primary defenses (e.g., decreased ciliary action); invasive procedures (e.g., intubation); chronic disease

Desired outcome: Patient is free of infection as evidenced by normothermia; WBC count within normal limits for patient; and sputum clear to white in color.

- Perform good hand-washing procedure before and after any patient contact (even though gloves were worn). Use special care with patient with tracheostomy or intubation. Inform visitors of effective precautions or pertinent isolation procedures.
- Identify presurgical candidate who is at increased risk for nosocomial pneumonia: age >70 yr; obesity; diabetes mellitus; COPD; history of smoking; abnormal pulmonary function tests (especially decreased forced expiratory flow rate); tracheostomy; prolonged intubation; abdominal or thoracic surgery.
  - ☐ Before surgery, provide patient and significant others with verbal and written instructions and demonstrations of turning, coughing, and deep-breathing exercises to perform after surgery to prevent respiratory tract infection. Make sure the patient verbalizes knowledge of the exercises and their rationale and *returns* the demonstrations appropriately.
  - ☐ Be aware that most patients can expand their lungs effectively after surgery but will not do so unless they are encouraged. At frequent intervals, encourage lung expansion: deep breathing; coughing if secretions are present; turning in bed; and walking (may not be possible in critical care). In addition, use of incentive spirometry promotes periodic, voluntary lung expansion greater than tidal volume. Educate significant others to encourage these activities.
  - ☐ If pain interferes with lung expansion, control it by administering prn analgesics ½ h before deep-breathing exercises and providing support of wound areas with hands or pillows placed firmly across site of incision.
  - ☐ For patients who cannot remove secretions effectively by coughing, perform procedures that stimulate coughing such as chest physiotherapy, which includes breathing exercises, postural drainage, and percussion.
  - ☐ If the patient has an endotracheal or tracheostomy tube, provide a fast, deep breath with a manual resuscitator to stimulate the cough receptors.
- Identify patients who are at high risk for aspiration: individuals who have a depressed LOC or dysphagia or who have a gastric tube in place.
- For patient with depressed LOC, consult physician regarding need for a method of feeding in which risk of aspiration is minimal (e.g., small-bore, weighted feeding tube that migrates to the duodenum; total parenteral nutrition [TPN]; or gastrostomy).
- For patient with a gastric tube in place, turn onto right side rather than back during feeding and provide continuous, rather than bolus, feedings. Elevate head of bed (HOB) to at least 30 degrees during feedings and for 1 h after any feeding or medication.
- Recognize the following ways in which nebulizer reservoirs can contaminate patient: introduction of nonsterile fluids or air; manipulation of nebulizer cup; or backflow of condensate into reservoir or into patient when delivery tubing is manipulated.
- Use only sterile fluids, and dispense them aseptically.
  - ☐ Replace (rather than replenish) solutions and equipment at frequent intervals (e.g., empty reservoir completely and refill with sterile solution q8-24h, according to agency protocol).
  - ☐ Change breathing circuits at regular intervals; if used for multiple patients, replace breathing circuit with sterilized or disinfected breathing circuit between patients.
  - ☐ Fill fluid reservoirs immediately before use.
  - ☐ Discard any fluid that has condensed in tubing; do not allow it to drain back into reservoir or into patient.
- Recognize risk factors for patients with tracheostomy or endotracheal (ET) tubes: presence of underlying lung disease or other serious illness;

colonization of oropharynx or trachea by aerobic gram-negative bacteria; greater access of bacteria to lower respiratory tract; and cross-contamination as a result of manipulation of these tubes.

☐ Employ "no-touch" technique or use sterile gloves on both hands until tracheostomy wound has healed or formed granulation tissue around the tube.

- Suction on an "as needed" rather than a routine basis, inasmuch as frequent suctioning increases the risk of trauma and cross-contamination. Consider use of an in-line suction device to reduce the risk of infection or contamination.
- Always wear gloves on both hands when suctioning to protect against transmission of the herpes simplex virus (HSV) from the patient's oral secretions; transmission of HSV into openings in the skin (e.g., a hangnail) can cause herpetic whitlow.

Risk for fluid volume deficit related to increased insensible loss secondary to hyperventilation, fever, and use of supplemental oxygen; reduced fluid intake
Desired outcome: Patient is normovolemic as evidenced by no clinical evidence of hypovolemia (such as furrowed tongue); stable weight; blood pressure (BP) within patient's normal range; central venous pressure (CVP) 2-6 mm Hg; pulmonary artery pressure (PAP) 20-30/8-15 mm Hg; cardiac output (CO) 4-7 L/min; mean arterial pressure (MAP) 70-105 mm Hg; HR 60-100 bpm; and systemic vascular resistance (SVR) 900-1200 dynes/sec/cm^{-5}.

- Monitor I&O hourly. Initially, intake should exceed output during volume replacement therapy. Consult physician for urine output <0.5 ml/kg/h for 2 consecutive hours.
- Monitor VS and hemodynamic pressures for signs of continued hypovolemia. Be alert to decreased values in BP, CVP, PAP, CO, and MAP, as well as increased HR and SVR.
- Weigh patient daily, at the same time of day (preferably before breakfast) on a balanced scale, with the patient wearing the same type of clothing.
- Administer fluids by mouth (PO) and IV as prescribed. Document patient's response to replacement therapy.
- Monitor for signs and symptoms of fluid overload or too-rapid fluid administration: crackles (rales); shortness of breath (SOB); tachypnea; tachycardia; increased CVP; increased pulmonary artery (PA) pressures; neck vein distention; and edema.

NIC Chest Physiotherapy; Cough Enhancement; Electrolyte Management; Electrolyte Monitoring; Environmental Management; Fluid/Electrolyte Management; Fluid Management; Fluid Monitoring; Hypovolemia Management; Infection Control; Intravenous Insertion; Intravenous Therapy; Nutrition Management; Positioning; Surveillance; Vital Signs Monitoring

ADDITIONAL NURSING DIAGNOSES

Also see "Near Drowning" for **Impaired gas exchange,** p. 139. See "Status Asthmaticus" for **Ineffective airway clearance,** p. 217, and **Activity intolerance,** p. 217. As appropriate, see nursing diagnoses and interventions in "Nutritional Support," p. 1; "Mechanical Ventilation," p. 17; "Prolonged Immobility," p. 74; "Psychosocial Support," p. 83; and "Psychosocial Support for the Patient's Family and Significant Others," p. 95.

Pulmonary hypertension

PATHOPHYSIOLOGY

Pulmonary hypertension is defined as a mean pulmonary artery pressure (MPAP) >20 mm Hg. Primary pulmonary hypertension (also known as *idiopathic* or *unexplained pulmonary hypertension*) occurs as a complication of disorders in pulmonary circulation such as recurrent pulmonary embolism or

T A B L E   3 - 4   Etiologic Factors in the Development of Pulmonary Hypertension

Cause	Clinical examples
Congenital heart disease with left-to-right shunt	Ventricular septal defect, atrial septal defect, patent ductus arteriosus
Congenital heart disease with diminished pulmonary blood flow	Tetralogy of Fallot, transposition of the great vessels
Obstruction to pulmonary venous outflow (congenital and acquired)	Mitral valve disease, left ventricular failure, stenosis of large pulmonary veins, portal hypertension
Pulmonary embolism	Thrombotic embolism, fat embolism
Chronic alveolar hypoxia	High-altitude hypoxia, COPD, obstructive sleep apnea, obesity (hypoventilation syndrome), neuromuscular disease processes
Diffuse pulmonary fibrosis	Lupus erythematosus, systemic sclerosis, sarcoidosis, idiopathic interstitial fibrosis

COPD, Chronic obstructive pulmonary disease.

vasoconstriction, and symptoms are characteristic of pulmonary vascular disease. Secondary pulmonary hypertension occurs as a result of complications of other underlying disorders such as chronic hypoxia secondary to COPD (see Table 3-4 for a discussion of etiologic factors).

Rising pulmonary artery pressure (PAP) increases pulmonary vascular resistance (PVR), which in turn causes two responses in the vasculature: standby vessels open to increase the surface area available for perfusion; and the capillaries distend to accommodate the increased blood flow. Although these responses reduce PVR initially, the system eventually fails if the increased pressure becomes chronic as a result of vasoconstriction that occurs in response to chronic alveolar hypoxia. Whereas most of the vascular system responds to hypoxia by dilating in an effort to increase blood flow to vital organs, the pulmonary vasculature responds to alveolar hypoxia by vasoconstriction, a beneficial mechanism that shunts blood away from underventilated areas in the lungs to better ventilated areas, thereby improving oxygenation. This regional mechanism is not strong enough to correct the ventilation/perfusion imbalance, however. Generally, Pao_2 decreases to ≤ 60 mm Hg before vasoconstriction occurs; the lower the Pao_2, the more severe the vasoconstriction.

The rise in PAP and the resulting increase in PVR from acute hypoxia are completely reversible after the hypoxia has been resolved. In the presence of chronic hypoxia, however, the pulmonary vasculature undergoes permanent changes (i.e., hypertrophy, hyperplasia), causing thickening of the vessel and narrowing of the lumen. In addition, polycythemia develops as a compensatory mechanism to increase oxygen transport; this condition increases blood viscosity, which in turn increases PVR.

The functions of the heart and lungs are interdependent. Increased PVR stimulates the right ventricle to increase the pumping force to maintain adequate cardiac output. The right ventricle dilates and hypertrophies under the constant strain and workload. Eventually, the right side of the heart weakens and is unable to accommodate venous blood returning to the heart. As a result, pressure in the systemic venous circulation increases, causing cor pulmonale, or right-sided heart failure. See "Right Ventricular Heart Failure/Pulmonary Edema," p. 265, for further discussion of right-sided heart failure.

ASSESSMENT
Because the low-resistance pulmonary vascular bed is clinically silent until late in the disease process, onset is insidious.

Clinical presentation

Early indicators: Hyperventilation, vague chest discomfort.

Late indicators: Tachypnea, dyspnea, orthopnea, chest congestion.

Physical assessment: Cyanosis of the lips and nail beds, edema of the hands and feet, anasarca (generalized, massive edema), distended jugular veins, right ventricular heave (visible left parasternal systolic lift), accentuated pulmonary component of the second heart sound, right ventricular diastolic gallop, pulmonary ejection click, distant breath sounds, basilar crackles.

Hemodynamic measurements: MPAP will be >20 mm Hg. Normally, PAP ranges from 8-15 mm Hg during diastole to 20-30 mm Hg during systole.

DIAGNOSTIC TESTS

ABG values: Will vary but are important to the differential diagnosis of the cause of pulmonary hypertension. Generally, Pao_2 will be <60 mm Hg, whereas $Paco_2$ will be within normal limits (35-45 mm Hg) unless COPD is the cause of the pulmonary hypertension, in which case $Paco_2$ is usually elevated.

Chest x-ray: Will confirm anatomic abnormalities associated with chronic right ventricular failure (right ventricular dilation or hypertrophy), enlarged pulmonary artery secondary to increased pressure, and diminished diaphragmatic excursion.

ECG: May show right-axis deviation, right bundle-branch block, and enlarged P waves.

Echocardiography: May reveal enlarged right atrium and right ventricle, diminished wall motion, and pulmonic valve malfunction (midsystolic closure or delayed opening).

Pulmonary function tests: Also important for the differential diagnosis of the underlying pathologic condition; will vary according to cause. For normal values, see Table 3-1.

Pulmonary angiography and perfusion scans: To rule out an embolic event as the underlying cause.

Hemodynamic monitoring: Pressures in the pulmonary vasculature are measured by way of the flow-directed pulmonary artery (e.g., Swan-Ganz) catheter. Data will differentiate or quantify the contribution of the left or right ventricular failure and measure the response to pharmacotherapy.

Open-lung biopsy: Usually avoided unless the cause of pulmonary hypertension cannot be diagnosed by less invasive studies. Data obtained from biopsy specimen may establish the type of pulmonary vascular disease and assess extent of the disease process.

RBC/Hct values: May be increased above normal.

COLLABORATIVE MANAGEMENT
The goal of medical management is to diagnose and treat the underlying disorder or process causing the pulmonary hypertension. Treatment is directed primarily toward increasing myocardial contractility or reducing right ventricular afterload caused by the high pulmonary vascular resistance.

Oxygen therapy: By eliminating hypoxia, pulmonary vascular vasoconstriction is reduced, which in turn may reduce right ventricular afterload.

Pharmacotherapy

Diuretics: Reduce circulating volume via loss of sodium and water, which may decrease PAP and right ventricular workload. In turn, this reduces leftward septal bulging seen with right ventricular overload.

Digitalis: Generally used only with biventricular failure. Otherwise, the

inotropic effects of digitalis can increase cardiac output and pulmonary resistance, which are deleterious in the presence of right ventricular failure. *Bronchodilators (e.g., aminophylline, isoproterenol, terbutaline):* Act as afterload reducers by decreasing pulmonary vascular resistance and increasing right ventricular ejection fraction. By improving gas exchange, bronchodilators may decrease hypoxic vasoconstriction of the pulmonary vascular bed.
Vasodilators (e.g., nitrates, hydralazine, calcium channel blockers, prostaglandins E_1 and I_2): Reverse pulmonary vasoconstriction, which will reduce right ventricular afterload and enhance pulmonary blood flow.

NURSING DIAGNOSES AND INTERVENTIONS

> **Note:**   See "Status Asthmaticus" for **Activity intolerance,** p. 217. Refer to "Heart Failure/Pulmonary Edema," p. 265, for nursing diagnoses and interventions related to the care of patients with heart failure. See "Near Drowning" for **Impaired gas exchange,** p. 139. As appropriate, see nursing diagnoses and interventions in "Prolonged Immobility," p. 74; "Psychosocial Support," p. 83; and "Psychosocial Support for the Patient's Family and Significant Others," p. 95.

Acute respiratory distress syndrome

PATHOPHYSIOLOGY

Acute respiratory distress syndrome (ARDS) is an often fatal condition, with a mortality approaching 60%. Although ARDS often is a result of a direct injury to the lung resulting from trauma or infection, it is more likely to occur as a sequela to an indirect insult to the lung. In either case, the hallmark of ARDS is multisystem organ failure and sepsis. Although the cause of ARDS is not understood completely, the site of injury is the alveolar-capillary membrane. Normally this membrane is permeable only to smaller molecules, such as water and electrolytes. The balance of the forces of hydrostatic pressure (pushing) and osmotic pressure (pulling) keeps fluids in their proper place and maintains the interstitium and alveoli in a relatively dry state. All of the etiologic factors that lead to the development of ARDS (see "History and Risk Factors," p. 229) cause an increase in the permeability of the alveolar-capillary membrane, either by altering hydrostatic or osmotic pressure or by injuring the alveolar epithelium or capillary endothelium. This enables the passing of larger molecules (e.g., albumin, globulin) across the membrane. Essentially, this altered permeability leads to a leaky membrane and an accumulation of protein-rich fluid in the interstitial and intraalveolar spaces, interfering with gas exchange at this critical level. As the leak grows larger, the interstitium, alveoli, and terminal airways become filled with fluid, blood, and protein. Surfactant activity is reduced, either because the cell producing the surfactant is destroyed or because the surfactant is inactivated. The alveoli tend to collapse and resist reexpansion in the absence of surfactant. Gas exchange no longer can occur, and these areas become a mass of interstitial and alveolar edema, hemorrhage, and focal atelectasis. Ventilation-perfusion mismatching, with resultant hypoxia, occurs as areas of the lung are perfused but not ventilated. Arterial oxygen tension (Pao_2) begins to fall, there is an increase in the shunt fraction (the amount of blood returning to the arterial system without passing through ventilated regions of the lung), and physiologic dead space increases. The patient becomes fatigued as the work of breathing increases in response to ever-stiffening lungs, and respiratory failure is possible.

ASSESSMENT

History and risk factors: Trauma, hemorrhagic shock, gram-negative sepsis, sepsis with disseminated intravascular coagulation (DIC), inhalation of toxic substances, severe pneumonitis, aspiration of gastric contents, near drowning, air or fat embolus, acute pancreatitis, postperfusion cardiopulmonary bypass, oxygen toxicity, drug overdose, neurologic injury, immunosuppression, and massive blood transfusion.

Clinical presentation: Will vary, depending on the pathophysiology contributing to the ARDS. The following are general early and late indicators. The goals are to diagnose ARDS in the early stages when treatment is much less complex and the patient is less critically ill and to reduce additional insults to the respiratory and other organ systems.

Early indicators: Dyspnea, restlessness, hyperventilation, cough, increased work of breathing, chest clear on auscultation.

Late indicators: Cyanosis, pallor, grunting respirations, adventitious breath sounds, rapid and shallow breathing, intercostal-suprasternal retractions, tachypnea, tachycardia, diaphoresis, mental obtundation.

DIAGNOSTIC TESTS

ABG analysis: Essential to the diagnosis of ARDS. Refractory hypoxemia is a key indicator (decreasing Pao_2 that is unresponsive to increasing Fio_2). Initially, the pH is above normal (>7.45) because the patient hyperventilates and exhales greater-than-normal levels of CO_2. As ARDS worsens, the pH falls below 7.35 because of respiratory acidosis, which may be further complicated by metabolic acidosis resulting from the anaerobic metabolism induced by hypoxia.

Pulse oximetry: Used for continuous monitoring of oxygenation (see discussion, p. 213).

Mixed venous oxygen saturation (Svo_2): Svo_2 is a more sensitive indicator of oxygen available for tissue oxygenation. Normal values range from 60%-80%. A value <50% is associated with impaired tissue oxygenation.

Serial chest x-rays: May be normal in the early stages. As ARDS progresses, the lung shows bilateral diffuse infiltrates. In later stages, few air spaces may be left in the lung—a condition that gives the lung a completely white appearance on x-ray.

Pulmonary function tests: Static and dynamic lung compliance will be decreased. Lung volumes also will be decreased, particularly functional residual capacity (FRC).

Hemodynamic monitoring: Measurements of pulmonary artery wedge pressure (PAWP) are important to the differential diagnosis. PAWP is normal in ARDS, but high (>12 mm Hg) in cardiogenic pulmonary edema. ARDS is sometimes referred to as *noncardiogenic pulmonary edema*. PAWP is a more sensitive indicator of fluid balance than is CVP and is obtained at frequent intervals in conjunction with fluid therapy.

Tracheal-protein/plasma-protein ratio: A relatively new diagnostic tool used to differentiate between cardiogenic and noncardiogenic pulmonary edema (ARDS). It compares total protein in tracheal aspirate with total protein in plasma. Ratio in cardiogenic pulmonary edema is <0.5, whereas the ratio in ARDS generally is >0.7.

Lactic acid level: Lactic acid is a byproduct of anaerobic metabolism and will accumulate in the serum in the presence of hypoxemia. The presence of arterial lactate contributes to acidosis.

$P(A-a)o_2$:   Alveolar-arterial oxygen tension difference or A-a gradient. Normally, it increases approximately 4 mm Hg with each decade of life. The value is greatly increased above the baseline in ARDS and reflects the intrapulmonary shunting that occurs secondary to alveolar flooding.

QS/QT: Ratio of shunt to cardiac output. Measures intrapulmonary shunting. Normal physiologic shunt is 3%-4%; may increase to 15%-20% with ARDS.

COLLABORATIVE MANAGEMENT

The goals for management are threefold: first, maintenance of adequate arterial oxygenation and pulmonary ventilation; next, treatment of the underlying pathophysiologic condition that caused the ARDS; third, therapy is initiated aimed at treating the lung injury.

Oxygen therapy: Goal is to provide acceptable Pao_2 levels (>60 mm Hg) with Fio_2 ≤0.50, but Fio_2 up to 1.00 may be necessary.

Mechanical ventilation: Indicated if the patient cannot receive adequate oxygen with acceptable concentrations of Fio_2 (≤0.50). Mechanical ventilation is indicated for nearly all patients with ARDS because decreased lung compliance significantly increases work of breathing and the increase in physiologic dead space causes a compensatory increase in ventilatory requirements. The goal of mechanical ventilation is to preserve arterial oxygen saturation while preventing complications of increased airway pressures and/or high concentration of oxygen.

Positive end-expiratory pressure: Used in conjunction with mechanical ventilation, PEEP or other means of maintaining positive airway pressure to allow better arterial oxygenation (Pao_2) with administration of lower levels of inspired oxygen tension (Fio_2). It also increases functional residual capacity by recruiting or maintaining open alveoli that are otherwise collapsed. High pressures (5-20 cm H_2O) are mechanically maintained at the end of the expiratory cycle, allowing alveoli to remain open and thus participate in gas exchange. For a more complete discussion of PEEP, see p. 18 in "Mechanical Ventilation."

Corticosteroids: Although use of steroids is controversial and their efficacy is not well established, short-term, high-dose corticosteroids may be useful in stabilizing the alveolar-capillary membrane to prevent further deterioration.

Fluid therapy: Primary goal is to maintain a minimal PAWP to provide adequate cardiac output. Usually, the patient's fluid volume is kept slightly depleted to minimize leakage of excess fluids into the interstitium through damaged capillary membrane. The use of crystalloid versus colloid fluids is controversial. Both types of fluid have been shown to leak across the alveolar-capillary membrane. Generally, colloids are reserved for those patients with hypoalbuminemia and crystalloids are used for all other patients.

Sedation: Most patients require sedation with medication such as morphine sulfate or anxiolytics. Those patients who are not able to cooperate with mechanical ventilation may be placed under heavy sedation with agents such as propofol (Diprivan) or paralyzed with a neuroblocking agent such as vecuronium bromide (Norcuron). The caregiver must recognize that, although the paralyzed patient may appear comatose, he or she may be alert and extremely anxious because of the total lack of muscle control. These patients must receive appropriate sedation (e.g., lorazepam [Ativan]) and analgesia (e.g., morphine), and they will require expert psychosocial nursing interventions. See "Sedating and Paralytic Agents," p. 38.

Nutritional support: Energy outlay with respiratory failure is high, in part because of the increased work of breathing. If the patient is unable to consume adequate calories with enteral feedings, total parenteral nutrition (TPN) is instituted.

NURSING DIAGNOSES AND INTERVENTIONS

Impaired gas exchange related to alveolar-capillary membrane changes secondary to increased permeability with alveolar injury and collapse

Desired outcomes: Within 12-24 h of initiation of therapy, patient has adequate gas exchange as evidenced by the following ABG values: Pao_2 >60 mm Hg; $Paco_2$ <45 mm Hg; pH 7.35-7.45. Within 4-6 days of initiation of

Research Brief 3-3   This study examined the relationship between age and mortality in patients with ARDS and examined the importance of factors that increase mortality. Over a 3½-year period, 256 patients were reviewed and data were compared regarding organ failure, sepsis, arterial oxygenation, and demographics. The data supported the conclusion that mortality is significantly higher in patients with ARDS who are older than 55 yr.

From Suchyta MR et al: Increased mortality of older patients with acute respiratory distress syndrome, *Chest* 111(5):1334-1339, 1997.

therapy, patient's RR is 12-20 breaths/min with a normal pattern and depth (eupnea) and there are no adventitious breath sounds.

- Assess and document character of respiratory effort: rate, depth, rhythm, and use of accessory muscles of respiration.
- Assess patient for signs and symptoms of respiratory distress: restlessness, anxiety, confusion, tachypnea (RR >20 breaths/min).
- Assess breath sounds with each vital signs (VS) check. Adventitious sounds, which usually are present in the later stages of ARDS, are not as likely to occur during the early stage.
- Monitor serial ABG values, and consult physician for significant changes. Explain need for frequent analysis to patient and significant others.
- Compare ABG saturation with pulse oximetry saturation for accuracy. Consult physician for pulse oximetry values <90%.
- Administer oxygen and monitor Fio_2 as prescribed.
- Monitor and record pulmonary function tests as prescribed, especially tidal volume and minute ventilation. Expect decreased tidal volume and increased minute ventilation with respiratory distress.
- Encourage patient to slow the rate of respirations by using pursed-lip breathing technique.
- Position patient for comfort and to promote adequate gas exchange. Usually, semi-Fowler's to high Fowler's position is therapeutic.
- Keep oral airway and self-inflating manual ventilating bag at the bedside for emergency use. Keep emergency intubation equipment at the bedside for use should patient's condition deteriorate.

NIC Acid-Base Management; Airway Management; Bedside Laboratory Testing; Laboratory Data Interpretation; Oxygen Therapy; Positioning; Respiratory Monitoring; Vital Signs Monitoring

ADDITIONAL NURSING DIAGNOSES

Also see "Status Asthmaticus" for **Activity intolerance,** p. 217. As indicated, see nursing diagnoses and interventions in "Nutritional Support," p 1; "Mechanical Ventilation," p. 17; "Prolonged Immobility," p. 74; "Psychosocial Support," p. 83; and "Psychosocial Support for the Patient's Family and Significant Others," p. 95.

Pulmonary emboli

PATHOPHYSIOLOGY

Pulmonary perfusion disorders are the result of any obstruction of blood flow in the pulmonary vasculature. The two most common abnormalities of pulmonary perfusion are thrombotic emboli and fat emboli. Venous air emboli are also discussed.

Thrombotic emboli (TE):   The most common pulmonary perfusion abnormality, TEs are caused by a dislodged blood clot from the systemic circulation, typically the deep veins of the legs or pelvis. Most often, the iliofemoral venous system is implicated. Thrombus formation is the result of one or more of the following factors: blood stasis; alterations in clotting factors; and injury to vessel walls. Many patients with TE do not exhibit signs and symptoms of deep vein thrombosis (DVT). The formed thrombus becomes dislodged and travels to the pulmonary circulation, where it obstructs one or both branches of the pulmonary artery or a subdivision. Total obstruction leading to pulmonary infarction is rare because the pulmonary circulation has multiple sources of blood supply. Early diagnosis and appropriate treatment reduce mortality to less than 10%. Although most thrombotic emboli resolve completely, leaving no residual deficits, some patients may be left with chronic pulmonary hypertension.

Fat emboli: The most common nonthrombotic cause of pulmonary perfusion disorders, fat emboli are generally the result of two events: the release of free fatty acids that cause a toxic vasculitis, followed by thrombosis and obstruction of small pulmonary arteries by fat. The syndrome occurs within 12-24 hours after skeletal trauma or major orthopedic surgery.

Venous air emboli: Almost always an iatrogenic complication with multiple causes, including surgical procedures, insertion of pulmonary artery catheters and central venous catheters, hemodialysis, endoscopy, and use of automatic injectors such as those used for contrast media. A large volume of air is introduced into the venous circulation and travels to the pulmonary circulation. Small amounts of air may be completely asymptomatic secondary to rapid reabsorption. A larger bolus of air into the right ventricle may completely obstruct pulmonary blood flow, leading to cardiac arrest. In severe cases, venous air embolus may have a mortality >50%. Rapid diagnosis and treatment are essential.

ASSESSMENT

Thrombotic emboli

History and risk factors

Prolonged immobilization: Especially significant when coexisting with surgical or nonsurgical trauma, carcinoma, or cardiopulmonary disease. Risk increases as length of immobilization increases.

Cardiac disorders: Atrial fibrillation, congestive heart failure, myocardial infarction, rheumatic heart disease, or any low cardiac output state.

Surgical intervention: Risk increases in postoperative period, especially for patients with pelvic, thoracic, and abdominal surgery and for those with extensive burns or musculoskeletal injuries of the hip or knee.

Pregnancy: Especially during the postpartum period.

Trauma: Especially fractures of the lower extremities, hip fracture in the older adult, burns, and acute head and spinal cord injuries. The degree of risk is related to the severity, site, and extent of trauma.

Carcinoma: Particularly neoplasms involving the breast, lung, pancreas, and genitourinary (GU) and gastrointestinal (GI) tracts.

Obesity: Patients with a ≥20% increase in ideal body weight have an increased incidence of TE.

Varicose veins or prior thromboembolic disease

Age: Risk of thromboembolism is greatest between 55 and 65 yr of age.

> **Note:** Low-dose heparin prophylaxis (e.g., 5000 U subcutaneously q8-12h) frequently is initiated in high-risk groups (except for neurosurgical patients). Low-molecular-weight (LMW) heparins, e.g., dalteparin (Fragmin) and enoxaparin (Lovenox), may be used for DVT prophylaxis in certain high-risk surgical patients, such as those with abdominal and orthopedic surgery.

Clinical presentation: Often nonspecific but may involve sudden onset of dyspnea, tachypnea, restlessness, and anxiety. The patient also may have a nonproductive cough, palpitations, nausea, and syncope. With a large embolism, oppressive substernal chest discomfort will be present. Fever, pleuritic chest pain, and hemoptysis are present with pulmonary infarction.

Physical assessment: RR >20 breaths/min, HR >100 bpm, crackles, decreased chest wall excursion secondary to splinting, S_3 and S_4 gallop rhythms, diaphoresis, edema, and cyanosis. Temperature may be elevated if pulmonary infarction has occurred, and transient pleural friction rub may be present.

Fat emboli
History and risk factors
Multiple long bone fractures: Especially fractures of the femur and pelvis (see p. 155).
Trauma to adipose tissue or liver
Burns: See p. 193.
Osteomyelitis
Sickle cell crisis: See p. 558.
Clinical presentation: Typically, patient is without symptoms for a period lasting 12-24 h after embolization; this period ends with sudden cardiopulmonary and neurologic deterioration: dyspnea, restlessness, confusion, delirium, and coma. Petechial rash may appear over the body, especially the upper body. This is secondary to thrombocytopenia, which may be related to platelet aggregation by circulating fats.
Physical assessment: RR >20 breaths/min; HR >100 bpm; increased BP; elevated temperature; petechiae, especially of the upper torso and axillae; inspiratory crowing; and expiratory wheezes.

Venous air emboli
History and risk factors
Recent surgical procedure
Pulmonary artery/central venous catheter insertion
Misuse of closed-wound suction unit
Cardiopulmonary bypass
Hemodialysis
Endoscopy
Clinical presentation: Depends on severity of the bolus. Agitation, confusion, cough, dyspnea, and chest pain.
Physical assessment: RR >20 breaths/min, HR >100 bpm, wheezing, hypotension, mill wheel heart murmur.

DIAGNOSTIC TESTS
Thrombotic emboli (TE)
ABG values: Hypoxemia (Pao_2 <80 mm Hg), hypocapnia ($Paco_2$ <35 mm Hg), and respiratory alkalosis (pH >7.45) usually are present. A normal Pao_2 does not rule out the presence of TE. Pulse oximetry is used for continuous monitoring of oxygen saturation (see p. 213).
Alveolar-arterial oxygen pressure difference: $P(A-a)o_2$ usually will be >10 mm Hg, depending on the severity of the perfusion disorder and the degree of ventilation-perfusion mismatch.
Chest x-ray: Initially, the chest x-ray shows normal findings or an elevated hemidiaphragm will be present. After 24 h the x-ray may reveal small infiltrates secondary to atelectasis from decrease in surfactant. More specific findings are abnormal blood vessel diameters (i.e., obstruction of right pulmonary artery would cause dilation of left pulmonary artery) and shapes (i.e., the affected blood vessel may taper to a sharp point and disappear). If pulmonary infarction is present, infiltrates and pleural effusions may be seen within 12-36 h.
ECG: If TE are extensive, signs of acute pulmonary hypertension may be present: right-shift QRS axes, tall and peaked P waves, ST-segment changes, and T-wave inversion in leads V_1-V_4.

Pulmonary ventilation-perfusion scan: A key diagnostic test used to detect the presence of abnormalities of ventilation or perfusion in the pulmonary system. The patient inhales radioactive-tagged gases, and radioactive particles are injected peripherally. If there is a mismatch of ventilation and perfusion (e.g., normal ventilation with decreased perfusion), vascular obstruction is likely. Results may not be definitive.

Pulmonary angiography: This is the definitive study for TEs. It is an invasive procedure involving catheterization of the right ventricle and injection of dye into the pulmonary artery (PA) to visualize pulmonary vessels. An abrupt vessel "cut off" may be seen at the site of embolization. Usually, filling defects are seen.

Hemodynamic studies: If TEs lead to increased pulmonary vascular resistance, PA pressure will be elevated. PA pressures increase significantly (>20 mm Hg) if 30%-50% of the pulmonary arterial tree is affected. If massive TEs are present and PA pressure increases to >40 mm Hg, right ventricular failure can develop, leading to a decrease in cardiac output and hypotension.

Fat emboli

ABG values: Hypoxemia (Pao_2 <80 mm Hg) and hypercapnia ($Paco_2$ >45 mm Hg) will be present with a respiratory acidosis (pH <7.35).

Chest x-ray: A pattern similar to ARDS is seen: diffuse, extensive, bilateral interstitial and alveolar infiltrates.

CBC count: May reveal decreased hemoglobin (Hgb) and Hct secondary to hemorrhage into the lung, in addition to thrombocytopenia.

Venous air emboli

ABG values: Hypoxemia (Pao_2 <80 mm Hg), hypercapnia ($Paco_2$ >45 mm Hg), and respiratory acidosis (pH <7.35) generally are present in severe cases.

Chest x-ray: Reveals changes consistent with pulmonary edema or air-fluid levels in the main pulmonary artery system.

Pulmonary artery pressure: Systolic, diastolic, and mean pressure are acutely elevated, but slight elevation of PAWP remains within normal limits (WNL).

COLLABORATIVE MANAGEMENT

Thrombotic emboli

Oxygen therapy: Delivered at appropriate concentration to maintain a Pao_2 of >60 mm Hg.

IV heparin therapy: Treatment of choice. It is started immediately in patients without bleeding or clotting disorders and in whom TE is strongly suspected.

Initial dose: IV bolus of 5,000-10,000 U.

Maintenance dose: 2-4 h after initial dose, a continuous IV infusion of approximately 1000 U/h is usually indicated; exact dose is adjusted according to the patient's weight. Maintenance continues for 7-14 days, during which time the patient is placed on bed rest to ensure that the thrombus is firmly attached to the vessel wall before ambulation is attempted.

Goals of therapy: To inhibit thrombus growth, promote resolution of the formed thrombus, and prevent further embolus formation. These goals are achieved by keeping activated partial thromboplastin time (aPTT) at 1½-2½ times the normal. In addition, platelet counts should be obtained q3days, because thrombocytopenia and paradoxic arterial thrombosis can occur as a result of heparin therapy. (See "Heparin-Induced Thrombocytopenia," p. 570.)

Protamine sulfate: Heparin antidote, which should be readily available during heparin therapy. Fatal hemorrhage occurs in 1%-2% of patients undergoing heparin therapy. Risk of bleeding is greatest in women >60 yr of age.

> **Research Brief 3-4**   Thrombolytic therapy for pulmonary embolism. The investigators attempted to determine the risk factors and frequency of intracranial hemorrhage in patients receiving thrombolysis for documented pulmonary embolism. There were 312 cases reviewed for incidence of intracranial hemorrhage as well as background information that might support or not support the use of such therapy. It was found that intracranial hemorrhage with thrombolytic therapy occurred infrequently but that risk factors such as diastolic hypertension or previous history of intracranial disease must be screened for in this population.

From Kanter DS et al:Thrombolytic therapy for pulmonary embolism: frequency of intracranial hemorrhage and associated risk factors, *Chest* 111(5):1241-1245, 1997.

Oral anticoagulants (warfarin sodium):   Started 48-72 h after initiation of heparin therapy. The two are given simultaneously for 4-6 days to allow time for warfarin to inhibit vitamin K-dependent clotting factors before heparin is discontinued. Daily dose is adjusted according to INR, and correct dosage is individualized per patient based on frequent INR determinations. An INR of 2.0-3.0 is desirable.

Prothrombin time (PT):   Monitored daily, with a goal of $1\frac{1}{4}$-$1\frac{1}{2}$ times normal. Once the patient's condition has stabilized and the heparin is discontinued, weekly monitoring of INR is acceptable. After hospital discharge the PT should be monitored q2wk for as long as the patient continues to take warfarin.

Maintenance: Usually 10 mg/day, continued for 3-6 months and based on the continued presence of risk factors. Certain tumors (e.g., Trousseau syndrome) necessitate lifetime therapy.

> **Note:**   Subcutaneous heparin therapy is an effective alternative to warfarin, with less risk of bleeding. The dose of heparin must be adjusted while the patient is hospitalized to ensure a PTT of $1\frac{1}{2}$ times that of normal.

Vitamin K: Reverses the effects of warfarin in 24-36 hours. Fresh frozen plasma may be required in cases of serious bleeding.

> *Caution:*   Warfarin crosses the placental barrier and can cause spontaneous abortion and birth defects.

Thrombolytic therapy: These drugs lyse clots via conversion of plasminogen to plasma and may be given in the first 24-72 h after TE to speed the process of clot lysis, especially when severe cardiopulmonary compromise has occurred. After the first 24 h of thrombolytic therapy, heparin therapy is initiated. Thrombolytic therapy may be preferred for initial treatment of TE in patients with hemodynamic compromise; in those with >30% occlusion of pulmonary vasculature; and in patients for whom therapy was initiated no later than 3 days after onset of TE.

> **Note:**   As many as 33% of patients who receive thrombolytic therapy have hemorrhagic complications. Discontinuing the drug and administering fresh-frozen plasma are the appropriate treatments.

Streptokinase: Loading dose of 250,000 IU in normal saline or D_5W given IV over a 30-min period. Maintenance dose is 100,000 IU/h given IV for 24-72 h.

Tissue plasminogen activator: Given 50 mg/h for 2 h. Followed by heparin therapy.

Thrombin time: Monitors therapy for both drugs. The test is repeated q4h during therapy to ensure adequate response, which should be 2-5 times normal. An aPTT can be used instead of thrombin time and should be 2-5 times control. Once thrombolytic therapy is stopped, thrombin time or aPTT should be checked frequently until values fall below 2 times normal. When the values are below 2 times normal, heparin is started.

Contraindications: Active internal bleeding, stroke, or intracranial bleeding within 2 months of TE. Other contraindications include trauma or surgery within 15 days of TE, diastolic hypertension >100 mm Hg, recent cardiopulmonary resuscitation, pregnancy, and <10 days postpartum.

Surgical interventions: Inferior vena caval interruption in severe or recurrent cases of pulmonary embolism. Inferior vena caval interruption most often involves the transvenous insertion of an umbrella filter (e.g., Greenfield filter) that prevents the passage of major emboli from deep venous thrombi in the lower extremities. Pulmonary embolectomy may be indicated in select cases of massive pulmonary embolism.

Fat emboli

Oxygen: Concentration of oxygen is based on clinical picture, ABG results, and patient's prior respiratory status. Intubation and mechanical ventilation may be required.

Steroids: Cortisone, 100 mg, or methylprednisolone, 30 mg/kg, is used to decrease local injury to pulmonary tissue and pulmonary edema.

Diuretics: Pulmonary edema develops in approximately 30% of patients with fat emboli, necessitating use of diuretics.

Venous air emboli

Emphasis is on prevention. Ensure that central venous catheter is inserted with the patient in Trendelenburg position. Use Luer-Lok connectors on all IV tubing to prevent a disconnection. Should venous air embolus occur despite precautions, the following are anticipated.

Oxygen therapy: 100% Fio_2 is initiated immediately.

Trendelenburg position with a left decubitus tilt: To minimize further movement of air bolus through the heart and into the pulmonary vasculature and beyond.

Aspiration of air: If a central venous catheter is in place near the right atrium, an attempt is made to aspirate the air.

NURSING DIAGNOSES AND INTERVENTIONS

Impaired gas exchange related to altered blood flow secondary to presence of pulmonary emboli

Desired outcomes: Within 12 h of initiation of therapy, patient has adequate gas exchange as evidenced by the following ABG values: Pao_2 ≥60 mm Hg; $Paco_2$ 35-45 mm Hg; and pH 7.35-7.45. Within 2-4 days of initiating therapy, patient's RR is 12-20 breaths/min with normal depth and pattern (eupnea).

- Monitor serial ABG values, assessing for the desired response to treatment: increased Pao_2 (≥60 mm Hg) and correction of respiratory alkalosis ($Paco_2$ ≥35 mm Hg and pH <7.45). Report lack of response to treatment or worsening ABG values. If pulse oximetry is present, monitor oxygen saturation.
- Monitor patient for signs and symptoms of increasing respiratory distress, and consult physician for significant findings: RR increased from baseline; increasing dyspnea; anxiety; cyanosis.
- Ensure delivery of prescribed concentrations of oxygen.

- Position patient for comfort and optimal gas exchange. Ensure that the area of the lung affected by the emboli is not dependent when patient is in the lateral decubitus position. Position patient with the unaffected side down, and elevate HOB 30 degrees. This will ensure a better ventilation-perfusion match, thereby improving Pao_2.
- Avoid positioning patient with knees bent (i.e., "gatching" the bed), because this impedes venous return from the legs and can increase the risk of TE.
- Ensure that patient performs deep-breathing exercises 3-5 times q2h.
- Decrease metabolic demands for oxygen by limiting or pacing patient's activities and procedures.
- Explain all procedures and offer support to minimize fear and anxiety, which can increase oxygen demands.
- Schedule rest times after meals to avoid competition for oxygen supply during digestion.

Altered protection related to risk of clotting anomalies secondary to anticoagulation or thrombolytic therapy
Desired outcome: Patient is free of bleeding signs, or if bleeding occurs, it is not prolonged.

- Monitor serial coagulation or thrombin times. Report values outside the desired therapeutic ranges. Optimal range for aPTT is 1½-2½ times that of control value. A therapeutic INR is 2.0-3.0. Optimal range for thrombin time is 2-5 times that of normal.
- Ensure easy access to antidotes for prescribed treatment:
  - ☐ *Protamine sulfate:* 1 mg counteracts 100 U of heparin. Usually, the initial dose is 50 mg.
  - ☐ *Vitamin K:* 20 mg given subcutaneously.
  - ☐ *Epsilon-aminocaproic acid* (e.g., Amicar): Reverses the fibrinolytic condition related to thrombolytic therapy.

Note: Although use of epsilon-aminocaproic acid as an antidote has not been approved, it has been used in some emergency situations.

- Inspect the following sites for evidence of bleeding: any entry site of an invasive procedure, oral mucous membranes, wounds, and nares; inspect the torso and extremities for evidence of petechiae or ecchymoses. Also check stool, urine, sputum, and vomitus for occult blood. Be alert to complaints of back pain or other site-specific pain (e.g., headache), which may signal occult bleeding.
- Apply pressure over puncture sites until bleeding stops—usually 5-10 min for venous site and 10-20 min for arterial site. Apply pressure dressing over arterial puncture sites to stop oozing of blood.
- To prevent hematoma formation, avoid giving intramuscular (IM) injections.
- Monitor Hgb and Hct. Consult physician for significant findings, including decreases in values or failure to see appropriate increases after transfusion.
- To avoid negative interactions with anticoagulants or thrombolytic therapy, establish compatibility of all drugs before administering them:
  - ☐ *Heparin:* Digitalis, tetracyclines, nicotine, and antihistamines decrease the effect of heparin therapy. Establish compatibility before infusing other IV drugs through heparin IV line.
  - ☐ *Warfarin sodium:* Numerous drugs result in a decrease or an increase in response to treatment with warfarin. Consult with pharmacist to obtain specific information about patient's medication profile.
  - ☐ *Thrombolytic therapy:* Do not infuse other medications through the same IV line.
- Because aspirin and nonsteroidal antiinflammatory drugs (e.g., ibuprofen) are platelet-aggregation inhibitors and can prolong episodes of bleeding, avoid use of *any* drug that contains these agents.

- Discuss with patient and significant others the importance of reporting promptly the presence of bleeding from any source.
- Teach patient the necessity of using sponge-tipped applicators (instead of toothbrush) and mouthwash for oral care to minimize the risk of gum bleeding during hospitalization when anticoagulant therapy is most intensive. Instruct patient to shave with an electric razor.
- If patient is restless and combative, provide a safe environment: pad the side rails; obtain prescription to restrain patient as necessary to prevent falls; and use extreme care when moving patient to avoid bumping extremities into side rails.

Knowledge deficit: Oral anticoagulant therapy: potential side effects and complications; foods and medications to avoid during therapy

Desired outcome: Within 24 h of initiation of oral anticoagulant therapy, patient and/or significant others verbalize knowledge of patient's prescribed anticoagulant drug, the potential side effects, and foods and medications to avoid during oral anticoagulant therapy.

- Determine patient's knowledge of oral anticoagulant therapy. As appropriate, discuss the drug name, purpose, dosage, schedule, potential side effects, and complications of therapy.
- Inform patient of the potential side effects and complications of anticoagulant therapy: easy bruising; prolonged bleeding from cuts; spontaneous nose bleeds; black and tarry stools; blood in urine and sputum.
- Teach the rationale and application procedure for antiembolism stockings. Explain that patient should put them on in the morning before getting out of bed.
- Stress the importance of preventing impairment of venous return from the lower extremities by avoiding prolonged sitting, avoiding crossing the legs, and avoiding wearing constrictive clothing.
- Teach patient about foods high in vitamin K (e.g., fish, bananas, dark-green vegetables, tomatoes, cauliflower), which can interfere with anticoagulation.
- Caution patient that a soft-bristle toothbrush, rather than a hard-bristle one, and an electric razor, rather than a safety razor, should be used during anticoagulant therapy while at home.
- Instruct patient to consult with physician before taking any new over–the-counter (OTC) or prescribed drugs. The following are among many drugs that enhance the response to warfarin: aspirin, ibuprofen, cimetidine, and trimethoprim. Drugs that decrease the response include antacids, diuretics, oral contraceptives, and barbiturates, among others.

NIC Acid-Base Management; Acid-Base Monitoring; Bedside Laboratory Testing; Bleeding Precautions; Health Education; Oxygen Therapy; Respiratory Monitoring; Surveillance; Teaching: Individual; Teaching: Prescribed Medication; Vital Signs Monitoring

ADDITIONAL NURSING DIAGNOSIS

See "Status Asthmaticus" for **Activity intolerance,** p. 217.

Pneumothorax

PATHOPHYSIOLOGY

Pneumothorax is an accumulation of air between the parietal and visceral pleura with secondary lung collapse. There are three types of pneumothorax.

Spontaneous: A type of closed pneumothorax in which the chest wall remains intact with no leak to the atmosphere. It results from the rupture of a bleb or bulla on the visceral pleural surface, usually near the apex. In a *primary* spontaneous pneumothorax, the cause of the rupture is unknown, although it may result from a weakness related to a respiratory infection. The affected individual is usually a young male (20-40 yr of age), previously healthy, and a smoker. Generally, onset of symptoms occurs at rest rather than with vigorous exercise or coughing. The potential for recurrence is great, with the second pneumothorax occurring an average of 2-3 yr after the first. A primary spontaneous pneumothorax is rarely life threatening. A *secondary* spontaneous pneumothorax results as a complication of an underlying lung disease (COPD, cystic fibrosis, tuberculosis, malignant neoplasm). The symptoms are more severe than with the primary spontaneous pneumothorax, and this disorder may be life threatening because of the underlying lung disease. In addition, recurrence rates are high in this population.

Traumatic: Can be open or closed. An *open* pneumothorax occurs when air enters the pleural space from the atmosphere through an opening in the chest wall, such as with a penetrating injury or an invasive medical procedure (e.g., lung biopsy, thoracentesis, placement of a central line into a subclavian vein). A *closed* pneumothorax occurs when the visceral pleura is penetrated but the chest wall remains intact, with no atmospheric leak. This usually occurs with blunt trauma that results in a fracture and dislocation of the ribs. It also may occur from the use of PEEP or after cardiopulmonary resuscitation (CPR). For more information about blunt chest injuries, see "Chest Trauma," p. 133.

Tension: Occurs when air enters the pleural space through a pleural tear during inspiration. Air continues to accumulate but cannot escape during expiration because of intrapleural pressure, which is greater than alveolar pressure. This leads to a one-way or flap-valve effect. As the pressure increases, it is transmitted to the mediastinum. This results in a mediastinal shift toward the unaffected side, which further impairs ventilatory efforts. The increase in pressure also compresses the vena cava, which impedes venous return, leading to a decrease in cardiac output and, ultimately, to circulatory collapse if it is not diagnosed and treated quickly. Tension pneumothorax is a life-threatening medical emergency. Although it can occur with a spontaneous pneumothorax, it most often is associated with trauma or infection or it can occur during mechanical ventilation in patients who require positive-pressure ventilation.

ASSESSMENT

The clinical presentation will vary in degree, depending on the type and size of pneumothorax.

Spontaneous or traumatic: Sudden onset of sharp, stabbing chest pain on the affected side, which may radiate to the shoulder; moderate to severe dyspnea; anxiety.

Inspection: Decreased chest wall movement on affected side.

Palpation: Tracheal shift toward unaffected side; subcutaneous emphysema (crepitus); tactile and vocal fremitus decreased or absent on affected side.

Percussion: Hyperresonance on affected side.

Auscultation: Absent or decreased breath sounds on affected side; increased RR. Moderate tachycardia (HR >140 bpm) may be present.

Tension: Severe dyspnea; chest pain on affected side; cool, clammy, mottled skin; anxiety and restlessness.

Inspection: Decreased chest wall movement on affected side; expansion of affected side throughout respiratory cycle; jugular vein distention.

Palpation: Tracheal shift toward unaffected side; subcutaneous emphysema in neck and chest.

Percussion: Hyperresonance on affected side.

Auscultation: Absent or decreased breath sounds on affected side; distant heart sounds; increased RR (>20 breaths/min); decreased BP; increased HR (may be >140 bpm).

> *Caution:* Tension pneumothorax is life threatening. Immediate medical intervention is critical.

DIAGNOSTIC TESTS

Chest x-ray: Will show size of the pneumothorax and any tracheal shift. The affected side will show air in the pleural space, expansion of the chest wall, lowering of the diaphragm, and partial to total collapse of the lung. A small pneumothorax (less than 20%) may not be detectable on physical examination.

ABG analysis: Hypoxemia (Pao_2 <80 mm Hg) will be evident immediately after a moderate to large pneumothorax that occupies ≥15% of the hemithorax. As the pneumothorax resolves, arterial oxygen saturation returns to normal. Hypoxemia may be accompanied by respiratory acidosis (pH <7.35) and hypercapnia ($Paco_2$ >45 mm Hg).

ECG: May reveal decrease in QRS amplitude, precordial T wave inversion, rightward shift of frontal QRS axis, and small precordial R voltage.

COLLABORATIVE MANAGEMENT

Oxygen therapy: Administered when ABG values demonstrate the presence of hypoxemia, which usually occurs with a large pneumothorax.

Analgesic: Provides relief of pain of pneumothorax or its treatment.

Thoracentesis: Performed immediately in tension pneumothorax to remove air from the chest cavity. A large-bore needle is inserted into the second intercostal space, midclavicular line, which correlates to the superior portion of the anterior axillary lobe. A sudden rushing out of air confirms the diagnosis of tension pneumothorax. To decrease the risk of further pleural laceration as the chest reexpands, a stylet introducer needle with a plastic sheath may be used. The needle is removed after penetration, and the plastic catheter sheath is left in place to allow decompression of the chest cavity. After air aspiration, chest tubes are inserted.

Chest tube placement: A chest tube may be inserted in a patient who has symptoms of a pneumothorax, depending on the severity of collapse. Chest tubes produce inflammation and, ultimately, scarring of the pleura and may help prevent recurrent spontaneous pneumothoraces. Patients with recurrent pneumothoraces require chest tubes because their visceral pleurae do not seal promptly. Chest tubes (26-30 Fr) are inserted in the second or third lateral intercostal space, midclavicular line. During insertion, the patient should be in an upright position so that the lung falls away from the chest wall. A small (1-2 cm) incision is made, and the chest tube is placed, sutured in place, and connected to an underwater-seal drainage system. Usually simple underwater-seal drainage is all that is necessary for 6-24 h. Suction may be used, depending on the size of the pneumothorax, the patient's condition, and the amount of drainage. A one-way flutter valve may be used with the chest tube instead of the underwater-seal drainage system. The flutter valve allows air to escape but prevents its reentry. The flutter valve (e.g., Heimlich valve) is placed on the end of the chest tube. Suction can be applied with the flutter valve in place. After chest tube insertion and removal of air from the pleural space, the lung begins to reexpand. A chest tube may produce inflammation of the pleura, causing pleuritic pain, slight temperature elevation, and pleuritic friction rub.

Thoracotomy: Often indicated because of the risk of continuous recurrence if patient has had two or more spontaneous pneumothoraces on one side or if resolution of the pneumothorax does not occur within 7 days. Thoracotomy may involve mechanical abrasion of the pleural surfaces with a dry, sterile sponge or chemical abrasion via an agent such as tetracycline solution or talc, both of which result in pleural adhesions to prevent recurrence. A partial pleurectomy may be performed instead of mechanical or chemical abrasion.

NURSING DIAGNOSES AND INTERVENTIONS

Impaired gas exchange related to decreased alveolar blood flow and decreased oxygen supply secondary to increased pleural pressure

Desired outcome: Within 2-6 h of initiation of treatment, patient exhibits adequate gas exchange as evidenced by Pao_2 ≥60 mm Hg and $Paco_2$ ≤45 mm Hg (or values within 10% of patient's baseline values, which depend on underlying pathophysiology); RR ≤20 breaths/min with normal depth and pattern (eupnea); and orientation to time, place, and person.

- Monitor serial ABG results to detect continued presence of hyper-capnia or hypoxemia. Monitor O_2 saturation via pulse oximetry as indicated. Consult physician for new or persistent hypoxemia or hypercapnia.
- Observe for indicators of hypoxia, including increased restlessness, anxiety, and changes in mental status.
- Assess patient for increasing respiratory distress: increased RR; diminished or absent movement of chest wall on affected side; complaints of increased dyspnea; cyanosis.
- Position patient to allow for full expansion of unaffected lung. Semi-Fowler's position usually provides comfort and allows adequate expansion of chest wall. The patient also can be turned unaffected side down with the HOB elevated to ensure a better ventilation-perfusion match.
- Change patient's position q2h to promote drainage and lung reexpansion and to facilitate alveolar perfusion.
- Encourage patient to take deep breaths, providing necessary analgesia to decrease discomfort during deep-breathing exercises. Deep breathing will promote full lung expansion and may decrease the risk of atelectasis.
- Ensure delivery of prescribed concentrations of oxygen.
- Assess and maintain closed chest-drainage system:
  - ☐ Tape all connections, and secure chest tube to thorax with tape.
  - ☐ Avoid all kinks in the tubing, and ensure that the bed and equipment are not compressing any component of the system.
  - ☐ Maintain fluid in underwater-seal chamber, and suction chamber at appropriate levels.
  - ☐ Be aware that the suction apparatus does not regulate the amount of suction applied to the closed drainage system. The amount of suction is determined by the water level in the suction control chamber. Minimal bubbling is optimal. Excessive bubbling causes rapid evaporative loss.

Note: Suction aids in the reexpansion of the lung, but removing suction for short periods, such as for transporting, will not be detrimental or disrupt the closed drainage system.

  - ☐ Be aware that fluctuations in the long tube of the underwater-seal chamber indicate a patent chest tube. Fluctuations stop when either the lung has reexpanded or there is a kink or obstruction in the chest tube.
  - ☐ Bubbling in the underwater-seal chamber occurs on expiration and is a sign that air is leaving the pleural space.
  - ☐ Continuous bubbling on both inspiration and expiration in the underwater-seal chamber is a signal that air is leaking into the drainage system. Locate and seal the system's air leak, if possible.
- Keep necessary emergency supplies at the bedside: (1) petrolatum gauze pad to apply over insertion site if the chest tube becomes dislodged; and (2) sterile water in which to submerge the chest tube if it becomes disconnected from the underwater-seal system. *Never* clamp a chest tube without a specific directive from the physician, inasmuch as clamping may lead to tension pneumothorax because the air can no longer escape.

Caution: Follow your agency's policy regarding chest tube stripping. Be aware that this mechanism for maintaining chest tube patency is controversial and has been associated with high negative pressures in the pleural space, which can damage fragile lung tissue. Chest tube stripping may be indicated when bloody drainage or clots are visible in the tubing. Squeezing alternately hand-over-hand along the drainage tube may generate sufficient pressure to move fluid along the tube.

Pain related to biophysical injury as a result of chest tube placement and pleural irritation

Desired outcomes: Within 1-2 h of initiating analgesic therapy, patient's subjective evaluation of discomfort improves as documented by a pain scale. Nonverbal indicators of discomfort, such as grimacing and splinting on inspiration, are absent.

- Give patient and significant others appropriate information regarding chest tube placement and maintenance.
- At frequent intervals, assess patient's degree of discomfort, using patient's verbal and nonverbal cues. Devise a pain scale with patient, rating discomfort on a scale of 0 (no pain) to 10 (worst pain). Medicate with analgesics as prescribed, evaluating and documenting the effectiveness of the medication on the basis of the pain scale.
- Position patient on unaffected side to minimize discomfort from chest tube insertion site. Administer medication 30 min before initiating movement.
- Teach patient to splint affected side during coughing, moving, or repositioning. Move patient as a unit to enhance stability and comfort.
- Schedule activities to provide for periods of rest, because fatigue may lower patient's pain threshold.
- Stabilize chest tube to reduce pull or drag on latex connector tubing. Tape chest tube securely to thorax, and loop latex tubing on bed beside patient.
- Teach patient to maintain active ROM on the involved side to prevent development of a stiff shoulder from the immobility.

NIC Acid-Base Management; Acid-Base Monitoring; Analgesic Administration; Environmental Management: Comfort; Exercise Promotion; Laboratory Data Interpretation; Medication Administration; Medication Management; Oxygen Therapy; Pain Management; Positioning; Respiratory Monitoring; Vital Signs Monitoring

ADDITIONAL NURSING DIAGNOSES

Also see "Status Asthmaticus" for **Activity intolerance,** p. 217. See appropriate nursing diagnoses and interventions in "Psychosocial Support," p. 83, and in "Psychosocial Support for the Patient's Family and Significant Others," p. 95.

Acute respiratory failure

PATHOPHYSIOLOGY

Acute respiratory failure is a clinical event in which either alveolar ventilation or pulmonary vascular perfusion or both are impaired. The accompanying increased work of breathing places demands on the cardiopulmonary system that exceed functional reserves. The result can be detrimental to respiratory homeostasis. Clinically, acute respiratory failure exists when Pao_2 is <50 mm Hg with the patient at rest and breathing room air. $Paco_2$ ≥50 mm Hg or pH <7.35 is significant for acute respiratory acidemia. Although a variety of disease processes can lead to respiratory failure, three basic mechanisms are involved.

Alveolar hypoventilation: Occurs as a result of reduction in alveolar minute ventilation. Because differential indicators (cyanosis and somnolence) occur late in the process, the condition may go unnoticed until hypoxia is severe.

Ventilation-perfusion mismatch: Considered the most common cause of hypoxia. Normal alveolar ventilation occurs at a rate of 4 L/min, with normal pulmonary vascular blood flow occurring at a rate of 5 L/min. The normal ventilation/perfusion ratio is 0.8 : 1. Any disease process that interferes with either side of the equation upsets the physiologic balance and can lead to respiratory failure as a result of reduction in arterial oxygen levels.

Diffusion disturbances: Processes that physically impair gas exchange across the alveolar-capillary membrane. Diffusion is impaired because of the increase in anatomic distance the gas must travel from the alveoli to the capillaries and from the capillaries to the alveoli.

Right-to-left shunting (intrapulmonary shunt): Occurs when the aforementioned processes go untreated. Large amounts of blood pass from the right side of the heart to the left and out into the general circulation without adequate ventilation; therefore blood is poorly oxygenated. This process occurs when alveoli are atelectatic or fluid filled, inasmuch as these conditions interfere with gas exchange. Unlike the first three responses, hypoxia secondary to right-to-left shunting does not improve with the administration of oxygen, because the additional Fio_2 is unable to cross the alveolar-capillary membrane.

> **Note:**   See Table 3-5 for a description of some of the disease processes that can lead to acute respiratory failure.

ASSESSMENT

Clinical presentation: Indicators of acute respiratory failure vary according to the underlying disease process and severity of the failure. Acute respiratory failure is one of the most common causes of impaired LOC. Often it is misdiagnosed as heart failure, pneumonia, or stroke. Sometimes the onset of

---

TABLE 3-5   Disease Processes Leading to the Development of Respiratory Failure

Impaired alveolar ventilation	*Ventilation or perfusion disturbances*
• COPD (emphysema, bronchitis, asthma, cystic fibrosis)	• Pulmonary emboli
• Restrictive pulmonary disease (interstitial fibrosis, pleural effusion, pneumothorax, kyphoscoliosis, obesity, diaphragmatic paralysis)	• Atelectasis
	• Pneumonia
	• Emphysema
	• Chronic bronchitis
	• Bronchiolitis
	• ARDS
• Neuromuscular defects (Guillain-Barré syndrome, myasthenia gravis, multiple sclerosis, muscular dystrophy, polio, brain/spinal injury)	*Diffusion disturbances*
	• Pulmonary/interstitial fibrosis
	• Pulmonary edema
	• ARDS
• Depression of respiratory control centers (drug-induced cerebral infarction, inappropriate use of high-dose oxygen therapy, drug/toxic agents)	• Anatomic loss of functioning lung tissue (pneumonectomy)
• Chest trauma (rib fractures)	

COPD, Chronic obstructive pulmonary disease; *ARDS,* acute respiratory distress syndrome.

acute respiratory failure is so insidious that it is missed because staff members do not want to disturb the patient who appears to be sleeping.

Early indicators: Dyspnea, restlessness, anxiety, headache, fatigue, cool and dry skin, increased BP, tachycardia, and cardiac dysrhythmias.

Intermediate indicators: Confusion, lethargy, tachypnea, hypotension caused by vasodilation, cardiac dysrhythmias.

Late indicators: Cyanosis, diaphoresis, coma, respiratory arrest.

DIAGNOSTIC TESTS

ABG analysis: Assesses adequacy of oxygenation and effectiveness of ventilation. Typical results are Pao_2 <60 mm Hg, $Paco_2$ ≥45 mm Hg, and pH <7.35, which are consistent with severe respiratory acidosis. Pulse oximetry is used for continuous monitoring of oxygen saturation (see p. 213).

Mixed venous oxygen saturation (Svo_2):   Mixed venous blood gases are drawn intermittently or measured continuously from the distal tip of the pulmonary artery catheter. A blood sample taken from this site ensures complete mixing of the blood returned from all parts of the body. Changes in Svo_2 provide an early indication of perfusion failure or increased tissue demands for oxygen. Svo_2 is a more sensitive indicator of oxygen available for tissue oxygenation than Spo_2. Normal values are 60%-80%. A value <50% is associated with impaired tissue oxygenation.

Chest x-ray: Ascertains presence of underlying pathophysiology or disease process that may be contributing to the failure.

COLLABORATIVE MANAGEMENT

Correction of hypoxemia: First treatment priority. Pao_2 levels <30 mm Hg for longer than 3-4 min may cause permanent brain damage or death. Oxygen therapy, in conjunction with pharmacotherapy (e.g., bronchodilators, steroids, antibiotics), often improve ABG levels sufficiently to remove the patient from danger.

Correction of abnormal pH level: Second treatment priority. Adequate cellular and metabolic functioning is hindered when pH level remains outside the normal range of 7.35-7.45. When the pH is <7.20, IV sodium bicarbonate may be used conservatively and usually only when the patient is mechanically ventilated. A pH >7.45 may be managed by placing a rebreathing mask on the patient or increasing dead space on mechanical ventilator circuitry.

Intubation and mechanical ventilation: The purposes of intubation and mechanical ventilation are to restore alveolar ventilation, restore pH level within normal limits, and decrease work of breathing. Early intubation can prevent further airway collapse and tissue injury. In most cases the patient will require intubation and mechanical ventilation to support adequate respiratory function and stabilize ABG levels. Mechanical support is used until the underlying cause of the failure can be corrected and the patient can resume ventilatory efforts independently. Mechanical ventilation is discussed in greater depth in Chapter 1.

Research Brief 3-5   The purpose of this prospective study was to assess whether pressure support ventilation (PSV) could successfully be used in place of the assist control ventilation mode in the treatment of respiratory failure. The respiratory parameters of 45 patients were measured while on conventional assist control and while on PSV. Results showed that respiratory parameters improved while patients were on PSV and that this would possibly be a good alternative in patients with respiratory failure.

From Tejeda M et al: Comparison of pressure support ventilation and assist-control ventilation in the treatment of respiratory failure, *Chest* 111(5):1322-1325, 1997.

NURSING DIAGNOSES AND INTERVENTIONS

See sections relating to patient's underlying pathologic condition (e.g., "Mechanical Ventilation," p. 17, and "Chest Trauma," p. 133).

Bibliography

Centers for Disease Control: Guideline for prevention of nosocomial pneumonia, *Am J Infect Control* 22:247-292, 1994.

Gowski D, Miro A: New ventilatory strategies in acute respiratory failure, *Crit Care Nurse Q* 19(3):1-22, 1996.

Grap MJ: Ventilator-associated pneumonia: clinical significance and implications for nursing, *Heart Lung* 26(6):419-429, 1997.

Horne M, Swearingen PL: *Pocket guide to fluid, electrolyte, and acid-base balance*, ed 2, St Louis, 1993, Mosby.

Howard C: Respiratory disorders. In Swearingen PL, Ross DG, editors: *Manual of medical-surgical nursing care: nursing interventions and collaborative management,* ed 4, St Louis, 1999, Mosby.

Keen JH, Swearingen PL, editors: *Mosby's critical care nursing consultant,* St Louis, 1997, Mosby.

Kirby RR, Taylor RW, Civetta JM: *Handbook of critical care,* ed 2, Philadelphia, 1997, Lippincott-Raven.

Lode H et al: Nosocomial pneumonia in the critical care unit, *Crit Care Clin* 14(1):119-133, 1998.

McCloskey JC, Bulechek GM: *Nursing interventions classification (NIC),* ed 2, St Louis, 1996, Mosby.

Misasi R, Keyes J: Matching and mismatching ventilation and perfusion in the lung, *Crit Care Nurse* 16(3):23-40, 1996.

North American Nursing Diagnosis Association: *Nursing diagnoses: definitions and classification, 1999-2000,* Philadelphia, 1999, NANDA.

Schuster DP, Kollef MH, Bone R: The acute respiratory distress syndrome (ARDS). In Bone R, editor: *Pulmonary and critical care medicine,* St Louis, 1997, Mosby.

St. John RE: The pulmonary system. In Alspach JG, editor: *American Association of Critical-Care Nurses core curriculum for critical care nursing,* ed 5, Philadelphia, 1998, Saunders.

Thelan LA et al: *Critical care nursing: diagnosis and management,* ed 3, St Louis, 1998, Mosby.

Yagan M: Hospital-acquired pneumonia and its management, *Crit Care Nurse Q* 20(3):36-43, 1997.

CHAPTER 4

Cardiovascular Dysfunctions

Acute coronary syndromes: chest pain—angina pectoris and myocardial infarction

PATHOPHYSIOLOGY

Acute or unstable coronary syndromes include patients with chest discomfort caused by angina pectoris and pain associated with myocardial infarction. Chest discomfort or pain associated with myocardial ischemia is called *angina pectoris*. If the pain has a predictable pattern, it is considered stable. Those with ischemic pain with an unpredictable pattern are considered unstable. It can occur at rest or with exercise and may result from a sudden decrease in coronary blood flow caused by coronary thrombosis or spasm or from the inability to increase coronary blood flow sufficiently to meet myocardial oxygen demands (e.g., during exercise). Acute chest pain caused by ischemia may occur when coronary perfusion pressure is low, as in sudden hypotension, or when oxygen demands are greatly elevated, as in aortic stenosis, wherein the heart's workload is significantly increased by pumping against tremendous resistance to ejection created by the narrowed valve. Dysrhythmias may lead to chest discomfort caused by either increased workload (e.g., with tachycardias) or coronary perfusion deficit (e.g., with bradycardias).

Acute myocardial infarction (AMI) is necrosis of myocardial tissue as a result of relative or absolute lack of blood supply to the myocardium. Most AMIs are caused by atherosclerosis (e.g., fat deposits, fibrosis, calcification, platelet aggregation), which results in a progressive narrowing of the coronary artery, thrombus formation, and ultimately, occlusion of blood flow. Occlusion can be caused also by coronary artery spasm. The site of infarction is determined by the location of the arterial occlusion.

Pathogenic mechanisms that can cause acute chest pain are not all related to myocardial ischemia. Differential diagnosis of cardiac versus other origins is critical and can challenge the most experienced clinicians. Extracardiac causes of chest pain include pulmonary embolus, pneumonia, bronchitis, pneumothorax, aortic arch or high thoracic aortic aneurysm, esophagitis, hiatal hernia, cholecystitis, cholelithiasis, gastroesophageal reflux disease (GERD), costochondritis, musculoskeletal strain, anemia, hypoglycemia, fractured ribs or sternum, thyroid disease, obstipation, and bowel obstruction. Cardiac causes of chest pain not directly related to ischemia include valvular disease, cardiac trauma, cardiac tamponade, pericarditis, and endocarditis.

The diagnostic process should initially focus on ruling out myocardial infarction (MI), because it is the most common cause of severe, unrelieved chest pain and requires immediate reperfusion therapy to minimize loss of myocardium. Left unchecked, patients with large areas of necrosis can progress to cardiogenic shock quickly if reperfusion is not initiated. The patient's history and physical examination provide the initial framework for treatment decisions, coupled with the initial diagnostic electrocardiogram (ECG) and serum enzymes to evaluate for MI. If MI does not appear likely from these findings, differential diagnosis of chest pain should then focus on identification of other life-threatening events such as dissecting thoracic or aortic arch aneurysms, large pulmonary embolus, or cardiac tamponade.

ASSESSMENT

History and risk factors: Familial history of coronary artery disease (CAD), age >65 yr, male sex (risk for females increases after menopause), cigarette smoking, hypercholesterolemia, hyperlipidemia, hypertension, diabetes, obesity, increased stress, sedentary life-style.

Clinical presentation

Angina pectoris

Chest pain caused by myocardial ischemia, which may result from exertion or emotional upset; usually subsides with rest; lasts for about 1-4 min but generally not longer than 30 min; should subside gradually when precipitating factor is removed; should be relieved by nitroglycerin, usually within 45-90 sec. Can be an abrupt or gradual onset of substernal discomfort described as deep, visceral, squeezing, choking, burning, heavy, tight, or aching. Many patients will deny the presence of chest "pain" but will admit to severe chest "discomfort" or "pressure." Pain may radiate to the jaw, neck, arms, or hands. Certain patients have pain in the teeth and may be referred from an emergent dental visit.

Forms of angina

Stable: Has not increased in frequency or severity over a period of several months.

Unstable: A broad category that includes several types. Usually the quality of pain has changed or increased in frequency, duration, or severity; can occur at rest.

☐ Wellens syndrome: unstable angina, usually associated with left anterior descending (LAD) coronary artery lesions.

☐ Rest angina.

☐ New-onset angina.

☐ Preinfarction or crescendo: unstable angina with the potential for progression to infarction.

Prinzmetal (variant):   May occur at rest, long after exercise, and during sleep; usually caused by coronary vasospasm.

Myocardial infarction

Chest pain with transmural (Q-wave) or nontransmural (non-Q-wave) infarction is generally more severe, of longer duration (i.e., >30 min), unrelieved by nitroglycerin. Patients with diabetic neuropathy may experience MI without pain (silent MI). Approximately 25% of AMIs are silent. Many characteristics of ischemic pain apply to infarct pain. Other associated signs and symptoms include nausea, vomiting, dyspnea, orthopnea, anxiety, apprehension, diaphoresis, unexplained weakness and fatigue, cyanosis, and denial. Sometimes the presentation can be vague, manifesting with symptoms of gastrointestinal (GI) upset such as heartburn; no chest discomfort, with only arm or shoulder pain, jaw/dental pain. The elderly with acute MI present more frequently with symptoms of fatigue, shortness of breath (SOB), nausea/vomiting, syncope, weakness, falls, congestive heart failure, and pain in areas other than the chest.

Older patients have a higher risk of stroke—both with and without thrombolytic therapy. Thrombolytic-eligible women have been offered reperfusion strategies significantly less frequently than men, which may indicate women are more difficult to diagnose, are older than men with acute MI, and may have more comorbidities.

Physical assessment: Blood pressure (BP) may be elevated related to the sympathetic response to the patient's pain experience. BP may also decrease when pain is caused by ischemia or infarction, because the loss of myocardial perfusion results in decreased myocardial contractile strength and decreased cardiac output. Heart rate (HR) may increase in response to hypoxia and enhanced sympathetic tone, or the patient may have other dysrhythmias such as sinus bradycardia, atrioventricular (AV) blocks, or ventricular ectopy. S_4 heart sound may be audible during ischemic and infarction episodes. Infarcting patients may have an elevated temperature because of inflammation and may develop abnormal heart sounds including split S_1 and S_2, as well as S_3 if left heart failure ensues. Other chest sounds may include a pericardial friction rub, crackles in lung fields, and new murmurs. Elders may manifest sensorimotor and cognitive deficits if stroke is also present.

DIAGNOSTIC TESTS

ECG

Angina pectoris: myocardial ischemia

Characteristic changes may establish diagnosis of ischemic heart disease, although the absence of abnormality does not rule out this disease. In the absence of pain and with the patient at rest, the 12/15/18-lead ECG may be normal; therefore this test must be obtained during an episode of chest pain. ST-segment and T-wave changes, which occur during spontaneous chest pain and disappear with relief of the pain, are significant. The most characteristic change is depression of the ST segment with or without T-wave inversion. In variant or Prinzmetal angina, the ST segments may be elevated during the chest pain episode. If chest pain persists for more than 30 min, serial ECGs should be repeated approximately every 30 min for 2 h to determine if the patient is having an MI.

With Wellens syndrome, characteristic changes include inverted symmetric T waves with little or no ST elevation.

Acute myocardial infarction

The first ECG is done immediately and is used as part of the process to differentiate AMI from angina pectoris or other causes of chest pain, to help determine suitability for thrombolytic therapy or other reperfusion strategy (e.g., coronary angioplasty). The standard 12-lead ECG is designed for evaluation of the anterior, inferior, and lateral walls of the left ventricle (LV). Infarcts that extend to the right ventricle (RV) and/or posterior wall of the LV cannot be clearly detected by the 12-lead. Indications for performing additional ECG evaluation with 15 or 18 leads include: ST-segment elevation suggestive of an inferior wall MI (II, III, aV_F); isolated ST-segment elevation in V_1 or ST-segment elevation in V_1 is greater than in V_2; borderline ST-segment elevation in V_5 and V_6 or in V_1 through V_3; and ST-segment depression or suspicious isoelectric ST segments in V_1 through V_3. ECGs are then done in a series (initially, and then every 30 min for the first 2 h). Characteristic changes in certain lead groups identify the area and evolution of infarct. After the initial evaluation phase, ECGs may be done every 8-24 h. Changes include:

Q waves: Are indicative of MI and meet one of two criteria: they are either wide (>.04 sec) or deep (>25% of the total voltage of the QRS). New literature indicates that patients with (Q-wave MI) and without Q waves (non-Q-wave MI) can have experienced a transmural MI (necrosis of all layers of the myocardium). In the past, patients without Q waves were thought to have a subendocardial MI (necrosis that did not progress through all layers of the myocardium), which was not considered as serious as a transmural event. Q waves have been used as one of the diagnostic criteria for acute MI that has determined if the patient is appropriate for thrombolytic therapy or other reperfusion strategy. Patients who initially are without Q waves may develop them later or may extend the tissue necrosis if a reperfusion strategy is withheld. Previously, non-Q-wave MIs often were untreated, because it was thought the risk of thrombolysis outweighed the benefits.

ST-segment changes: Will be elevated in the lead over or facing the infarcted area. Reciprocal changes (ST-segment depressions) will be found in leads 180 degrees from the area of infarction.

Note: Fewer than 42% of patients with acute MI have diagnostic ST-segment elevation on their emergency department admission 12-lead ECG.

For posterior wall MI, ECG diagnosis is made only by notation of the reciprocal changes apparent in the anterior leads, so diagnosis of this type MI is difficult with a 12-lead ECG. For right ventricular MI, only changes in the V_1 lead suggest a problem in this area. Use of 15/18-lead ECGs that provide a more direct view of the posterior and right ventricular walls of the heart is recommended for more accurate diagnosis of both posterior wall and right ventricular MI.

T-wave changes: May occur hours to weeks after infarction. Within the early hours of infarction, "giant," upright T waves may be seen in leads over the infarct. Within several hours to days, the T wave becomes inverted. Gradually over time, the ST segment becomes isoelectric and the T wave may remain inverted. T-wave changes may last for weeks and return to normal or remain inverted for the rest of the patient's life. T-wave changes reflective of posterior and right ventricular MI are not clearly seen in the 12-lead ECG. Use of 15/18-lead ECG should provide clearer information about these areas.

Serial cardiac enzyme levels: Serum cardiac enzymes should be measured on all patients who experience chest pain of any etiology at the onset of pain and at least q8h ×3 to assess for signs of MI. Elevation of creatine kinase (CK) or creatine phosphokinase (CPK) will begin at about 2 h post-MI and peak within 24 h. Other enzymes such as serum myoglobin or troponin levels may provide better information regarding whether infarction is present in the earlier stages (30 min-2 h) of tissue necrosis. CK and/or myoglobin elevation alone are not indicative of an MI because they can be elevated for a variety of reasons, such as trauma or surgery. Creatine kinase-myocardial band isoenzyme (CK-MB) and troponin levels are more specific indicators of cardiac muscle damage. Generally, a CK-MB level that is >10% of the total CK is indicative of myocardial muscle damage. The ratio of the MB2 (cardiac) to MB1 (all muscle) types of CK-MB is also diagnostic for MI if the ratio becomes >2.5. Normal levels vary from one institution to another. If MI·is strongly suspected and CK total and MB are within normal limits (WNL), testing for lactic dehydrogenase (LD) isoenzyme may be helpful. If the total LD is elevated and LD_1 is the predominant isoenzyme, this is diagnostic of MI. With the availability of myoglobin troponin testing, the use of LD has decreased.

Chest x-ray: May reveal cardiac enlargement or new infiltrates indicative of heart failure in MI patients. In patients with ischemic heart disease, cardiomegaly signals the presence of myocardial ischemia and decreased myocardial contractility. May also provide information regarding other anomalies that cause chest pain, such as pneumonia, pneumothorax, thoracic fractures, and aortic aneurysm.

Echocardiography (ECHO): Ultrasound technique of the area above the heart on the chest wall used to detect abnormalities of left ventricular wall motion, measure ejection fraction, evaluate valve function, and estimate left ventricular end-diastolic pressure (LVEDP). Normal ejection fraction is >60% (approximate). Wall motion abnormalities or reduced ejection fraction may indicate an MI and will help define any risk of heart failure.

Transesophageal echocardiography (TEE): Ultrasound technique done via a high-frequency transducer on an endoscope that is inserted into the esophagus as the patient swallows. Provides clearer ultrasonic images of the heart.

Complete blood cell count (CBC): May provide useful information regarding possible anemia or infection/inflammation. Can assist in differential diagnosis of chest discomfort.

Serum electrolytes: May provide information regarding potential for development of dysrhythmias or the cause of dysrhythmias occurring with chest discomfort.

Coagulation studies: Obtained as part of screening for thrombolytic therapy in acute MI patients, wherein a question exists about potential for bleeding. More extensive coagulation studies may provide information about hematologic problems associated with an increased risk of thrombosis formation.

Multiple-gated acquisition (MUGA) scanning: Intravenous (IV) injection of the isotope *technetium pertechnetate* to evaluate left ventricular function and detect aneurysms, wall-motion abnormalities, and intracardiac shunting. In the stress MUGA test, the same test is performed at rest and after exercise.

Stress test: Patient exercises while being monitored by electrocardiography. Its purpose is to elicit chest pain and document any associated ECG changes. Positive stress test results elicit at least 1-mm horizontal depression or downsloping ST segment in one or more leads that lasts 0.08 sec. In addition, frequent premature ventricular complexes (PVCs) or runs of ventricular tachycardia are suggestive of ischemia. Not indicated if acute MI is suspected.

Thallium treadmill stress test: Normal myocardial tissue will accumulate thallium, whereas infarcted or ischemic areas will have decreased uptake, appearing as "cold spots" on the scan. To identify areas of decreased uptake, the patient exercises after an injection of thallium. A scan is obtained both immediately after exercise and 4 h later to determine if areas with decreased uptake fill in after 4 h. Ischemic areas that fill in are considered to have viable tissue and reversible damage, whereas areas that remain as "cold spots" are diagnosed as infarcted. For MI patients, generally used after the acute phase of MI.

Dipyridamole (Persantine) thallium stress test: Used when exercise is not possible because of physical disabilities or exercise intolerance. Dipyridamole is a coronary vasodilator that simulates the effect of exercise on the heart while scanning is done to assess for decreased blood flow through the coronary arteries. Not generally used for patients at high risk for infarction or those who are experiencing acute MI, because the test can prompt MI.

Technetium-99m pyrophosphate radionuclide imaging: May help to localize area of infarction and demonstrate necrotic tissue. IV pyrophosphate will bind with calcium, which is found in high concentrations within the cells of necrotic tissue, and appears as a darkened area or "hot spot" on the scan up to 10 days after MI.

Technetium-99m sestamibi radionuclide imaging: Enhances nuclear imaging to allow clearer views of myocardial tissue perfusion, ventricular function, and gated pool ejection fractions.

Coronary angiocardiography or cardiac catheterization: To determine presence and extent of coronary artery disease or valvular disease as the cause of the chest pain or myocardial infarction. Reliably determines the status of coronary perfusion to the left and right sides of the heart. A radiopaque catheter is inserted through a peripheral vessel and advanced to the heart, where measurements are done of ejection fraction, degree of stenosis of vessels and valves, status of pressures in the major vessels and chambers (atria and ventricles), and wall motion. Characteristics of lesions can be described for prescription of most appropriate treatment. Cardiac catheterization also allows for direct injection of thrombolytics (e.g., streptokinase, t-PA) into the coronary system during acute MI.

Positron emission tomography (PET): Use of isotopes to assess metabolic activity of areas of infarction to determine if viable, but jeopardized, myocardial tissue is present. Viable tissue has metabolic activity as seen by increased uptake of the glucose tracer and decreased uptake of the blood flow tracer, which is ammonia.

Indium-111 antimyosin imaging: Technique in which antibodies (antimyosin) are labeled with radioactive indium-111 and injected to permit visualization of damaged areas. The antibody is taken up by damaged myocardial cells as white blood cells rush to the area as part of the inflammatory process.

Serum lipid tests

Cholesterol analysis: A total cholesterol test measures the circulating levels of free cholesterol and cholesterol esters. Concentrations vary with age. Most cardiologists prefer patients to have a total cholesterol level of <200 mg/dl.

Lipoprotein-cholesterol fractionation: Measures the major lipids in the serum. These include very-low-density lipoproteins (VLDL), low-density lipoproteins (LDL), and high-density lipoproteins (HDL). Cholesterol in HDL is inversely related to the incidence of CAD: the higher the HDL, the lower the incidence of CAD. Normal HDL levels range from 29 to 77 mg/dl; normal LDL levels range from 62 to 185 mg/dl. High LDL levels increase the risk of CAD.

Triglyceride analysis: This test analyzes the storage form of lipids, which constitute 95% of fatty tissue. Although not in itself diagnostic of CAD, serum triglyceride analysis enables early identification of those individuals who may have increased risk of CAD. Triglyceride values are age related, but a generally accepted range is 40-150 mg/dl in individuals age 50-59 yr.

Serum magnesium level: Often drops in AMI. Low levels are associated with dysrhythmias.

COLLABORATIVE MANAGEMENT

Relief of acute pain: Drugs are administered and titrated to reduce or eliminate chest pain.

Oxygen: Usually 2-4 L/min by nasal cannula, or mode and rate as directed by arterial blood gas (ABG) values. Used to promote both myocardial and generalized increases in oxygenation. As oxygen (O_2) delivery to the heart is enhanced, pain can be relieved. If the patient deteriorates, other methods of O_2 delivery may be implemented (e.g., non-rebreathing mask with reservoir and mechanical ventilation for those who markedly deteriorate).

> **Note:** Patients with chest discomfort that is unrelieved by O_2 and nitrates are in all probability having an acute MI and should be evaluated immediately for a reperfusion strategy.

Oral, sublingual, and other forms of nitrates/nitroglycerin (NTG): Can be used for short-term therapy or longer-lasting prophylactic effects. These non-IV medications are used for management of myocardial ischemia or angina pectoris rather than for myocardial infarction.

IV nitrates/NTG: For unstable angina or evolving MI, it is titrated until relief is obtained, generally up to 200 μg/min as long as the patient maintains a systolic blood pressure of at least 80 mm Hg.

IV morphine sulfate: Given in small increments (e.g., 2 mg) until relief is obtained. This medication is usually not necessary unless an MI is occurring.

Calcium channel blockers (e.g., nifedipine, diltiazem):   Block the movement of calcium into the cells, causing vasodilation of the coronary and peripheral arteries to relieve chest pain caused by coronary artery spasm. In addition, they can control a rapid heart rate (e.g., supraventricular tachycardias) and decrease the force of contraction, resulting in reduced oxygen demand. For patients with acute MI, these medications are no longer recommended as part of primary therapies but may be used as an adjunct for dysrhythmia management per advanced cardiac life support (ACLS) guidelines.

Reduction of cardiac workload to decrease oxygen demand

Beta-(β-)adrenergic blocking agents (e.g., metoprolol, carvedilol, propranolol):   To decrease HR, BP, and myocardial contractility. Strongly recommended as part of primary pharmacologic therapy for acute MI patients.

Angiotensin-converting enzyme (ACE) inhibitors (e.g., enalapril, ramipril, quinapril):   To decrease BP and thus reduce the resistance to ventricular ejection. Used for patients with myocardial ischemia and after MI if patients need long-term BP control. Effective in prevention of heart failure.

Prevention, recognition, and treatment of dysrhythmias: ACLS algorithms (see Appendix 1) or agency protocol used.

> *Caution:*   Caution should be exercised in use of antidysrhythmic agents in acute MI patients, especially with management of reperfusion dysrhythmias.

Instability of the conduction system with acute MI is sometimes aggravated by use of antidysrhythmic agents. Electrical therapies such as synchronized cardioversion, defibrillation, external/transthoracic pacing, or transvenous pacing may provide a safer management strategy for these patients.

Limit activities: Restrictions based on patient's activity tolerance. Bed rest with bedside commode privileges generally is recommended for patients with acute MI for up to 12 h after symptom onset. Longer periods of bed rest can promote development of orthostatic intolerance, which is preventable by elevation of the head of the bed, dangling, and other low exertion activities. Patients should be instructed to avoid the Valsalva maneuver when toileting, because it may predispose them to ventricular dysrhythmias.

Management of unstable angina and myocardial infarction

Prevention of coronary thrombus formation: May include administration of an anticoagulant (heparin infusion) and antiplatelet drugs (aspirin, ticlopidine, GPIIb/IIIa inhibitors such as abciximab, eptifibatide, tirofiban) to prevent thrombus formation. In acute MI patients, these agents are thought to abate complete closure of the coronary arteries or to prevent more extensive clot formation.

Hemodynamic monitoring: Used in a patient with a complicated MI that results in ventricular failure with threat of cardiogenic shock. Pulmonary artery (PA) and capillary pressures are measured, along with cardiac output and systemic vascular resistance (SVR). With AMI, the following are likely to be found: increased pulmonary artery pressure (PAP), increased pulmonary artery wedge pressure (PAWP), decreased cardiac output (CO), and increased SVR.

Percutaneous transluminal coronary angioplasty (PTCA):   Invasive procedure for improving blood flow through stenotic coronary arteries. A balloon-tipped catheter is inserted into the coronary arterial lesion, and the balloon is inflated to compress the plaque material against the vessel wall, thereby opening the narrowed lumen. PTCA is indicated for the surgical candidate whose angina is refractory to medical treatment. It also is performed on individuals with acute MI, postinfarction angina, postbypass angina, and chronic stable angina. The ideal candidate has single-vessel disease with a discrete, proximal, noncalcified lesion. As technology has improved, patients with more complex conditions have become routine candidates for the procedure if performed by an experienced invasive cardiologist.

During the procedure the patient is sedated lightly and is given a local anesthetic at the insertion site—usually the femoral artery; ECG electrodes are placed on the chest. A PA catheter is passed through the vena cava and right atrium into the heart for pressure measurements. A pacing wire may be inserted as well. An introducer sheath is inserted into the femoral artery, a guidewire is passed into the aorta and coronary artery, and the balloon catheter is passed over the guidewire to the stenotic site. The patient may be asked to take deep breaths and cough to facilitate passage of the catheter. Heparin is given to prevent clot formation. The balloon is inflated repeatedly for 60-90 sec at a pressure of 4-15 atmosphere (atm). Subsequently, radiopaque dye is injected to determine whether the stenosis has been reduced to less than 50% of the vessel diameter, which is the goal of the procedure. The introducer sheath is left in the femoral artery for up to 12 h after PTCA for heparin infusion or in the event of the need for repeat angiography.

Complications after PTCA include acute coronary artery occlusion, reocclusion in acute MI patients, acute myocardial infarction (AMI), coronary artery spasm, bleeding, circulatory insufficiency, renal hypersensitivity to contrast material, hypokalemia, vasovagal reaction, dysrhythmias, and hypotension. Restenosis can occur 6 wk-6 mo after PTCA, although the patient may not experience angina.

Coronary artery atherectomy: Removes atherosclerotic plaque from coronary arteries using special catheter equipped with a cutting device that shaves the lesion. Fragments from the technique are collected into the "nose cone" of the device (directional atherectomy); pulverized and dispersed into the circulation (rotational or "rotoblade" atherectomy); or aspirated (transluminal extraction catheterization [TEC]). May be used for patients with myocardial ischemia and during or after an acute MI.

Intracoronary stent procedure: Endovascular stents are metal-mesh tubes used to keep arteries open. A variety of designs, materials, and deployment procedures are available. Balloon-expanded stents are most commonly used in the United States and are inserted during PTCA. May be used for stenosed coronary arteries or to reopen stenotic coronary artery bypass graft (CABG) replacement vessels (grafts).

Laser coronary angioplasty: Enables debulking of distal coronary lesions in tortuous arteries to allow for reperfusion. The laser is a part of the coronary artery catheter (similar to the device used in PTCA) and ablates only the tissue it contacts.

Additional interventions for management of acute myocardial infarction
Thrombolytic therapy (lysis of coronary arterial clot):   Used for reperfusion of the occluded coronary vessel(s) that cause AMI. Drugs include alteplase (r-TPA, Activase); reteplase (Retavase); streptokinase; urokinase; and anisoylated plasminogen streptokinase activator complex (APSAC, Eminase). Thrombolytic therapy is an American Heart Association (AHA) and American College of Cardiology (ACC) class I intervention for patients with ST-segment elevation in two or more contiguous leads, bundle branch block (obscuring ST-segment analysis), and history suggestive of acute MI who present within 12 h of symptom onset and are <75 years of age. Patients must be carefully screened for risk of bleeding before administration of these IV medications. Time from the entry of the patient into the emergency department of the hospital to treatment with thrombolytics should be no longer than 1 h and, ideally, within 30 min of arrival. Thrombolytics are also used for direct injection into the coronary arteries as part of coronary angiography during cardiac catheterization and angioplasty.

Surgical revascularization: Revascularization procedures are seldom used as the primary management strategy for acute MI. Several approaches are available for myocardial revascularization, including CABG via median sternotomy or minimally invasive technique. Patients with multivessel or diffuse coronary artery disease are the most appropriate candidates for these procedures. Surgical indications include (1) stable angina with 50% stenosis of the left main coronary artery, (2) stable angina with three-vessel coronary artery disease, (3) unstable angina with three-vessel disease or severe two-vessel disease, (4) recent MI, (5) ischemic heart failure with cardiogenic shock, and (6) signs of ischemia or impending MI after angiography procedure.

Cardiac surgery should be readily available for patients who experience complications undergoing any diagnostic or treatment procedures in the cardiac catheterization laboratory.

NURSING DIAGNOSES AND INTERVENTIONS

Pain (chest) related to biophysiologic injury secondary to decreased oxygen supply to the myocardium

Desired outcomes: Within 1 h of intervention, patient's subjective evaluation of discomfort improves, as documented by a pain scale. Nonverbal indicators, such as grimacing, are absent. Vital signs return to baseline. ECG changes present during event resolve.

- Assess and document the character of the patient's chest pain, including location, duration, quality, intensity, precipitating and alleviating factors, presence or absence of radiation, and associated symptoms. Devise a pain scale with patient, rating discomfort from 0 (no pain) to 10.
- Measure BP and HR with each episode of chest pain. BP and HR may increase because of sympathetic stimulation as a result of pain. If the chest pain is caused by ischemia, the heart muscle may not be functioning normally and cardiac output may decrease, resulting in a low BP. In addition, dysrhythmias such as bradycardia and ventricular ectopy may be noted with ischemia.
- Obtain a 12/15/18-lead ECG during patient's episode of chest pain. During angina, ischemia usually is demonstrated on the ECG by ST-segment depression and T-wave inversion.
- Administer nitrates as prescribed, titrating IV NTG so that chest pain is relieved yet systolic BP remains >90 mm Hg. NTG drip is usually 100 mg NTG in 250 ml D_5W. Begin with 3 ml/min, which is 19.8 μg/min. Titrate by increments of 3 ml q5min (or 19.8 μg/min q5min) up to a maximum dosage determined by agency protocol or physician.
- After each titration of IV NTG, evaluate patient's BP and the effects of therapy in relieving patient's chest pain. If slight hypotension occurs (80-90 mm Hg systolic), reduce the flow rate to 1/2 or less of the infusing dose. If severe hypotension (<80 mm Hg systolic) occurs, stop the infusion and contact the physician for further directions. In either situation the physician may prescribe a low-dose positive inotropic agent (e.g., dopamine, dobutamine) to enhance cardiac contractility. For additional information, see "Inotropic and Vasoactive Agents," Appendix 7.
- Monitor for side effects of NTG, including headache, hypotension, syncope, facial flushing, and nausea. If side effects occur, place patient in a supine position and consult physician for further interventions.
- As prescribed, administer β-blockers and calcium channel blockers, which relieve chest pain by (1) diminishing coronary artery spasm, causing coronary and peripheral vasodilation and (2) decreasing myocardial contractility and oxygen demand. Monitor for side effects, including bradycardia and hypotension. Be alert to indicators of heart failure, including fatigue, SOB, weight gain, and edema, and to indicators of heart block, such as syncope and dizziness.
- Administer heparin, GPIIb/IIIa inhibitors (abciximab, tirofiban, eptifibatide),

and ASA as prescribed. Heparin infusion usually should be administered using a weight-based protocol, which is titrated according to partial thromboplastin time (PTT) results. These patients are predisposed to bleeding and may need to be placed on bleeding precautions.

- Administer oxygen per nasal cannula at 2-4 L/min, as prescribed.
- Position patient according to his or her comfort level.
- Provide care in a calm and efficient manner; reassure and support patient during chest pain episodes. Offer healing touch therapy, relaxation exercises, or music therapy, as appropriate.
- Maintain a quiet environment and group patient care activities to allow for periods of uninterrupted rest.
- Ensure that activity restrictions and bed rest are maintained; teach patient about activity limitation and its rationale: to minimize oxygen requirements and thus decrease chest pain. Reassure patient that activities are allowed based on individual response. Often, patients may be afraid to engage in activities for fear of further deterioration.
- Instruct patient to report any further episodes of chest pain.

You may also wish to refer to the following interventions from the Nursing Interventions Classification (NIC):

NIC Pain Management; Analgesic Administration; Cardiac Care: Acute; Hemodynamic Regulation; Oxygen Therapy
- For more information about pain, see p. 61.

Decreased cardiac output (or risk for same) related to negative inotropic changes secondary to vessel occlusion, infarction, coronary artery spasm, and cardiac tamponade; electrical factors secondary to dysrhythmias

Desired outcomes: Within 24 h of this diagnosis, patient exhibits adequate cardiac output, as evidenced by BP within normal limits for patient; HR 60-100 beats per minute (bpm); normal sinus rhythm on ECG; peripheral pulses >2+ on a 0-4+ scale; warm and dry skin; hourly urine output ≥0.5 ml/kg; measured CO 4-7 L/min; right atrial pressure (RAP) 4-6 mm Hg; PAP 20-30/8-15 mm Hg; PAWP 6-12 mm Hg; and patient awake, alert, oriented, and free from anginal pain.

- Monitor BP, RAP/CVP, and PAP continuously; monitor PAWP and CO hourly. Be alert to the following indicators of decreased CO: decreased BP, increased HR, increased PAP, increased PAWP, decreased measured CO, and decreased RAP.
- Monitor ECG continuously for evidence of dysrhythmias and ST and T-wave changes. Observe for bradydysrhythmias during sheath removal. Run a 12/15/18-lead ECG daily.
- Monitor urinary output hourly for the first 4 h, and thereafter according to agency protocol. Consult physician for hourly output <0.5 ml/kg/h for 2 consecutive hours.
- Measure creatine kinase-myocardial band (CK-MB) immediately after PTCA and then q8h for 24 h; report elevations. Optimally, CK-MB will be 0%-5% of total CK.
- Monitor patient for hypotension caused by antianginal and coronary vasodilator medications. As a result of vessel occlusion, consult physician and treat hypotension immediately, as prescribed. Usually, fluids are given and the patient is placed in supine position. If the patient has left ventricular heart failure and pulmonary congestion, the supine position may prompt respiratory distress.
- When patient first sits up, ensure that it is done in stages to minimize the likelihood of postural hypotension. Monitor VS at frequent intervals during this stage.
- Monitor patient continuously for bleeding at sheath insertion site. Monitor hematocrit (Hct) level for decrease from baseline values.
- Monitor patient for evidence of cardiac tamponade: hypotension, tachycardia, pulsus paradoxus, jugular venous distention, elevation and plateau

pressuring of PAWP and RAP, and possibly an enlarged heart silhouette on chest x-ray.

- When heparin and antiplatelet drugs are discontinued, monitor patient closely for indicators of coronary occlusion: ST-segment elevation on ECG, angina, hypotension, tachycardia, dysrhythmias, and diaphoresis.
- Monitor peripheral pulses (radial and pedal) and color and temperature of extremities q4h for first 4 h.
- Monitor patient's mental alertness on an ongoing basis.

Additional interventions for decreased cardiac output for myocardial infarction
- Assess for and document the following as evidence of myocardial dysfunction with decreasing cardiac output: presence of jugular venous distention, dependent edema (e.g., sacral), hepatomegaly, fatigue, weakness, decreased activity level, and SOB with activity. In addition, assess and document the following:
  □ *Mental status:* Be alert to restlessness, decreased responsiveness.
  □ *Lung sounds:* Monitor for crackles, rhonchi.
  □ *Heart sounds:* Note presence of gallop, murmur, increased HR.
  □ *Urinary output:* Be alert to output <0.5 ml/kg/h.
  □ *Skin:* Monitor for pallor, mottling, cyanosis, coolness, diaphoresis.
  □ *Vital signs:* Note BP <90 mm Hg systolic, HR >100 bpm, RR >20 breaths/min, and temperature >38.5° C (101.3° F). The temperature of patients with MI may spike as a result of the body's reaction to necrotic tissue.
- Keep accurate intake and output (I&O) records, and weigh patient daily. Be alert to fluid volume excess. A 1-kg acute weight gain can signal retention of 1 L of fluid.
- Help minimize cardiac workload by administering prescribed β-blockers, positioning patient in Fowler's or semi-Fowler's position, and encouraging bed rest.
- Have patient perform active range-of-motion (ROM) exercises, along with level I activities (see Table 4-1) to help prevent deleterious effects of bed rest on oxygen supplies.
- If a PA catheter is present, record hemodynamic readings q1-2h and prn. Be alert to PAWP >18 mm Hg, CO <4 L/min, and cardiac index (CI) <2.5 L/min/m^2.
- Administer and titrate prescribed medications: nitrates and afterload reducing agents, such as nitroprusside, and preload reducing agents, such as nitroglycerin, to maintain SVR within 900-1200 dynes/sec/cm^{-5} and PAWP ≤18 mm Hg; diuretics, such as furosemide and metolazone, to keep PAWP ≤18 mm Hg and urine output ≥0.5 ml/kg/h; and inotropic agents, such as milrinone, dobutamine and dopamine, to keep systolic BP >90 mm Hg.
- Monitor patient continuously in modified chest lead (MCL) V$_1$ to detect ventricular ectopy versus aberrancy. Monitor on V$_2$ if supraventricular dysrhythmias are present or if it is imperative to identify axis deviations. Keep alarms on at all times (e.g., 50-100).
- Assess apical HR hourly. Monitor for irregularities in rhythm.
- Document rhythm strip every shift and prn if dysrhythmias occur. Measure PR segment, QRS complex, and QT interval with each strip. Note and report any deviations from the patient's baseline. Normal intervals are PR 0.10-0.20 sec and QRS 0.10 sec. The QT interval is rate related, and the upper limits of normal usually correspond to approximately one-half the RR interval.
- Monitor serum potassium for levels >5 mEq/L or <3.5 mEq/L. Hypokalemia or hyperkalemia can cause dysrhythmias. Replace potassium as prescribed.

NIC Cardiac Care; Cardiac Care: Acute; Shock Prevention; Hemodynamic Regulation; Dysrhythmia Management

Activity intolerance related to imbalance between oxygen supply and demand secondary to decreased cardiac output associated with coronary artery disease

TABLE 4-1	Activity Level Progression for Hospitalized Patients*	
Level		**Activity**
I	Bed rest	Flexion and extension of extremities qid, 15 times each extremity; deep breathing qid, 15 breaths; position change from side to side q2h
II	OOB to chair	As tolerated, tid for 20-30 min
III	Ambulate in room	As tolerated, tid for 20-30 min
IV	Ambulate in hall	Initially, 50-200 ft bid; progressing to 50-200 ft qid

OOB, Out of bed; *BP,* blood pressure; *HR,* heart rate; *bpm,* beats per minute.
Signs of activity intolerance: Decrease in BP >20 mm Hg; increase in HR to >120 bpm (or >20 bpm above resting HR in patients receiving β-blocker therapy).

Desired Outcome: Within the 12- to 24-h period before discharge from CCU, patient exhibits cardiac tolerance to increasing levels of activity as evidenced by respiratory rate (RR) <24 breaths/min; normal sinus rhythm on ECG; BP within 20 mm Hg of patient's normal range; HR <120 bpm (or within 20 bpm of resting HR for patients on β-blocker therapy); and absence of chest pain.

- Assist patient with identifying activities that precipitate chest pain, and teach patient to use NTG prophylactically before the activity.
- Assist patient as needed in progressive activity program, beginning with level I and progressing to level IV, as tolerated (Table 4-1).
- Assess patient's response to activity progression. Be alert to presence of chest pain, SOB, excessive fatigue, and dysrhythmias. Monitor for a decrease in BP >20 mm Hg and an increase in HR to >120 bpm (>20 bpm above resting HR in patients receiving β-blocker therapy).
- Teach patient about measures that prevent complications of decreased mobility, such as active ROM exercises. (For additional details, see "Prolonged Immobility," p. 74).

NIC Activity Therapy; Energy Management

Knowledge deficit: disease process and its life-style implications

Desired outcome: Within the 24-h period before discharge from the step-down unit, patient verbalizes understanding of his or her disease, as well as the necessary life-style changes that may modify risk factors.

- Teach patient about ischemia and its resultant chest pain, referred to as *angina pectoris.*
- Discuss the pathophysiologic process underlying patient's angina, using drawings or heart models as indicated.
- Assist patient in identifying his or her own risk factors (e.g., cigarette smoking, high-stress life-style).
- Teach patient about risk-factor modification:
  - ☐ *Diet low in cholesterol and saturated fat:* Provide sample diet plan for meals that are low in cholesterol and saturated fat. Teach patient about foods that are high in cholesterol and low in cholesterol and saturated fat (see Tables 4-3 and 4-4). Stress the importance of reading food labels.
  - ☐ *Smoking cessation:* Teach patient that smoking causes the coronary arteries to constrict, thus decreasing blood flow to the heart.
  - ☐ *Stress management:* Discuss the role that stress plays in angina. Explain that stress increases sympathetic tone, which can cause the BP and HR to increase, resulting in increased oxygen demand. By employing relaxation techniques such as imagery, meditation, or biofeedback, one can decrease the effects of stress on the heart. For a sample relaxation technique, see **Health-seeking behavior,** p. 302.

TABLE 4-2   Guidelines for a Progressive At-Home Walking Program

Week	Distance	Time
1	100-200 ft	2×/day
2	200-400 ft	2×/day
3	¼ mi	8-10 min
4	½ mi	15 min
5	1 mi	30 min
6	1¾ mi	30 min
7	2 mi	40 min

- Teach patient about the prescribed medications, including name, purpose, dosage, action, schedule, precautions, and potential side effects.
- Teach patient the actions that should be taken if chest pain is unrelieved or increases in intensity. If chest pain occurs:
  1. Stop and rest.
  2. Take one NTG; wait 5 min. If pain is not relieved, take a second NTG; wait 5 min. If pain is not relieved, take a third NTG.
  3. Lie down if headache occurs. Explain that the vasodilation effect of NTG causes a decrease in BP, which may result in orthostatic hypotension and transient headache.
  4. If the pain is not relieved after three NTGs taken over a 15-min period, call physician or dial 911 or local emergency number.
- Explain to patient that it is no more beneficial to be in the emergency department than it is to be at home during episodes of chest pain caused by angina and therefore traveling to a hospital at the first sign of chest pain usually is unnecessary.
- Review activity limitations and prescribed progressions (Tables 4-1 and 4-2). Provide the following information:
  When you are discharged from the hospital, it is important that you continue your walking program. The guidelines in Table 4-2 are to help you plan a program that is right for you. Don't overestimate your ability; rather, start off slowly and build up. Depending on how you feel, you may only be able to stay at one level or you may progress to 2 mi quickly. Remember to warm up and cool down with stretches for 5-7 min and to walk 3-5 times each week. In addition:
  ☐ Avoid sudden energetic activities.
  ☐ Plan for regular rest periods in the afternoon.
  ☐ Let your body guide you regarding whether to increase or decrease activity.
  ☐ Inform your physician of any changes in activity tolerance, such as the development of new symptoms with the same activity.
  ☐ Avoid exercising outdoors in very cold, hot, or humid weather. Extreme weather places an additional stress on the heart. If you do exercise in extremes of weather, decrease the pace and monitor your response carefully.
- Pulse monitoring: Teach patient how to take pulse, including parameters for target heart rates and limits.
- Sexual activity guidelines: Because sexual activity is a physical activity, certain guidelines can help the patient and his or her partner enjoy a satisfying sexual relationship while minimizing the workload of the heart:
  ☐ Rest is beneficial before engaging in intercourse.

- ☐ Find a position that is comfortable for you and your partner. Assuming a different position that is uncomfortable to both may increase the workload of the heart.
- ☐ Medications such as NTG may be taken prophylactically by the patient before intercourse to prevent chest pain.
- ☐ Postpone intercourse for 1-1½ h after eating a heavy meal.
- ☐ Report the following symptoms to your physician if they are experienced after sexual relations: SOB, increased HR that persists for more than 15 min, unrelieved chest pain.

▉NIC Teaching: Disease Process; Teaching: Prescribed Activity/Exercise; Teaching: Prescribed Medication; Teaching: Sexuality

For patients undergoing percutaneous transluminal coronary angioplasty
Knowledge deficit: angioplasty procedure and postprocedure care
Desired outcomes: Within the 24-h period before the procedure, patient describes the rationale for the procedure, how it is performed, and postprocedure care. Patient relates discharge instructions within the 24-h period before discharge from the CCU.
- Assess patient's understanding of CAD and the purpose of angioplasty. Evaluate patient's style of coping and degree of information desired.
- As appropriate for coping style, discuss the following with patient and significant others:
  - ☐ Location of patient's CAD, using heart drawing.
  - ☐ Use of local anesthesia and sedation during procedure.
  - ☐ Insertion site of catheter: groin or arm.
  - ☐ Sensations that may occur: mild chest discomfort; a feeling of heat as the dye is injected.
  - ☐ Use of fluoroscopy during procedure. Determine patient's history of sensitivity to contrast material.
  - ☐ Ongoing observations made by nurse after procedure: BP, HR, ECG, leg or arm pulses, blood tests.
  - ☐ Importance of lying flat in bed for 6-12 h after procedure.
  - ☐ Necessity for nursing assistance with eating, drinking, and toileting needs after procedure.
  - ☐ Need for increased fluid intake after procedure to flush dye from system.
  - ☐ Discharge instructions: importance of taking antiplatelet drugs to prevent restenosis, avoidance of strenuous activity during first few weeks at home, follow-up visit with cardiologist 1 wk after hospital discharge, signs and symptoms to report to physician (e.g., GI upset, repeat of angina, fainting).
- If patient and significant others express or exhibit evidence of anxiety regarding the procedure, try to arrange for them to meet with another patient who has had a successful angioplasty.

▉NIC Teaching: Procedure/Treatment; Anxiety Reduction; Support Group
Altered tissue perfusion (or risk for same): peripheral: involved limb, related to interruption of arterial blood flow secondary to presence of angioplasty sheath; risk of clot formation in vessel after sheath removal
Desired outcome: Upon admission to CCU and continuously thereafter, patient has adequate tissue perfusion in the involved limb as evidenced by warm skin; peripheral pulses >2+ on a 0-4+ scale; normal skin color; ability to move the toes; and complete sensation.
- Monitor circulation to affected limb q30min for 2 h and then q2h thereafter. Assess pulses, temperature, color, sensation, and mobility of toes. Be alert to weak or thready pulses, coolness and pallor of the extremity, and patient complaints of numbness and tingling. Consult physician immediately if any of these signs or symptoms are present.
- Inspect sheath site for signs of external or subcutaneous bleeding.
- Keep sandbag at insertion site until discontinued by physician.

- Maintain immobilization of limb for at least 6 h or until discontinued by physician. *Requirements may differ per institutional protocols.*
- Keep head of bed (HOB) no higher than 15 degrees to prevent kinking of sheath.
- Monitor sheath patency by evaluating for continuous IV infusion into the involved vessel.
- Instruct patient to notify staff immediately if numbness, tingling, or pain occurs at the affected extremity.

NIC Peripheral Sensation Management; Surveillance

Knowledge deficit: myocardial infarction and its implications for life-style changes

Desired outcome: Within the 24-h period before discharge from CCU, patient and significant others verbalize an understanding of heart attack and the necessary life-style changes that must be made.

- Discuss the following with patient and significant others, providing both oral instructions and written materials:
  ☐ Anatomy and functions of the heart muscle.
  ☐ Coronary arteries and the atherosclerotic process.
  ☐ Definition of "heart attack."
  ☐ Healing process of the heart and the role of collateral circulation.
- Assist patient with identifying his or her own risk factors.
- Assist patient with devising a plan for risk-factor modification (e.g., diet, smoking cessation, stress-reduction techniques).
- Provide guidelines for a diet low in cholesterol and saturated fat (Tables 4-3 and 4-4); refer patient to nutritionist.
- Discuss post-MI activity progression (e.g., a progressive walking program). See Tables 4-1 and 4-2.
- Discuss guidelines for resuming post-MI sexual activity. Explain that sexual activity requires the same amount of oxygen as that needed to walk briskly up two flights of stairs; consequently, patients usually are instructed to wait 2 wk after hospital discharge before resuming sexual activity.
- Teach patient about medications that will be taken after hospital discharge, including name, purpose, dosage, schedule, precautions, and potential side effects.

NIC Teaching: Prescribed Diet; Anxiety Reduction; Support Group; Teaching: Disease Process; Teaching: Prescribed Activity/Exercise; Teaching: Prescribed Medication; Teaching: Sexuality

For patients undergoing coronary artery bypass grafting (CABG) for myocardial revascularization
Risk for fluid volume deficit related to loss of fluid through normal and abnormal routes secondary to postoperative diuresis and excessive bleeding

> **Note:**   Diuresis is common in the early postoperative period because of the hormonal changes that accompany surgery.

Desired outcome: Patient is normovolemic as evidenced by intake equal to output plus insensible losses; RAP ≥4 mm Hg; PAWP ≥6 mm Hg; and urinary output between 30 and 120 ml/h.

- Measure I&O hourly. Consult physician for imbalance in I&O ratio (i.e., urinary output ≥120 ml/h and chest tube drainage ≥100 ml/h). Replace excessive chest tube drainage with packed red blood cells (RBCs) as prescribed.
- Monitor RAP and PAP mean hourly. Correlate PAP mean to PAWP. Consult physician for PAP/PAWP <6 mm Hg and RAP <4 mm Hg.
- As prescribed, administer IV fluids in the early postoperative period to equal the amount of diuresis.

TABLE 4-3   Low-Cholesterol Dietary Guidelines

Foods to avoid	Foods allowed
Egg yolks (no more than 3/wk)	Egg whites; cholesterol-free egg substitutes
Foods made with many egg yolks (e.g., sponge cakes)	Lean, well-trimmed meats; minimize servings of beef, lamb, and pork
Fatty cuts of meat, fat on meats	Fish (except shellfish), chicken, and turkey (without the skin)
Skin on chicken and turkey	Dried peas and beans as meat substitutes
Luncheon meats or cold cuts	Nonfat (skim) or low-fat (2%) milk
Sausage, frankfurters	Low-fat cheeses
Shellfish (e.g., lobster, shrimp, crab)	Ice milk and sherbet
Whole milk, cream, whole milk cheese	Polyunsaturated oils for cooking and food preparation: canola, corn, safflower, cottonseed, sesame, and sunflower
Ice cream	Margarines that list one of the above oils as their first ingredient
Commercially prepared foods with hydrogenated shortening, which is saturated fat	Foods prepared "from scratch" with the above suggested oils
Coconut and palm oils and products made with them (e.g., cream substitutes)	Meats (in acceptable quantity) and vegetables prepared by broiling, steaming, or baking (never frying)
Butter, lard, hydrogenated shortening	Spices, herbs, lemon juice, wine, flavored wine vinegars
Meats and vegetables prepared by frying	
Seasonings containing large amounts of sugar and saturated fats	
Sauces and gravies	
Salad dressings containing cream, cheeses, or mayonnaise	

TABLE 4-4   Guidelines for a Diet Low in Saturated Fat

Foods to avoid	Foods to choose
Red meat, especially when highly "marbled"; salami, sausages, bacon	Lean cuts of meat, fresh fish, poultry from which skin was removed before cooking; meats that have been grilled
Whole milk, whipping cream	Low-fat or skim milk
Tropical oils (coconut, palm oils; cocoa butter)	Monosaturated cooking oils, such as olive or canola oil
Candy	Fresh fruit, vegetables
Sweet rolls, donuts	Whole grain breads, cereals
Ice cream	Nonfat yogurt, sherbet
Salad dressings	Vinegar, lemon juice
Peanut butter, peanuts, hot dogs, potato chips	Unbuttered popcorn
Butter	Margarine (safflower oil listed as the first ingredient)

- Monitor clotting studies (i.e., prothrombin time [PT], PTT, activated clotting time [ACT], platelet count) immediately postoperatively and then q12h for 24 h. Be alert to prolongation of PT, PTT, ACT; decreased platelet count; and low fibrinogen value. Optimal values are: PT 11-15 sec; PTT 30-40 sec (activated); ACT ≤120 sec; platelet count 150,000-400,000/mm^3; and fibrinogen 200-400 mg/dl.
- Replace clotting factors as prescribed with platelets, fresh frozen plasma, cryoprecipitate; administer protamine or aminocaproic acid as prescribed.
- Assess chest x-ray immediately after surgery and daily for signs of bleeding into the pericardial sac and mediastinum, as evidenced by an increase in the cardiac silhouette.

NIC Fluid Management; Fluid Monitoring; Blood Products Administration; Shock Management: Volume; Hypovolemia Management

Hypothermia related to prolonged cooling of body during surgery

Desired outcomes: Patient's body temperature is returned to normal at a rate not greater than 1° C/h as evidenced by warm extremities and absence of shivering. Within 8 h of treatment, oxygen saturation is ≥95%; CO is 4-7 L/min; SVR is ≥900 dynes/ sec/cm^{-5}; HR is 60-100 bpm; and BP is within patient's normal range.

> **Note:** The danger of postoperative hypothermia in heart surgery is that the patient will warm too quickly and shiver, causing hypertension or hypotension, increased or decreased SVR, metabolic acidosis, and hypoxia. Each of these problems can increase cardiac workload and may potentiate ischemia, dysrhythmias, or hemorrhage in the early postoperative period.

- On a continuous basis, measure core temperature via rectal, tympanic, or thermodilution catheter. If temperature is <36° C (96.8° F), initiate warming measures such as warm blankets, thermal garment, heating lamps, heating blankets, or warm inspired gases.
- Continue to monitor patient during rewarming phase, maintaining rewarming rate at 1° C/h.
- Monitor skin temperature, particularly that of the extremities, q30min-1h during rewarming. Once extremities are warm, patient should be close to normothermia and warming measures should be discontinued.
- Monitor BP, pulse, CO, and SVR continuously during rewarming for sudden changes related to rewarming. SVR may fall along with BP as the peripheral vascular bed dilates. This can precipitate sudden hypotension.
- If shivering caused by hypothermia develops, treat immediately with warming measures and drug therapy as prescribed. Drugs used to treat shivering may include morphine sulfate, diazepam or other benzodiazepines, or, in extreme instances, a neuromuscular blocking agent (e.g., vecuronium). During shivering episodes, monitor VS for changes and assess oxygen saturation continuously with oximeter.

NIC Hypothermia Treatment; Temperature Regulation; Vital Signs Monitoring

Impaired gas exchange (or risk for same) related to altered oxygen supply, alveolar-capillary membrane changes, and altered oxygen-carrying capacity of the blood secondary to central nervous system (CNS) depression from anesthesia, atelectasis, and decreased hemoglobin

Desired outcomes: Within 12-24 h of treatment, patient has adequate gas exchange as evidenced by Pao$_2$ ≥80 mm Hg; Paco$_2$ 35-45 mm Hg; pH 7.35-7.45; presence of normal breath sounds; and absence of adventitious breath sounds. RR is 12-20 breaths/min with normal pattern and depth (eupnea).

- During intubation period, provide supportive measures to ensure optimal aeration: perform suctioning when its need is determined by auscultatory findings, turn patient q2h, and maintain HOB at an elevation of 45 degrees, if tolerated.

- Assess breath sounds, RR, and amount and character of mucus production hourly during the first 12 h after surgery. Be alert to crackles and rhonchi, labored breathing, and subjective complaints of breathing difficulties. Copious, tenacious secretions place the patient at risk for airway obstruction caused by mucus plugging.
- Monitor SpO_2. Be alert to sustained levels <90%.
- Assess ABG values upon admission and prn during periods of respiratory distress. Consult physician for significant findings, including a decreasing PaO_2, increased $PaCO_2$, and the presence of acidosis or alkalosis.
- Consult physician regarding need for ventilation changes if the aforementioned assessments suggest the need.
- As prescribed, perform weaning and extubation as early as possible. Use nonopiate analgesics (e.g., ketorolac [Toradol]), and closely monitor the effects of incremental doses of opiate analgesics and sedatives to avoid excessive sedation during the weaning process.
  - ☐ Explain weaning procedure to patient. Stay with patient during first 15 min after each ventilatory change, and reassure patient about his or her ability to breathe independently. Instruct patient to take slow, deep breaths.
  - ☐ Monitor patient's RR, tidal volume, expiratory pressure, BP, HR, and ECG during weaning. Consult physician for changes, inasmuch as they may be indicative of weaning intolerance.
  - ☐ Assess for indicators that suggest hypoxemia during weaning: agitation, irritability, tachycardia, and diaphoresis.
- After extubation, turn patient q2h. Have patient deep breathe and cough q2h, and use incentive spirometry hourly. As prescribed, perform chest physiotherapy qid.
- As soon as tolerated, have patient dangle lower extremities over the side of bed and sit in chair.
- Instruct patient to sit upright as much as possible and to perform deep-breathing exercises. In addition, teach patient the following procedure for basal expansion exercises, which are indicated for patients recovering from chest surgery for whom pain on the surgical side inhibits bilateral chest expansion:
  1. With patient sitting upright, position your palms on the midaxillary lines in the area of the eighth ribs. Instruct patient to inhale as you apply moderate pressure.
  2. Instruct patient to attempt to move your hands outward while expanding the lower ribs.
  3. Instruct patient to maintain maximum inspiration for 1-2 sec to achieve optimal aeration of the alveoli.
  4. Have patient exhale in a relaxed, passive manner.
  5. Teach patients to perform this exercise independently by positioning their own palms against the eighth ribs.
- Explain that performing this technique correctly and at frequent intervals will promote mobility of the lower portion of the chest wall.

NIC Airway Management; Acid-Base Monitoring; Acid-Base Management; Oxygen Therapy; Respiratory Monitoring

ADDITIONAL NURSING DIAGNOSES

Also see nursing diagnoses and interventions as appropriate in "Nutritional Support," p. 1; "Mechanical Ventilation," p. 17; "Hemodynamic Monitoring," p. 28; "Prolonged Immobility," p. 74; "Psychosocial Support," p. 83; "Psychosocial Support for the Patient's Family and Significant Others," p. 95; "Acute Cardiac Tamponade," p. 144; "Heart Failure/Pulmonary edema," p. 265; "Dysrhythmias and Conduction Disturbances," p. 277; "Acute Pericarditis," p. 325; "Cardiogenic Shock," p. 343.

Heart failure/pulmonary edema

PATHOPHYSIOLOGY

Any form of cardiovascular disease may lead to heart failure. Effective pumping of the heart depends on the cardiac cycle: preload (end diastolic volume in the ventricles), which stretches the myocardial fibers; afterload (resistance to ejection); and contractility of the myocardium. Myocardial contractility heavily depends on the delivery of oxygen and nutrients to the heart. Patients with cardiomyopathy, valvular disease, hypertension, or coronary artery disease may have oxygen deprivation to a portion of the myocardium (local) or across the entire ventricle (global), resulting in ventricular wall motion or contractility alterations. Deprived areas can become hypokinetic (weakly contractile), akinetic (noncontractile), or dyskinetic (moving opposite from the normal tissues). Compromised patients may also have dysrhythmias that disturb the cardiac cycle, resulting from damage to the conduction pathways. Less frequently, the heart cannot compensate for greatly increased metabolic demands, such as with thyroid storm or pheochromocytoma. These metabolically deranged patients manifest symptoms of heart failure as a result of insufficient oxygen delivery to compensate for an elevated metabolic rate. One ventricle typically fails before the other, so pump failure is discussed as either the left or right heart/ventricular or both ventricles (biventricular). Failure caused by problems with contractility results from CAD (ischemia) and cardiomyopathy. As blood fails to be effectively ejected, preload increases when the volume of blood in the ventricles increases. Heart failure also results from elevated arterial pressure (hypertension, aortic stenosis) or elevated diastolic volume (i.e., aortic stenosis), which both increase afterload.

Heart failure is the leading cause of death in the United States. The incidence more than doubles each decade among the population who are 45-75 years old, and the disease is the most common nonsurgical medical discharge diagnosis for patients 65 years and older. Approximately 75% of the ambulatory patients with heart failure are at least 60 years old. Nearly 50% of patients with heart failure die within 5 years of initial diagnosis. The annual medical cost is $10-$15 billion, with certain estimates 2-3 times higher when including the debilitating, life-changing nature of the disease.

Left heart failure: Patients may have left heart failure resulting from problems with either ventricular systole or diastole. With inadequate contraction of the heart during systole, blood cannot move forward effectively through the arterial system to deliver oxygen and nutrients to the rest of the body systems. Problems with diastole are related to failure of the ventricle to effectively "relax" during diastole, resulting in inadequate filling. Either cause of heart failure can result in pulmonary vascular congestion and edema.

Right heart failure: Failure of the right heart results from increased resistance to right ventricular ejection, owing to either left heart failure or lung disease (e.g., pulmonary hypertension). Right ventricular MI, cardiomyopathy, or trauma often result in ineffective, abnormal right ventricular wall motion, resulting in reduced ejection into the pulmonary circulation with subsequent congestion in the venous system (inferior and superior vena cava and branching vessels). Perfusion to the left ventricle is also compromised because blood does not flow at the normal rate from the right ventricle through the pulmonary vasculature into the left side of the heart.

Biventricular failure: Patients who experience a left ventricular MI coupled with a right ventricular MI experience hemodynamics that are extremely complex to manage. The impaired right ventricle needs volume infusion to promote better expansion, or "more stretch," of the ventricle, whereas the left ventricle may be unable to accommodate a normal or pre-MI volume and requires volume reduction. Deviation of the intraventricular septum associated with right heart failure caused by distention of the ventricle can significantly reduce the size of the left ventricle. Ultimately, failure in either side of the heart will affect both sides, because the ventricles are interdependent.

ASSESSMENT

History and risk factors: Familial history of CAD, age >65 yr, male sex (risk for females increases after menopause), cigarette smoking, hypercholesterolemia, hypertension, diabetes, obesity, increased stress, and sedentary life-style. Other important data include noncompliance with low-sodium diet or medications and a decreased exercise tolerance.

Left heart failure (pulmonary edema/congestion)
Clinical presentation: Anxiety, air hunger, increased respiratory rate, nocturnal dyspnea, dyspnea on exertion (DOE), orthopnea, moist cough with frothy sputum, tachycardia, diaphoresis, cyanosis or pallor, insomnia, palpitations, weakness, fatigue, anorexia, and changes in mentation.
Physical assessment: Decreased BP, tachycardia, dysrhythmias, tachypnea, crackles or bibasilar rales, S_3 or summation gallop, and pulsus alternans (alternating strength of the peripheral pulse caused by the failing heart muscle).
Monitoring parameters: Decreased CO/CI; elevated PAP, PAWP, and SVR.

Right heart failure (cor pulmonale/systemic congestion)
Clinical presentation: Fluid retention, peripheral edema, decreased urinary output, abdominal tenderness, nausea, vomiting, constipation, and anorexia.
Physical assessment: Hepatomegaly, splenomegaly, dependent pitting edema, jugular venous distention, positive hepatojugular reflex, and ascites.
Monitoring parameters: Elevated RAP and central venous pressure (CVP). Possibly decreased CO/CI, caused by failure of right ventricle to pump adequate blood through the pulmonary vasculature to maintain adequate left ventricular filling volumes for normal cardiac output.

Biventricular failure (systemic and pulmonary congestion)
Clinical presentation: All signs of both right and left heart failure, as stated, along with probable signs of cardiogenic shock in acutely ill patients. Peripheral cyanosis, fatigue, decreased tissue perfusion, decrease in metabolism, and low urinary output.
Physical assessment: Hypotension, tachycardia, tachypnea, pulmonary edema, pitting peripheral edema, hepatosplenomegaly, distended neck veins, pallor, and cyanosis.
Monitoring parameters: Decreased CO/CI; elevated PAP, PAWP, SVR, pulmonary vascular resistance (PVR), RAP, and CVP.

DIAGNOSTIC TESTS

Chest x-ray: May reveal pulmonary edema, increased interstitial density, infiltrates, engorged pulmonary vasculature, and cardiomegaly.
Serum electrolyte levels: May reveal hyponatremia (dilutional); hyperkalemia if glomerular filtration is decreased; or hypokalemia, which can result from use of diuretics.
Hepatic enzymes: Serum glutamate oxaloacetate transaminase/aspartate aminotransferase (SGOT/AST) and serum glutamate pyruvate transaminase/alanine aminotransferase (SGPT/ALT) levels may be elevated because of hepatic venous congestion.
Serum bilirubin levels: May reveal hyperbilirubinemia if there is liver congestion.
CBC: May reveal decreased Hgb and Hct levels in the presence of anemia or dilution.
ABG values: May reveal hypoxemia caused by the decreased oxygen available from fluid-filled alveoli and respiratory alkalosis because of the

compensatory increase in respiratory rate, causing patient to exhale more carbon dioxide (CO_2).

Digitalis levels: The patient with heart failure may have been treated with digitalis. Chronic heart failure predisposes the patient to digitalis toxicity because of the low cardiac output state, which also causes decreased renal excretion of the drug.

Echocardiogram: May reveal a reduced ejection fraction, ventricular wall motion disorders, valvular dysfunction, or other cardiac dysfunction related to the reduced ejection fraction.

Holter monitoring: Continuous, portable cardiac monitoring technique used for assessment of heart rate changes as patient is placed on β-adrenergic blocking agent or other heart rate–altering agent to assess for efficacy of the medication while the person engages in routine daily activities. Typically not used in management of acutely ill, hospitalized patients.

COLLABORATIVE MANAGEMENT

Treatment of underlying cause and precipitating factors: Therapy for heart failure has changed from focusing on the weakened heart to a broader focus wherein peripheral and myocardial factors are important. In the past, therapy included mainly digitalis glycosides and diuretics. Current goals of therapy focus on improvement of the quality of the patient's life and strive to manage the compensatory mechanisms causing the patient's symptoms in an attempt to reduce mortality.

Diseases/conditions causing left heart failure: Atherosclerotic heart disease, AMI, dysrhythmias, cardiomyopathy, increased circulating volume, systemic hypertension, aortic stenosis, aortic regurgitation, mitral regurgitation, coarctation of the aorta, atrial septal defect, ventricular septal defect, cardiac tamponade, and constrictive pericarditis.

Diseases/conditions causing right heart failure: Left-sided heart failure, pulmonary hypertension, atherosclerotic heart disease, AMI, dysrhythmias, pulmonary embolism, fluid overload or excess sodium intake, chronic obstructive pulmonary disease (COPD), mitral stenosis, pulmonary stenosis, and myocardial contusion.

Diseases/conditions causing biventricular failure: Any combination of the diseases that cause either right or left heart failure.

Oxygen therapy: Supplemental oxygen delivered by an appropriate device to assist with oxygenation. May include use of a nasal cannula, face mask, Venturi mask (for pulmonary-impaired patients), partial-rebreathing mask, or nonrebreathing mask. The device is chosen based on the patient's oxygen saturation determined by pulse oximetry.

Pulse oximetry: Device placed on the patient's finger or ear to determine efficacy of ventilation through measurement of oxygen saturation.

Pharmacotherapy

Diuretics: To reduce blood volume and decrease preload.

Morphine: To induce vasodilation and decrease venous return, preload, sympathetic tone, anxiety, myocardial oxygen consumption, and pain.

Inotropic agents: Digitalis to strengthen contractions; dopamine or dobutamine to support BP and enhance contractility (see Appendix 7).

Vasodilators: Nitrates (oral, topical, or IV) to dilate venous or capacitance vessels, thereby reducing preload and cardiac and pulmonary congestion. Nitroprusside, hydralazine, captopril, or prazosin hydrochloride will dilate the arterial or resistant vessels and reduce afterload, thus increasing forward flow (see Appendix 7).

Inodilators: Phosphodiesterase-inhibiting drugs such as amrinone (Inocor) and milrinone (Primacor), which both increase contractility of the heart and lower systemic vascular resistance by vasodilation. In this manner, the failing heart is able to most effectively pump against less pressure (reduced afterload), resulting in increased cardiac output.

ACE inhibitors (benazepril, captopril, enalapril, fosinopril, lisinopril, moex-ipril, quinapril, ramipril):   Affect the renin-angiotensin system by inhibiting the conversion of circulating angiotensin I into angiotensin II. Reduce both preload and afterload to decrease the work of the ventricles while resulting in increased cardiac output and systemic perfusion/oxygenation.

β-Adrenergic blocking agents: Drugs such as metoprolol, carvedilol, pro-pranolol, which block the effects of circulating catecholamines released during heart failure. Catecholamines cause peripheral vasoconstriction, increased resistance to ventricular ejection, and increased myocardial oxygen consumption and may precipitate myocardial ischemia and ventricular dysrhythmias. β-Adrenergic blocking agents also reduce contractility, resulting in decreased myocardial oxygen consumption and demand and can prevent ventricular dysrhythmias.

AT$_1$ receptor antagonists: Include losartan and similar drugs that have effects similar to ACE inhibitors. AT$_1$ receptor blocking agents may offer some advantage over conventional ACE inhibitor therapy by avoiding persistent renal dysfunction sometimes associated with use of ACE inhibitors.

Treatment of acute pulmonary edema: Immediate interventions include:
- High concentrations of supplemental oxygen and possible endotracheal (ET) intubation with mechanical ventilation.
- Diuretic therapy: in severely ill patients, furosemide and bumetanide may be used as continuous IV infusions to assist with constant fluid removal. Patients with renal impairment/failure may require infusions of appropriate diuretics or ultrafiltration if other efforts to remove fluid fail.
- Pharmacologic therapy, including continuous IV infusions of inotropic agents, vasodilators, β-adrenergic blocking agents, and IV morphine. If cardiogenic shock ensues, vasopressors and intraaortic balloon pumping may also be necessary. If the person has evidence of renal insufficiency or failure, ACE inhibitors should be discontinued.

Bed rest and stress reduction

Low-calorie diet (if weight control is necessary) and low-sodium diet: Extra salt and water are held in the circulatory system, causing increased strain on the heart. Limiting sodium (Table 4-5) will reduce the amount of fluid retained by the body. In addition, fluids may be limited to 1500 ml/day.

NURSING DIAGNOSES AND INTERVENTIONS

Fluid volume excess related to compromised regulatory mechanism secondary to decreased cardiac output

Desired outcome: Within 24 h of treatment, patient becomes normovolemic as evidenced by absence of adventitious lung sounds; decreased peripheral edema; increased urine output; weight loss; PAWP ≤18 mm Hg (reasonable outcome for these patients); SVR ≤1200 dynes/sec/cm^{-5}; and CO ≥4 L/min.
- Auscultate lung fields for presence of crackles and rhonchi or other adventitious sounds.
- Monitor I&O closely. Report positive fluid state or decrease in urine output to <0.5 mg/kg/h.
- Weigh patient daily; report increases in weight. An acute gain in weight of 1 kg can signal a 1-L gain in fluid.
- Note changes from baseline assessment to detect worsening of heart failure, such as increased pedal edema, increased jugular venous distention, development of S$_3$ heart sound or new murmur, and dysrhythmias.
- Monitor hemodynamic status q1-2h and prn. Note response to drug therapy as well as indicators of the need for more aggressive therapy, including increasing PAWP and SVR and decreasing CO.
- Administer diuretics (furosemide), positive inotropes (dopamine), inodilators (amrinone and milrinone), β-adrenergic blocking agents, and vasodilators (nitroprusside) as prescribed. (See Appendix 7 for more information about inotropic and vasoactive drugs.)

TABLE 4-5   Low-Sodium Dietary Guidelines

Foods high in sodium*	Foods low in sodium
Beans and frankfurters	Bread
Bouillon cubes	Cereal (dry or hot); read labels
Canned or packaged soups	Fresh fish, chicken, turkey, veal, beef,
Canned, smoked, or salted meats; salted fish	and lamb (if limiting fats, avoid the latter two)
Dill pickles	Fresh fruits and vegetables
Fried chicken dinners and other fast foods	Fresh or dried herbs
Monosodium glutamate (e.g., Accent)	Gelatin desserts
Olives	Oil, salt-free margarine
Packaged snack foods	Peanut butter
Pancake or waffle mix	Tabasco sauce
Processed cheese	Low-salt tuna packed in water
Seasoned salts (e.g., celery, onion, garlic)	
Sauerkraut	
Soy sauce	
Vegetables in brine or cans	

Additional suggestions
- Do not add table salt to foods.
- Season with fresh or dried herbs.
- Avoid salts or powders that contain salt.
- Do not buy convenience foods; remember that fresh is best.
- Read all labels for salt, sodium, or sodium chloride content.

*Many of these foods now are available in low-salt or salt-free versions.

- Watch for signs and symptoms of renal insufficiency to assess whether the physician may need to discontinue ACE inhibitors and initiate aggressive diuretic infusions or consider hemodialysis with ultrafiltration therapy.
- Limit oral fluids as prescribed, and offer patient ice chips or frozen juice pops to decrease thirst and relieve discomfort of dry mouth.
- Maintain bed rest restrictions to facilitate fluid movement from interstitial spaces in dependent extremities to the intravascular spaces.

NIC Fluid/Electrolyte Management; Invasive Hemodynamic Monitoring; Medication Management; Nutrition Counseling; Surveillance; Teaching: Disease Process; Hemodialysis Therapy

Cardiac output: decreased, related to disease process that has resulted in decreased ability of the heart to provide adequate pumping to maintain effective oxygenation and nutrition of body systems

Desired outcomes: Within 24 h of initiating treatment, the patient has attained a CI of at least 2.0; PAP is reduced to within 10% of patient's normal baseline; BP has stabilized to within 10% of baseline; and HR is controlled to within 10% of normal baseline.

- Monitor cardiac rhythm and rate continuously.
- Monitor CO, CI, pulmonary and systemic vascular pressures, and other hemodynamic values at least hourly, as appropriate. Implement continuous CO monitoring if available.
- Monitor neurologic status to assess for adequate cerebral perfusion.

- Monitor renal function (blood urea nitrogen [BUN] and creatinine) daily, as appropriate.
- Monitor liver studies (SGOT/AST, SGPT/ALT, and/or bilirubin) daily, as appropriate.
- Monitor the other determinants of oxygen delivery, including level of Hgb and oxygen saturation.
- Refrain from taking rectal temperatures, to prevent bradycardias.
- Control tachycardia as soon as possible with β-adrenergic blocking agents or other appropriate measure as determined by the physician and ACLS guidelines.
- Obtain 12/15/18-lead ECG to assess new dysrhythmias or profound instability.
- Intraaortic balloon pumping may be necessary; prepare needed equipment for insertion of the balloon catheter and implementation of pumping.
- If patient has atrial fibrillation, ensure that patient has been receiving appropriate anticoagulants or antiplatelet agents to prevent thrombus formation.

NIC Cardiac Care: Acute; Circulatory Care: Mechanical Assist Device; Hemodynamic Regulation; Shock Management: Cardiac; Neurologic Monitoring; Medication Management; Dysrhythmia Management

Impaired gas exchange related to alveolar-capillary membrane changes secondary to fluid collection in the alveoli and interstitial spaces

Desired outcome: Within 24 h of initiation of treatment, patient has improved gas exchange as evidenced by Pao_2 ≥80 mm Hg; RR 12-20 breaths/min with normal pattern and depth (eupnea); and absence of adventitious breath sounds.

- Monitor respiratory rate, rhythm, and character q1-2h. Be alert to RR >20 breaths/min, irregular rhythm, use of accessory muscles of respiration, or cough.
- Auscultate breath sounds, noting presence of crackles, wheezes, and other adventitious sounds.
- Provide supplemental oxygen as prescribed.
- Monitor Spo_2 for decreases to <90%-92%.
- Assess ABG findings; note changes in response to oxygen supplementation or treatment of altered hemodynamics.
- Suction patient's secretions as needed.
- Establish a protocol for deep breathing, coughing, and turning q2h.
- Place patient in semi-Fowler's or high Fowler's position to maximize chest excursion.
- If mechanical ventilation is necessary, monitor ventilator settings, ET tube function, and respiratory status.

NIC Airway Management; Anxiety Reduction; Cardiac Care: Acute; Medication Management; Oxygen Therapy; Respiratory Monitoring

Activity intolerance related to imbalance between oxygen supply and demand secondary to decreased functioning of the myocardium

Desired outcome: Within the 12- to 24-h period before discharge from CCU, patient exhibits cardiac tolerance to increasing levels of activity as evidenced by RR <24 breaths/min; normal sinus rhythm on ECG; HR ≤120 bpm (or within 20 bpm of resting HR); BP within 20 mm Hg of patient's normal range; and absence of chest pain.

- Maintain prescribed activity level, and teach patient the rationale for activity limitation.
- Organize nursing care so that periods of activity are interspersed with extended periods of uninterrupted rest.
- To help prevent complications of immobility, assist patient with active/passive ROM exercises, as appropriate. Encourage patient to do as much as possible within prescribed activity allowances.
- Note patient's physiologic response to activity, including BP, HR, RR, and heart rhythm. Signs of activity intolerance include chest pain, increasing

SOB, excessive fatigue, increased dysrhythmias, palpitations, HR response >120 bpm, systolic BP >20 mm Hg from baseline or >160 mm Hg, and ST-segment changes. If activity intolerance is noted, instruct patient to stop the activity and rest.

- Administer medications as prescribed, and note their effect on patient's activity tolerance. Examples of medications include prophylactic NTG tablets, paste, or patch to reduce preload.
- As needed to help prevent muscle loss and wasting, refer patient to physical therapy department.

NIC Activity Therapy; Energy Management; Teaching: Prescribed Activity/ Exercise; Dysrhythmia Management; Pain Management; Medication Management

Knowledge deficit: disease process with heart failure and the prescribed diet and medications

Desired outcome: Within the 24-h period before discharge from CCU, patient and significant others verbalize understanding of patient's disease, as well as the prescribed diet and medication regimens.

- Teach patient the physiologic process of heart failure, discussing in terms appropriate to the patient how fluid volume increases because of poor heart functioning.
- Teach the patient about the adverse effects of smoking and how smoking cessation may benefit him or her.
- Teach patient about the importance of a low-sodium diet and medications to help reduce volume overload. Provide patient with a list of foods that are high and low in sodium. Teach patient how to read and evaluate food labels.
- Teach patient the signs and symptoms of fluid volume excess that necessitate medical attention: irregular or slow pulse, increased SOB, orthopnea, decreased exercise tolerance, and steady weight gain (≥1 kg/day for 2 successive days).
- Advise patient about the need to keep a journal of daily weight. Explain that an increase of ≥1 kg/day on 2 successive days of normal eating necessitates notification of physician.
- If patient is taking digitalis, teach the technique for measuring pulse rate. Provide parameters for withholding digitalis (usually for pulse rate <60/min) and notifying the physician.
- Instruct patient regarding the prescribed activity progression after hospital discharge and signs of activity intolerance that signal the need for rest and use of prophylactic NTG to reduce congestion of the heart and lungs. General activity guidelines are as follows:
  - ☐ Get up and get dressed every morning.
  - ☐ Space your meals and activities to allow time for rest and relaxation.
  - ☐ Perform activities at a comfortable, moderate pace. If you get tired during any activity, stop to rest for 15 min before resuming.
  - ☐ Avoid activities that require straining or lifting.
  - ☐ Plan at least two periods a day of walking, following the guidelines in Table 4-6.
  - ☐ Warning signals to stop your activity and rest: chest pain, SOB, dizziness or faintness, unusual weakness.

NIC Cardiac Care: Rehabilitation; Exercise Promotion; Smoking Cessation Assistance; Teaching: Prescribed Activity/Exercise; Emotional Support; Progressive Muscle Relaxation; Weight Management; Mutual Goal Setting; Teaching: Prescribed Diet; Teaching: Prescribed Medication

ADDITIONAL NURSING DIAGNOSES

Also see nursing diagnoses and interventions in "Hemodynamic Monitoring," p. 28; "Prolonged Immobility," p. 74; "Psychosocial Support," p. 83; and "Psychosocial Support for the Patient's Family and Significant Others," p. 95.

TABLE 4-6   Activity Progression After Hospital Discharge

Week	Distance walked	Time
1-2	¼ mi	Leisurely; twice daily
2-3	½ mi	15 min
3-4	1 mi	30 min
4-5	1½ mi	30 min
5-6	2 mi	40 min

Cardiomyopathy

PATHOPHYSIOLOGY

Cardiomyopathy (CM) is a disease process that affects the myocardial structure and function. CM may occur as a primary (idiopathic) or secondary disease process (Table 4-7). The three classifications of cardiomyopathy are based on the functional effect on the heart muscle. All three classifications can ultimately lead to the clinical syndrome of heart failure.

Functional classification

Dilated cardiomyopathy (DCM) (previously referred to as congestive): DCM is characterized by marked, progressive dilation of the ventricles, resulting in decreased myocardial contractility and reduced systolic ejection fraction (<40%). Heart failure occurs secondary to decreased systolic ejection fraction. There is little or no hypertrophy of the ventricles. DCM is the most common cardiomyopathy. In the United States, *ischemic cardiomyopathy* is the most common cause of DCM. Ischemic cardiomyopathy is associated with a history of AMI or >70% luminal narrowing of a major coronary artery.

Hypertrophic cardiomyopathy (HCM):   The significant feature of this disease process is the hypertrophy of the ventricular muscle, which leads to left ventricular diastolic dysfunction. The hypertrophy affects the ventricular septum as well as the ventricular free wall. Though the hypertrophy results in a decreased left ventricular volume, the ejection fraction may actually increase. Obstructive HCM can occur when the hypertrophy obstructs the ventricular outflow channel, but nonobstructive HCM is more common. Although cardiac function may remain normal for varying periods of time, deterioration and poor ventricular compliance usually occur. This is also referred to as *idiopathic hypertrophic subaortic stenosis (IHSS).*

Restrictive cardiomyopathy (RCM):   The ventricular walls become rigid from fibrosis, resulting in inadequate left ventricular filling. LV diastolic dysfunction occurs, often associated with very high end-diastolic pressures. Systolic function remains normal. Treatment is difficult, and prognosis is poor. It is important to discern the difference between RCM and constrictive pericarditis, since the clinical picture is similar but the treatment is very different. RCM is the least common cardiomyopathy.

ASSESSMENT

Clinical presentation: Will vary based on classification, extent, and severity of CM.

Physical assessment: Decreased BP, increased HR, and presence of dysrhythmias. Mild to severe cardiomegaly may be present, causing a displaced and diffuse point of maximal impulse (PMI). Peripheral hypoperfusion may be

TABLE 4-7   Secondary Causes of Cardiomyopathy

Dilated	Hypertrophic	Restrictive
Ischemic insult	Inherited: autosomal dominant trait	Amyloidosis
Infection: viral and bacterial		Cardiac transplant
Chronic alcohol consumption		Endocardial fibroelastosis
Childbirth/postpartum period		
Drug therapy (daunorubicin, doxorubicin)		
Kawasaki syndrome		

present, manifested as diminished pulses, cool skin, and mottling or cyanosis. Hepatomegaly and ascites may be present (Table 4-8).
Monitoring parameters: See Table 4-9.

DIAGNOSTIC TESTS

Cardiac catheterization: Does not confirm cardiomyopathy but can be used to rule out other disorders, such as ischemic heart disease. Findings in DCM may include decreased cardiac output, abnormal ventricular wall motion, and decreased ejection fraction; increased filling pressure; and valvular regurgitation.

Endocardial biopsy: Used to determine the classification and/or cause of CM through histologic studies, identification of the pathologic agent, and in some cases, to identify genetic disorders. May be performed during cardiac catheterization.

Chest x-ray: For *DCM:* may detect cardiomegaly with enlarged left ventricle, pulmonary venous congestion, and characteristic lines of interstitial edema; for *HCM:* normal cardiac silhouette, may have pulmonary venous hypertension; for *RCM:* may have mild cardiac enlargement.

ECG: Dysrhythmias, such as supraventricular tachycardias, atrial fibrillation, and ventricular dysrhythmia occur with all three cardiomyopathies. Other changes may include left ventricular hypertrophy, left bundle-branch block, left anterior hemiblock, left axis deviation, AV conduction delays, nonspecific ST-segment changes, and Q waves that resemble those that occur with myocardial infarction.

Echocardiography: Assesses degree of left ventricular impairment and dilation of the cardiac chambers. Ventricular wall and septal contractility can be evaluated, as well as valvular motion. Two-dimensional echo can detect thrombus formation, estimate ejection fraction, and detect the location and degree of hypertrophy.

Radionuclide studies: For *DCM:* may show diffuse left ventricular hypokinesis, left ventricular ejection fraction <40%, and elevated end-diastolic and systolic volumes; for *HCM:* reveal vigorous systolic function, hypertrophy, and a small LV volume; for *RCM:* reveal normal systolic function and a small to normal LV.

COLLABORATIVE MANAGEMENT

Pharmacotherapy: To maintain or reestablish hemodynamic stability.
ACE inhibitors: For *DCM:* to block the compensatory response of the renin-angiotensin system to heart failure, decreasing preload and afterload.
Diuretics: For *DCM:* to reduce preload and pulmonary congestion; for *HCM:* may be contraindicated or given cautiously in obstructed *HCM.*

TABLE 4-8   Signs and Symptoms of Cardiomyopathy

	Dilated	Hypertrophic	Restrictive
Source of initial dysfunction **Clinical presentation**	Systolic dysfunction S&S caused by biventricular failure: exertional dyspnea, fatigue, weakness, orthopnea, PND, ascites, peripheral edema. May have changes in mentation, i.e., confusion, restlessness.	Diastolic dysfunction Wide spectrum of S&S, depending on extent and severity of dysfunction. *Most common: dyspnea* (caused by increasing LV diastolic pressure) and *angina* (caused by hypertrophy and relative ischemia). *Also:* decreased exercise tolerance, fatigue, syncope, exertional dyspnea, orthopnea, palpitations.	Diastolic dysfunction Exercise intolerance, exertional dyspnea, fatigue, nocturnal dyspnea, plus other signs of pulmonary edema and heart failure.
Physical assessment	PMI: displaced down and to left, heave palpated; S_3 and S_4 gallops, systolic murmur of AV valves; basilar rales; hepatomegaly; extremities cool, mottled, cyanotic; peripheral pulses weak with pulsus alternans; BP normal or low; sinus tachycardia, atrial fibrillation, ventricular dysrhythmias.	Harsh systolic murmur, S_4 gallop; basilar rales; supraventricular dysrhythmias, especially atrial ventricular dysrhythmias are common, and sudden death can be the first symptom.	Jugular venous distention; PMI: typically in normal position and of normal character; S_3 gallop; peripheral edema; ascites; hepatomegaly

S&S, Signs and symptoms; *PND,* paroxysmal nocturnal dyspnea; *PMI,* point of maximal impulse; *AV,* atrioventricular; *BP,* blood pressure; *LV,* left ventricle.

TABLE 4 - 9 Hemodynamic Presentation With Cardiomyopathy

Pressure	Effect	Normal values
Right atrial pressure	Increased	4-6 mm Hg
Pulmonary artery pressure	Increased	20-30/8-15 mm Hg
Pulmonary wedge pressure	Increased	6-12 mm Hg
Cardiac output	Decreased	4-7 L/min
Cardiac index	Decreased	2.5-4 L/min/m^2
Pulmonary vascular resistance	Unchanged or increased	60-100 dynes/sec/cm^{-5}
Systemic vascular resistance	Increased	900-1200 dynes/sec/cm^{-5}

Inotropic therapy: For *DMC:* to enhance contractility (see Appendix 7). NOTE: Digitalis is contraindicated in the treatment of obstructive *HCM.*

Vasodilators: To decrease preload and afterload, thus improving cardiac output.

β-*Blockers:* For *DCM:* to block the compensatory response of the adrenergic system to heart failure. Though exact mechanism is not known, left ventricular ejection fraction is improved, symptoms are reduced, and survival rate is increased. For *HCM:* to decrease outflow obstruction during exercise and reduce sympathetic cardiac stimulation.

Antidysrhythmic agents: To control atrial and ventricular dysrhythmias (see Table 4-10) common to *DCM* and *HCM.*

Calcium channel blockers: For *DCM:* to produce vasodilation and decrease cardiac workload; for *HCM:* to improve diastolic filling and increase exercise capacity.

Anticoagulants: To prevent thrombus formation related to decreased ventricular contraction and emptying, as well as atrial fibrillation.

Potassium supplements: To replace potassium lost in the urine as a result of diuresis. Maintenance of serum levels in the high normal range (4.3-5 meq/L) is optimal.

Hemodynamic monitoring: To guide and evaluate therapeutic interventions.

Activity level: Initially reduced to decrease oxygen demand, but then increased gradually to prevent complications of immobility.

Dual chamber pacemakers: To improve CO and treat cardiac dysrhythmias

Implantable cardioverter-defibrillator (ICD): To treat life-threatening ventricular dysrhythmias (see discussion, p. 297).

Intraaortic balloon pump: In the presence of a failing myocardium, may be used to decrease afterload and increase coronary artery perfusion (see discussion, p. 346).

Surgical interventions

Ventricular septal myotomy-myectomy: For removal of the hypertrophied ventricular septum in obstructive HCM.

Heart transplantation: For advanced CM that is refractory to medical therapy to manage progression and symptoms of heart failure. Each institution has criteria that must be met before transplantation is considered as alternative treatment. (See discussion, p. 354.)

NURSING DIAGNOSES AND INTERVENTIONS

Note: Care must be based on the type of cardiomyopathy, its associated pathology, and the patient's clinical manifestations. Because DCM is the most commonly occurring cardiomyopathy, the primary aspects of care related to DCM are outlined.

Decreased cardiac output related to negative inotropic changes in the heart secondary to myocardial cellular destruction and dilation

Desired outcomes: Within the 24-h period before discharge from CCU, patient has adequate cardiac output as evidenced by systolic BP ≥90 mm Hg; CO 4-7 L/min; CI 2.5-4 L/min/m^2; RR 12-20 breaths/min; HR ≤100 bpm; urinary output ≥0.5 ml/kg/h; warm and dry skin; peripheral pulses >2+ on a 0-4+ scale; and orientation to time, place, and person. PAWP is ≤18 mm Hg, and RAP is 4-6 mm Hg.

- Assess for and document the following factors as evidence of decreasing CO: the degree of exertional dyspnea, jugular venous distention, dependent edema, and hepatomegaly. In addition, assess and document the following:
  - ☐ *Mental status:* Be alert to restlessness, decreased responsiveness.
  - ☐ *Lung sounds:* Auscultate for crackles, rhonchi, wheezes.
  - ☐ *Heart sounds:* Note presence of S$_3$ gallop, murmur.
  - ☐ *Urinary output:* Be alert to output <0.5 ml/kg/h.
  - ☐ *Skin:* Monitor for pallor, mottling, cyanosis, coolness, diaphoresis.
  - ☐ *Vital signs:* Note BP <90 mm Hg systolic, HR >100 bpm, RR >20 breaths/min, and elevated temperature. Increasing HR and BP may reflect compensatory mechanisms in response to sodium and water retention.
- If a PA catheter is present, record hemodynamic readings q1-2h and prn. Be alert to PAWP >18 mm Hg and RAP >6 mm Hg. Although normal PAWP is 6-12 mm Hg, these patients may need increased filling pressures for adequate preload, with wedge pressure at 15-18 mm Hg.
- Measure CO/CI q2-4h and prn. Optimally, CO should be 4-7 L/min and CI should be 2.5-4 L/min/m^2; for some patients the best CO/CI will be below expected normal values.
- Keep accurate I&O records and weigh patient daily, noting trends. Individuals with cardiomyopathy may be on strict fluid restriction (e.g., 1000 ml/day).
- Assess peripheral pulses and rate on a scale of 0-4+.
- Monitor cardiac rhythm continuously for dysrhythmias that may further decrease CO, such as sinus or atrial tachycardias, atrial fibrillation, or ventricular ectopy.
- Assist patient with activities of daily living (ADL) when necessary to minimize patient's cardiac workload.
- Administer medications as prescribed. Observe for the following desired effects:
  - ☐ *Vasodilators:* Decreased BP, decreased SVR, increased CO/CI.
  - ☐ *Diuretics:* Decreased PAWP.
  - ☐ *ACE inhibitors:* Decreased SVR, RAP, PAWP.
  - ☐ *Inotropes:* Increased CO/CI, increased BP.
  - ☐ β-*blockers:* Increased CO/CI, decreased PAWP. NOTE: These effects are not immediate and may take days to weeks for positive effects to be noted.
- Be alert to the following undesirable effects:
  - ☐ *Vasodilators:* Postural hypotension, dizziness, headache, nausea, vomiting.
  - ☐ *Diuretics:* Weakness, postural hypotension, hypokalemia (see p. 649).
  - ☐ *ACE inhibitors:* Headache, dizziness, postural hypotension.
  - ☐ *Inotropes:* Dysrhythmias, headache, angina.
  - ☐ β-*Blockers:* Initial or increased dosing may cause bradycardia and vasodilation and worsen symptoms of heart failure, such as increased dyspnea and edema. The vasodilator and heart failure side effects are typically transient and can be managed by adjusting diuretic and vasodilator medications until the patient is stabilized on the β-blocker. Bradycardia side effects are not transient and will not resolve with time. Not all patients with cardiomyopathy can tolerate β-blockers.

NIC Cardiac Care; Dysrhythmia Management; Electrolyte management: Hypokalemia; Fluid Monitoring; Fluid Management; Hemodynamic Regulation; Medication Management; Shock Management: Cardiac

Activity intolerance related to imbalance between oxygen supply and demand secondary to decreased myocardial contractility

Desired outcome: Within the 12- to 24-h period before discharge from CCU, patient exhibits cardiac tolerance to increasing levels of activity as evidenced by RR <24 breaths/min; normal sinus rhythm on ECG; BP within 20 mm Hg of patient's normal range; HR within 20 bpm of patient's resting HR; and patient report of decreased fatigue level and absence of chest pain.

- Monitor patient's physiologic response to activity, reporting any symptoms of chest pain, new or increasing SOB, increases in HR >20 bpm above resting HR, and increase or decrease in systolic BP >20 mm Hg.
- Monitor cardiac rhythm for the occurrence of dysrhythmias during activity.
- Observe for and report any signs of decreased cardiac output, e.g., changes in mentation.
- Plan nursing care so that patient is assured of extended periods of rest (at least 90 min).
- To prevent complications of immobility, perform or teach patient and significant others active, passive, and assistive range-of-motion (ROM) exercises. For a discussion of an in-bed exercise program, see Table 4-1 and interventions in "Prolonged Immobility," p. 74. Consult physician to ensure that exercises are within patient's prescribed limitations.

NIC Energy Management; Cardiac Care: Rehabilitative

ADDITIONAL NURSING DIAGNOSES

Also see nursing diagnoses and interventions in "Hemodynamic Monitoring," p. 28; "Heart Failure/Pulmonary Edema," p 265; "Prolonged Immobility," p. 74; "Patients With Implantable Cardioverter-Defibrillator," p. 292; "Psychosocial Support," p. 83; and "Psychosocial Support for the Patient's Family and Significant Others," p. 95.

Dysrhythmias and conduction disturbances

PATHOPHYSIOLOGY

Cardiac dysrhythmias reflect abnormal function of the heart's electrical system. Cardiac electrophysiology involves studying the electrical impulses and their conduction across the atria and throughout the ventricles to provide power and coordination for the cardiac cycle. Electrical dysfunction can markedly change the cardiac output and prompt deterioration in the patient's vital signs. (See Figure 4-1.)

Dysrhythmias may originate in any part of the electrical system, from the pacing cells (SA node, AV junction) to any portion of the conduction system (atria, His-Purkinje system, bundle branches, and ventricles). Myocardial ischemia, electrolyte or other chemical imbalance, and an abnormally configured electrical system are factors likely to stimulate dysrhythmias. The normal flow of impulses depends on properly nourished, well-oxygenated electrical tissues with an anatomically correct pacing and conduction system. The cardiac cycle depends on a balance of basic regulatory substances: electrolytes such as sodium, potassium, calcium, glucose; and appropriate amounts of catecholamines. Imbalance of these regulators can cause a disturbance in pacing (automaticity), conduction, or myocardial contractility. (See Figure 4-2.)

Disturbances in automaticity: May involve an increase or decrease in the pacing function (automaticity) in the sinus node, such as sinus tachycardia (HR >100 bpm) or sinus bradycardia (HR <60 bpm). Premature beats or possibly an escape or compensatory heart rhythm may arise from the atria, junction, or ventricles. Escape rhythms occur when the sinus node ceases to function or arrests. Abnormal rhythms, such as atrial or ventricular tachycardia, also may occur, especially if there is an excess of catecholamines. Without excessive catecholamines, escape rhythms generated from the AV junction or ventricles are usually bradycardic (HR <60 bpm).

Disturbances in conduction: Conduction may be too rapid, as in conditions that prompt excessive catecholamines (e.g., severe/critical illness, certain endocrine diseases, profound emotional stress) or in the presence of an accessory pathway (e.g., Wolff-Parkinson-White syndrome). Accessory pathways are extra conduction fibers that provide a direct connection between the atria and ventricles, which circumvent the AV node. Rhythms generated from these anatomically incorrect conduction systems are called *AV reciprocating tachycardias* and may have rates >250 bpm. Impulse conduction may be delayed or too slow (e.g., first- and second-degree AV block). Reentry is a situation in which a misdirected electrical impulse reexcites a conduction pathway through which it already has passed. Once started, this impulse may circulate through the same area repeatedly, which prompts an AV reentrant tachycardia. The trapped impulse becomes the pacemaker in this circumstance. Impulses may also be totally blocked from continuing down the pathway by abnormal electrical tissues (e.g., third-degree or complete heart block). (See Figure 4-3, p. 282.)

Combinations of disturbed automaticity and conduction: Observed when several dysrhythmias are noted (e.g., first-degree AV block [disturbance in conductivity]; premature atrial complexes [PACs] [disturbance in automaticity]).

ASSESSMENT

History and risk factors: Coronary atherosclerotic heart disease (CASHD), acute MI, recent MI, current use of antidysrhythmic or bronchodilating drugs, electrolyte disturbances (especially potassium, glucose, magnesium), endocrine disease (thyroid, adrenal, pancreas), low blood pressure/shock, increased intracranial pressure, valvular heart disease, cardiomyopathy, unstable angina, acid-base imbalance, hypoxemia, pulmonary disease, respiratory failure, anemia, drug overdose.

Clinical presentation: Varies from absence of symptoms to complete cardiopulmonary arrest. Most commonly: activity intolerance, weakness, hypotension, dizziness, SOB, dyspnea, palpitations, chest discomfort or pressure, sensation of "racing heart" or "skipped beats." More serious symptoms include: altered mental status, anxiety, respiratory insufficiency, syncope, and seizures, which may lead to heart failure and cardiopulmonary arrest. Pulseless ventricular tachycardia, ventricular fibrillation, asystole, and electromechanical dissociation result in immediate cardiac arrest.

Physical assessment: Symptomatic dysrhythmias most often result in a very rapid, slow, or irregular pulse, changed pulse quality, hypotension, pallor, possibly a variable heart rate (fast, then slow), and tachypnea. If the cardiac output is markedly decreased, shocklike symptoms ensue including cold, clammy skin, dusky or cyanotic appearance, decreased urine output, feeling of impending doom or imminent death. If heart failure is present, heart sounds may include S_3, S_4; basilar crackles or rales are audible with lung auscultation; jugular veins are distended; and peripheral edema and a wet cough with frothy sputum may be present.

ECG and hemodynamic measurements: Hemodynamic measurements will vary depending on the effect of the dysrhythmia on the cardiac output. If patient has heart failure, CO is decreased and PAP is elevated. Tachycardias usually increase CO initially unless the rate is too fast to allow adequate ventricular filling, wherein CO decreases and may lead to heart failure. Some ECG findings seen with various dysrhythmias include abnormalities in rate such as sinus bradycardia or sinus tachycardia; irregular rhythm such as atrial fibrillation;

Text continued on p. 283

Sinoatrial (SA) node

Interatrial conduction tract
(Bachmann bundle)

Internodal atrial conduction tracts

Atrioventricular
(AV) node

Bundle of His

Atrioventricular
(AV) junction

Left bundle branch

Left posterior fascicle

Left anterior fascicle

Right bundle branch

Purkinje network

Purkinje fibers

1. Superior vena cava
2. Inlet of the superior vena cava
3. Right atrium
4. Inlet of the inferior vena cava
5. Coronary sinus
6. Inferior vena cava

7. Tricuspid valve
8. Right ventricle
9. Interatrial septum
10. Interventricular septum
11. Left atrium
12. Mitral valve
13. Left ventricle

Figure 4-1: Electrical conduction system.
From Huszar RJ: *Basic dysrhythmias: interpretation and management*, ed 2, St Louis, 1994, Mosby.

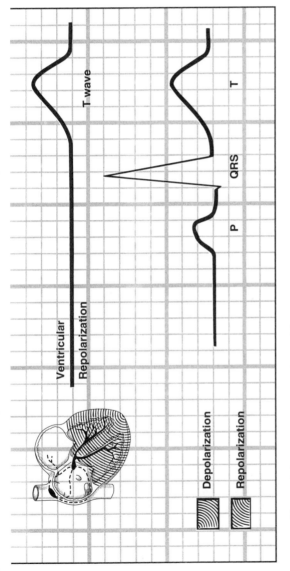

Figure 4-2:   Electrical basis of the ECG.
From Huszar RJ: *Basic dysrhythmias: interpretation and management*, ed 2, St Louis, 1994, Mosby.

1. Prolonged PR interval (>0.20 sec)
(first-degree AV block)

Delay of
conduction of the
electrical impulse
through the:

AV node or
bundle of His

\ Electrical impulse
■ Conduction delay

2. Absence of a QRS after a P wave
(second- and third-degree AV block)

Blockage of
conduction of the
electrical impulse
through the:

AV node or
bundle of His,
or bundle branches

\ Electrical impulse
■ Conduction delay

3. Short PR interval (<0.12 sec)

a. Ectopic
pacemaker in
the atria or
AV junction

OR

b. Conduction of the
electrical impulse
through abnormal
AV conduction
pathways

\ Electrical impulse

Figure 4-3:   Anomalous AV conduction.
From Huszar RJ: *Basic dysrhythmias: interpretation and management,* ed 2,
St Louis, 1994, Mosby.

extra beats such as PACs and premature junctional complexes (PJCs); wide and bizarre-looking beats such as premature ventricular complexes (PVCs) and ventricular tachycardia (VT); a fibrillating baseline such as ventricular fibrillation (VF); and a straight line as with asystole. (See Figure 4-4.) Figures 4-5 through 4-25 give an overview of common rhythms, dysrhythmias, and conduction disturbances and their treatment. Occasionally, patients have an electrical rhythm without corresponding mechanical pumping. This condition is known as *electrical-mechanical dissociation (EMD)* or *pulseless electrical activity (PEA)*. Initially, the rhythm may appear nearly normal but rapidly deteriorates as the conduction pathway becomes hypoxic.

DIAGNOSTIC TESTS

12-lead ECG: Accepted standard method used to detect and analyze dysrhythmias, including those associated with myocardial ischemia, injury, and infarction. Leads are attached to the patient's limbs and on the chest over the left ventricle. (See Figure 4-26.)

15/18-lead ECG: Expanded method used to detect and analyze dysrhythmias, in which leads are added to the 12-lead ECG on the right side of the chest and/or left posterior subscapular area to better detect problems with the perfusion to the right ventricle and posterior wall of the left ventricle.

Serum electrolyte levels: Identify key chemical imbalances that may precipitate dysrhythmias. Both elevations and deficits of electrolytes can create an electrically unstable environment.

Therapeutic drug levels: Toxic levels of many cardiac, pulmonary, neurologic, and antidysrhythmic medications may prompt development of new, possibly more dangerous dysrhythmias. All antidysrhythmic agents are proarrhythmic in toxic amounts or when certain electrolyte imbalances are present, especially the class I agents (e.g., quinidine, mexiletine, disopyramide).

Stress testing: Continuous ECG monitoring of the patient while a stressor (e.g., exercise on the treadmill, Persantine or adenosine injection) is induced. The test continues until the patient reaches the target heart rate or becomes symptomatic (e.g., chest pain, severe fatigue, dysrhythmias). Results determine the ability of the heart to compensate for various amounts of stress.

Electrophysiologic studies (EPS): Invasive test in which two or three catheters are placed into the heart at suspected proarrhythmic sites, to give a pacing stimulus at those sites with various voltages of electricity to induce dysrhythmias. Various medications and electrical therapies are then implemented to terminate the induced dysrhythmias. Results help to determine the type of device and medications the patient may need to maintain cardiac electrical stability.

Toxicology screening: Toxic levels of "recreational" or "street" drugs (e.g., "crack," cocaine, amphetamines, barbiturates) or mood-altering drugs (e.g., tricyclic antidepressants, sedative/hypnotics) can induce lethal dysrhythmias.

Ambulatory monitoring (e.g., 24-h Holter monitor or cardiac event recorder): Continuous cardiac monitor worn for 24 h by the patient so that ECG changes that occur during normal daily activities (including sleeping) can be determined. The patient keeps a timed log of all activities/events/symptoms,which is later compared with the ECG recording to analyze the relationship of dysrhythmias to symptoms and activities.

Atrial electrogram (AEG): Specialized and somewhat invasive ECG used to diagnose atrial dysrhythmias, wherein a needle is inserted into the patient's chest over the right atrium and through a single wire, the atrial activity can be more thoroughly analyzed by an atrial ECG.

ABG values: May reflect hypoxemia or pH abnormality that can interfere with electrolyte balance, both of which can cause dysrhythmias. Hypoxemia can also result from dysrhythmias that significantly decrease cardiac output.

Text continued on p. 288

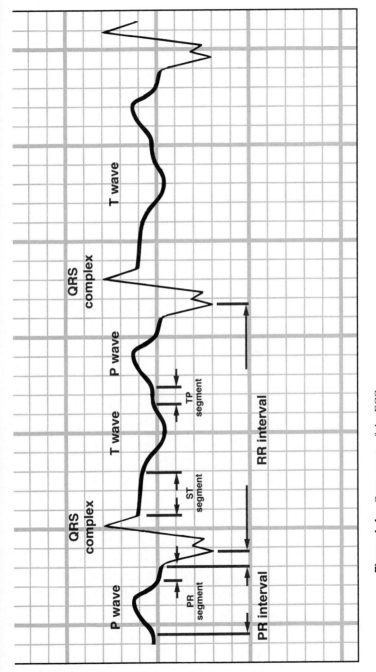

Figure 4-4:   Components of the ECG.
From Huszar RJ: *Basic dysrhythmias: interpretation and management*, ed 2, St Louis, 1994, Mosby.

Normal Sinus Rhythm

- Rhythm: regular
- Atrial rate: 60-100 bpm
- Ventricular rate: 60-100 bpm
- P waves: before each QRS
- QRS: normal and of normal width
- PR interval: normal
- P: QRS: 1:1

Significance: Usual, normal rhythm and conduction.
Intervention: None.

Figure 4-5: Normal sinus rhythm.
Illustration from Huszar RJ: *Basic dysrhythmias: interpretation and management,* ed 2, St Louis, 1994, Mosby.

Sinus Tachycardia

- Rhythm: regular
- Atrial rate: >100 bpm; usually <160 bpm
- Ventricular rate: >100 bpm; usually <160 bpm
- P waves: before each QRS
- QRS: normal duration
- PR interval: normal
- P: QRS: 1:1

Significance: Increased rate usually caused by sympathetic stimulation.
            Causes may include pain, fever, anxiety, hypovolemia, heart
            failure, caffeine intake, use of theophylline or sympatho-
            mimetic agents.
Intervention: Treat cause.

Figure 4-6: Sinus tachycardia.
Illustration from Huszar RJ: *Basic dysrhythmias: interpretation and management,* ed 2, St Louis, 1994, Mosby.

Sinus Bradycardia

- Rhythm: regular
- Atrial rate: <60 bpm
- Ventricular rate: <60 bpm
- P waves: before each QRS
- QRS: normal duration
- PR interval: normal
- P: QRS: 1:1

Significance: Slow rate usually caused by increased parasympathetic stimulation. Causes may include vagal stimulation, β-adrenergic blocking agents and other drugs, AMI, increased intracranial pressure (IICP). This rhythm may be "normal" in some people.

Intervention: No treatment necessary unless patient's BP drops and/or LOC is altered or PVCs occur. Initial treatment is atropine and oxygen. See "Bradycardia Algorithm" in Appendix 1.

Figure 4-7: Sinus bradycardia.
Illustration from Huszar RJ: *Basic dysrhythmias: interpretation and management,* ed 2, St Louis, 1994, Mosby.

Sinus Dysrhythmia

- Rhythm: regular
- Atrial rate: 60-100 bpm
- Ventricular rate: 60-100 bpm
- P waves: before each QRS
- QRS: normal duration
- PR interval: normal
- P: QRS: 1:1

Significance: This rhythm usually increases in rate with respiration and decreases with expiration. It can be a normal finding in children. As an abnormal finding, it may be caused by drugs, IICP, or heart disease.

Intervention: Observation; usually no treatment necessary.

Figure 4-8: Sinus dysrhythmia.
Illustration from Huszar RJ: *Basic dysrhythmias: interpretation and management,* ed 2, St Louis, 1994, Mosby.

Atrial origin of
abnormal impulse

Premature Atrial Complexes (PACs)

- Rhythm: irregular
- Atrial rate: depends on underlying rhythm
- Ventricular rate: depends on underlying rhythm
- P waves: early beat P looks different from sinus P
- QRS: normal duration
- PR interval: variable in premature complexes
- P: QRS: 1:1

Significance: PACs come from an ectopic atrial focus. Causes often are the same as sinus tachycardia. May progress to atrial fibrillation or atrial tachycardia.

Intervention: Observation. Limit caffeine, alcohol, and smoking. If symptoms occur (decreased BP, dizziness), treatment may include β-blockers, verapamil, or diltiazem.

Figure 4-9: Premature atrial complexes (PACs).
Top illustration modified from Sheehy SB, Lenehan GP: *Manual of emergency care,* ed 5, St Louis, 1999, Mosby. Bottom illustration from Huszar RJ: *Basic dysrhythmias: interpretation and management,* ed 2, St Louis, 1994, Mosby.

COLLABORATIVE MANAGEMENT

Antidysrhythmic drugs: Pharmacologic management of dysrhythmias is based on providing and/or balancing electrolytes, catecholamines, and other regulators of the cardiac cycle. Provision of these substances is the basis of the antidysrhythmic drug classification system, which has evolved from the original Vaughan Williams classification system. Toxic levels of any antidysrhythmic medication can prompt development of different and sometimes lethal

Atrial Tachycardia

Paroxysmal atrial tachycardia (PAT) ⟶ NSR

- Rhythm: mostly regular
- Atrial rate: 160-240 bpm
- Ventricular rate: depends on AV conduction ratio
- P waves: may be difficult to identify because of fast rate
- QRS: normal; may be wide if aberrant conduction is present

Significance: Can precipitate chest pain and ischemia. Patients often experience dizziness, diaphoresis, and nausea. Many patients diagnosed with wide-complex atrial tachycardia (SVT) are found to have ventricular tachycardia when electrophysiology studies are done.

Intervention: Vagal maneuvers, verapamil, adenosine. Other agents include digoxin, β-blockers, and procainamide. See "Tachycardia Algorithm" in Appendix 1. If the patient has an accessory pathway with AV reciprocating tachycardia, catheter ablation may be necessary to correct the problem.

Figure 4-10: Atrial tachycardia.
Illustration from Huszar RJ: *Basic dysrhythmias: interpretation and management,* ed 2, St Louis, 1994, Mosby.

Wandering Atrial Pacemaker

P   T/P'   P   P   P'   P'   P'   P'   P'   P'
PAC

- Rhythm: irregular
- Atrial rate: usually 60-100 bpm
- Ventricular rate: usually 60-100 bpm
- P waves: before each QRS
- QRS: normal duration
- PR interval: usually normal; some variation
- P: QRS: 1:1

Significance: An ectopic atrial focus. Causes may include drugs, COPD, inflammatory disorders.

Intervention: Observation. If cause can be determined, treat cause. If patient is receiving digoxin, check serum level.

Figure 4-11: Wandering atrial pacemaker.
Illustration from Huszar RJ: *Basic dysrhythmias: interpretation and management,* ed 2, St Louis, 1994, Mosby.

Atrial Flutter (Type I)

- Rhythm: regular if block is regular; may be irregular
- Atrial rate: 240-340 bpm (type I); 340-430 bpm (type II)
- Ventricular rate: depends on AV conduction
- P waves: saw-toothed; F waves
- QRS: normal
- PR interval: not measurable
- P: QRS: P > QRS

Significance: An atrial ectopic focus. AV conduction ratios can be variable, usually at least 2:1. The ineffective contraction can cause thrombus formation in the atria, which may subsequently embolize to the lungs, brain, and possibly other distal vessels.

Intervention: IV diltiazem, verapamil, or β-blockers. For type I, rapid atrial pacing or cardioversion if unstable. Other agents may include ibutilide or procainamide. PO flecainide, propafenone, or sotalol may also be used.
Patients with an atrial rate of >240 may need to be anticoagulated to prevent atrial thrombus formation. See "Tachycardia Algorithm" in Appendix 1.

Figure 4-12: Atrial flutter (type I).
Illustration from Huszar RJ: *Basic dysrhythmias: interpretation and management,* ed 2, St Louis, 1994, Mosby.

---

dysrhythmias. All antidysrhythmic agents have the potential for proarrhythmic effects. See Table 4-10, p. 303.
Defibrillation and cardioversion: Delivery of electrical shocks to the heart through the chest wall via use of an external defibrillator. Shocks may be synchronized with the patient's R waves (QRS complexes) or may be given as random/unsynchronized countershocks. Used to convert symptomatic, rapid atrial or ventricular rhythms to sinus rhythm. The operator must set the desired amount of electricity, apply the defibrillator paddles with conductive gel or gel pads to protect the patient from electrical burns, apply at least 80 lb of pressure, and discharge the device. Defibrillators may include "hands off" capability, wherein the device has a special cable and defibrillator pads that are used instead of the conventional paddles. The operator is not required to apply the paddles with pressure if "hands off" is available but, rather, applies one pad near the right sternal border and the other to the anterior axillary line, 5th intercostal space (ICS)—the same position as is used with paddles.
Automatic external defibrillation (AED): Defibrillation technique designed for families of patients and others (including health care providers untrained in ECG interpretation), in which the device is programmed to interpret the patient's dysrhythmia and deliver an unsynchronized countershock if deemed necessary. The operator must be able to assess for pulselessness and apnea, along with applying "hands off" defibrillator pads in the proper position (see

Abnormal chaotic and incomplete atrial depolarizations

Atrial Fibrillation

- Rhythm: irregularly irregular
- Atrial rate: >350 bpm
- Ventricular rate: variable
- P waves: coarse or fine fibrillatory waves
- QRS: normal
- PR interval: not measurable
- P: QRS: P > QRS

Significance: Chaotic atrial firing and ineffective atrial contraction. Cardiac output usually drops because of loss of atrial "kick." Ineffective atrial contraction makes clot formation a danger.

Intervention: Patients in chronic AF with controlled ventricular response may not require intervention. For new-onset AF with a rapid ventricular response, use the same protocol as recommended for atrial flutter. See "Tachycardia Algorithm" in Appendix 1. Patients should be anticoagulated to prevent atrial thrombus formation, unless contraindication because of other medical problems.

Figure 4-13:   Atrial fibrillation (AF).
Illustrations from Huszar RJ: *Basic dysrhythmias: interpretation and management,* ed 2, St Louis, 1994, Mosby.

AV Junctional Rhythm or Junctional Escape Rhythm

- Rhythm: regular
- Atrial rate: cannot determine
- Ventricular rate: 40-60 bpm
- P waves: inverted before or after QRS or not present
- QRS: normal
- PR interval: <0.2 sec if P precedes QRS
- P: QRS: P ≤ QRS

Significance: AV node assumes primary pacing function from atria.
Intervention: Usually no specific therapy indicated. If patient becomes symptomatic because of a slow rate, see "Bradycardia Algorithm" in Appendix 1.

Figure 4-14: AV junctional rhythm or junctional escape rhythm.
Illustration from Huszar RJ: *Basic dysrhythmias: interpretation and management,* ed 2, St Louis, 1994, Mosby.

---

defibrillation and cardioversion, p. 290). Devices may be semiautomatic or fully automatic.
Cardiac pacing (internal): Temporarily inserted or permanently placed, battery-powered device that provides an artificial pacing or electrical pacing stimulus for the heart. Used in situations where the heart is unable to either generate pacing impulses or appropriately conduct the impulses, or both. Most often used for management of symptomatic bradycardias including second- and third-degree heart block. Specialized devices may also be used to correct rapid atrial and ventricular rhythms via antitachycardia pacing. Third-generation implantable cardioverter defibrillators (ICDs) may also be programmed for cardiac pacing. Temporary pacing can be done via transvenous catheter insertion with positioning of leads into the endocardium or via surgically inserting epicardial wires with leads during open heart surgery. Pacemakers are named or coded based on the functions they are able to perform. (See Table 4-11, p. 304, for various pacing options.)
Transthoracic cardiac pacing (external): Cardiac pacing done by a device that delivers electrical stimulation to the heart via two conductive pads positioned over the anterior and posterior walls of the heart. One pad is near the left sternal border and the other near the left paraspinal line beneath the scapula. The device includes an ECG monitor so that efficacy of pacing can be assessed. Resistance of all muscles and bones of the chest wall must be overcome for impulses to reach the heart. The technique is usually quite uncomfortable for the patient, and sedation may be required. Certain defibrillators include capability for transthoracic cardiac pacing.
Implantable cardioverter-defibrillator (ICD): A battery-powered pulse generator (electrical device) implanted into either the umbilical or pectoral area, with lead systems (one or two leads) positioned inside the heart and superior vena cava, which can recognize and terminate potentially lethal dysrhythmias. Older devices required thoracotomy to attach epicardial screw-in leads. Newer, third generation devices do not require thoracotomy for insertion and may also

Premature Junctional Complexes

- Rhythm: irregular
- Atrial rate: cannot determine
- Ventricular rate: depends on underlying rhythm
- P waves: before, during, and after QRS
- QRS: normal
- PR interval: <0.2 sec if present
- P: QRS: P ≤ QRS

Significance: Less common than PACs; may precede blocks.
Intervention: Observation. Usually no treatment is necessary. If indicated, therapy is similar to that for PACs.

Figure 4-15: Premature junctional complexes.
Top illustration modified from Sheehy SB, Lenehan GP: *Manual of emergency care,* ed 5, St Louis, 1999, Mosby. Bottom illustration from Huszar RJ: *Basic dysrhythmias: interpretation and management,* ed 2, St Louis, 1994, Mosby.

---

provide antitachycardia pacing (ATP), low-energy cardioversion, antibradycardia pacing, and ability to score performance data. Algorithms for treatment of recognized dysrhythmias are programmed into the device. Maximal energy output is 30-40 joules, which can defibrillate malignant or lethal rhythms such as pulseless ventricular tachycardia and ventricular fibrillation. Magnets may be used for emergency deactivation/activation or suppression of all or part of programmed therapies in newer devices.

Risks and complications of thoracotomy (T) versus non-thoracotomy (NT) approaches are outlined in Table 4-12, p. 305.

Catheter ablation: A procedure in which a catheter is placed in the heart via cardiac catheterization and an electrical heat stimulus is applied to the area in

Junctional Tachycardia

- Rhythm: regular
- Atrial rate: cannot determine
- Ventricular rate: 100-250 bpm
- P waves: inverted before or after QRS
- QRS: normal
- PR interval: cannot determine
- P: QRS: P < QRS

Significance: This rhythm is essentially the same as junctional rhythm (JR), except that an increase in sympathetic stimulation results in increased HR. Causes may include heart disease, electrolyte disturbances, COPD, or hypoxia.

Intervention: See "Tachycardia Algorithm" in Appendix 1.

Figure 4-16:   Junctional tachycardia (JT).
Illustration from Huszar RJ: *Basic dysrhythmias: interpretation and management,* ed 2, St Louis, 1994, Mosby.

---

which the dysrhythmia originates. The heat stimulus causes controlled, localized necrosis of the area.

Transesophageal echocardiography (TEE):   Ultrasound technique to monitor atrial and ventricular wall motion through a sound-sensitive lead that the patient swallows. Can also detect clots that are present in the heart as a result of stasis of blood secondary to dysrhythmias (e.g., atrial fibrillation).

Anticoagulation: Use of warfarin (Coumadin) and/or platelet inhibitors may be recommended for patients at higher risk for development of blood clots within the heart secondary to dysrhythmias that decrease either atrial or ventricular wall motion.

Dietary guidelines: Patients with recurrent dysrhythmias are usually placed on a diet that restricts or reduces caffeine and is low in fat and cholesterol (see Tables 4-3 and 4-4).

Surgical procedures

Left ventricular aneurysmectomy and infarctectomy: Excision of possible focal spots of ventricular dysrhythmias.

Myocardial revascularization: Performed alone or in conjunction with electrophysiologic mapping, with excision or cryoablation of the dysrhythmia focus. Newer surgical techniques are less invasive than the more standard median sternotomy approach.

Encircling ventriculotomy: Excises the diseased portion of the ventricle without compromising myocardial blood supply.

Stellate ganglionectomy and block: Alters the electrical stability of the myocardium and predisposition to ventricular dysrhythmias.

NURSING DIAGNOSES AND INTERVENTIONS

Decreased cardiac output related to altered rate, rhythm, or conduction or negative inotropic changes secondary to cardiac disease

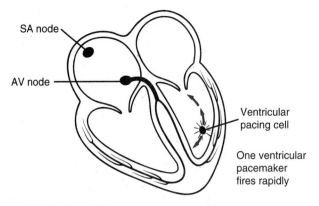

SA node

AV node

Ventricular
pacing cell

One ventricular
pacemaker
fires rapidly

Ventricular Tachycardia

- Rhythm: slightly irregular
- Atrial rate: cannot determine
- Ventricular rate: 150-250 bpm
- P waves: not visible
- QRS: wide (>0.12 sec)
- PR interval: cannot determine
- P: QRS: absent

Significance: Cardiac output falls significantly, cannot be tolerated for long, and will deteriorate into VF and asystole. May be monomorphic (same form repeated) or polymorphic (more than one type present).

Intervention: If pulseless, patient requires immediate defibrillation. Recent studies indicate patients who survive sudden cardiac death and those with sustained VT should be considered for an implantable cardioverter-defibrillator (ICD). See "Tachycardia Algorithm" and "Ventricular Fibrillation/Pulseless Ventricular Tachycardia (VF/VT) Algorithm" in Appendix 1.

Figure 4-17:   Ventricular tachycardia.
Top illustration modified from Sheehy SB, Lenehan GP: *Manual of emergency care,* ed 5, St Louis, 1999, Mosby. Bottom illustration from Huszar RJ: *Basic dysrhythmias: interpretation and management,* ed 2, St Louis, 1994, Mosby.

Desired outcomes: Within 15 min of development of serious dysrhythmias, patient has adequate cardiac output as evidenced by BP ≥90/60 mm Hg; HR 60-100 bpm; and normal sinus rhythm on ECG. PAP is 20-30/8-15 mm Hg; PAWP is ≤18 mm Hg (a reasonable outcome for these patients); RAP is ≤7 mm Hg; and CO is 4-7 L/min.

Premature Ventricular Complexes (PVCs)

- Rhythm: irregular
- Atrial rate: not determined with PVCs
- Ventricular rate: depends on underlying rhythm
- P waves: not seen
- QRS: wide (>0.12 sec); bizarre
- PR interval: not determined
- P: QRS: P < QRS

Significance: PVCs signal an irritable focus in the ventricle. Causes may include AMI, hypoxia, hypovolemia, electrolyte imbalance. PVCs may be monomorphic (same form repeated) or polymorphic (more than one type present) and may occur in patterns. They may precipitate lethal dysrhythmias.

Intervention: PVCs are common in AMI, and there is controversy regarding treatment. Antidysrhythmic agents may not be used for asymptomatic patients. Treatment should include correction of electrolyte abnormality, specifically hypokalemia and hypomagnesemia.

Figure 4-18: Premature ventricular complexes (PVCs).
Illustration from Huszar RJ: *Basic dysrhythmias: interpretation and management,* ed 2, St Louis, 1994, Mosby.

- Monitor patient's heart rhythm continuously; note BP and symptoms if dysrhythmias occur or increase in occurrence.
- If a PA catheter is present, note PAP, PAWP, and RAP; monitor for a reduced CO in response to dysrhythmias.
- Document dysrhythmias with rhythm strip. Use a 12/15/18-lead ECG as necessary to identify the dysrhythmia.
- Monitor patient's laboratory data, particularly K^+, Mg^{++}, glucose, and digoxin levels.
- Administer antidysrhythmic agents as prescribed; note patient's response to therapy.
- Provide oxygen as prescribed. Oxygen may be beneficial if dysrhythmias are related to ischemia.
- Maintain a quiet environment, and administer pain medications promptly. Both stress and pain can increase sympathetic tone and cause dysrhythmias.
- If life-threatening dysrhythmias occur, initiate immediate unit protocols or standing orders for treatment, as well as CPR and ACLS algorithms (see Appendix 1) as necessary.
- When dysrhythmias occur, stay with patient; provide support and reassurance while performing assessments and administering treatment.
- Administer inotropic agents (see Appendix 7) as prescribed to support patient's BP and CO.

■NIC Cardiac Care; Hemodynamic Regulation; Medication Management; Oxygen Therapy; Respiratory Monitoring; Vital Signs Monitoring

Multiple ectopic pacemaker in the ventricles

Abnormal, chaotic, and incomplete ventricular depolarizations

Ventricular Fibrillation

- Rhythm: irregular
- Atrial rate: cannot determine
- Ventricular rate: rapid
- P waves: not seen
- QRS: absent; fibrillatory waves
- PR interval: none
- P: QRS: none

Significance: Most common cause of sudden cardiac death. VF produces no cardiac output.

Intervention: Current research indicates Amiodarone is useful in conversion of unstable VT to sinus rhythm. Patients who survive sudden cardiac death (VF) should be considered for an implantable cardioverter-defibrillator (ICD). See "Ventricular Fibrillation/Pulseless Ventricular Tachycardia (VF/VT) Algorithm" and "Automatic External Defibrillator (AED) Algorithm" in Appendix 1.

Figure 4-19: Ventricular fibrillation.
Illustrations from Huszar RJ: *Basic dysrhythmias: interpretation and management*, ed 2, St Louis, 1994, Mosby.

Idioventricular Rhythm

- Rhythm: regular or irregular
- Atrial rate: none
- Ventricular rate: <40 bpm
- P waves: none
- QRS: wide (>0.12 sec); bizarre
- PR interval: none
- P: QRS: none

Significance: Usually lethal. Pulse may be present but usually is not.
Intervention: See "Pulseless Electrical Activity (PEA) Algorithm" in Appendix 1.

Figure 4-20:   Idioventricular rhythm.
Illustration from Huszar RJ: *Basic dysrhythmias: interpretation and management,* ed 2, St Louis, 1994, Mosby.

Asystole

- No electrical activity
- May see a rare, wide, bizarre QRS

Significance: Mortality >95%. Always confirm asystole in 2 leads.
Intervention: See "Asystole Algorithm" in Appendix 1.

Figure 4-21:   Asystole.
Illustration from Huszar RJ: *Basic dysrhythmias: interpretation and management,* ed 2, St Louis, 1994, Mosby.

Risk for activity intolerance related to imbalance between oxygen supply and demand secondary to dysrhythmias that reduce cardiac output
Desired outcomes: During activity, patient rates exertion <3 on a scale of 0-10 and exhibits tolerance of the dysrhythmia by a RR <20 breaths/min; systolic BP within 20 mm Hg of baseline; HR within 20 bpm of resting HR; and absence of chest discomfort and/or new dysrhythmias.
- Monitor patient's response to activity. Instruct patient to report chest discomfort and SOB. Note new dysrhythmias associated with activity or other stressors.

First-Degree AV Block

- Rhythm: regular
- Atrial rate: 60-100 bpm
- Ventricular rate: 60-100 bpm
- P waves: present; precede each QRS
- QRS: normal
- PR interval: prolonged (>0.2 sec)
- P: QRS: 1:1

Significance: Impulse conduction is delayed through the AV node. Causes are varied and may include heart disease, ischemia, digitalis toxicity, other drug effect, and myocarditis.

Intervention: Observation; usually no treatment needed.

Figure 4-22:   First-degree AV block.
Illustration from Huszar RJ: *Basic dysrhythmias: interpretation and management,* ed 2, St Louis, 1994, Mosby.

Second-Degree AV Block Type I (Wenckebach)

- Rhythm: irregular
- Atrial rate: exceeds ventricular rate
- Ventricular rate: less than sinus rate
- P waves: one P wave precedes each QRS except during nonconducted P waves, which occur regularly
- QRS: normal
- PR interval: lengthens progressively with each cycle until one is nonconducted

Significance: Usually a transient block that does not progress to complete heart block.

Intervention: Observation; treatment usually not necessary.

Figure 4-23:   Second-degree AV block (type I) (Wenckebach).
Illustration from Huszar RJ: *Basic dysrhythmias: interpretation and management,* ed 2, St Louis, 1994, Mosby.

Second-Degree AV Block Type II

- Rhythm: irregular
- Atrial rate: exceeds ventricular rate
- Ventricular rate: depends on degree of block
- P waves: 2 or more for each QRS
- QRS: normal duration
- PR interval: normal or prolonged on the conducted complex
- P: QRS: P > QRS

Significance: This block may occur with anterior wall AMI and may progress rapidly to complete heart block.

Intervention: Observation if patient is asymptomatic. If symptoms occur, see "Bradycardia Algorithm" in Appendix 1.

Figure 4-24:   Second-degree AV block (type II).
Illustration from Huszar RJ: *Basic dysrhythmias: interpretation and management,* ed 2, St Louis, 1994, Mosby.

- Administer medications as prescribed.
- Observe and report signs of acute decreased CO, including oliguria, decreasing BP, and altered mentation, and dizziness.
- Monitor BP and other vital signs frequently as necessary, and report changes such as irregular HR, HR >120 bpm, or decreasing BP to the physician as soon as possible.
- Assess integrity of peripheral perfusion by monitoring peripheral pulses, distal extremity skin color, and urinary output. Report changes such as decreased pulse amplitude, pallor or cyanosis, and decreased urine output.

NIC Activity Therapy; Cardiac Care; Energy management; Surveillance

Knowledge deficit: mechanism by which dysrhythmias occur; life-style implications

Desired outcome: Within the 24-h period before discharge from CCU, patient and significant others verbalize knowledge about causes of dysrhythmias and the implications for modification of patient's life-style.

- Discuss causal mechanisms for dysrhythmias, including resulting symptoms. Use a heart model or diagrams as necessary.
- Teach the signs and symptoms of dysrhythmias that necessitate medical attention: unrelieved and prolonged palpitations, chest pain, SOB, rapid pulse (>150 bpm), dizziness, and syncope. Teach patient and significant others how to check pulse rate for a full minute.
- Teach patient and significant others about medications that will be taken after hospital discharge, including drug name, purpose, dosage, schedule, precautions, and potential side effects. Stress that patient will be maintained on long-term antidysrhythmic therapy and that it could be life threatening to stop or skip these medications without physician approval, because doing so may decrease blood levels effective for dysrhythmia suppression.
- Advise patient and significant others about the availability of support groups and counseling; provide appropriate community referrals. Patients who

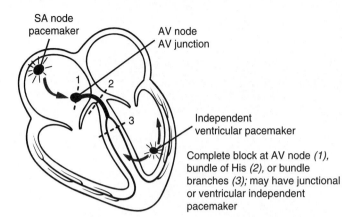

Complete block at AV node *(1),* bundle of His *(2),* or bundle branches *(3);* may have junctional or ventricular independent pacemaker

Complete Heart Block

- Rhythm: usually regular
- Atrial rate: exceeds ventricular rate
- Ventricular rate: <60 bpm
- P waves: occur at regular intervals
- QRS: <0.12 sec if pacemaker is in the AV node; >0.12 sec if ventricular pacemaker
- PR interval: no relationship between P and QRS
- P: QRS: no relationship

Significance: No conduction of SA node impulses. The atria and ventricles beat independently of each other. The slow rate can cause myocardial ischemia.

Intervention: Pacemaker insertion necessary. See "Bradycardia Algorithm" in Appendix 1.

Figure 4-25: Complete (third-degree) AV block.
Top illustration modified from Sheehy SB, Lenehan GP: *Manual of emergency care,* ed 5, St Louis, 1999, Mosby. Bottom illustration from Huszar RJ: *Basic dysrhythmias: interpretation and management,* ed 2, St Louis, 1994, Mosby.

---

survive sudden cardiac arrest may experience nightmares or other sleep disturbances at home. Explain that anxiety and fear, along with periodic feelings of denial, depression, anger, and confusion, are normal following this experience.
- Stress the importance of leading a normal and productive life, even though patient may fear breakthrough of life-threatening dysrhythmias. If patient is going on vacation, advise him or her to take along sufficient medication and to investigate health care facilities in the vacation area.

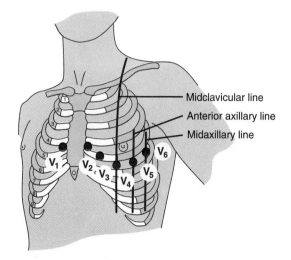

Figure 4-26: Placement of precordial electrodes.
From Huszar RJ: *Basic dysrhythmias: interpretation and management,* ed 2,
St Louis, 1994, Mosby.

- Advise patient and significant others to take CPR classes; provide addresses of community programs.
- Teach the importance of follow-up care; confirm date and time of next appointment, if known. Explain that outpatient Holter monitoring is performed periodically.
- Explain that individuals with recurrent dysrhythmias should follow a general low-fat and low-cholesterol diet (see Tables 4-3 and 4-4) and reduce intake of products containing caffeine, including coffee, tea, chocolate, and colas.
- As indicated, teach patient relaxation techniques, which will reduce stress and enable patient to decrease sympathetic tone (see next nursing diagnosis).

NIC Surveillance; Teaching: Individual; Teaching: Prescribed Medication; Vital Signs Monitoring

Health-seeking behavior: relaxation technique effective for stress reduction and facilitation of decreased sympathetic tone
Desired outcome: Within the 24-h period after instruction, patient verbalizes and demonstrates the following relaxation technique.

- Explain that to decrease sympathetic tone, some patients with dysrhythmias may benefit from practicing a relaxation response. Many different techniques can be used, including use of breathing alone or in conjunction with muscle group contraction and relaxation. Other techniques incorporate use of imagery. The following is a relaxation response that can facilitate a state of decreased sympathetic nervous system outflow. Give patient the following instructions:
  1. Sit quietly in a comfortable position. Close your eyes.
  2. Relax all your muscles, starting at your feet and progressing to your facial muscles.

TABLE 4-10 Antidysrhythmic Drugs

Class I (sodium channel blockers)

Block the rapid, inward sodium current. Local anesthetics and other drugs that decrease automaticity of ventricular conduction, delay ventricular repolarization, decrease conduction velocity, increase conduction via AV node, and suppress ventricular automaticity. Class IA decreases depolarization moderately and prolongs repolarization. Class IB decreases depolarization and shortens repolarization. Class IC significantly decreases depolarization with minimal effect on repolarization.

Class IA	Class IB	Class IC
Disopyramide (PO)	Lidocaine (IV, IM)	Encainide (PO)
Procainamide (PO, IV, IM)	Mexiletine (PO)	Flecainide (PO)
Quinidine (PO, IV)	Phenytoin (PO)	Propafenone (PO)
	Tocainide (PO)	

Class II (β-adrenergic blockers)

Block stimulation of β_1- and β_2-receptors by catecholamines. Slow sinus node automaticity, slow conduction via AV node, control ventricular response to supraventricular tachycardias, and shorten the action potential of Purkinje fibers.

Acebutolol (PO)
Atenolol (PO)
Carvedilol (PO)
Esmolol (IV)
Metoprolol (PO, IV)
Propranolol (PO, IV)

Class III (potassium channel/IK1 blockers)

Block the outward current of potassium. Increase the action potential and refractory period of Purkinje fibers, increase ventricular fibrillation threshold, restore injured myocardial cell electrophysiology toward normal, and suppress reentrant dysrhythmias.

Amiodarone (PO, IV)	*Final stages of clinical trials*
Bretylium (IV, IM)	Dofetilide
Ibutelide (IV)	Azimilide
Sotalol (PO, IV)	

Class IV (calcium channel blockers)

Depress automaticity in the SA and AV nodes, block the slow calcium current in the AV junctional tissue, reduce conduction via the AV node, and are useful in treating tachydysrhythmias due to AV junctional reentry.

Diltiazem (PO, IV)
Verapamil (PO, IV)

Unclassified

Depress activity of the AV node.
Adenosine (IV)

SA, Sinoatrial; *AV,* atrioventricular; *PO,* by mouth; *IV,* intravenous; *IM,* intramuscular; β, beta.

3. Breathe through your nose. As you breathe out, say the word "one" silently to yourself. Become aware of your breathing, and continue this process for approximately 20 min.
4. Do not worry whether you are achieving a deep level of relaxation. Maintain a passive attitude, and permit relaxation to occur at its own

TABLE 4-11 Five-Position Pacemaker Code

Position	I	II	III	IV	V
Category	Chamber(s) paced	Chamber(s) sensed	Mode of response(s)	Programmable functions	Special tachyarrhythmia functions
Letters used	V—Ventricle A—Atrium D—Double	V—Ventricle A—Atrium D—Double	T—Triggered I—Inhibited D—Double* O—None R—Reverse	P—Programmable (rate and/or output) M—Multiprogrammable O—None	B—Bursts N—Normal rate C—Competition S—Scanning E—External
Manufacturer's designation only	S—Single chamber	S—Single chamber			

From Dunn MI, Lipman BS: *Lipman-Massie clinical electrocardiography*, Chicago, 1989, Year Book.
*Atrial triggered, and ventricular inhibited.

T A B L E 4 - 1 2 Implications for Patient Care and Costs: Implantable Cardioverter Defibrillators (ICD)

NOTE:
Magnetic fields are measured in units (gauss) or 1000th of a gauss, or milligauss (MG). 10 gauss will affect an ICD or some programmable pacemakers. Common household electrical appliances (interferences) are less than 50 MG. Electrical fields are measured in volts per meter. 750 volts is approximately 30 joules.

Complication	Thoracotomy (T)	Non-Thoracotomy (NT)	Patient care implications
Pneumothorax or hemothorax	Higher risk	Lower risk	ICU monitoring required for **T**. ICU unnecessary for **NT**. Length of hospital stay decreases with **NT**.
Pocket hematoma, seroma, wound adhesions	Higher risk	Lower risk	Wound care and home care less complex for **NT**.
Wound infection	Higher risk	Lower risk	If wound infection, **T** more likely to require IV antibiotics, which will increase costs and length of hospital stay.
Blood loss/bleeding	Higher risk	Lower risk	**T** may need type and screen for blood products. **NT** does not.
Pneumonia	Higher risk	Lower risk	**T** may have decreased activity tolerance and requires pulmonary toilet.
Pain	Higher risk	Lower risk	**NT** requires less analgesia to manage pain.

pace. Expect distractions to occur, but just ignore them. Continue breathing and repeating the word "one."

- Encourage patient to practice this technique once or twice a day. Reassure him or her that relaxation is a learned skill that takes practice and becomes easier over time.

NIC Anxiety Reduction; Calming Technique; Meditation; Music Therapy; Simple Guided Imagery; Simple Relaxation Therapy; Teaching: Prescribed Activity/Exercise

For patients with an implantable cardioverter-defibrillator and permanent pacemaker
Knowledge deficit: ICD or pacemaker insertion procedure and follow-up care
Desired outcomes: Within the 24-h period before the procedure, patient and significant others describe rationale for the procedure and method of insertion. Within the 24-h period before discharge from CCU, patient and significant others describe postinsertion care and need for continued physician and nurse follow-up.

- Assess patient's understanding of his or her medical condition (dysrhythmias) and the amount of detailed information desired.
- Discuss the following with the patient and significant others:
  - ☐ Type of dysrhythmia patient has, using rhythm strip and heart model or drawings/illustrations/charts to promote understanding.
  - ☐ Possible need for temporary transvenous pacemaker insertion before ICD or permanent pacemaker procedure.
  - ☐ Use of appropriate anesthesia throughout procedure.
  - ☐ Testing of the ability of the device to control lethal dysrhythmias, which will occur in the operating room/catheterization lab after implantation, before the incision is closed.
  - ☐ Reassurance that should the mechanism fail to control the dysrhythmia, the device can be adjusted or reprogrammed to control the dysrhythmia.
  - ☐ Continuous observation of patient in a cardiac care unit for ~24 h, with ongoing monitoring of BP, HR, and RR.
  - ☐ Importance of deep breathing, coughing (as necessary), and incentive spirometry exercises as appropriate. Explain that patient is at increased risk for respiratory tract and incisional infection if thoracic surgery was done, which tends to cause patient to avoid deep breathing and coughing to guard against pain. Have patient return demonstrations of breathing exercises. Reassure patient that analgesics can be administered before pulmonary toilet exercises, if needed.
  - ☐ Discharge instructions: Follow-up visit within 10-14 days, need for obtaining an automatic external defibrillator (AED)/"home defibrillator," and importance of CPR/defibrillator classes for significant others.
- Describe the procedure should ICD device deliver a "shock." If the patient is aware of the shocks, the physician should be notified as soon as possible that the device is firing. With newer devices, patients may be unaware of shocks but may become symptomatic (e.g., become intolerant of activity, dizzy, have chest discomfort) with prolonged or serious dysrhythmias. Teach patient to record the number of "shocks" experienced.
- Explain use of the AED/ "home defibrillator," which is available commercially from several companies. It is designed to allow the nonmedical person or care providers untrained in dysrhythmia interpretation to effect defibrillation, and its purpose is to convert lethal dysrhythmias should the ICD fail.
- Explain that "shocks" during sinus rhythm may indicate a lead fracture in the ICD system. Usually this is detected while the patient is being monitored (e.g., by ECG in physician's office, hospital monitor, or Holter monitor).

NIC Learning Facilitation; Learning Readiness Enhancement; Risk Identification; Teaching: Disease Process; Teaching: Prescribed Medication; Teaching: Psychomotor Skill

Risk for infection related to invasive procedure into thorax

Desired outcome: Patient is free of infection as evidenced by normothermia; WBC count ≤11,000/mm^3; negative culture results; and absence of the clinical indicators of infection at the incision site and of the respiratory tract.

- Encourage and assist with deep breathing, coughing (if needed), and incentive spirometry exercises q2h, and encourage early ambulation to the chair. As indicated, assist patient with splinting the incision site with hands or pillow to promote pain control. Administer prescribed analgesics 20 min before scheduled breathing exercises. For more information, see this nursing diagnosis in "Acute Pneumonia," p. 224.
- Assess incision site q2h for warmth, erythema, swelling, and drainage. The presence of a seroma, which has the same symptoms as incision site infection, is confirmed by decubitus chest x-rays or CT.
- Monitor patient's temperature q2-4h, being alert to elevation >38.6° C (101.5° F).
- Monitor CBC for elevation of WBCs.
- Consult physician for significant findings.

   Teach patient and significant others the signs and symptoms of infection, both of the incision site and respiratory tract: cough, sputum production, fever, dyspnea, chills, headache, myalgia. Explain that the older adult may be confused and disoriented and may run low-grade fevers but few other indicators are present.

NIC Infection Control; Infection Protection; Cough Enhancement; Exercise Promotion; Surveillance; Medication Prescribing; Home Maintenance Assistance

For patients with a pacemaker (temporary or permanent) or patients with third-generation ICDs with cardiac pacing

Decreased cardiac output related to malfunction of cardiac pacemaker

Desired outcome: Within the 24-h period preceding hospital discharge or throughout the duration of temporary cardiac pacing, patient has adequate CO as evidenced by systolic BP >90 mm Hg; RR 12-20 breaths/min; HR <100 bpm; urinary output >0.5ml/kg/h; warm and dry skin; and ECG indicative of effective capture, sensing, response to sensing, and function of antitachycardia pacing (if operational).

- Recognize and document paced rhythms. Events to document include: (1) recognition of pacing spike preceding P wave and /or QRS complex as appropriate for settings; (2) sensing of patient's inherent pacing; (3) response of pacemaker when triggering and/or inhibiting pacing; (4) response of heart rate to activity if pacemaker is programmed "rate responsive"; and (5) initiation of antitachycardia pacing or electric shock (with ICD) for dysrhythmias.
- Promptly detect problems with pacemaker functions. Include assessment of potential electromagnetic interference (EMI) (Table 4-13). Ensure that temporary pacemaker battery is still functional or changed as needed and that cable connectors for temporary pacemakers are appropriately connected to the pulse generator (pacemaker box). For problems with functions of permanent pacemakers and ICDs, the physician should be notified immediately.
- Provide electrical safety measures for temporary cardiac pacing to include proper grounding, protection of exposed catheter tips and/or heart wires. Caregiver must wear rubber/non-conductive gloves when handling pacing lead wires/catheter so that microshocks are avoided. Microshocks can induce lethal dysrhythmias.
- Observe for complications of temporary pacing, which include dysrhythmias, lead displacement or fracture, lead perforation of the heart possibly leading to cardiac tamponade, pericarditis, infection, and bleeding.

TABLE 4-13   Electromagnetic Interference and the Third-Generation ICD and Some Programmable Pacemakers

Unsafe hospital procedures/ equipment	Unsafe home equipment: use caution	Safe home equipment
MRI (magnetic resonance imaging)	Large magnets: junkyards, construction sites, other areas that may have large magnets	Microwave ovens
Nerve stimulator		Refrigerator magnets
Electrocautery		Electric blankets
Diathermy		Tanning bed
Lithotripsy	Hand-held wands at airport security	Riding lawnmower
	Bingo wands	Jacuzzi
	Certain slot machines	CB radio
	Large stereo speakers (unsafe to carry)	HAM radio (except for antennas)
	Cellular telephones	Table saw
	High-tension wires	Gas welder
	Industrial transformers	Electric drill
	Robotic jacks	Weed Eater™
	Arc welders	Small boat motors
	Power generators in dams	
	Industrial motors	
	Large boat motors	

ICD, Implantable cardioverter defibrillator.

NIC Cardiac Care; Dysrhythmia Management; Vital Signs Management; Surveillance; Environmental Management: Safety

For patients with an implantable cardioverter-defibrillator
Altered sexuality patterns (or risk for same) related to fear of inducing dysrhythmias during sexual activity
Desired outcome: Within the 24-h period before discharge from CCU, patient and significant other verbalize understanding of interventions during and alternatives for sexual intercourse.
- Ask patient to describe any symptoms of dysrhythmias during presurgical sexual experiences.
- Explain the following interventions or alternatives that can be made if patient continues to experience dysrhythmias during sexual intercourse:
  ☐ Patient may need to take a less active role.
  ☐ Patient may find that taking a prescribed vasodilator before engaging in sexual intercourse will prevent dysrhythmias.
  ☐ Suggest that during periods when dysrhythmias are a problem, less stressful forms of sexual activity, such as caressing and hugging, are positive alternatives.
- As appropriate, advise patient that stressful situations, such as extramarital relations or unfamiliar environment, may contribute to symptoms during sexual activity.
- Explain that the device may "shock" at any time. If the patient's significant other is in contact with the patient's body at that time, the shock may be experienced as a tingling sensation by the significant other.

NIC Sexual Counseling; Teaching: Sexuality; Anxiety Reduction; Coping Enhancement; Support Group

ADDITIONAL NURSING DIAGNOSES

The patient with ICD is at risk for pneumothorax. As indicated, also see "Pneumothorax," p. 239, for information related to this disorder. Also see nursing diagnoses and interventions in "Hemodynamic Monitoring," p. 28; "Psychosocial Support," p. 83; and "Psychosocial Support for the Patient's Family and Significant Others," p. 95.

Valvular heart disease

PATHOPHYSIOLOGY

Valvular heart disease involves obstruction to forward flow (stenosis) or insufficiency of the valve, allowing backward flow (regurgitation). One or more valves may be affected by one or both processes. When the effectiveness of a valve is compromised, symptoms of valvular incompetence may develop or the heart may begin to show signs of failure.

Usually, stenosis of a valve is caused by sclerosing, thickening, and calcification of the valve leaflets. A stenotic valve obstructs blood flow from the affected atrium or ventricle, which leads to hypertrophy of the chamber with the fluid overload. With a stenotic aortic or pulmonic valve, intramyocardial wall tension increases; this increase enables the heart to compensate by pumping more blood through the highly resistant valve opening. If the stenosis is unrelieved, the ventricle eventually fails. When the left ventricle fails, blood backs up into the left atrium and pulmonary capillary bed, leading to pulmonary congestion or peripheral edema, depending on the side of the heart that is involved. In addition, with ventricular hypertrophy and high intramyocardial wall tension, blood flow to the endocardium may be diminished. These patients therefore may have angina and ventricular dysrhythmias. Both mitral and tricuspid stenosis can be severely debilitating, causing easy fatigability and limited activity.

Regurgitation of a valve may be caused by rheumatic heart disease, dilation of the valve ring, or damage to the nearby valve structures. Regurgitation results in increased volume into the affected chamber. (See Figure 4-27.)

ASSESSMENT

See Table 4-15, p. 318.

Many people with long-standing valvular disease that results in atrial enlargement eventually develop atrial fibrillation. Observe the cardiac monitor for this dysrhythmia, and note any irregularly irregular heart sounds on auscultation or heart beat noted on palpation. Syncope during activity is often the presenting symptom for aortic valve stenosis. In addition, cardiac cachexia may be seen in persons with long-standing valvular dysfunction. Hepatic tenderness and enlargement may be present with tricuspid or pulmonic valve disease.

DIAGNOSTIC TESTS

Cardiac catheterization: A ventriculogram may assist in visualization of blood flow. Measurement of chamber pressures assists in determining type of disorder present and the degree of severity.
Echocardiography: To determine ventricular function, chamber size, and valve function.
- *Doppler flow studies:* Continuous wave or pulsed wave frequencies used to determine blood flow.
- *Color flow mapping studies:* Uses colors (red and blue) to enhance the image of blood flowing through the heart.

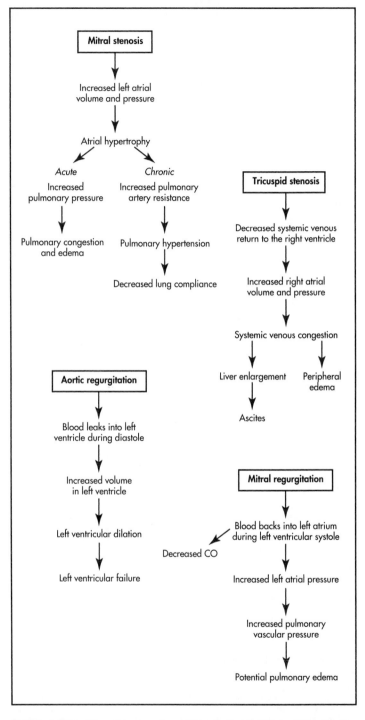

Figure 4-27: Disease progression with valvular disorders. (*CO,* Cardiac output.)

Research Brief 4-1 A study of 109 persons undergoing cardiac surgery for either valvular disease or coronary artery disease was conducted to determine if age, duration of aortic cross-clamping, smoking habit, preoperative respiratory rehabilitation, and abdominal wall problems had an effect on the occurrence of respiratory complications. Complications rates were: pleural effusion, 39%; atelectasis, 34%; retained secretions, 13%; infection, 6%; ARDS, 4.9%; thromboembolism, 1.2%; pneumothorax, 1.2%; and phrenic nerve paralysis, 1.2%. There was no significant difference in complications between those with risk factors and those without.

From Rico DP et al: Respiratory complications after open heart surgery, *Rehabilitation* 32(2): 105-108, 1998.

- *TEE:* Uses an endoscope that produces an image unimpeded by the chest wall. Because the esophagus is close to the heart, the images are clear and undistorted.

ECG: See Table 4-16, p. 321.

SURGICAL INTERVENTIONS

Methods of surgical treatment include valve repair (valvuloplasty), commissurotomy, and replacement.

Valve replacement: Performed in patients with moderate to severe calcification, mixed stenosis and insufficiency, and pure insufficiency; procedure has a mortality of about 6%. Three types of valves are used for replacement: homografts, heterografts, and artificial grafts. Homografts are human cadaver valves that have been specially treated for surgical use. Because they are not readily available, they seldom are used. A heterograft is a valve from an animal, usually a pig or cow, that has been prepared for surgical use. These valves are readily available and in common use. Artificial valves are made from stainless steel, carbon, and other durable materials, such as plastic. Tissue grafts are advantageous because they are natural and thus blood elements do not tend to form on them. Their disadvantage is their short duration of use, which is about 5-8 yr. There is a tendency for clots to form on artificial valves, and therefore the patient must receive lifetime anticoagulant therapy; however, the valve can be used for 10-15 yr. Postoperative care of the patient who has had valve surgery is similar to that of the patient who has undergone CABG (see p. 261). It is important to note, however, that patients undergoing valve surgery are at increased risk for thrombosis and embolism (particularly with mechanical mitral valves and in patients with atrial fibrillation) and for valvular endocarditis.

Postoperative considerations specific to these patients are discussed in "Nursing Diagnoses and Interventions."

Percutaneous balloon valvuloplasty: For dilation of stenotic heart valves. Candidates for this procedure (1) are at high risk for surgery, (2) refuse surgery, (3) are older adults (often >80 yr of age), or (4) are informed of treatment choices and choose this procedure over others. The procedure parallels the technique for PTCA (see p. 253). The femoral artery and vein are cannulated, and the patient receives anticoagulation therapy with heparin. For aortic valve dilation, a catheter is passed into the femoral artery to measure supravalvular and left ventricular pressures before valvuloplasty. A balloon valvuloplasty catheter is then passed over a guidewire into the left ventricle. It is inflated three times for 12-30 sec at a pressure of 12 atm. Additional heparin is administered, and the valve gradient is remeasured. To reach the mitral valve, the balloon valvuloplasty catheter is passed via the femoral vein and through the atrial septum to the mitral valve opening. The inflation procedure is the same.

With both aortic and mitral dilation, significant improvement has been demonstrated in the valve gradient and in blood flow across the valve.

Complications that have been observed include embolization to the brain, disruption of the valve ring, acute valve regurgitation, valvular restenosis, hemorrhage at the catheter insertion site, guidewire perforation of the left ventricle, and dysrhythmias.

Commissurotomy: A procedure in which the stenotic valve is opened by a dilating instrument. When performed early in the course of the disease, chances of success are good, although the procedure may result in valve regurgitation and recurrent stenosis.

NURSING DIAGNOSES AND INTERVENTIONS

Altered protection related to risk of bleeding/hemorrhage secondary to anticoagulation

> **Note:** Patients undergoing aortic valve replacement are at a higher risk for postoperative hemorrhage than those undergoing CABG.

Desired outcome: Throughout hospitalization, patient is free of symptoms of bleeding or hemorrhage as evidenced by RAP ≥4 mm Hg; PAWP ≥6 mm Hg; BP within patient's normal range; CO ≥4 L/min; CI ≥2.5 L/min/m^2; urine output ≥0.5 ml/kg/h; urine specific gravity 1.010-1.030; and chest tube drainage ≤100 ml/h.

- Measure chest tube drainage hourly. Report chest tube drainage >100 ml/h. Maintain patency of chest tubes at all times.
- Monitor clotting studies. Be alert to and report prolonged PT, PTT, and ACT and decreased platelet count. Optimal values are as follows: PT 11-15 sec; PTT 30-40 sec (activated); and ACT ≤120 sec. For patient with prolonged PT, PTT, or ACT, administer IV protamine sulfate as prescribed.
- Assess VS hourly, and monitor patient for physical indicators of hemorrhage or hypovolemia: RAP <4 mm Hg; PAWP <6 mm Hg; decreased BP; decreased measured CO/CI; urine output <0.5 ml/kg/h; increased urine specific gravity; and excessive chest tube drainage (>100 ml/h). Be alert to a decreased Hct. Optimal values are: Hct ≥37% (female) and ≥40% (male).
- Assess postoperative chest x-ray for a widened mediastinum, which may indicate hemorrhage and possible cardiac tamponade.
- As prescribed, administer platelets, fresh-frozen plasma, or cryoprecipitate to replace clotting factors and blood volume.
- Administer packed RBCs as prescribed to replace blood volume, or use chest tube drainage for autotransfusion.
- To correct hyperfibrinolytic state (increased fibrin degradation products), administer aminocaproic acid slowly per IV bolus as prescribed (see Table 6-4).

NIC Bleeding Reduction; Autotransfusion; Hemorrhage Control

Decreased cardiac output (or risk for same) related to negative inotropic changes secondary to intraoperative subendocardial ischemia and administration of myocardial depressant drugs

> **Note:** After cardiac surgery some myocardial depression is always present, usually lasting 48-72 h. Patients with long-standing aortic stenosis or ventricular failure caused by mitral valve disease are at an even greater risk for postoperative low cardiac output.

Desired outcomes: Within 48-72 h of this diagnosis, patient has adequate cardiac output as evidenced by normal sinus rhythm on ECG; measured CO of 4-7 L/min; CI ≥2.5 L/min/m^2; BP within patient's normal range; PAP 20-30/8-15 mm Hg; PAWP 6-12 mm Hg (or range specified by physician); Svo$_2$ 60%-80%; SVR 900-1200 dynes/sec/cm^{-5}; peripheral pulses >2+ on a 0-4+ scale; warm and dry skin; and hourly urine output ≥0.5 ml/kg/h. Patient is awake, alert, and oriented.

- Monitor BP, PAP, RAP, Svo$_2$, HR, and heart rhythm continuously. Monitor

PAWP, SVR, and CO hourly. Be alert to and report the following: elevated PAWP; decreased CO; decreased Svo_2; or elevated SVR.
- Monitor urinary output, noting output that is <0.5 ml/kg/h for 2 consecutive hours.
- Monitor peripheral pulses and color and temperature of extremities q2h.
- Provide oxygen therapy as prescribed.
- Maintain an adequate preload (i.e., PAWP >6 mm Hg; RAP >4-6 mm Hg) via administration of IV fluids.

> **Note:** With aortic stenosis and severe left ventricular hypertrophy, a high filling pressure (i.e., PAWP >18 mm Hg) may be necessary to ensure an adequate cardiac output.

- Maintain a normal or reduced afterload (SVR <1200 dynes/sec/cm^{-5}) by administering prescribed IV vasodilating drugs, such as nitroprusside and NTG.
- Maintain normal sinus rhythm by administering antidysrhythmic agents as prescribed. Atrial fibrillation is common in aortic and mitral valve disease and may result in a 20% decrease in CO. If a junctional rhythm or bradycardia occurs, a pacemaker usually becomes necessary.
- Administer inotropic agents as prescribed to maintain CI ≥2.5 L/min/m^2 and systolic BP >90 mm Hg. Commonly used agents include dobutamine, dopamine, milrinone, and amrinone. Monitor for side effects, including tachydysrhythmias, ventricular ectopy, headache, and angina.

NIC Cardiac Care; Hemodynamic Regulation

Altered tissue perfusion (or risk for same): cerebral, related to impaired blood flow to the brain secondary to embolization resulting from cardiac surgery

> **Note:** Air embolism, particulate embolism from calcified valves, and thrombotic emboli from prosthetic valves may lodge in the brain, leading to varying degrees of stroke.

Desired outcome: Throughout hospitalization, patient has adequate or baseline brain perfusion as evidenced by orientation to time, place, and person; equal and normoreactive pupils; and ability to move all extremities, communicate, and respond to requests (or comparable to patient's preoperative baseline).
- Monitor patient immediately after surgery and hourly for signs of neurologic impairment: diminished LOC, pupillary response, ability to move all extremities, and response to verbal stimuli.
- Assess patient's orientation and ability to communicate, answer yes-no questions, point to objects, write responses and requests, identify family members, and state his or her location. Inform other health care personnel about patient's LOC and communication deficits.
- Assess patient's PT, PTT, international normalized ratio (INR) as heparin is tapered off and Coumadin therapy is instituted.
- If CNS impairment is suspected, administer urea solutions, mannitol, and corticosteroids as prescribed.
- In the presence of CNS impairment, implement the following measures:
  - ☐ Assist patient with turning and moving as needed. Teach patient to use unaffected extremities to assist with moving.
  - ☐ Perform ROM to all extremities qid. Have patient assist as much as possible.
  - ☐ Progress patient's activity level, as tolerated, with the assistance of a physical therapist.
- When patient is able to take oral foods and fluids, assess patient's ability to swallow. If patient's voice is hoarse or patient coughs when swallowing,

consult physician. Patient may require NPO status and an enteric tube until the swallowing reflex has improved.

NIC Surveillance; Cerebral Perfusion Promotion

Knowledge deficit: risk of infective endocarditis after valve surgery and precautions that must be taken to prevent it

> **Note:** All patients with valve surgery are at risk for infective endocarditis (IE) as a result of bacteria entering the bloodstream and traveling to the heart, leading to destruction of a new tissue valve or obstruction of a new artificial valve.

Desired outcome: Within the 24-h period before discharge from CCU, patient verbalizes knowledge about the risk of IE after valve surgery and the precautions that must be taken to prevent it.

- Teach patient about IE (see "Acute Infective Endocarditis," p. 316), describing what it is, how it develops, and how it may affect the repaired valve.
- Teach patient that antibiotics are prescribed as a prophylaxis against endocarditis after valve surgery. Explain that they must be taken before any dental work or examination by instrument is undertaken, including teeth cleaning, fillings, extractions, cystoscopy, endoscopy, or sigmoidoscopy. Caution patient to notify dentists and all health care providers about the valve surgery so that antibiotics can be prescribed before any invasive procedure.
- Instruct patient to cleanse all wounds and apply antibiotic ointments to help prevent infection.

NIC Teaching: Prescribed Medication; Surveillance

Knowledge deficit: risk of hemorrhage or embolus caused by excessive or insufficient anticoagulation therapy with Coumadin

> **Note:** Finding and maintaining the dose of Coumadin that results in the target INR can be difficult. Also, foods, medications, vitamins, and food supplements can enhance or inhibit the efficacy of Coumadin.

Desired outcome: Within the 24-h period before discharge from the hospital, patient or significant others verbalize knowledge about the risk of Coumadin therapy after valve surgery and the precautions that must be taken to prevent embolus or hemorrhage.

- Teach patient how to institute bleeding precautions after discharge. Shave with an electric razor. Take care when handling sharp objects. Prevent injury through a fall safety home check. Use soft-bristle toothbrush.
- Teach patient to call physician if bleeding or bruising noted.
- Teach patient and significant others to report all changes in medication to health care provider who is managing Coumadin therapy.
- Teach patient and significant others to avoid altering the intake of foods that may be high in vitamin K. Excessive intake of vitamin K can block Coumadin and lower the INR.

NIC Teaching: Prescribed Medication; Teaching: Prescribed Diet; Surveillance

For patients undergoing percutaneous balloon valvuloplasty

Knowledge deficit: procedure for percutaneous balloon valvuloplasty (PBV) and postprocedural assessment

Desired outcome: Within the 24-h period before PBV, patient verbalizes rationale for the procedure, the technique, and postprocedural care.

- Assess patient's understanding of aortic stenosis and the purpose of valvuloplasty. Evaluate patient's style of coping and the degree of information desired.

- As appropriate for patient's coping style, discuss with patient and significant others the valvuloplasty procedure, including:
  - ☐ Location of diseased valve, using heart drawing.
  - ☐ Use of local anesthesia and sedation during procedure.
  - ☐ Insertion site of catheter: femoral artery and vein.
  - ☐ Use of fluoroscopy during procedure. Evaluate patient for a history of sensitivity to contrast material.
  - ☐ Postprocedural observations made by nurse: BP, HR, ECG, pulses, and catheter insertion site.
  - ☐ Importance of lying flat for 6-12 h postprocedure to minimize the risk of bleeding.

NIC Teaching: Procedure/Treatment

Decreased cardiac output (or risk for same) related to altered preload and negative inotropic changes associated with valve regurgitation or hemorrhage secondary to PBV; altered rate, rhythm, or conduction associated with dysrhythmias secondary to PBV

Desired outcome: Throughout the postoperative course, patient has adequate cardiac output as evidenced by normal sinus rhythm; CO 4-7 L/min; CI ≥2.5 L/min/m^2; HR 60-100 bpm; RAP 4-6 mm Hg; PAWP 6-12 mm Hg; PAP 20-30/8-15 mm Hg; BP within patient's normal range; urinary output ≥0.5 ml/kg/h; peripheral pulses >2+ on a 0-4+ scale; orientation to time, place, and person; and absence of new murmurs, pulsus paradoxus, or jugular vein distention.

- Monitor ECG continuously after procedure. Document any changes. Consult physician for dysrhythmias, and treat according to type of dysrhythmia and hospital protocol.
- Monitor CO/CI, HR, RAP, PAWP, and PAP hourly or as prescribed. Report a fall in CO/CI, change in HR, and increase or decrease in RAP, PAWP, or PAP.
- Monitor Hct and electrolyte values. Observe for a decrease in Hct or any change in electrolyte levels (particularly potassium) that could precipitate dysrhythmias. Optimal values are: Hct >37% (female) or >40% (male); and serum potassium 3.5-5 mEq/L.
- Assess heart sounds immediately after procedure and q4h. Report the development of a new murmur.
- Monitor patient for evidence of cardiac tamponade: hypotension, tachycardia, pulsus paradoxus, jugular vein distention, elevation and plateau pressuring of PAWP and RAP, and possibly an enlarged heart silhouette on chest x-ray. For more information, see "Acute Cardiac Tamponade," p. 144.

NIC Cardiac Care; Hemodynamic Regulation

Altered protection related to risk of hemorrhage or hematoma formation secondary to heparinization with PBV

Desired outcomes: Throughout the postoperative course, patient has minimal or absent bleeding or hematoma formation at the catheter insertion site. PTT is within therapeutic anticoagulation range (per physician or agency protocol).

- Monitor catheter insertion site for evidence of bleeding. Report hematoma formation, and outline the bleeding on the dressing for subsequent comparison.
- Keep patient's catheterized leg straight for the prescribed amount of time.
- Monitor heparin drip as prescribed. Usually heparin drip is maintained until 1-2 h before the sheaths are removed.
- Monitor PTT for therapeutic range, which is usually 1½ times that of normal.
- When IV or invasive lines (arterial or venous sheaths) are removed, apply firm pressure either manually or with a mechanical clamp for 30 min.

NIC Surveillance; Bleeding Reduction: Wound

ADDITIONAL NURSING DIAGNOSES

Also see "Pulmonary Emboli" for **Knowledge deficit,** p. 239. Also see "Percutaneous Transluminal Coronary Angioplasty" in "Acute Coronary Syndromes" for **Altered peripheral tissue perfusion (or risk for same),** p. 260. See all nursing diagnoses in the discussion of "Coronary Artery Bypass Graft" in "Acute Coronary Syndrome," p. 247. Also see nursing diagnoses and interventions in "Hemodynamic Monitoring," p. 28; "Prolonged Immobility," p. 74; "Psychosocial Support," p. 83; and "Psychosocial Support for the Patient's Family and Significant Others," p. 95.

Acute infective endocarditis

PATHOPHYSIOLOGY

Infective endocarditis (IE) is infection of the endocardium (the innermost layer of the heart), which often involves the natural or prosthetic valve. It is caused by bacteria, viruses, fungi, or rickettsiae. Four mechanisms are known to contribute to the development of IE. One is a congenital or acquired defect of the heart valve or the septum (i.e., septal defect, stenotic or insufficient valve). Frequently it is accompanied by a jet-Venturi stream of blood flowing from a high- to low-pressure area through a narrow opening. The low-pressure sink beyond the narrowed jet-flow site provides an area that is ideal for colonization by any infecting organism. The second mechanism is the formation of a sterile platelet fibrin thrombus at the low-pressure site, which gives rise to vegetation. Third, a bacteremia occurs as a result of colonization in the vegetation. Finally, a high level of agglutinating antibodies promotes the growth of the vegetation.

Portals of entry for the infecting organism include the mouth and GI tract, upper airway, skin, and external genitourinary (GU) tract. Any heart valve can become infected, but the aortic and mitral valves are more common sites than the right-sided pulmonic and tricuspid valves. Once the infection process begins, valvular dysfunction, manifested by insufficiency with regurgitant blood flow, can occur, ultimately resulting in a decrease in cardiac output. The vegetation may become so large that it obstructs the valve orifice, further reducing cardiac output. At times, pieces of the vegetation may break off and embolize to vital organs. In severe cases, the affected valve may necrose, develop an aneurysm, and rupture or the infection may extend through the myocardium and epicardium to cause a pericarditis (see "Acute Pericarditis," p. 325). If the conduction system is affected by the spreading infection, bundle-branch block may occur. Most complications of IE occur suddenly, with a dramatic change in the clinical picture. Mortality rates between 20% and 50% have been reported with IE. Recurrence of the infection occurs at a rate of 10%-20%.

ASSESSMENT

History and risk factors: Invasive procedures, such as temporary pacemaker insertion, PA catheter insertion, transurethral resection, endoscopy, surgery, or dental work, place the patient with a preexisting valvular disorder at greater risk for bacteremia, which can lead to IE. Recent increases in injection drug use have led to increased incidences in IE, especially IE involving the tricuspid valve. An immunosuppressed patient (e.g., one with a transplant, carcinoma, burns, or diabetes mellitus) also is at risk for IE.

To prevent recurrence of IE or reduce the risk of initial occurrence in the individual with an abnormal heart valve, the American Heart Association recommends prophylactic antibiotics before and after some types of invasive procedures and certain forms of dental work. See Table 4-14.

Clinical presentation (acute infective stage): Fever, diaphoresis, fatigue, anorexia, joint pain, weight loss, and abdominal pain. The severity of symptoms

TABLE 4-14 Antibiotic Prophylaxis With Infective Endocarditis

Regimen for dental, oral, or upper respiratory tract procedures
Standard regimen for those at risk who can take oral medications

Amoxicillin	3 g PO 1 h before procedure*

If allergic to amoxicillin/penicillin

Erythromycin ethylsuccinate	800 mg PO 2 h before procedure* *or*
Erythromycin stearate	1 g PO 2 h before procedure* *or*
Clindamycin	300 mg PO 1 h before procedure*

Alternate regimen for those unable to take oral medications

Ampicillin	2 g IV or IM 30 min before procedure

If allergic to amoxicillin/penicillin

Clindamycin	300 mg IV 30 min before procedure* *or*
Vancomycin	1 g IV 1 h before procedure (no repeat dose needed)

Regimen for those considered at high risk but not candidates for standard regimen

Ampicillin	2 g IV or IM† *and*
Gentamicin	1.5 mg/kg (not >80 mg) IV 30 min before procedure† *and*
Amoxicillin	1.5 mg orally q6h after initial dose of other medications

Regimen for genitourinary/gastrointestinal procedures
Standard regimen

Ampicillin	2 g IM or IV† *and*
Gentamicin	1.5 mg/kg (not >80 mg) IV 30 min before procedure† *and*
Amoxicillin	1.5 g orally q6h after initial dose of other medications

If allergic to ampicillin/amoxicillin/penicillin

Vancomycin	1 g IV over 1 h before procedure† *and*
Gentamicin	1.5 mg/kg (not >80 mg) 1 h before procedure‡

Alternative low-risk patient regimen

Amoxicillin	3 g PO 1 h before procedure*

Modified from Dajani AS et al: Prevention of bacterial endocarditis: recommendations by the American Heart Association, *JAMA* 264:2919-2922, 1990.
PO, By mouth; *IV,* intravenous; *IM,* intramuscular.
*Give half of original dose q6h after initial dose.
†Optional to give same dose IV or IM q8h after initial dose.
‡May repeat once, 8 h after initial dose.

varies, depending on the infective organism. For example, *Staphylococcus aureus* will produce more severe symptoms than will *Streptococcus viridans.* **Physical assessment:** A new or changed murmur may be heard as a result of the valvular dysfunction. (See Table 4-15 for a description of the types of murmurs that can be heard, depending on the valve affected and the type of dysfunction present.) If heart failure has resulted from the valvular disorder, fine crackles may be auscultated at the bases of the lungs and an S_3 or S_4 heart sound may be heard. The skin is often pale, but if right-sided heart failure is present because of valvular insufficiency, jaundice of the skin and sclera may occur, as well as edema, neck vein distention, a positive hepatojugular reflex,

TABLE 4-15   Assessment Findings With Valvular Heart Disease

Valve dysfunction	Murmur	Pathology	Hemodynamic changes
Aortic stenosis	Systolic, blowing murmur at second ICS, RSB; may radiate to the neck	Reduced flow across aortic valve with ↑ LV volume and pressure, with diminished CO; LV hypertrophy eventually occurs	↑ LV pressure; ↑ PAEDP; ↓ CO and aortic pressure with a narrow pulse pressure reflecting the decreased stroke volume
Aortic insufficiency	Diastolic blowing murmur at second ICS, RSB, beginning immediately with S_2	Regurgitant blood flow from aorta to LV during diastole	↑ LV pressure and PAEDP; ↓ CO; ↑ systolic BP and widened pulse pressure
Mitral stenosis	Loud, long, diastolic rumbling murmur at fifth ICS, MCL; may radiate to axilla; S_1 is loud and there is an opening snap with S_2	Reduced flow across mitral valve with left atrial and pulmonary congestion	↑ Mean PAP; ↓ CO
Mitral insufficiency	Systolic murmur at fifth ICS, MCL	Regurgitant blood flow from LV to left atrium, resulting in pulmonary congestion	Giant V waves in the PA occlusive tracing; ↑ systolic PAP; ↓ CO; mean PAP may be normal

Condition	Murmur	Pathophysiology	Hemodynamic findings
Pulmonic stenosis	Systolic blowing murmur at second ICS, LSB; may radiate to neck	Reduced flow across pulmonic valve with ↑ RV volume and pressure, with diminished LV return, resulting in ↓ CO	↑ RV systolic pressure, mean RAP, PAEDP, and mean PAP
Pulmonic insufficiency	Diastolic murmur at second ICS, LSB that starts later and is lower pitched than aortic murmur	Regurgitant blood flow from pulmonary artery to RV during diastole, resulting in RV overload	↑ Systolic RV pressure with wide pulse pressure; LVEDP and CO often normal but may ↓ if disorder is severe
Tricuspid stenosis	Diastolic murmur at fourth ICS	Reduced flow across tricuspid valve with ↑ right atrial and venous congestion	CVP ↑ with accentuated A wave on the RA waveform
Tricuspid insufficiency	Pansystolic murmur at fourth ICS, LSB that increases in intensity with inspiration	Regurgitant blood flow from RV to RA; right atrial and venous congestion occurs	↑ CVP with prominent V wave on the RA tracing; normal or low PAP, LVEDP, and CO

BP, Blood pressure; *CO*, cardiac output; *CVP*, central venous pressure; *ICS*, intercostal space; *LSB*, left sternal border; *LV*, left ventricle/ventricular; *LVEDP*, left ventricular end-diastolic pressure; *MCL*, midclavicular line; *PA*, pulmonary artery; *PAP*, pulmonary artery pressure; *PAEDP*, pulmonary artery end-diastolic pressure; *RA*, right atrium; *RAP*, right atrial pressure; *RSB*, right sternal border; *RV*, right ventricle/ventricular.

and ascites. Late assessment findings include anemia, petechiae, and clubbing of the fingers.

Classic findings

Splinter hemorrhages: Small red streaks on the distal third of the fingernails or toenails.

Janeway lesions: Painless, small, hemorrhagic lesions found on the fingers, toes, nose, or earlobes, probably occurring as the result of immune complex deposition with inflammation.

Osler nodes: Painful, red, subcutaneous nodules found on the pads of the fingers or on the feet, probably occurring as a result of emboli producing small areas of gangrene or vasculitis.

Roth spots: Retinal hemorrhages with pale centers seen on funduscopic examination.

> **Note:** If emboli of the vegetations occur in other areas, signs and symptoms of stroke or peripheral, myocardial, renal, or mesenteric insufficiency or infarct will be seen.

Hemodynamic measurements: Invasive monitoring devices are used cautiously with these patients to prevent further valvular dysfunction, embolization, and infection. However, when warranted, a PA catheter may be used to assess hemodynamic function. Elevations of PAP or RAP can be expected in most patients with IE. In addition, CO is usually reduced.

DIAGNOSTIC TESTS

Blood cultures: Provide the definitive diagnosis of the infecting organism. Organism sensitivity to various antibiotics is essential in guiding therapy. The most common bacteria found in native valve IE are: *Streptococcus viridans* (50%), *Staphylococcus aureus* (20%), and the HACEK group (*Haemophilus, Actinobacillus, Cardiobacterium, Eikenella,* and *Kingella* species). Manipulations of the GI or GU tract may result in *Enterococcus faecalis* IE. Early prosthetic valve infections are often the result of *Staphylococcus epidermidis.* Candida is the most common fungal source of IE.

Echocardiography: Reveals valvular involvement and vegetation size and defines the severity of the valvular dysfunction. M-mode, two-dimensional, or Doppler echocardiograms may be used. Transesophageal echocardiograms may be more useful in detecting vegetation, especially with prosthetic valves.

ECG: Although ECG is not useful in diagnosing IE, it frequently is performed to determine if conduction system defects are present. AV node or bundle of His may be affected as the area of infection spreads. Right or left atrial or ventricular enlargement may be seen as a result of prolonged hemodynamic effects on chamber size or muscle wall thickness (Table 4-16). Atrial dysrhythmias (PAC, paroxysmal atrial tachycardia [PAT], atrial fibrillation [AF]) frequently are seen as that chamber enlarges from volume overload. Also see Figures 4-5 through 4-25.

Hematology studies: Will show an increase in the WBC count and eosinophil rate. Frequently, anemia is present.

Cardiac enzyme levels: Will be elevated if an MI occurs as a result of emboli of vegetations that migrate to the coronary arteries.

ABG values: Evaluated to determine the degree of pulmonary dysfunction as a result of the cardiac disorder.

Additional studies: May be performed to assess for embolization to other organs. Studies such as renal, mesenteric, or peripheral arteriograms or CT may be done.

COLLABORATIVE MANAGEMENT

Antibiotic treatment: Patients usually require 4-6 wk of IV antibiotics. Antibiotic selection is based on the results of the blood or tissue culture and sensitivity studies.

TABLE 4-16   ECG Changes Frequently Found With Ventricular and Atrial Hypertrophy

Chamber	ECG change
Left ventricular enlargement	"R" voltage increases in V_{4-6}; "S" voltage increases (deeper inflection) in V_{1-2}; the sum of "S" in V_1 or V_2 and "R" in V_5 or V_6 will be >35 mm, or "R" in any V lead will be >25 mm
Left atrial enlargement	"P mitrale" in leads II, III, aV_F, and V_1; P wave is m-shaped with a duration >0.1 sec
Right ventricular enlargement	"R" voltage increases in V_1, V_2; "S" voltage increases in V_5, V_6; sum of "R" in V_1 or V_2 and "S" in V_5 or V_6 will be ≥35 mm
Right atrial enlargement	"P pulmonale" in leads II, III, aV_F, and V_1; P wave is >2.5 mm voltage and <0.1 sec duration

Fluid and sodium limitations: Often required to promote optimal hemodynamics. Specific restrictions must be individualized and based on severity of symptoms and impairment of hemodynamic function.

Bed rest: Recommended initially, with activity limitations throughout the remainder of the treatment.

Diet: High in protein and calories to prevent cardiac cachexia.

Pharmacotherapy

Diuretics and vasodilators: May be required to decrease the symptoms of heart failure by decreasing preload.

Positive inotropic agents (e.g., digoxin, dobutamine, milrinone, amrinone): May be needed to increase contractility and cardiac output. For more information, see Appendix 7.

Nitroprusside, nitroglycerin: To reduce afterload.

Sedation: May be necessary to allay patient's anxiety during this long period of hospitalization.

Oxygen therapy: Administered as needed at an Fio_2 rate that maintains Pao_2 >60 mm Hg and oxygen saturation at >95%. Pulse oximetry is used continuously or intermittently to verify satisfactory oxygen saturation.

Treatment of other signs and symptoms: If heart failure has resulted from the valvular disorder, see "Heart Failure," p. 265, for treatment of those signs and symptoms. See "Cardiogenic Shock," p. 343, for the medical treatment that may be necessary if the valvular dysfunction deteriorates to the point that it is life threatening.

Prophylaxis regimen: Provides prophylactic antibiotics for those individuals at risk who undergo dental, oral, upper respiratory tract, genitourinary, or gastrointestinal procedures. See Table 4-14, p. 317.

Surgical valve replacement: Required when hemodynamic function deteriorates or if the infection does not respond to antibiotic therapy. See "Valvular Heart Disease," p. 309. An abscess or infected tissue may be surgically removed if there is no response to long-term antibiotics. If the patient is hemodynamically stable, the role of surgery is less clear. A surgeon is usually consulted in case emergency surgery is needed because of signs of heart failure.

Research Brief 4-2 According to recent guidelines published by the American Heart Association, persons with no prior history of cardiac disease who also have a murmur of mitral valve prolapse may not need antibiotic prophylaxis. An echocardiogram should be obtained. If the mitral valve is myxomatous, prophylaxis should be used. If the valve does not demonstrate this abnormality, prophylaxis is not necessarily needed because the risk of developing IE is no greater than what occurs generally in the population of persons without heart disease and without a murmur.

From Dajani ADD et al: Prevention of bacterial endocarditis: recommendations by the American Heart Association, *Circulation* 96:358-366, 1997.

NURSING DIAGNOSES AND INTERVENTIONS

Decreased cardiac output related to altered preload, afterload, or contractility secondary to valvular dysfunction

Desired outcomes: Within 72 h after initiation of therapy, patient has adequate hemodynamic function with controlled atrial fibrillation as evidenced by normal sinus rhythm; HR $\leq$100 bpm; BP $\geq$90/60 mm Hg; stable weight; intake equal to output plus insensible losses; RR $\leq$20 breaths/min with normal depth and pattern (eupnea); and absence of S_3 or S_4 heart sounds, crackles, distended neck veins, and other clinical signs of heart failure. Optimally, the following normal parameters will be achieved: CO 4-7 L/min; CVP 2-6 mm Hg; PAP 20-30/8-15 mm Hg; RAP 4-6 mm Hg; and MAP 60-105 mm Hg.

- Assess heart sounds q2-4h. A change in the characteristics of a heart murmur may signal progression of valvular dysfunction, which can occur with insufficiency, stenosis, dislodgment of vegetation, or unseating of a prosthetic valve.
- Assess for the presence of an extra heart sound. A new S_3 or S_4 sound may signal heart failure.
- Monitor heart rhythm continuously. Report dysrhythmias or conduction defects, which may indicate the spread of infection to the conduction system or atrial volume overload.
- Monitor for signs of left-sided heart failure secondary to valvular dysfunction: crackles; S_3 or S_4 sounds; dyspnea; tachypnea; digital clubbing; decreased BP; increased pulse pressure; increased LVEDP; and decreased CO.
- Monitor for signs of right-sided heart failure secondary to valvular dysfunction: increased CVP; distended neck veins; positive hepatojugular reflex; edema; jaundice; and ascites.
- Monitor I&O hourly, and measure weight daily. To help prevent miscalculations of patient's weight, use the same scale and amount of clothing and weigh patient at the same time of day. Consult physician if patient's weight increases by more than 1 kg (2.2 lb) per day.
- If patient's PAP or RAP is high, decrease preload by limiting fluid and sodium intake and administering diuretics and venous dilators as prescribed.
- If patient's MAP is high, decrease afterload with prescribed arterial dilators.
- If afterload is low, increase afterload with vasopressors, as prescribed.

Note: See "Cardiogenic Shock," p. 343, for a discussion of preload and afterload medications.

- If afterload is low, prevent further reductions caused by vasodilation (e.g., by avoiding administration of morphine sulfate or rapid warming of the hypothermic patient). Increase contractility with positive inotropes, as prescribed.
- Limit patient's activities to reduce myocardial oxygen needs; schedule patient care activities to patient's tolerance.

- Help patient reduce stress by teaching stress-reduction techniques, such as imagery, meditation, or progressive muscle relaxation. For description of a relaxation technique, see **Health-seeking behavior,** p. 302.
- Provide sedation as needed.
- Prevent orthostatic hypotension by changing patient's position slowly.

NIC Energy Management; Cardiac Care

Impaired gas exchange related to alveolar-capillary membrane changes with decreased diffusion of oxygen secondary to pulmonary congestion

Desired outcome: Within 24 h of initiation of oxygen therapy and during the weaning process, patient has adequate gas exchange as evidenced by RR ≤20 breaths/min with normal pattern and depth (eupnea); Svo_2 60%-80%; Pao_2 ≥80 mm Hg; Sao_2 ≥95%; and natural skin color.

- Assess rate, effort, and depth of patient's respirations. Tachypnea may indicate pulmonary congestion, inasmuch as the RR increases to compensate for the decreased depth caused by pulmonary congestion or airway obstruction.
- Assess color of skin and mucous membranes, being alert to pallor as a signal of impaired oxygenation.
- Auscultate lungs q2h. Report presence of crackles, rhonchi, and wheezing.
- If hemodynamic monitoring with oximetry is used, assess Svo_2. Svo_2 will fall below normal levels if oxygen uptake is increased as a result of increased metabolic demands or if extraction is increased as a result of reduced oxygen delivery. This change occurs before symptoms change, and it correlates with cardiac output.
- Monitor ABG values for evidence of hypoxemia (Pao_2 <80 mm Hg), respiratory acidosis ($Paco_2$ >45 mm Hg, pH <7.35), or respiratory alkalosis ($Paco_2$ <35 mm Hg, pH >7.45), which may be present with pulmonary congestion.
- Deliver humidified oxygen as prescribed.
- Assess arterial oxygen saturation with a transcutaneous pulse oximeter. Normal oxygen saturation is 95%-99%. Levels of 90%-95% necessitate frequent assessment. Levels <90% require aggressive interventions to increase oxygen saturation. This is accomplished by increasing Fio_2, decreasing preload, and taking measures to improve ventilation.
- Unless contraindicated, place patient in high Fowler's position to facilitate gas exchange.
- Schedule coughing, deep breathing, and incentive spirometry q2-4h to prevent atelectasis.

NIC Invasive Hemodynamic Monitoring; Oxygen Therapy; Respiratory Monitoring

Risk for infection related to presence of invasive catheters and lines; inadequate secondary defenses secondary to prolonged antibiotic use

Desired outcomes: Patient is free of secondary infection as evidenced by urine that is clear with characteristic odor; wound healing within acceptable time frame; and absence of erythema, warmth, and purulent drainage at insertion sites for IV lines. On resolution of acute stage of IE, patient remains normothermic with WBC count ≤11,000/mm³; negative culture results; and HR ≤100 bpm. SVR is ≥900 dynes/sec/cm⁻⁵; CO is ≤7 L/min; and Svo_2 is 60%-80%. Patient and significant others verbalize rationale for antibiotic therapy and identify where and how to obtain guidelines.

- Ensure strict aseptic technique for insertion site care for all invasive monitoring devices and IV lines. Rotate central line catheter insertion sites at frequent/agency-recommended intervals. Check with physician regarding feasibility of tunneled catheter for patients with long-term antimicrobial therapy.
- Change tubing, containers, and peripheral insertion sites q48-72h, per agency protocol. Inspect all catheter insertion sites daily for redness, drainage, or other evidence of infection. Rotate site immediately if infection is suspected.

> **Research Brief 4-3** Embolization of fragments of valvular vegetation has been reported to occur in 22%-50% of the cases of IE. Emboli can lodge in major arterial beds such as the brain, lungs, coronary arteries, spleen, bowel, or extremities. The use of transesophageal and transthoracic echocardiography may be useful in predicting embolic events.

From DeCastro S et al: Role of transthoracic and transesophageal echocardiography in predicting embolic events in patients with active infective endocarditis involving native cardiac valves, *Am J Cardiol* 80:1030-1034, 1997.

- Provide mouth care q4h to minimize the potential for fungal and other infections.
- For patients with indwelling urinary catheters, cleanse urinary meatus with soap and water during the daily bath. Inspect urine for evidence of infection, such as casts, cloudiness, or foul odor. Be alert to patient complaints of burning with urination after catheter is removed.
- Monitor temperature, WBC count, and HR. Increases may be signs of infection.
- Calculate SVR whenever CO measurements are obtained. Septic shock is demonstrated by an increase in CO, a drop in SVR, and increased Svo_2 during the early stages.
- Teach patient and significant others the importance of reporting signs and symptoms of recurring infections (e.g., fever, malaise, flushing, anorexia) or heart failure (e.g., dyspnea, tachypnea, tachycardia, weight gain, peripheral edema).
- Stress the importance of prophylactic antibiotics before invasive procedures such as dental examinations or surgery. The American Heart Association publishes general guidelines for prophylactic antibiotic treatment for preventing IE (see Table 4-9).

NIC Fever Treatment; Surveillance; Infection Control

Altered tissue perfusion (or risk for same): renal, gastrointestinal, peripheral, cardiopulmonary, and cerebral, related to interrupted arterial blood flow secondary to emboli caused by vegetations

Desired outcome: Patient has adequate perfusion as evidenced by urine output ≥0.5 ml/kg/h; 5-34 bowel sounds/min; peripheral pulses >2+ on a 0-4+ scale; warm and dry skin; BP ≥90/60 mm Hg; RR 12-20 breaths/min with normal pattern and depth (eupnea); normal sinus rhythm on ECG; and orientation to time, place, and person.

> **Note:** Unlike peripheral venous emboli, these emboli are caused by the vegetations; therefore prevention is difficult. Interventions are aimed at early detection of embolization and supportive therapies.

- Monitor I&O at frequent intervals. Be alert to urinary output <0.5 ml/kg/h for 2 consecutive hours. Report oliguria, because it may be a sign of renal infarct.
- Monitor bowel sounds q2h. Report hypoactive or absent bowel sounds, because they may be the result of mesenteric infarct.
- Assess peripheral pulses, color, and temperature of extremities. Be alert to pulses ≤2+ (on a 0-4+ scale) and extremities that are pale and cool, inasmuch as these findings may denote embolization to the extremities.
- Monitor patient for confusion, changes in sensorimotor capabilities, or changes in cognition. Alterations can occur with cerebral emboli.
- Assess for chest pain, decreased BP, SOB, ischemic or injury pattern on 12-lead ECG, or elevated cardiac enzyme levels. These may be signs of MI caused by emboli of vegetations that have migrated to the coronary arteries (see "Acute Coronary Syndromes," p. 247).

TABLE 4-17	Conditions Associated With the Development of Pericarditis
Autoimmune cardiac injury	Neoplasms
• Dressler syndrome (post-MI)	Radiation injury
• Postpericardiotomy syndrome	Rheumatologic disease
Drug induced	• Rheumatic fever
• Procainamide, hydralazine	• Rheumatoid arthritis
Idiopathic	• Systemic lupus erythematosus
Infection	Trauma
Myocardial infarction	Uremia

MI, Myocardial infarction.

- Assess for and report appearance of splinter hemorrhages, Osler nodes, Janeway lesions, and Roth spots (see "Assessment," p. 316).

NIC Circulatory Care; Cardiac Care: Acute

ADDITIONAL NURSING DIAGNOSES

As appropriate, also see nursing diagnoses and interventions in "Nutritional Support," p. 1; "Hemodynamic Monitoring," p. 28; "Prolonged Immobility," p. 74; "Psychosocial Support," p. 83; "Psychosocial Support for the Patient's Family and Significant Others," p. 95; "Heart Failure," p. 265; and "Cardiogenic Shock," p. 343.

Acute pericarditis

PATHOPHYSIOLOGY

Pericarditis is the general term for an inflammatory process involving the epicardial surface of the heart and the protective covering, the pericardium. The inflammatory process can occur as the result of a myocardial infarction, an infection, chronic renal failure, or an immunologic, chemical, or mechanical event. Often early pericarditis manifests as a dry irritation, whereas late pericarditis (after 6 wk) involves pericardial effusions that can lead to cardiac tamponade if severe. Most often, pericarditis is seen in the ICU as a secondary finding in the critically ill patient. Because symptoms can be masked by the primary condition, astute assessment and recognition are essential for appropriate treatment. Occasionally patients are admitted to the ICU with cardiac decompensation caused by the effusions.

The initial pathophysiologic findings of pericarditis include infiltration of polymorphonuclear leukocytes, increased vascularity, and fibrin deposit. The inflammation may spread from the pericardium to the epicardium or pleura. Eventually, the visceral layer develops exudates, and in some cases adhesions may develop. (See Table 4-17 for conditions that are associated with the development of pericarditis.) Large effusions can lead to cardiac tamponade (see p. 144). The excess fluid compresses the heart and impairs filling of the chambers. In addition, ejection of the left ventricle is impaired.

ASSESSMENT

Clinical presentation: The chief complaint is chest pain, but location and quality can vary. Usually the pain is aggravated by a supine position, coughing, deep inspiration, and swallowing. Dyspnea develops because of shallow breathing to prevent pain.

Early indicators: Fatigue, pallor, fever, and anorexia.

TABLE 4-18   ECG Changes With Pericarditis

Stage	Time of change	Pattern
1	Onset of pain	ST segments have a concave elevation in all leads except aV_L and V_1; T waves are upright
2	1-7 days	Return of ST segments to baseline with T-wave flattening
3	1-2 wk	Inversion of T waves without R or Q changes
4	Weeks to months	Normalization of T waves

Research Brief 4-4   The 12-lead ECG plays an important role in making the diagnosis of pericarditis. Accurate lead placement is essential to make the appropriate differential diagnosis when a patient presents with chest pain caused by coronary artery disease or pericarditis. A study was conducted to assess the written knowledge, simulated clinical practice, and actual clinical practice of 44 telemetry and ICU nurses regarding the placement of ECG leads. Few nurses were able to place the leads correctly in any of the three methods of testing (18%, 25%, and 9%, respectively). There were no significant differences between telemetry and ICU nurses. This study supports the need for routine training and competency testing of 12-lead ECG lead placement for nurses who are required to perform this test.

From Bupp JE: Placement of cardiac electrodes: written, simulated, and actual accuracy, *Am J Crit Care* 6:457-462, 1997.

Late indicators (evident after development of effusions):   Increased dyspnea, crackles, and neck vein distention. Heart sounds will be distant, and the pulmonic component of the second heart sound will be accentuated. Joint pain may be present when inflammation is generalized.

Physical assessment: Auscultation of heart sounds often will reveal an intermittent friction rub composed of one, two, or three components: atrial systole, ventricular systole, and rapid ventricular filling. The rub is heard best with the patient sitting and leaning forward and the diaphragm of the stethoscope positioned at the left lower sternal border.

Note: A friction rub may not be heard, even in the presence of pericarditis.

Pulsus paradoxus: BP should be checked for a paradox >10 mm Hg pressure. Normally the systolic pressure is slightly higher during the inspiratory portion of the respiratory cycle. When effusions are present, arterial systolic BP will be decreased during inspiration and the difference will be >10 mm Hg. For procedure, see "Acute Cardiac Tamponade," p. 144.

ECG findings: During acute episodes, atrial dysrhythmias such as PAT, PACs, atrial flutter, or atrial fibrillation may occur. Late dysrhythmias include ventricular ectopy or bundle-branch blocks if the inflammatory process involves the ventricles. Pericardial effusion may decrease the voltage of the QRS complex on the ECG. Diffuse ST-segment elevation can be documented as described in Table 4-18.

Hemodynamic measurements: If a PA catheter is in place, it will reveal elevated CVP, PAP, and PAWP. As effusions increase, cardiac output will decrease. If adhesions are present, the filling of the chambers may be restricted, resulting in low volumes and pressures.

DIAGNOSTIC TESTS

ECG: Will show ST or T-wave changes, which often are confused with ischemic changes. In pericarditis they are more diffuse and follow a four-stage pattern (see Table 4-18).

Echocardiography: Will show absence of echoes in the areas of effusion. This test, which is essential for quantifying and evaluating the trend of effusions, will appear normal if the pericarditis is present without effusions. TEE may be helpful in identifying some areas of effusion.

Computed tomography (CT):   Will differentiate restrictive pericarditis from constrictive cardiomyopathy via the appearance of thickened pericardium on the cross-sectional views of the thorax, which occurs with pericarditis.

Cardiac enzyme levels: May reveal elevation of the CK and MB bands if the epicardium is inflamed.

Cardiac technetium pyrophosphate scan: May show a diffuse regional uptake ("hot spot") in an area of epicardial inflammation.

Hematologic studies: Antistreptolysin O (ASO) titer is elevated when the cause of the pericarditis is an immunologic disorder. If the pericarditis is the result of an infection, blood cultures will identify the infecting organism.

COLLABORATIVE MANAGEMENT

Bed rest: Until pain and fever have disappeared. Activity limitations continue if effusions are present.

Pharmacotherapy

Nonsteroidal antiinflammatory drugs (NSAIDs):   Preferred for reducing inflammation, particularly if the patient has had MI or cardiac surgery, inasmuch as these medications do not delay healing as do corticosteroids. In addition, these medications have fewer side effects than do steroids. Examples include aspirin, indomethacin, and ibuprofen.

Prednisone: Given if there is no response to NSAIDs. It is begun at 60-80 mg qd for 5-7 days and then tapered gradually.

> **Note:** In the presence of effusions, anticoagulants are contraindicated because of the high risk of cardiac tamponade, which can result from bleeding into the pericardium.

Subxiphoid pericardiocentesis: Performed if effusions persist and cardiac status begins to decompensate. It removes fluid that is compressing the heart. Echocardiography is used to guide the catheter tip and assess the amount of effusion remaining. The pericardial catheter may be removed after the fluid has been withdrawn or may be left in place for several days to allow for gradual removal of fluid. Usually ≥100 ml is withdrawn q4-6h. The catheter is flushed with saline q4-6h after withdrawal of the effusion to prevent clotting. Strict aseptic technique is essential for preventing infection.

Pericardiectomy: To prevent cardiac compression or relieve the restriction. It may be necessary in chronic pericarditis for patients with recurrent effusions or adhesions.

NURSING DIAGNOSES AND INTERVENTIONS

Ineffective breathing pattern related to guarding as a result of chest pain
Desired outcome: Within 48 h of this diagnosis, patient demonstrates RR 12-20 breaths/min with normal depth and pattern (eupnea) and verbalizes that chest pain is controlled.

- Assess the character and intensity of the chest pain. Provide prescribed pain medication as needed.
- Teach patient to avoid aggravating factors such as a supine position. Encourage patient to alter his or her position to minimize the chest pain. The following positions may be helpful: side-lying, high Fowler's, or sitting and leaning forward.
- Assess lung sounds q4h. If breath sounds are decreased, encourage patient to perform incentive spirometry exercises q2-4h along with coughing and deep-breathing exercises.
- To facilitate coughing and deep breathing, support patient's chest by splinting with pillows, or teach patient to press his or her arms against the chest for added support.

NIC Positioning; Pain Management

Activity intolerance related to bed rest, weakness, and fatigue secondary to impaired cardiac function, ineffective breathing pattern, or deconditioning

Desired outcome: Within 72 h of this diagnosis, patient exhibits cardiac tolerance to increasing levels of exercise as evidenced by peak HR ≤20 bpm over patient's resting HR; peak systolic BP ≤20 mm Hg over patient's resting systolic BP; Svo_2 ≥60%; RR <24 breaths/min; normal sinus rhythm; warm and dry skin; and absence of crackles, murmurs, and chest pain during or immediately after activity.

> **Note:** Steroid myopathy may develop in patients who receive high doses or long-term treatment with steroids. Muscle weakness occurs predominantly in the large proximal muscles. Patients experience difficulty in lifting objects and moving from a sitting position to a standing position.

- Assess the patient for evidence of muscle weakness; assist with activities as needed.
- Modify the activity plan for the patient with post-MI pericarditis who is receiving steroids. A lower activity level may help prevent thinning of the ventricular wall and reduce the risk of an aneurysm or rupture of the ventricle.
- Teach patient to resume activities gradually, as prescribed, allowing for adequate periods of rest between activities.
- For other interventions, see this nursing diagnosis in "Prolonged Immobility," p. 74.

NIC Energy Management; Cardiac Care: Rehabilitative; Teaching: Prescribed Activity/Exercise

ADDITIONAL NURSING DIAGNOSES

Also see "Acute Cardiac Tamponade" for **Decreased cardiac output,** p. 146. See "Renal Transplantation" for **Knowledge deficit: immunosuppressive medications and their side effects,** p. 392; **Impaired skin integrity,** p. 394; and **Risk for infection,** p. 393. For other nursing diagnoses and interventions, see "Prolonged Immobility," p. 74.

Hypertensive emergencies

PATHOPHYSIOLOGY

Hypertension is sustained elevation of the resting arterial pressure. In 1998 the American Heart Association (AHA) estimated that more than 63 million Americans have hypertension defined as elevation of BP above 140/90 mm Hg. Because fatal stroke or other cardiac event can occur as a result of hypertension, the impact of this disease on mortality is greater than that of any other health problem. Table 4-19 describes the blood pressure classifications and the recommendations for follow-up.

TABLE 4-19 Classification of Blood Pressure for Adults Age 18 and Older*; Recommendations for Follow-up

Category	Systolic pressure (mm Hg)		Diastolic pressure (mm Hg)	Follow-up
Optimal†	<120	and	<80	
Normal	<130	and	<85	Recheck in 2 yr
High-normal	130-139	or	85-89	Recheck in 1 yr‡
Hypertension§				
Stage I	140-159	or	90-99	Confirm within 2 mo
Stage II	160-179	or	100-109	Evaluate or refer to source of care within 1 mo
Stage III	≥180		≥110	Evaluate or refer to source of care within 1 wk or immediately

Modified from National Institutes of Health: the Sixth Report of the Joint National Committee on Prevention, Detection, Evaluation, and Treatment of High Blood Pressure (JNCVI). NIH Pub. No. 98-4080. November, 1997.

*Not taking hypertensive drugs and not actually ill.

†Optimal blood pressure with respect to cardiovascular risk is below 120/80 mm Hg. However, unusually low readings should be evaluated for clinical significance.

‡Begin instructions on life-style modification, including:

1. Lose weight if overweight.
2. Limit alcohol intake <1 oz ethanol/day (24 oz beer, 8 oz wine, or 2 oz whiskey).
3. Reduce sodium intake to <100 mmol/day (2.3 g sodium or 6 g sodium chloride).
4. Maintain adequate dietary potassium, calcium, and magnesium intake.
5. Stop smoking.
6. Reduce dietary saturated fat and cholesterol intake for general cardiovascular health.

§Based on the average of two or more readings taken at each of two or more visits after an initial screening.

Most often, hypertension occurs as a primary disorder of unknown etiology. Secondary hypertension is the result of other disorders that alter the mechanisms that control BP. Many factors contribute to the development of secondary hypertension: (1) increase in secretion of catecholamines; (2) increase in secretion of renin by the kidneys; (3) increase in serum sodium and blood volume; (4) increase in plasma and extracellular fluid volume; (5) reduction in kidney perfusion pressure; (6) impairment of control mechanisms in the kidney; and (7) alteration in adrenal cortical hormone secretion. Table 4-20 lists the causes of secondary hypertension.

Hypertensive crisis is seen in about 1% of the population with hypertension. When it occurs, immediate vascular necrosis is a threat, which can occur if the diastolic pressure exceeds 120 mm Hg, although necrosis also has been seen with mean arterial pressures (MAP) ≥150 mm Hg.

The rapidity of the rise in pressure may be more destructive than the actual BP level recorded. If left untreated, hypertensive crisis is fatal in 75% of affected persons within 1 yr. With current treatment techniques, 1-year mortality is 30% and 5-yr mortality is 50%. Hypertensive crisis can lead to hypertensive encephalopathy as cerebral blood vessels dilate because of their inability to effect autoregulation. Blood flow is increased, and the excessive pressure drives fluid into the perivascular tissue, resulting in cerebral edema. The extreme pressure can cause arteriolar damage, as demonstrated by fibrinoid necrosis of the intima and media of the vessel wall. Although any organ is

TABLE 4-20   Causes of Secondary Hypertension

Renal disease	Endocrine disorders	Congenital disorders	Pregnancy-induced disorders	Drug-induced disorders
Acute glomerulonephritis	Cushing syndrome	Adrenal hyperplasia	Pregnancy-induced hypertension (PIH)	Cyclosporine
Chronic pyelonephritis	Hyperparathyroidism	Coarctation of the aorta	Preeclampsia	Oral contraceptives
Hydronephrosis	Pheochromocytoma		Eclampsia	Steroids
Renal tumors	Primary aldosteronism			
Renovascular hypertension				

vulnerable, the eyes and kidneys are most likely to suffer damage, leading to blindness and renal failure.

Patients with hypertension who are admitted to the ICU may have a rebound elevation of the BP if their usual antihypertensive regimen is interrupted. In addition, a loss of BP control can occur because of the nature of the primary disorder, trauma, or the stress of the ICU. Complications of hypertension include nephrosclerosis, aortic dissection, coronary artery disease, heart failure, stroke, and peripheral vascular disease.

Pheochromocytoma is a chromaffin-cell tumor of the adrenal medulla that causes secretion of high levels of catecholamines (epinephrine and norepinephrine). The surge of catecholamines causes episodic elevations of blood pressure, increased metabolism, and hyperglycemia. These surges can occur as often as 25 times a day or as infrequently as every 2 mo. Although pheochromocytoma accounts for only 0.5% of all new cases of hypertension, it is found in a much larger proportion of individuals who experience hypertensive crisis. The tumor is most often benign (90% of cases).

ASSESSMENT

History and risk factors: Psychologic stress, diet high in sodium, and cigarette smoking increase the risk of developing high BP. Hypertension is a familial disease; genetic and environmental factors contribute to its etiology. Hypertension is a risk factor for angina and MI. See "Acute Coronary Syndromes," p. 247.

Clinical presentation

Early indicators: Although most patients are free of symptoms, vague discomfort, fatigue, dizziness, and headache can occur.

Late indicators (nearly always present during a hypertensive crisis): Throbbing suboccipital headache, irritability, confusion, somnolence, stupor, visual loss, focal deficits, and coma. The patient also may have signs of heart failure, including dyspnea on exertion, orthopnea, and paroxysmal nocturnal dyspnea. If coronary artery disease is present, angina may occur as a result of increased myocardial oxygen consumption caused by the high vascular resistance, which is evidenced by high BP. Renal symptoms include hematuria, nocturia, and azotemia. Nausea and vomiting also may occur.

Physical assessment: An accurate cuff pressure must be obtained after 5 min of rest, with two or more measurements taken at least 2 min apart. Average these readings unless there is a 5 mm Hg or greater difference. Greater differences warrant additional readings . A well-calibrated manometer with a properly fitting cuff or an automatic blood pressure recorder should be selected for use. The bladder of the cuff must encircle 80% of the arm and cover two thirds of the length of the upper portion of the arm. Note when the patient last smoked or used any nicotine product, how much caffeine was consumed during the previous 4 h, and whether adrenergic stimulants (e.g., over-the-counter [OTC] decongestants or bronchodilators) have been used within the past 24 h, because these substances elevate BP.

Cardiac assessment: Evaluates for left ventricular hypertrophy, which results from the need of the heart to pump against the high SVR or afterload. A left ventricular heave may be palpated with the palm of the hand at the mitral area (5th ICS at the MCL). A fourth heart sound or S_4 gallop may be auscultated in the same site with the stethoscope bell. If cardiac failure is present or the left ventricle is enlarged, the apical impulse will be felt nearer to the anterior axillary line (AAL) instead of the MCL. In addition, crackles may be auscultated in the presence of cardiac failure. Pulsus alternans, an alteration in pulse pressure with a regular rhythm, may be palpated at any of the major pulse points. All peripheral pulses should be palpated bilaterally. With coarctation of the aorta, the femoral pulses will be bilaterally weak with a slow up-stroke, whereas the radial and brachial pulses will be normal or bounding.

Eye assessment: A funduscope is used to determine whether hemorrhage, fluffy cotton exudates, or arterial-venous nicking of the vessels has occurred. When these changes occur, visual perception is decreased. Nurses should assess the patient's ability to read and recognize objects and people.

Neurologic assessment: May reveal evidence of a residual neurologic deficit from a cerebral infarct or ischemic event, as manifested by a positive Babinski reflex (up-going toe), hemiparesis, hemiplegia, ataxia, confusion, or cognitive alterations.

Pheochromocytoma assessment: Paroxysmal elevations of BP associated with palpitations, tachycardia, headache, diaphoresis, pallor, warmth or flushing, tremor, excitation, fright, nervousness, feelings of impending doom, tachypnea, abdominal pain, nausea, and vomiting. Episodes also are associated with hyperglycemia and hypermetabolism. Postural hypotension and paradoxic response to antihypertensive medications may occur.

DIAGNOSTIC TESTS

The definitive test for hypertension is BP measurement. Once hypertension has been documented, many tests may be performed to determine the amount of end-organ damage or to diagnose the condition responsible for the development of secondary hypertension.

ECG: Left ventricular hypertrophy (LVH) is demonstrated by an increase in voltage in the LV precordial lead (V_{5-6}). In addition, a strain pattern of ST-segment depression and T-wave inversion reflects repolarization abnormalities caused by the endocardial fibrosis that accompanies hypertrophy. General voltage criteria for LVH are (1) "R" in V_5 or V_6 plus "S" in V_1 >35 mm or (2) voltage of "R" in any precordial lead >25 mm.

Echocardiography: LVH with or without dilation will be demonstrated on echo by an increase in the wall thickness with or without increased chamber size.

Chest x-ray: If dilation of the left ventricle is present, the cardiac silhouette will be enlarged. If failure is present, there will be evidence of pulmonary congestion and pleural effusions. Notching of the aorta and a distended aortic root are indicative of coarctation of the aorta. If widening of the aorta is seen, dissection is suspected (see p. 341).

Urinalysis/urine culture: Urinalysis results will be normal until hypertension causes renal impairment. Specific gravity may be low (<1.010), and proteinuria may be present. Glomerulonephritis is suspected if the urine contains granular or red cell casts or if the patient has hematuria. Pyelonephritis is suspected if there is bacterial growth in the urine. Elevations of the 24-h urine vanillylmandelic acid (VMA) and urinary catecholamines (10-50 times normal) are indicative of pheochromocytoma. The VMA level is elevated only during episodes of hypertension. If the patient has Cushing disease, the urine cortisol or ACTH level will be elevated.

Blood studies: If renal parenchymal disease is present, the patient may have serum creatinine >1.3 mg/dl and BUN >20 mg/dl. The RBC count may fall because of hematuria caused by renal parenchymal disease.

Radiographic studies to detect pheochromocytoma: Angiography may identify an adrenal medullary tumor. An intravenous pyelogram (IVP) with nephrotomography or CT may identify the adrenal tumor.

COLLABORATIVE MANAGEMENT

Treatment of hypertensive crisis: Necessitates immediate and rapid reduction in pressure. Goal is to lower MAP no more than 25% within 2 h and then reach 160/100 within 2-6 h.

Nitroprusside: Frequently used because of its rapid vasodilation effects. Usual initial dose is 10-25 µg/min, with increases of 5-10 µg q5min. Until oral treatment is effective, the maintenance dose for nitroprusside ranges from

0.25-10 µg/kg/min. This drug has a short action time, and BP will rise almost immediately if the drip is stopped. Direct arterial pressure monitoring is essential for the titration of this drug, with constant vigilance to prevent hypotension. When oral antihypertensives begin to affect the BP, nitroprusside weaning requires care to prevent hypotensive episodes. Nitroprusside is metabolized to thiocyanate, which can cause fatigue, nausea, tinnitus, blurred vision, and delirium. Serum thiocyanate levels should be drawn after 48 h of use and regularly thereafter. Levels <10 mg/dl are considered safe.

Labetalol hydrochloride: A fast-acting alpha- (α-) and β-blocker, which also can be used to treat the patient in hypertensive crisis. It is less likely to cause hypotension than is diazoxide. It is administered by IV push slowly, beginning with a 20- to 80-mg dose. This can be repeated q10min, or a continuous infusion of 2 mg/min can be administered. The usual cumulative dose is 50-200 mg. Keep the patient supine during the injection and for as long as 1 h afterward. Maintain BP checks q5min × 6 and then q30min × 4. Monitor for bronchospasm, heart block, or orthostatic hypotension.

Esmolol: A fast-acting β-blocker with an onset of action of 1-2 min and duration of 10-20 min. Initial dose is 250-500 µg/kg/min for 1 min; then 50-100 µg/kg/min for 4 min. May repeat the sequence but watch for hypotension and nausea and vomiting. May cause bronchospasms so avoid in persons with asthma.

Nicardipine: A potent calcium channel blocker that is given 5-15 mg/h. Onset of action is 5-10 min, and duration is 1-4 h. May cause tachycardia, headache, and flushing.

Enalaprilat: An ACE inhibitor. Usual dose is 1.25-5 mg IV bolus, administered over a 5-min period. Thereafter, the initial dose may be repeated q6h. Patients on diuretics should receive the lower standard dose. Peak effect from the first IV dose will be observed at 4 h, but for subsequent doses, the peak effect occurs 1 h after administration. Enalaprilat should be used with caution in individuals with renal failure or bilateral renal artery stenosis due to high renin states. Avoid in acute MI.

Hydralazine: A potent vasodilator. It is administered as a 10- to 20-mg IV bolus or a 10- to 40-mg IM injection. The onset of action is 10-30 min, with a duration of 2-6 h. Adverse effects include tachycardia, headache, vomiting, and aggravation of angina.

Nitroglycerin: A coronary and peripheral vasodilator. It is supplied in a 50-mg vial, which is added to a 250-ml glass bottle of D_5W. The solution may be concentrated to prevent fluid overload if higher doses are needed to control the BP. Nitroglycerin is administered via an infusion controller starting at 5 µg/min. Onset of action is rapid, so BP must be monitored closely during titration of the drug. Increase by 5-10 µg q3-5 min. Headache is the most common side effect and requires analgesic administration.

Phentolamine: An α-adrenergic blocking agent. Although this drug reduces afterload, it has minimal effect in reducing BP except for secondary hypertension caused by pheochromocytoma. A dose of 5-15 mg is administered via IV push. Onset of action is 1-2 min. Use this drug with caution in individuals with coronary artery disease.

Nifedipine

Caution: Nifedipine has been given sublingually by piercing the capsule to provide rapid treatment for hypertension. This is no longer recommended because the effects are variable and several serious side effects have been reported. Do not use this as treatment for hypertensive emergency.

Oral antihypertensive medications: These drugs are added as soon as the patient is able to take oral medications. Examples include captopril, clonidine, and labetalol.

Research Brief 4-5 Although salt intake and hypertension have been repeatedly linked in many studies, the nature of the relationship is relatively weak. It is hypothesized that a stronger link exists between sodium and the degree of target organ disease. In a meta-analysis of nine studies of 24-h urinary sodium excretion and left ventricular hypertrophy, a stronger link was found. These findings support the need to teach patients with hypertension ways to reduce dietary sodium intake.

From Messerli FH, Schmieder RE, Weir MR: Salt: a perpetrator of hypertensive target organ disease? *Arch Intern Med* 157:2449-2452, 1997.

Life-style alterations: Behavioral changes are the cornerstones of medical treatment for early and established hypertension. Normal body weight should be maintained. Alcohol consumption should be <1 oz ethanol a day. Daily intake of sodium for the average adult should be modified to 2 to 3 g for the person with hypertension. Smoking cessation is imperative (1) to halt the injury to the intima of the coronary and peripheral vessels and (2) to reduce the workload of the heart. A regular aerobic program has been proved beneficial in maintaining better control of blood pressure. This should consist of 30 min of exercise 3-5 times per week at a target heart rate of 60%-80% maximum. Maintenance of adequate potassium, calcium, and magnesium intake is important.

Pharmacotherapy: Maintenance pharmacotherapy for hypertension is now approached by individually evaluating the best treatment option based on the patient's other disease states or demographic factors. This approach has been accepted and promoted by the Joint National Committee VI (JNC VI) and American Heart Association. After an adequate trial of the first drug, a second drug from a different category may be tried. Figure 4-28 identifies the algorithm, and Table 4-21 lists the medications, usual dosage, schedule, and potential side effects of the antihypertensive agents commonly used.

Surgical treatment: Although there is no surgical intervention for primary hypertension, several forms of secondary hypertension respond well to the surgical correction of the primary problem. A coarctation of the aorta can be repaired via removal of the narrowed area of the vessel with insertion of a Teflon aortic graft. Renal artery stenosis may be corrected by grafting or by renal artery angioplasty. For patients with pheochromocytoma, surgical removal of the tumor(s) will return the patient to a normotensive state.

NURSING DIAGNOSES AND INTERVENTIONS

Altered tissue perfusion: cardiopulmonary, cerebral, and renal, related to interruption of arterial flow secondary to vasoconstriction that occurs with interruption of the normal BP control mechanism; interruption of venous flow secondary to vasodilation or tissue edema that occurs with loss of autoregulation

Desired outcomes: Tissue perfusion is established within 24 h as evidenced by systemic arterial BP 110-160/70-110 mm Hg (or within patient's normal range); MAP 70-105 mm Hg; equal and normoreactive pupils; strength and tone of the extremities bilaterally equal and normal for patient; orientation to time, place, and person; urinary output ≥0.5 ml/kg/h; and stable weight. Within 48 h systolic BP is <140 mm Hg and diastolic BP is <90 mm Hg, with MAP 70-105 mm Hg.

* Monitor BP and MAP q1-5min during titration of the medications. As patient's condition stabilizes, perform these assessments q15min-1h. Be alert to sudden drops or elevations in BP. As the oral medications begin to affect BP, gradually wean IV nitroprusside and other potent vasodilators to prevent hypotensive episodes. Continuous monitoring by arterial cannulation or automatic BP apparatus is recommended.

Text continued on p. 339

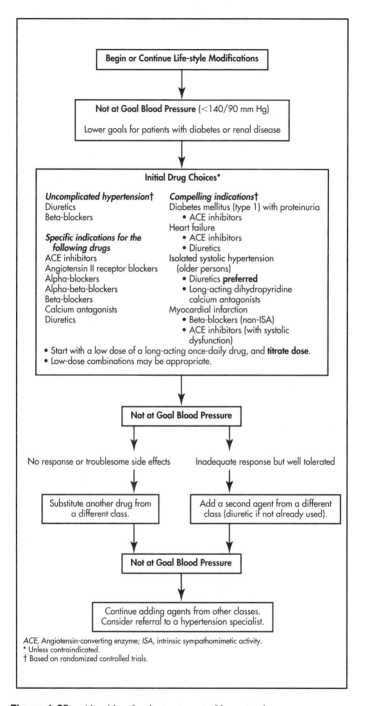

Figure 4-28: Algorithm for the treatment of hypertension.
Modified from the National Institutes of Health: The Sixth Report of the Joint National Committee on Prevention, Detection, Evaluation, and Treatment of High Blood Pressure (JNC VI), NIH Pub. No. 98-4080, Nov, 1997.

TABLE 4-21   Medications Used in the Treatment of Hypertension

Drug type	Medication	Dosage/schedule	Side effects
Diuretics			
Thiazides/related compounds	Bendroflumethiazide	2.5-5 mg; qd	Hypokalemia and hyperuricemia in the first two categories; hypercholesterolemia, hypoglycemia, impotence, and indigestion in all categories of diuretics
	Benzthiazide	12.5-50 mg; qd	
	Chlorothiazide	125-500 mg; q6-12h	
	Chlorthalidone	12.5-50 mg; q24-72h	
	Cyclothiazide	1-2 mg; qd	
	Hydrochlorothiazide	12.5-50 mg; q12-24h	
	Hydroflumethiazide	12.5-50 mg; qd	
	Indapamide	2.5-5 mg; qd	
	Methyclothiazide	2.5-5 mg; qd	
	Metolazone	0.5-5 mg; qd	
	Polythiazide	1-4 mg; qd	
	Trichlormethiazide	1-4 mg, qd	
Loop diuretics	Bumetanide	0.25-2.5 mg; q12h	
	Ethacrynic acid	25-200 mg; q12h	
	Furosemide	20-320 mg; q6-24h	
Potassium-sparing agents	Amiloride	5-10 mg; q12-24 h	Gynecomastia, menstrual abnormalities
	Spironolactone	25-200 mg; q8-12h	
	Triamterene	100-300 mg; q12h	
Adrenergic-inhibiting agents			
β-Blockers	Atenolol*	25-200 mg; qd	Fatigue, drowsiness, depression, fluid retention, heart failure, impotence, hypoglycemia, flushing, bronchospasm (for all β-blockers); bronchospasm is diminished with cardioselective (β₁-blockers)
	Betaxolol*	5-40 mg; qd	
	Bisoprolol*	5-20 mg; qd	
	Metaprolol*	50-200 mg; qd-bid	

Continued

	Nadolol	20-240 mg; qd
	Propranolol	40-120 mg; q6-24h
	Timolol	20-40 mg; bid
β-Blockers with ISA	Acebutolol*	100-600 mg; bid
	Carteolol	2.5-10 mg; qd
	Penbutolol	20-80 mg; qd
	Pindolol	5-30 mg; bid
α- and β-Blocker	Labetalol	100-600 mg; bid	May cause severe postural hypotension; dose adjustments should be made based on standing BP
α-Receptor blockers	Doxazosin	1-16 mg; qd	Hypoglycemia, diarrhea, hypotension, flushing
	Phentolamine	50 mg; qid	First-dose syncope, blurred vision
	Prazosin HCl	1-7 mg; tid	
	Terazosin	1-20 mg; qd	
ACE inhibitors	Benazepril	10-40 mg; qd-bid	To prevent severe hypotension, reduce dose of patient's diuretic; may cause hyperkalemia in persons with renal failure; may cause acute renal failure in bilateral renal artery stenosis; also may cause profound postural hypotension; dose adjustments should be made based on standing BP
	Captopril	6.25-75 mg; bid-tid	
	Enalapril	2.5-40 mg; qd-bid	
	Fosinopril	10-40 mg; qd-bid	
	Lisinopril	5-40 mg; qd-bid	
	Perindopril erbumine	1-16 mg; qd-bid	
	Quinapril HCl	5-80 mg; qd-bid	
	Ramipril	1.25-20 mg; qd-bid	

ACE, Angiotensin-converting enzyme; *ISA*, intrinsic sympathomimetic activity; *BP*, blood pressure.
*Cardioselective.

TABLE 4-21   Medications Used in the Treatment of Hypertension—cont'd

Drug type	Medication	Dosage/schedule	Side effects
Calcium channel blockers			
	Diltiazem	20-90 mg; tid-qid	Constipation, peripheral edema
	Verapamil	30-90 mg; tid-qid	
Dihydropyridines	Amlodipine	2.5-10 mg; qd	Dihydropyridines are more potent peripheral vasodilators than diltiazem and verapamil and may cause more flushing, peripheral edema, tachycardia, dizziness, and headache
	Felodipine	5-20 mg; qd	
	Isradipine	1.25-5 mg; bid	
	Nicardipine	20-40 mg; bid	
	Nifedipine	10-40 mg; tid	
Supplemental antihypertensive agents			
Central α-receptor blockers			
	Clonidine HCl	0.1-6 mg; bid *or* 0.1-0.3 mg patch/week	Hypotension
	Guanabenz	2-32 mg; bid	
	Guanfacine	1-3 mg; qd	
	Methyldopa	250 mg-1 g; bid-qid	Hemolytic anemia, depression, dry mouth, nasal stuffiness, impotence
Peripheral neuronal inhibitors			
	Guanethidine	10-50 mg; qd	Hypotension, impotence, weight gain
	Reserpine	0.1-0.5 mg; qd	Hypotension, hyperacidity, depression
Vasodilators			
	Diazoxide	50-300 mg IV push	Hypotension, fluid retention
	Hydralazine	20-40 mg IV push; 10-50 mg PO q6-12h	Lupus syndrome, angina, sodium retention
	Minoxidil	2.5-80 mg PO; q12-24h	Edema, pericardial effusions, increased hair growth
	Nitroprusside	0.5 μg/kg/min IV (immediate effects last only 1-5 min)	Hypotension; thiocyanate toxicity (if >20 mg/dl) as evidenced by fatigue, anorexia, weakness, delirium

IV, Intravenous; *PO,* by mouth.

☐ Correlate cuff pressure with pressure from arterial cannulation.
☐ Determine ideal range for BP control and maximal nitroprusside dose with physician. Usually the following guidelines are used: systolic BP <140-160 mm Hg; MAP <110 mm Hg; diastolic BP <90 mm Hg.
☐ If hypotension develops, decrease or stop nitroprusside infusion until the pressure rises.

- Assess patient for neurologic deficit by performing hourly neurostatus checks. Be alert to sensorimotor deficit if MAP is >140 mm Hg. As patient's condition stabilizes and BP becomes controlled, perform neurostatus checks at least q4h.
- Monitor patient for changes in funduscopic examination. Consult physician if hemorrhages or fluffy cotton exudates are present.
- Assess patient for evidence of decreasing renal perfusion by monitoring I&O and weighing patient daily. Consult physician if urinary output is <0.5 ml/kg/h for 2 consecutive hours or if weight gain ≥1 kg (2.2 lb). Also be alert to azotemia (increasing BUN), decreasing creatinine clearance, and increasing serum creatinine. Optimal laboratory values are: BUN ≤20 mg/dl; creatinine clearance ≥9.5 ml/min; and serum creatinine ≤1.5 mg/dl.

NIC Hemodynamic Regulation; Medication Administration; Cardiac Care; Circulatory Care

Pain related to headache secondary to cerebral edema occurring with high perfusion pressures
Desired outcomes: Patient's subjective evaluation of pain improves within 12-24 h, as documented by a pain scale. Nonverbal indicators, such as grimacing, are absent or diminished.

- Monitor patient for headache pain at frequent intervals. Devise a pain scale with patient, rating discomfort from 0 (no pain) to 10 (severe pain).
- Provide pain medications as prescribed. A variety of analgesics may be used, ranging from acetaminophen with codeine to morphine, depending on the severity of the symptoms. Assess effectiveness of the pain medication, using the pain scale to determine degree of relief obtained.
- Teach patient relaxation techniques to use in conjunction with the medications. Guided imagery, meditation, progressive muscle relaxation, and music therapy often are effective. See **Health-seeking behavior,** p. 302.
- Maintain a quiet, low-lit environment that is free of extensive distraction and stimulation. Limit visitations as indicated.

NIC Analgesic Administration; Pain Management; Environmental Management: Comfort; Progressive Muscle Relaxation

Sensory/perceptual alterations related to decreased visual acuity secondary to retinal damage occurring with high perfusion pressures; pain secondary to cerebral edema
Desired outcome: Within 24-48 h of this diagnosis, patient reads print, recognizes objects or people, and demonstrates coordination of movement.

- Assess patient for signs of decreased visual acuity by monitoring patient's ability to read and recognize objects or people. Evaluate patient's coordination of movement to determine depth perception. Perform a funduscopic examination q8h for evidence of findings discussed on p. 332. Consult physician for significant findings.
- If patient has decreased visual acuity, assist with feeding and other ADL and keep patient's personal effects within his or her visual field.
- Reassure patient and significant others that visual problems usually resolve when the BP is lowered sufficiently.

NIC Surveillance: Safety

ADDITIONAL NURSING DIAGNOSES

For other nursing diagnoses and interventions, see the following as appropriate: "Hemodynamic Monitoring," p. 28; "Psychosocial Support," p. 83;

and "Psychosocial Support for the Patient's Family and Significant Others," p. 95.

Aortic aneurysm/dissection

PATHOPHYSIOLOGY

An aneurysm is any abnormal dilation of an artery. When the aorta is involved, the complications can be life threatening, owing to the potential for disruption of blood flow to a large portion of the body, including vital organs such as the brain, heart, kidneys, and GI tract. A true aneurysm involves all three layers of the arterial wall (intima, media, adventitia). The two forms of true aneurysm are: fusiform (a concentric, spindle-shaped deformity); and saccular (an eccentric, balloon-shaped deformity). A false aneurysm is a pulsatile hematoma caused by disruption of the intimal layer or the intimal and medial layers only.

Most often, aneurysms develop at the site of an atherosclerotic lesion, which initially involves only the intimal layer of the aorta. As the lesion becomes more complicated, there is hemorrhage into the media, which weakens and dilates the arterial wall. With advancing age, the elastin in the aorta is decreased, which further weakens the vessel wall. Acute hypertension may decrease flow into the media, leading to ischemia, which further weakens this layer. The abdominal, thoracic, or ascending arch of the aorta may be affected. The rate at which the aneurysm increases is not predictable; however, the likelihood of rupture or dissection increases dramatically when the size exceeds 6 cm.

Rupture of an abdominal aneurysm may lead to extravasation of blood either anteriorly into the peritoneal cavity or posteriorly into the retroperitoneal space. Anterior bleeds often occur rapidly and are associated with a high mortality because of rapid circulatory collapse. Posterior bleeds may lead to tamponade on the spinal cord, with neurologic deficits. Either form of rupture can lead to mesenteric ischemia. Surgical repair is the only treatment for rupture.

An *aortic dissection* is a longitudinal tear in the medial layer of the aortic wall caused by the driving pressure of a column of blood. The column of blood drives the dissection distally with the force of systole, and the diastolic recoil within the aorta forces the dissection in the proximal direction. Precipitating factors include medial necrosis from other disorders, trauma, or hypertension (see p. 328). The three types of aortic dissections first described by DeBakey are differentiated by the site of the intimal tear and the direction of dissection. In type I, which accounts for 60%-80% of all cases, the tear begins in the ascending aorta and the dissection extends beyond the aortic arch. Type II is the rarest form, with the intimal tear and entire dissection confined to the ascending aorta. Type III occurs in 20%-30% of all cases and involves a tear in the descending aorta, with distal dissection only.

Aortic dissection is a sudden and very serious threat to life because the disruption of the vessel may continue along any arterial branch of the aorta, compromising organs such as the heart, brain, and kidneys if the coronary, subclavian, innominate, and renal arteries are involved. Approximately 2000 episodes occur annually, with a mortality approaching 100% if the dissection is left untreated.

ASSESSMENT

History and risk factors: Hypertension and related risk factors, connective tissue disorders, coarctation of the aorta, blunt chest trauma, medial necrosis of the aorta, pregnancy, family history of aortic aneurysm.

Clinical presentation: The major symptom is a sudden onset of severe, tearing chest or abdominal pain that is unrelieved by position or respiratory change. The pain may radiate to the back if the dissection is moving distally or to the neck if the dissection is moving proximally. With rupture of an abdominal aneurysm, pain will occur along the flank or lumbar back. Vasovagal responses

Research Brief 4-6 A quasi-experimental study was conducted to assess the effect of a nurse-delivered smoking cessation program for hospitalized patients with cardiac disorders. Two structured contacts were made while in the hospital, and follow-up surveys were completed 3 and 6 mo after discharge. Those in the control group were three times more likely to relapse and resume smoking after discharge than those in the treatment group. Self-efficacy scores related to positive social situations and habit/addictive situations were significantly higher in the intervention group when background variables were included as covariables. This emphasizes how brief interventions can play an important role in smoking cessation. Persons with aortic dissection/aneurysm can reduce the risk of redissection by stopping smoking, and this intervention may assist them in making this behavioral change.

From Johnson JL et al: Evaluation of a nurse-delivered smoking cessation intervention for hospitalized patients with cardiac disease, *Heart Lung* 28:55-64, 1999.

such as diaphoresis, apprehension, nausea, vomiting, and faintness may occur. Signs of acute left ventricular failure may be seen if the dissection involves the coronary arteries or the aortic valve. Neurologic deficits such as confusion, sensorimotor changes, and lethargy may be the result of a dissection along the branches of the ascending aorta. Urine output will fall if the dissection extends to the renal arteries.

Physical assessment: Pulse deficits or BP differences between extremities are classic findings. A drop in BP or pulse at a site helps identify the location of the dissection, inasmuch as both will be decreased beyond the area of dissection. Usually the skin is pale and cool and capillary refill is sluggish as a result of poor tissue perfusion. If bleeding extends to the pericardium, cardiac tamponade can occur (see p. 256).

DIAGNOSTIC TESTS

Chest/abdominal x-ray: Will demonstrate widening of the aortic arch or descending aorta. Film taken with patient in upright position is necessary to demonstrate widening of the mediastinum.

Echocardiography of the aortic arch or descending aorta or TEE: Will locate the site of dissection, inasmuch as the hemorrhage within the vessel will be an area of absent echoes and the total diameter of the vessel will be enlarged.

Aortography or digital subtraction angiography: Will locate actual site of the tear and dissection via use of contrast material.

CT: Often as useful as an aortogram in locating the dissection; its advantage over an aortogram is that it is noninvasive.

COLLABORATIVE MANAGEMENT

Antihypertensive therapy: Initiated as soon as possible to prevent further aortic dissection. Usually nitroprusside is started, as described in "Hypertensive Crisis," p. 328. A MAP of 70-80 mm Hg is desired. After control of the pressure is achieved, oral antihypertensive therapy is begun, along with gradual weaning from the IV infusion.

Propranolol therapy: To reduce velocity of the left ventricular ejection, HR, and BP. Usually it is administered intravenously in increments of 1 mg at 5-min intervals until the HR is reduced to 60-80 bpm. The maximal initial dosage should not exceed 0.15 mg/kg body weight. Additional dosages of 2-6 mg q4-6h then are administered until the condition can be managed with oral medications.

Absolute bed rest: To prevent further dissection. This may continue for days to weeks until the dissection has stabilized. A gradual resumption of activity is recommended.

Pain relief: Usually achieved with IV morphine sulfate, 2-10 mg.

Sedation: To prevent sympathetic stimulation, which can increase BP. Lorazepam or midazolam used for sedation.

Long-term medical management: Aimed at maintaining systolic BP under 130 mm Hg to prevent redissection. It is important to instruct patients to stop smoking to prevent the increases in blood pressure that can result from nicotine.

Surgical treatment: Recommended for proximal dissection, distal dissection when vital organ compromise occurs, impending rupture, or when pain and BP are refractory to medications. The surgery involves removal of the dissected vessel sections and replacement of the vessel sections with Teflon grafts.

NURSING DIAGNOSES AND INTERVENTIONS

Altered tissue perfusion: peripheral, cardiopulmonary, renal, and cerebral, related to interruption of arterial blood flow secondary to narrowed aortic lumen
Desired outcome: Within 48 h of this diagnosis, patient has adequate tissue perfusion as evidenced by distal pulses bilaterally equal and >2+ on a 0-4+ scale; brisk capillary refill (<2 sec); warm skin; bilaterally equal sensations in the extremities; bilaterally equal systolic BP; BP within patient's normal range; HR ≤100 bpm; normal sinus rhythm on ECG; urine output ≥0.5 ml/kg/h; equal and normoreactive pupils; and orientation to time, place, and person.

- Perform bilateral assessment of BP and distal pulses (particularly radial, femoral, dorsalis pedis) hourly during initial phase of dissection and then q4h as the patient's condition stabilizes. Note changes in strength or symmetry of distal pulses. Correlate cuff pressures with arterial monitor recordings. Be alert to any change in color, capillary refill, and temperature of each extremity. Report significant findings.
- If the difference in systolic BP between the extremities exceeds 10 mm Hg, consult physician immediately.
- Monitor for paresthesias of the extremities—a sign of decreased peripheral perfusion.
- Assess for signs of pericardial tamponade: distended neck veins; muffled heart sounds; decreased systolic BP (<90 mm Hg or >20 mm Hg drop in systolic trend); and paradoxic pulse.
- Assess cardiovascular status by monitoring heart rate and rhythm, ECG, and cardiac enzyme levels. A dissection along the coronary arteries will result in an MI.
- Monitor urine output hourly. Consult physician if urine output is <0.5 ml/kg/h for 2 consecutive hours.
- Assess neurologic status hourly. Report restlessness and changes in level of consciousness (LOC), pupil size, or reaction to light.
- Use relaxation techniques such as guided imagery or meditation to reduce BP. Avoid techniques that involve exercise, such as progressive muscle relaxation.

NIC Hemodynamic Regulation; Cardiac Care: Acute; Circulatory Care; Surveillance
Pain related to biophysical injury secondary to necrosis at the aortic media and distal tissue hypoperfusion
Desired outcomes: Within 24-48 h of this diagnosis, patient's subjective evaluation of pain improves, as documented by a pain scale. Nonverbal indicators, such as grimacing, are decreased or absent.

- Monitor patient at frequent intervals for the presence of discomfort. Devise a pain scale with patient, rating discomfort from 0 (no pain) to 10 (severe pain). Medicate with analgesics as prescribed, and rate relief obtained, using the pain scale.
- Teach patient relaxation techniques to use in conjunction with analgesics. Examples include guided imagery and meditation. Avoid progressive muscle relaxation, which may increase cardiac and aortic workload. For guidelines, see **Health-seeking behavior,** p. 302.
- During episodes of pain, assess for a change in peripheral pulses or altered

hemodynamics (i.e., BP, PAP, PAWP, CO, SVR), because such changes often are associated with an increase in aortic dissection.

- Control BP during episodes of pain by titrating nitroprusside to maintain specified parameters.
- Immediately consult physician for any increase in the severity of pain, because it may indicate the need for emergency surgery.

NIC Pain Management; Anxiety Reduction; Simple Relaxation Therapy

ADDITIONAL NURSING DIAGNOSES

For other nursing diagnoses and interventions, also see the following as appropriate: "Hemodynamic Monitoring," p. 28; "Prolonged Immobility," p. 74; "Psychosocial Support," p. 83; "Psychosocial Support for the Patient's Family and Significant Others," p. 95; and "Chest Trauma," p. 133.

Cardiogenic shock

PATHOPHYSIOLOGY

Cardiogenic shock is a state in which impaired cardiac function results in a profound reduction in peripheral blood flow that is incompatible with life. Usually, cardiogenic shock is caused by a massive MI that renders 40% or more of the myocardium dysfunctional because of necrosis or ischemia. As a result, cardiac output is reduced and all tissues suffer from inadequate perfusion. With decreased perfusion to the heart, coronary flow is reduced, which further impairs cardiac function, decreasing cardiac output even more. Cardiogenic shock occurs with 15%-20% of all MIs and carries a mortality of 80% or more. Other causes of cardiogenic shock include depressed cardiac function, post–cardiac surgery, massive pulmonary embolus, severe valvular dysfunction, end-stage cardiomyopathy, congestive heart failure, and cardiac tamponade.

The first stage of shock is characterized by increased sympathetic discharge as the baroreceptors at the carotid sinus and aortic arch become stimulated by the drop in BP. The release of epinephrine and norepinephrine is a compensatory mechanism that increases cardiac output by increasing the heart rate and contractility of the uninjured myocardium. Vasoconstriction, a mechanism that increases BP, occurs. The second, or middle, stage of shock is characterized by decreased perfusion to the brain, kidney, and heart. Lactate and pyruvic acid accumulate in the tissues, and metabolic acidosis occurs because of anaerobic metabolism. Blood is diverted from the skin, gut, and skeletal muscles to the vital organs: brain, heart, and kidneys. In the late stage of shock, which usually is irreversible, compensatory mechanisms become ineffective and multiple organ failure occurs.

At the cellular level, injury begins with hypoxia and loss of adenosine triphosphate (ATP), the energy source for all cellular functions. This leads to condensations in the mitochondria and swelling of the endoplasmic reticulum. The final phase of cellular damage is marked by swelling, rupture of the membrane, and complete cellular degradation. Cellular changes are similar in all body organs and types of tissue.

ASSESSMENT

Clinical presentation: The assessment section in "Acute Coronary Syndromes" (see p. 248) describes the early stage of cardiogenic shock. As cardiogenic shock progresses, mentation is decreased because of poor cerebral perfusion. This is evidenced by agitation, restlessness, lethargy, confusion, or unresponsiveness. Urine output drops to <0.5 ml/kg/h as renal perfusion pressure drops and the kidneys attempt to compensate by triggering the renin-angiotensin system to retain more fluid.

Physical assessment: HR is elevated, and the pulses are equal bilaterally, but they are weak and often irregular. Pulsus alternans may be palpated. Systolic BP

Research Brief 4-7 In 60 ICU patients with established low cardiac output (CO), two measures of this marker of cardiac function were compared. Continuous CO readings were recorded, and then iced injectate bolus CO measures were obtained. Mean paired differences were not significant; however, 23 paired measurements differed by more than 15%. Of those with the greatest difference, 78% had higher bolus readings. Results suggest that continuous CO measurement may be more accurate than bolus in persons with depressed cardiac function.

From Albert NM, Spear BT, Hammel J: Agreement and clinical utility of two techniques for measuring cardiac output in patients with low cardiac output, *Am J Crit Care* 8:464-474, 1999.

is <90 mm Hg or at least 30 mm Hg below the patient's normal resting level. The skin is cold, clammy, and mottled because of compromised peripheral perfusion. Cardiac auscultation usually reveals S_3 or S_4 sounds because of the overdistended and noncompliant ventricle. Crackles are auscultated over the lung fields because of pulmonary congestion; hyperventilation is common.

Hemodynamic measurements: Cuff pressures are unreliable during shock, mandating the use of arterial pressure monitoring. PAP monitoring is essential for guiding therapy during cardiogenic shock. Arterial systolic and mean arterial pressures are decreased, with a decreased or narrow pulse pressure. Because contractility is greatly reduced, the stroke volume, ejection fraction, and cardiac output are decreased. CVP, RAP, PAP, and PAWP all are elevated as evidence of increased preload secondary to pulmonary congestion. SVR is increased because of vasoconstriction, which occurs as a compensatory mechanism when flow to an organ is reduced. Coronary perfusion pressure (diastolic BP minus PAWP) will be less than the normal 60 mm Hg.

An oximetric catheter may be used to provide continuous measurement of Svo_2 in the pulmonary artery. The Svo_2 reflects the adequacy of oxygen supply in meeting tissue demands. When tissue demand is increased (as in exercise) or supply is decreased (as in cardiogenic shock), the Svo_2 will fall below the normal range of 60%-80%. The Svo_2 has a positive correlation with CO; thus continuous monitoring of Svo_2 provides an indirect but continuous assessment of CO. For detailed parameters for assessment, see Table 4-22.

DIAGNOSTIC TESTS

The diagnosis of cardiogenic shock is made by physical assessment and analysis of the hemodynamic profile. The primary problem, MI, is diagnosed by enzyme changes and ECG (see discussion, p. 248). Other diagnostic tests are useful in assessing the effect of hypoperfusion on other organs.

ABG values: Hypoxemia (Pao_2 <80 mm Hg) and metabolic acidosis (pH <7.35; $Paco_2$ usually <35 mm Hg) are seen because of impaired oxygen diffusion in the alveoli and tissue lactic acidosis from anaerobic metabolism.

Serum chemistry values: Moderate hyperglycemia may be found as a result of epinephrine-induced glycogenolysis. Because the pancreas is hypoperfused, inadequate insulin is released to meet this need. Serum lactate levels may be elevated as a result of anaerobic metabolism. Electrolyte studies may reveal hypernatremia, which is reflective of a water deficit; hypokalemia, which may be associated with the cause of shock; or hyperkalemia, which may be seen with renal failure secondary to the shock state.

Urinalysis: Urine sodium, osmolality, and creatinine levels are reflective of the patient's renal status.

Coagulation profile: Although coagulation studies often are abnormal, there is no established pattern with cardiogenic shock.

ECG: Although not specific for cardiogenic shock, dysrhythmias may occur as a result of infarction or injury to areas of the conduction system and/or myocardium or as a result of electrolyte imbalance.

TABLE 4-22 Hemodynamic Profile of Shock

Values	RAP (mm Hg)	RVP (mm Hg)	PAP (mm Hg)	PAWP (mm Hg)	SVR (dynes/sec/cm^{-5})	Svo$_2$ (%)	CO (L/min)	CI (L/min/m^2)
Normal	4-6	25/0-5	20-30/8-15	6-12	900-1200	60-80	4-7	2.5-4
Shock values								
Cardiogenic	6-10	40-50/6-15	50/25-30	25-40	>1200	≤50	<4	≤1.5
Hypovolemic	0-2	15-20/0-2	15-20/2-8	2-6	>1200	65	<4	2.5
Neurogenic	0-2	20-25/0-2	20-25/0-8	0-6	≤1000	60-80	≥4-7	2.5
Septic								
Early	0-2	20-25/0-2	20-25/0-8	0-6	≤900	≥60	>7	≥4
Late	0-4	25/0-4	25/4-10	>12	>1200	≤60	<4	<2.5

RAP, Right atrial pressure; *RVP*, right ventricular pressure; *PAP*, positive airway pressure; *PAWP*, pulmonary artery wedge pressure; *SVR*, systemic vascular resistance; *Svo$_2$*, mixed venous oxygen saturation; *CO*, cardiac output; *CI*, cardiac index.

COLLABORATIVE MANAGEMENT

Oxygen therapy: To maximize tissue oxygenation, since perfusion is impaired. If dyspnea, hypoxemia, acidosis, or pulmonary congestion worsens, intubation and mechanical ventilation will be necessary. Morphine sulfate 2 mg IV push may assist in reducing pulmonary congestion, thereby relieving dyspnea and increasing Pao_2.

Correction of acidosis: Sodium bicarbonate delivered by IV push and guided by serial ABG checks to assess effectiveness of treatment.

Correction of electrolyte imbalance: Replacement of potassium, sodium, chloride, or calcium as indicated by serum chemistry findings.

Diuretics: To decrease preload and improve stroke volume and cardiac output. Diuretics such as furosemide 40-200 mg IV push or ethacrynic acid 25-100 mg IV push may be given. Bumetanide (Bumex) is another frequently used diuretic similar in action to furosemide. One mg of bumetanide is equal to 40 mg of furosemide. Morphine sulfate also reduces preload. Nitrates such as oral, topical, or IV nitroglycerin and IV nitroprusside (Nipride) may be used to decrease filling pressures via venous dilation.

> **Note:** It may be necessary to increase preload if the patient is hypovolemic. In this situation, fluids are increased cautiously, the patient's hemodynamics are monitored carefully, and diuretics are avoided.

Positive inotropic agents: To improve contractility of the uninjured myocardium and to increase CO. Dopamine infusions at 2-20 µg/kg/min are titrated to accomplish the desired effect. Higher doses increase HR and SVR, which increase the myocardial workload. Dobutamine infusions of 2-20 µg/kg/min increase contractility and decrease preload with less of an increase in HR, but renal perfusion may decrease at the higher dose range. Amrinone infusions of 5-15 µg/kg/min or milrinone 0.375 to 0.75 µg/kg/min provide similar inotropic effects.

Vasopressors: To increase BP to an adequate mean level (usually ≥70 mm Hg) that will perfuse the tissues. This is accomplished by stimulating the α-adrenergic receptors in the blood vessels, which causes vasoconstriction. Vasopressors that may be used include dopamine, norepinephrine, epinephrine, phenylephrine, and methoxamine (see Appendix 7).

Intraaortic balloon pump (IABP): A counterpulsation device that assists the failing heart by decreasing afterload and increasing coronary artery perfusion. It may be used in cardiogenic shock, heart failure, unstable angina, pre–cardiac surgery and post–cardiac surgery, refractory ventricular dysrhythmias, cardiomyopathy, and post-PTCA complications, as well as in patients awaiting heart transplantation. IABP is a temporary measure that supports the heart and circulation for up to 30 days. It is used as an adjunct to medical therapy.

Balloon insertion can be performed emergently at the bedside or under controlled conditions during fluoroscopic examination. A local anesthetic agent is injected over the femoral artery, the introducer sheath is inserted, and the balloon is passed through the sheath into the thoracic aorta. The catheter is placed so that the balloon is below the left subclavian artery and above the renal artery. If the balloon migrates in either direction, arterial flow can be obstructed. The balloon is then unwrapped and connected to the pump console. Pumping is timed according to the ECG or arterial pressure waveform. Balloon inflation occurs with diastole, and deflation occurs with systole.

The patient derives benefits from both phases of balloon pumping. Balloon inflation, the first phase, is termed *diastolic augmentation.* During this phase, blood flow is increased antegrade and retrograde within the aorta. Coronary artery blood flow is increased, resulting in increased oxygen supply to the myocardium. Also, blood flow to the kidneys is increased, improving urinary output. Systolic unloading or balloon deflation is the second phase. Aortic pressure decreases rapidly, reducing afterload and resistance to blood flow out of the left ventricle and decreasing ventricular wall tension. With reduced afterload the ventricle empties more completely, stroke volume rises, and myocardial oxygen use diminishes. Clinical signs of the balloon's benefits include increased BP, increased cardiac output, increased urinary flow, improved mental alertness, warm extremities, palpable peripheral pulses, decreased chest pain, and improvement of the ECG changes that denote ischemia.

Complications of IABP therapy include aortic dissection, thrombus formation, impaired circulation to the involved leg, sepsis, obstruction to the left subclavian artery blood flow, obstruction to the renal and mesenteric arteries, and paraplegia (caused by spinal artery thrombosis). In addition, problems such as pneumonia and dermal ulcers can occur as a result of prolonged immobility.

> **Note:** Pulmonary artery balloon counterpulsation (intrapulmonary artery balloon pump) is available for support of the right ventricle after cardiac surgery. The catheter usually is inserted during surgery and involves creation of an artificial diverticulum on the pulmonary artery. During systole, the balloon is deflated and right ventricle stroke volume is directed into the diverticulum, which reduces afterload. During diastole, the balloon inflates and the cardiac output is propelled into the pulmonary vessels.

Ventricular assist device: A mechanical ventricular assist device (VAD) is used to support the patient with massive left ventricular and/or right ventricular dysfunction. The VAD provides a conduit that diverts blood from the ventricle to an artificial pump. The VAD can maintain circulation and decreased myocardial workload to promote ventricular recovery. Candidates for this device include individuals with acute ventricular dysfunction; shock after cardiotomy, angioplasty, or myocardial infarction; cardiac arrest; or massive pulmonary embolism.

In general, the right ventricle recovers within 5 days and the left ventricle recovers within 10 days. This device is used as a temporary measure to promote rest and healing of the damaged myocardium. Left ventricular assistance is provided through either percutaneous cannulation of the femoral artery or direct cannulation of the atrium and ascending aorta, whereas a right VAD is used in the right atrium and the main pulmonary artery. In individuals with right and left ventricular failure, biventricular assistance is available. As the patient's overall condition improves, the goal is to gradually wean the patient from the device by decreasing the flow rate. Some devices are implanted for prolonged periods and used as a bridge to transplant. Studies of permanent assist devices for severe heart failure are in progress.

Complications of the assist device include coagulopathy, bleeding, embolization, infection, sepsis, right ventricular failure (with left-sided heart assist only), and renal failure. Because of the critical nature of these patients' condition and their need for constant monitoring by means of multiple assessment modalities, highly specialized nursing care is imperative.

Emergency cardiac catheterization: To determine patient's suitability for emergency PTCA, CABG, or arthrectomy.

Emergency CABG: To reperfuse areas with reversible injury patterns. This procedure will not be as beneficial if the tissue already is necrotic as evidenced by Q waves on the ECG (see discussion, p. 250). At the time of surgery a left ventricular aneurysmectomy may be performed to remove the thin-walled, dysfunctional sac.

Emergency PTCA: To reperfuse areas of the myocardium with reversible injury pattern (see discussion, p. 253).

Thrombolytic therapy: To reperfuse the injured and uninfarcted myocardium (see discussion, p. 254).

TABLE 4-23   Fluid Challenge Guidelines in Cardiogenic Shock

Assessment	PAWP (mm Hg)	Fluids
CO low, and PAWP low or normal	<6	200 ml infused over 10 min
	6-12	100 ml infused over 10 min
	≥12	50 ml infused over 10 min
PAWP increases during infusion	>6	Return to KVO rate
	≤3	Continue infusion
Assess PAWP after 10 min	If >3 or <6	Repeat challenge

KVO, Keep vein open; *PAWP,* pulmonary artery wedge pressure; *CO,* cardiac output.

Heart transplantation: To replace the failing heart with a suitably matched donor organ. The recipient is screened carefully to ensure that all other organs are still functional. Refer to "Cardiac Transplantation," p. 354.

NURSING DIAGNOSES AND INTERVENTIONS

Decreased cardiac output related to increased afterload, increased preload, or decreased contractility secondary to loss of ≥40% of myocardial functional mass

Desired outcome: Before weaning from assist device or pharmacologic agents is attempted, the patient's hemodynamic function is as near the acceptable limits as possible as evidenced by CO ≥4 L/min; BP ≥90/60 mm Hg; SVR ≤1200 dynes/sec/cm^{-5}; and PAWP ≤12 mm Hg.

- On a continuous basis, monitor arterial BP, PAP, Svo$_2$, and heart rate and rhythm. Titrate vasoactive drugs to achieve a CO between 4-7 L/min; arterial BP ≥90/60; and PAWP ≤12 mm Hg.
- Assess CO and SVR q1-4h and after every change in pharmacologic therapy. Consult physician if SVR increases (>1200 dynes/sec/cm^{-5}), inasmuch as nitroprusside or similar medication may be needed to decrease excessive afterload.
- Auscultate lung sounds q1-2h, and monitor urinary output. Report changes, including an increase in crackles and decreased urine output, because additional diuretics may be necessary.
- To prevent further decreases in BP, do not increase the angle of the HOB more than 30 degrees.
- Treat ventricular dysrhythmias with prescribed lidocaine, procainamide hydrochloride, or bretylium infusions.
- Be prepared to employ pacing if bradycardia or a second- or third-degree heart block is found. Either temporary transcutaneous or transvenous pacing may be used.
- If preload is low, administer prescribed crystalloid IV fluids according to fluid challenge protocol (see Table 4-23 for sample protocol). Document patient's hemodynamic response.
- If medical management is ineffective, prepare patient for insertion of IABP (see p. 346) or left VAD (see "Ventricular Assist Device," p. 347).

NIC Cardiac Care: Acute; Circulatory Care: Mechanical Assist Device; Hemodynamic Regulation; Shock Management: Cardiac

Altered tissue perfusion: cardiopulmonary, cerebral, peripheral, and renal, related to interrupted arterial blood flow to vital organs secondary to inadequate arterial pressure

Desired outcome: Within 96 h of this diagnosis, patient has adequate tissue perfusion as evidenced by orientation to time, place, and person; equal and normoreactive pupils; normal reflexes; urine output ≥0.5 ml/kg/h; warm and dry skin; peripheral pulses >2+ on a 0-4+ scale; brisk capillary refill (<2 sec); and BP >90/60 mm Hg or within patient's normal range.

- Check neurologic status q1-2h to assess cerebral perfusion. Be alert to changes in LOC, orientation, perception, motor activity, reflexes, and pupillary response to light. Consult physician for any changes.
- Monitor I&O hourly to assess renal perfusion; report urine output <0.5 ml/kg/h for 2 consecutive hours. Assess extremities q1-2h, noting changes in skin color, temperature, capillary refill, BP, and distal pulses.
- Titrate vasoactive drugs to maintain systolic BP >90 mm Hg.

NIC Circulatory Care: Peripheral, Cerebral, Cardiac, Gastrointestinal

Impaired gas exchange related to alveolar-capillary membrane changes secondary to pulmonary congestion; altered oxygen-carrying capacity of the blood secondary to acidosis occurring with anaerobic metabolism

Desired outcome: Before weaning from supplemental oxygen or ventilatory assistance is attempted, the patient has adequate gas exchange as evidenced by Pao_2 ≥80 mm Hg; RR 12-20 breaths/min with normal depth and pattern (eupnea); oxygen saturation ≥95%; and Svo_2 60%-80%.

- At least hourly, assess rate, depth, and effort of patient's respirations for tachypnea or labored breaths. Also inspect skin and mucous membranes for pallor or cyanosis (a late sign of hypoxia). Consult physician promptly for significant findings.
- Auscultate lung fields q1-2h. Be alert to crackles, rhonchi, or wheezes.
- Monitor ABG values for hypoxemia (Pao_2 <80 mm Hg) or metabolic acidosis (pH <7.35 and HCO_3^-<24 mEq/L).
- Deliver humidified oxygen as prescribed.
- Monitor transcutaneous oxygen saturation with a pulse oximeter. Consult physician if oxygen saturation falls below 90%.
- Monitor Svo_2. When cardiac output drops, Svo_2 will decrease, indicating increased oxygen extraction, which occurs when perfusion is decreased. Alert physician to Svo_2<60%.
- If patient's condition continues to deteriorate, prepare patient for intubation and mechanical ventilation.

NIC Acid-Base Management; Airway Management; Oxygen Therapy; Mechanical Ventilation

For patients undergoing intraaortic balloon pump procedure

Decreased cardiac output (or risk for same) related to negative inotropic changes and rate, rhythm, and conduction alterations secondary to ischemia or injury

Desired outcomes: Within 24 h of this diagnosis, patient has adequate cardiac output as evidenced by BP within patient's normal range; normal sinus rhythm on ECG; HR 60-100 bpm; peripheral pulses >2+ on a 0-4+ scale; warm and dry skin; hourly urinary output ≥0.5 ml/kg/h; measured CO 4-7 L/min; CI ≥2.5 $L/min/m^2$; PAWP ≤12 mm Hg; SVR ≤1200 dynes/sec/cm^{-5}; Svo_2 60%-80%; and patient awake, alert, oriented, and free from anginal pain.

- Monitor BP, PAP, RAP, Svo_2, and heart rate and rhythm on a continuous basis. Monitor PAWP, SVR, and CO/CI hourly. Be alert to and report to physician the following: elevation in PAWP; decreased CO; ST-segment changes; ectopic heartbeats; decreased Svo_2; or elevated SVR.
- Monitor hourly urinary output, noting output that is <0.5 ml/kg/h for 2 consecutive hours. Monitor BUN and creatinine values daily. Be alert to increased BUN (>20 mg/dl) and serum creatinine (>1.5 mg/dl), which can occur with low urinary output and acute tubular necrosis.
- Monitor bilateral peripheral pulses and color and temperature of extremities q2h.
- Provide oxygen therapy or maintain ventilator settings as prescribed.

- Regulate IV inotropic agents, such as dobutamine, dopamine, and amrinone, to maintain CI ≥ 2.5-4 L/min/m^2. Monitor for side effects, including tachyarrhythmias, ventricular ectopy, headache, and angina. (See Appendix 7 for more information.)
- Regulate afterload-reducing agents such as nitroprusside and nitroglycerin to maintain SVR <1200 dynes/sec/cm^{-5}. Monitor for drug side effects, including hypotension, headache, dizziness, nausea, vomiting, and cutaneous flushing.
- Administer diuretic agents as prescribed for elevated PAWP (>12 mm Hg). Monitor for signs and symptoms of hypokalemia (e.g., weakness, dysrhythmias), a potential side effect of diuretics.
- Provide a quiet environment conducive to stress reduction.
- Administer prescribed pain medications as needed to reduce sympathetic response, which increases afterload.
- Monitor Hgb and Hct values daily for decrease, which may signal bleeding and reduced blood volume, along with reduced oxygen-carrying capacity of the blood.

NIC Circulatory Care: Mechanical Assist Device; Surveillance

Altered tissue perfusion (or risk for same): peripheral: involved leg, related to interrupted arterial blood flow secondary to arterial wall dissection by sheath; thrombus formation

Desired outcome: Throughout duration of hospitalization, patient has adequate perfusion in the involved leg as evidenced by peripheral pulses >2+ on a 0-4+ scale; normal color and sensation; warmth; full motor function; and absence of bleeding, abdominal pain, and tingling in the involved leg.

- Monitor circulation in affected leg q30min × 4 and q2h thereafter if assessment is within normal limits. Assess pulses, temperature, color, sensation, and mobility of the toes in the involved leg. Consult physician immediately for significant changes.
- Instruct patient to notify staff member if pain, numbness, or tingling occurs in the involved leg.
- Provide protection to heel of involved foot, using sheepskin, occlusive opaque dressing, or heel protector. Place lamb's wool between the toes to minimize the pressure of the toes against each other.
- To enhance perfusion in the involved leg, have patient perform passive foot exercises without bending leg at the hip. The following should be performed qid: foot flexion/extension, foot circles, quadriceps setting. A pneumatic compression device may be beneficial.
- Administer IV dextran or heparin as prescribed to prevent clots from forming on the balloon. Monitor patient for signs of bleeding, including decreased Hct (optimal values are $\geq 37\%$ [female] or $\geq 40\%$ [male]), abdominal pain, hematuria, oral bleeding, or blood-tinged mucus.
- Monitor PTT if heparin is used (optimal value is 30-40 sec [activated]). Therapeutic anticoagulation is usually 1½ times that of normal. Maintain adequate hydration (2-3 L/day) to minimize risk of clot formation.
- Keep HOB at 30 degrees or less to prevent upward migration of catheter, which would occlude subclavian artery.
- Assess for the following signs of balloon migration: decreased left radial pulse, sudden decrease in urine output (<0.5 ml/kg/h), flank pain, and dizziness.
- When the balloon is no longer needed, maintain regular balloon inflation to prevent clot formation until balloon can be removed.

NIC Positioning; Circulatory Care: Peripheral

Impaired tissue integrity (or risk for same) related to external factors (pressure and immobilization); internal factors (altered circulation and decreased protein intake because of NPO status)

Desired outcome: Throughout hospitalization, patient's tissue remains intact.

- Position patient on low-pressure protective bed. These beds reduce the capillary pressure to less than closing pressure, thereby enhancing blood flow to dependent areas. In addition, they also circulate air around the patient to promote evaporation of moisture.

- Reposition patient q2h, particularly at night when spontaneous movement is diminished. When turning patient, keep involved leg extended and log roll patient onto side.
- Ensure meticulous skin care to keep skin clean and dry. Inspect vulnerable areas (e.g., coccyx, ischial tuberosity, calcaneus, malleolus) at least tid.
- Ensure that patient's diet is high in protein and calories to promote nitrogen balance. If patient's oral intake is inadequate or in the event of intubation, confer with physician regarding need for nutritional support such as enteral feedings or parenteral nutrition.
- As patient's condition improves, teach patient how to move in bed while minimizing flexion of involved hip.
- See "Wound and Skin Care," p. 55, for more information.

NIC Bedrest Care; Positioning; Self-Care Assistance

Ineffective breathing pattern related to fatigue and decreased energy secondary to heart failure; decreased lung expansion secondary to medically imposed position (HOB no higher than 30 degrees)

Desired outcome: Within 4 h of this diagnosis, patient has an effective breathing pattern as evidenced by Pao_2 ≥80 mm Hg; Spo_2 >90%; absence of adventitious breath sounds; and RR 12-20 breaths/min with normal pattern and depth (eupnea).

- Monitor breath sounds q2h. Assess anterior and posterior lung fields for adventitious (e.g., crackles, rhonchi) or absent sounds.
- Monitor oxygen saturation by pulse oximetry. Be alert to levels <90%.
- Monitor respiratory rate, rhythm, and breathing pattern hourly.
- Be alert to indicators of atelectasis (e.g., dyspnea, elevated temperature, weakness, absent or decreased breath sounds) and respiratory infection (elevated temperature, SOB, increased sputum production or coughing, altered color of sputum).
- Monitor temperature q4h and WBC count daily for signs of infection. Be alert to low-grade fever of ≤37.8° C (≤100° F) and increased WBC count.
- Provide supplemental oxygen and chest physiotherapy as prescribed.
- Encourage patient to perform deep-breathing exercises or incentive spirometry q1-2h while awake to promote gas exchange, followed by coughing to raise secretions, if indicated.
- If coughing is ineffective in raising secretions, suction as indicated, using aseptic technique.
- Reposition patient at least q2h to minimize stasis of lung secretions.
- Monitor patient's fluid volume status to ensure that hydration is adequate to keep secretions thin and mobile. Unless contraindicated, maintain patient's fluid intake at 2-3 L/day.
- As often as it is allowed, elevate HOB 30 degrees to promote effective breathing pattern.
- If patient continues to exhibit ineffective breathing pattern in spite of these measures, prepare for ET intubation and mechanical ventilation.

NIC Airway Management; Oxygen Therapy; Respiratory Monitoring; Mechanical Ventilation

Altered protection related to risk of bleeding/hemorrhage secondary to mechanical coagulopathy and IV anticoagulants

Desired outcome: Throughout hospitalization, patient has no symptoms of bleeding as evidenced by secretions and excretions negative for blood and absence of abdominal pain or ecchymoses. Hct is ≥37% (female) or ≥40% (male); PTT is in the range of therapeutic anticoagulation established by physician or protocol; ACT is ≤120 sec; and platelet count is 150,000-400,000/mm³.

- Monitor PTT, ACT, and platelet level daily. Be alert to levels not within

therapeutic range. Note that anticoagulation and decreased platelet level increase the risk of bleeding and hemorrhage.
- Monitor Hct and Hgb daily. Decreased levels may signal the presence of bleeding.
- Test GI drainage and stool daily for blood.
- Protect patient from injury. Pad side rails, if necessary, and turn patient carefully. Use sponge-tipped applicators for oral care.
- Test gastric pH q4h. Administer gastric acid-neutralizing drugs, such as antacids or histamine H_2-receptor antagonists as prescribed to maintain gastric pH >5.

NIC Bleeding Precautions
NOTE: Also see **Risk for infection,** which appears in the next section, "For Patients with a Ventricular Assist Device," p. 353.

For patients with a ventricular assist device
Altered protection related to risk of bleeding secondary to therapeutic anticoagulation and effects of cardiopulmonary bypass or VAD on blood components
Desired outcome: Throughout duration of hospitalization, patient has no symptoms of internal or external bleeding as evidenced by secretions and excretions negative for blood; chest tube drainage within acceptable amounts (<100 ml/h); and absence of ecchymoses and abdominal or back pain.
- Monitor Hct daily for a decrease in value. Optimal values are as follows: Hct ≥37% (female) or ≥40% (male).
- Test gastric drainage and stool daily for blood; report positive results.
- Monitor daily clotting studies (PT, PTT), platelets, and ACT. Report elevations of PT (>11-15 sec), PTT (>30-40 sec), or ACT above desired range, which will depend on whether patient has received anticoagulants. Anticoagulation of patients with a heart assist device in place is desirable but may not be feasible if the patient is bleeding actively from the surgical site. Monitor platelets, and be alert to a decrease to <100,000/mm³, which represents a significant drop and the increased risk of bleeding.
- Inspect all drainage for evidence of bleeding.
- Administer coagulation factors as prescribed (e.g., platelets, fresh-frozen plasma, cryoprecipitate, vitamin K, protamine sulfate, and amino-caproic acid).
- Test gastric pH q4h, and administer prescribed antacids to maintain pH >5.
- Administer prophylactic acid-neutralizing drugs (i.e., antacids) as prescribed, as well as H_2-receptor antagonists, which block the release of histamine.

NIC Bleeding Precautions
Risk for disuse syndrome related to imposed restrictions against movement secondary to presence of assist device or debilitated state
Desired outcome: Patient maintains baseline ROM without evidence of muscle atrophy or contracture formation.
- Be aware that patient can be turned gently from side to side when the heart assist device is in place. Do this q2h, observing assist device cannulas closely to ensure that tension is not placed on them during patient repositioning.
- Provide passive ROM to extremities qid.
- See "Prolonged Immobility," p. 74, for more information.

NIC Energy Management
Decreased cardiac output (or risk for same) related to altered preload and negative inotropic changes secondary to reduced right ventricular contraction occurring with left heart assist device

> **Note:** This is a complication of the left heart assist device, particularly when the outflow cannula is located in the left ventricle. When the left ventricle is decompressed, septal wall motion is diminished, thereby reducing right ventricular contraction. Patients who have pulmonary hypertension or impaired right ventricular function caused by AMI or cardiopulmonary bypass are especially prone to this problem.

Desired outcome: Within 24 h of this diagnosis, patient's cardiac output is adequate as evidenced by measured CO 4-7 L/min; RAP 4-6 mm Hg; PVR 60-100 dynes/sec/cm^{-5}; and LAP ≥10 mm Hg.
- Monitor patient for a decrease in CO with associated increases in RAP and PVR, which are diagnostic of the complication just described.
- Ensure that patient attains prescribed IV fluid intake to maintain a minimal LAP of 10 mm Hg. An adequate preload is necessary to prevent a vacuum effect from the device, which would aggravate this problem.

NIC Circulatory Care: Mechanical Assist Device; Hemodynamic Regulation

Risk for infection related to inadequate primary defenses secondary to presence of multiple invasive lines, movement restrictions, and stasis of body fluids

Desired outcome: Patient is free of infection as evidenced by normothermia; WBC count ≤11,000/mm^3; negative culture results; and absence of erythema, swelling, warmth, tenderness, and purulent drainage at incision or cannulation sites.
- On a daily basis, monitor temperature, WBC count, and all incisions and cannulation sites for evidence of infection. Be alert to low-grade fever of approximately 37.8° C (100° F); WBC count >11,000/mm^3; and incision that is erythematous, warm, swollen, and tender to the touch or that has purulent discharge.
- Culture any suspicious drainage or secretions; report positive findings.
- Change IV tubing q72h (or per agency protocol), using aseptic technique.
- Change all dressings over catheter insertion sites per agency protocol, using aseptic technique. Apply antimicrobial ointment (e.g., povidone-iodine).
- Administer prophylactic IV antibiotics as prescribed.
- Provide nutritional support to ensure that nitrogen balance is attained.
- Monitor breath sounds q2h. Assess for the presence of crackles, rhonchi, or signs of consolidation. If extubation has occurred, establish hourly deep-breathing and coughing exercises.
- If patient is incapable of raising secretions independently, suction as often as need is determined by auscultation. Inspect the mucus, noting color and consistency. Be alert to secretions that are yellow, green, or thickened.
- Provide gentle chest physiotherapy as prescribed. Percussion and vibration can be performed over the posterior and lateral lung lobes during every positioning change, or at least qid.

NIC Infection Protection

Altered nutrition: less than body requirements, related to decreased intake secondary to oral intubation; increased need secondary to debilitated state and impaired tissue perfusion with concomitant nitrogen malabsorption

Desired outcome: Within the 24- to 48-h period before discharge from ICU, patient has adequate nutrition as evidenced by a balanced nitrogen state; stable weight; urine nitrogen 10-20 g/24 h; thyroxine-binding prealbumin 20-30 mg/dl; and retinol-binding protein 4-5 mg/dl.
- Provide nutrition via tube feedings or total parenteral nutrition to ensure minimum of 1-5 g protein/kg/day and a calorie intake of 100 kcal/kg/day, along with other essential elements. Ask dietitian to monitor daily calorie and protein intake.
- Weigh patient daily for trend. Report continuing decreases in weight.
- Monitor 24-h urinary nitrogen q3days for increase in excretion.

- Monitor I&O hourly. Report positive or negative fluid state of 300 ml/h.
- Assess patient for signs of cardiac cachexia: muscle atrophy, weakness, anorexia, and weight loss.
- For more information, see "Nutritional Support," p. 1.

NIC Nutritional Monitoring; Nutrition Therapy

ADDITIONAL NURSING DIAGNOSES

Also see the following, as appropriate: "Mechanical Ventilation," p. 17; "Hemodynamic Monitoring," p. 28; "Prolonged Immobility," p. 74; "Psychosocial Support," p. 83; and "Psychosocial Support for the Patient's Family and Significant Others," p. 95.

Cardiac transplantation

PATHOPHYSIOLOGY

Cardiac transplantation is the selected treatment choice for patients with end-stage heart failure. Since the discovery of cyclosporine in 1980, patient outcomes and success rates have supported growing numbers of transplant centers. In the USA alone, 20,000-30,000 patients could benefit from cardiac transplantation. However, 20%-40% of the actual transplant candidates die, waiting for the only 2500 available donors annually.

The three transplant procedures are *orthotopic, heterotopic,* and *xenotransplantation.*

- *Orthotopic/homotopic/allotransplantation:* recipient's heart, except for the posterior atria, is replaced with a donor heart. This is the most common procedure and the focus of this chapter.
- *Heterotopic:* donor heart is "piggy backed" to the right of the recipient's heart. An anastomosis allows for both hearts to function.
- *Xenotransplantation:* donor heart is from a different species.

Functional classifications for the etiologies of heart failure or cardiomyopathy are numerous but can be categorized as follows:

- *Idiopathic dilated:* gross dilation of the heart as a result of damaged myofibrils causing cellular hypertrophy and fibrosis. The precise etiology is unclear, but related factors include alcohol abuse, pregnancy, viral infection, ischemia, immunologic disorders, muscular dystrophy, myocarditis, and a positive family history.
- *Hypertrophic/obstructive:* abnormal muscle fiber organization. There is thickening and hypertrophy of the interventricular septum with ventricular wall rigidity. The stiff ventricular wall results in poor ventricular filling (diastole) and sometimes obstruction of the outflow tract (systole). Etiology: unknown but probably genetically transmitted.
- *Restrictive/constrictive:* endocardial scarring of ventricle. Impairment of diastolic function. Least common. Etiology: amyloid, hemochromatosis, glycogen deposition, and others.

Although the primary indication for cardiac transplantation is cardiomyopathy, additional indications include valvular disease and congenital heart defects.

With the imbalance between supply and demand, patients must meet selection criteria before they can be considered for transplantation (Table 4-24). Once the patient has been determined as a candidate for cardiac transplantation, he or she is placed on a waiting list and given a status code. The status code is assigned to all transplant candidates and identifies the level of urgency for transplantation (Table 4-25).

TABLE 4-24   **Patient Selection Criteria for Cardiac Transplantation**

Inclusion criteria	Exclusion criteria
End-stage heart failure	*Relative*
Refractory and intolerable symptoms; New York Heart Association classes III-IV	Active substance abuse
	Psychologic-social issues related to support, finances
Failure of maximal medical treatment (e.g., digoxin, diuretics, vasodilators, ACE inhibitors, β-blockers)	Age >70 yr
	Absolute
	Complicated IDDM with end-organ damage
One-year survival expectancy <50% and poor short-term prognosis or poor functional capacity	Active infection (until resolved)
	Irreversible liver or kidney dysfunction
Age <65-70 yr	Pulmonary hypertension; PVR >6-8 Wood units
Left ventricular ejection fraction 20%-35%	Comorbid diseases
Chronic, unstable angina	Active peptic ulcer disease
Peak O_2 consumption 14 ml/kg/min	Poor compliance
Onset of atrial fibrillation	Coexisting cancer
Decreasing cardiac output	Severe obesity
Cachexia	Symptomatic peripheral and cerebral vascular disease
Refractory ventricular arrhythmias	
Otherwise good health	Severe osteoporosis

IDDM, Insulin-dependent diabetes mellitus; *PVR,* pulmonary vascular resistance.

LEFT VENTRICULAR ASSIST DEVICES

Implantation, as a bridge to transplant, is becoming more prevalent for patients awaiting transplantation. Not only does the bridge provide more time to wait for a donor, patients have experienced better health, physical fitness, and increase in their quality of life.

DONOR PROCUREMENT

During surgery, the donor heart is exposed and then is inspected to assess viability. The heart is cooled with a high-potassium cardioplegic agent, excised, and protected in plastic bags containing ice-cold normal saline. It is then transferred via an ice chest to the waiting recipient.

POSTOPERATIVE CLINICAL PRESENTATION

Physical assessment: Varies depending on time of postoperative assessment.
Neurologic: Initially somnolent related to anesthesia. As cerebral perfusion improves, alertness increases and neurologic status improves relative to baseline.
Cardiovascular: Initially maintained on isoproterenol (Isuprel) to increase heart rate and decrease PVR. HR maintained at 110 bpm, usually atrially paced at 110/min; SBP maintained at >100 mm Hg; MAP >65; CI should be >2.5, and CI will improve as heart is warmed and perfused. Skin warm, dry, and intact; color appropriate for race; mucous membranes pink. All pulses palpable. S_1, S_2 without murmur. If rejecting, CI will be <2.2; BP will be decreased; and atrial

TABLE 4-25   Allocation of Thoracic Organs*

Status 1A

A patient is admitted to the transplant center and has at least one of the following:

A Mechanical circulatory support for acute hemodynamic decompensation that includes at least one of the following:

- Left or right ventricular assist device implanted <30 days
- Total artificial heart
- Intraaortic balloon pump
- Extracorporeal membrane oxygenator

B Mechanical circulatory support for >30 days with significant device-related complications such as thromboembolism, device infection, mechanical failure, or life-threatening ventricular arrhythmias

C Mechanical ventilation

D Continuous infusion of a single high-dose inotrope or multiple inotropes with hemodynamic monitoring

E Patient does not meet the above criteria but has a life expectancy without a heart transplant of <7 days

Status 1B

A patient listed as status 1B has at least one of the following devices or therapies in place:

A Left and/or right ventricular assist device implanted for >30 days

B Continuous infusion of inotropes

Status 2

A patient who does not meet the criteria for status 1A or 1B is listed as a status 2.

Status 7

A patient listed as status 7 is considered temporarily unsuitable to receive a thoracic organ transplant.

From United Network for Organ Sharing (UNOS) for allocation of Thoracic Organs.
*For complete detailed criteria, see actual policy at www.UNOS.org.

(most common) or other dysrhythmias may be present. Generalized edema expected until postoperative diuresis.

Respiratory: Clear throughout unless in rejection; then rales, rhonchi are possible. Chest tubes to 20-cm suction for first 24 h or until output <100 ml/8h. Ventilator initially with extubation expected 4-6 h postoperative. RR 12-20/min and unlabored.

Gastrointestinal: Initially bowel sounds (BS) inactive because of anesthesia, with gradual resumption of normal BS. May have some nausea and vomiting related to anesthetic agent and medications.

Genitourinary: Urine output initially decreased and then increased after warming as diuresis ensues.

Musculoskeletal: Weak but may experience more energy because of increase in cardiac output from new heart. HOB should be flat until extubated because of potential air trapped in the circulatory system when the donor heart was attached.

Pain: Incisional pain is expected.

Vital signs/hemodynamics: BP initially decreased and then normal (nl); HR maintained at ≥110. Temperature initially decreased and then nl with rewarming. CVP/PAWP initially increased or decreased and then nl. CO initially may be decreased and then nl. ECG nl sinus tachycardia with possible native P wave along with donor P wave.

Diagnostic studies

Laboratory studies: immediate postoperative period
- CBC: watch for increase in WBC count indicative of infection. Imuran can cause leukopenia.
- Hgb, Hct, platelets: may be decreased as a result of postoperative bleeding.
- Chemistry panel: assess electrolyte balance. Carefully monitor potassium (prevent dysrhythmias) and glucose (promote tissue healing).
- BUN/creatinine: assess renal function, especially with cyclosporine use.
- ABGs: initially, then pulse oximetry and end-tidal CO_2 for weaning purposes from ventilator.
- 12-Lead ECG: watch for atrial dysrhythmias and ventricular hypertrophy.

Daily laboratory studies
- Chemistry panels: electrolytes, liver and renal function. Steroids bind with albumin; may need less steroids if albumin low.
- PT and PTT: assessment of coagulation status.
- Chest x-ray: assessment of cardiac enlargement and pulmonary complications.
- Electrolytes plus BUN/creatinine or BUN/creatinine alone every afternoon to adjust PM dose of cyclosporine.
- Urine and sputum culture and sensitivity 1-3 times a week to monitor for infection.
- Cytomegalovirus (CMV) and toxoplasmosis cultures.
- Cyclosporine level daily.

COLLABORATIVE MANAGEMENT

Infection control: Infection control is paramount because of immunosuppression therapy.
- Betadine scrub for 5 min to initially enter room; then good hand washing thereafter.
- Keep door closed, and limit visitors; no employees or visitors with active infection; avoid taking care of other patients with infections.
- Leukocyte filter for blood administration.
- Remove lines and tubes as soon as possible.
- Sterile dressing changes for lines and wounds q24h and PRN.
- Clean large equipment brought into room with hospital disinfectant.
- Monitor temperature: >99.2° F may be sign of infection.

Rejection: The major complication of organ transplantation is the threat of rejection. When the recipient's body detects the new heart as a foreign object (antigen), the immune response is triggered. This inflammatory response causes infiltrates with fibrosis and scar formation in the heart muscle. Untreated rejection results in complete destruction of the heart (see p. 615 for more details). Signs of rejection include fever (>99.5° F); atrial dysrhythmias; decreased cardiac output/heart failure with syncope; peripheral edema; S_3, S_4; decreased urine output; jugular vein distention (JVD); hypotension; rales. Patient symptoms might include malaise, weakness, anorexia, nausea, vomiting, SOB, decreased activity tolerance.

Myocardial biopsy: Tiny pieces of muscle tissue are removed from the endocardium for pathologic examination to assess for tissue rejection. Performed in a cardiac cath lab/biopsy lab. Prophylactic antibiotics may be given. The cannulation site is generally the right internal jugular or sometimes the femoral vein. Biopsies are graded according to one of several grading systems (see pp. 617-618 in "Organ Rejection"). Biopsies are performed generally at 7 and 14 days postoperatively and at specified intervals thereafter.

Oxygenation: Extubate as soon as tolerated; prolonged mechanical ventilation is avoided. Supplemental O_2 PRN. Encourage frequent coughing and deep breathing.

Fluid management: I&O q1-2h. Evaluate urine output to assess volume status and kidney function. Fluid retention is common because of steroids and cyclosporine therapy, which may cause renal failure. Restrict fluids to 2000-3000 ml/day. Weigh daily.

Other

- Initially NPO with nasogastric tube (NGT) to low intermittent suction. Clear liquids after extubation if bowel sounds present. Advance to a low-fat, 4-gm sodium diet as tolerated.
- Activity: turn patient from side to side q2h if stable. On first postoperative day or after extubation up in chair. Advance activity as tolerated.
- Chest tubes to 20 cm suction. Assess for bleeding. Discontinue when drainage less than 100 ml in an 8-h period.
- Atrial/ventricular pacing PRN to keep heart rate >110/min. Commonly used to improve cardiac output and to avoid bradycardia as a result of an anoxic heart during transport. In addition, mild tachycardia reduces filling time, keeps the heart from excessive stretching, prevents right-sided failure, and decreases tension on suture lines.

Pharmacotherapy

Postoperative immunosuppression

Steroids: Solu-Medrol and prednisone: antiinflammatory agents used to suppress both T- and B-lymphocyte function, to reduce or prevent edema, promote normal capillary permeability, and prevent vasodilation. Can be used for maintenance to prevent rejection or as part of an acute rejection protocol. Side effects are numerous, including mood changes, sodium retention, blurred vision, fragile skin, bleeding, glucose intolerance, increase in appetite and subsequent weight gain, osteoporosis, "Moon face" appearance from an accumulation of fatty tissue on cheeks and upper back.

- Solu-Medrol—dosage: 125 mg IV q12h for 3 doses.
- Prednisone—30-35 mg PO q12h. Taper to as low a dose as tolerated.

Cyclosporine: Immunosuppressant. Dose adjusted according to daily blood levels and body weight. Dosage: 0.5 mg/kg/day is adjusted to maintain blood levels between 300 and 500 ng/ml. Side effects include kidney and renal dysfunction, excessive hair growth, hypertension, diarrhea, swelling and tenderness in gums, hand tremors, and increased risk of infections and tumors.

Azathioprine (Imuran): Immunosuppressant. WBC counts monitored, and dose adjusted accordingly. Taken once a day at bedtime. Maintenance dose is 2 mg/kg/day, maximum of 150-175 mg/day. Side effects include decreased WBC count, bone marrow suppression, toxic hepatitis, hair loss, mouth sores, and muscle wasting. Decrease or hold if WBC is <5.0.

OKT3: Orthoclone OKT®3 substituted for cyclosporine if patient is in perioperative hepatorenal dysfunction. Strong immunosuppressant used in acute rejection. 5-mg dose IV for 10 days. CD3 levels are measured daily to maintain adequate levels of OKT3. Side effects, usually seen after the first 1-3 days, include alterations in temperature control, bronchial smooth muscle tone, and GI tract. Fever, chills, nausea, vomiting, diarrhea, and pulmonary edema can result. During the first 1-3 days of OKT3 therapy, steroids are given at much higher doses. Imuran is continued and cyclosporine is added once the serum creatinine has decreased. When receiving OKT3, patients are premedicated with acetaminophen, H_2-receptor antagonist, and hydrocortisone (before) and diphenhydramine (after)

Tacrolimus: Prograf FK 506: Immunosuppressant similar but more potent than cyclosporine. Replaces cyclosporine if multiple rejections while on cyclosporine. Inhibits T-lymphocyte activation. Dosage depends on trough blood levels, organ function, and rejection status. Cleared through the liver and depends on liver function. Dosage 0.15mg/kg/day IV given in two divided doses 12 h apart, followed by a PO dose of 0.3 mg/kg/day after GI function has

Research Brief 4-8   Research conducted by Grady, Jalowiec, and White-Williams (1999) studied 232 patients 1 year after heart transplant and found that patients do fairly well and, generally, would do it all over again. These patients were most satisfied with their social interactions and family relationships and least satisfied with the psychologic aspects of their life related to their appearance and what they could accomplish. The authors further identified predictors of better quality of life, which include less stress, more helpfulness of information, better health perception, better compliance with the transplant regimen, more effective coping, less functional disability, less symptom distress, older age, and fewer complications. The understanding of these predictors can assist the health care professional to identify patients at risk and assist those who may experience a less-than-optimal quality of life.

Grady K, Jalowiec A, White-Williams C: Predictors of quality of life in patients at one year after heart transplantation, *J Heart Lung Transplant* 18(3):202-210, 1999.

returned. Should be given on an empty stomach without other medications. Side effects are dose related and diminish when dose is decreased. They include hyperkalemia, nephrotoxicity, glucose intolerance, hypertension, nausea, diarrhea, infections, and lymphoproliferative disorders. Consult pharmacist before administering.

Others
Antibiotics: Kefzol or similar antibiotic is given until chest tubes are removed. Ganciclovir: prophylaxis and treatment for CMV. Given IV postoperatively and changed to PO when tolerated. CMV remains the major cause of morbidity and mortality with cardiac transplantation patients.
Mycostatin: 5 ml swish and swallow or Mycelex troche tid beginning after extubation, for potential secondary candida infections related to immunosuppression.
H_2-blocker: For gastric secretion suppression.
Inotropic medications: Nitroglycerin to decrease preload; nitroprusside (Nipride) to decrease afterload; dobutamine to increase contractility/CO; epinephrine to increase heart rate and contractility; norepinephrine to increase BP; milrinone (Primacor) to increase contractility/CO and decrease afterload; dopamine for renal perfusion in smaller doses, and increase HR and BP at higher doses; and isoproterenol (Isuprel) (very common to increase heart rate and decrease pulmonary vascular resistance).
Calcium channel blockers: Used to control hypertension.
Pain: Fentanyl is commonly used because it is short acting and does not cause histamine-mediated hypotension as morphine does.
Pretransplant and posttransplant sensitization: Poor outcomes, such as coronary artery disease, and an increased incidence of rejection have been associated with pretransplant sensitization. Positive panel-reactive antibody (PRA) levels detect circulating human leukocyte antigens (HLA) and reflect level of sensitization. Pregnancy, blood transfusion, or previous transplants can trigger sensitization. Elevated PRA levels increase the difficulty of finding an HLA-compatible donor heart. HLA-compatible hearts will enhance graft survival and reduce infection and malignancies related to aggressive immunosuppression. Plasmapheresis may decrease sensitization and reduce PRA levels.

NURSING DIAGNOSES AND INTERVENTIONS
Risk for injury: (rejection) related to inadequate immunosuppressant drug levels
Desired outcomes: No signs of rejection (clinical or with biopsy); patient and staff are compliant with immunosuppression therapy.

- Assess patient's knowledge of drug therapy.
- Monitor blood levels as appropriate for drug.
- Instruct patient to take medication at designated time(s) each day. Never withhold immunosuppressant without consulting with physician.
- Monitor for signs of rejection: atrial fibrillation or other dysrhythmias; hypotension; increase in temperature; decrease in cardiac output; or malaise.
- Reinforce necessity of regularly scheduled appointments with transplant coordinator. Encourage patient to bring a significant other to the visit.

Risk for infection related to immunosuppression

Desired outcomes: Infections will be absent or minimized; if signs and symptoms occur, the patient will report within 1-4 h.

- Patient is to wear mask when outside immediate living area, in public areas, or near construction.
- Notify physician/transplant coordinator immediately if temperature >99.5° F; WBC increasing; patient complaints of malaise; or any obvious infection.
- Avoid placement of indwelling catheters; if necessary, remove as soon as possible.

NIC Infection Control; Infection Protection

Decreased cardiac output related to rejection; inadequate donor pump/long ischemic time

Desired outcomes: The patient will have an adequate cardiac output as evidenced by a systolic BP >90-100; MAP 65-85; CI >2.2 L/min; RR 12-20 breaths/min; and HR >100 bpm; regular sinus rhythm without ectopy; urinary output >0.5 ml/kg/h; intake equals output; and ejection fraction >60%.

- Consult MD for:
  - ☐ Signs and symptoms of infection: temperature >99.5° F; increased WBC count; or changes in drainage from incisions.
  - ☐ Signs and symptoms of rejection: atrial or ventricular dysrhythmias; temperature >99.5° F; decreased BP; decreased CO/CI; malaise; anorexia; nausea and vomiting, activity intolerance, or SOB.
  - ☐ Increase in chest tube output to >400 ml/h or sudden cessation of chest tube output.
  - ☐ Svo_2 <60%; SBP <90; CI <2.2.
  - ☐ Any other abnormal lab results.

NIC Hemodynamic Regulation

Caring for patients undergoing coronary artery thrombolysis

PATHOPHYSIOLOGY

Acute thrombus formation with coronary artery occlusion is the most common cause of AMI. During the initial phase of injury, the development of necrosis typically starts with the subendocardial layer and spreads to the epicardial layer of heart muscle. Early reperfusion of an ischemic myocardium can prevent or reduce myocardial injury. Therefore the ability to dissolve (lyse) fresh coronary thromboses early in the course of infarction is essential to salvage myocardial tissue and preserve ventricular function. The goal of thrombolysis is to reduce infarct size, improve left ventricular function, and minimize morbidity and mortality. Thrombolytic therapy is a safe and effective way to establish reperfusion for patients with AMI secondary to complete or partial coronary arterial thrombotic occlusion.

Thrombolytic agents act to dissolve or lyse existing clots. A clot, or thrombus, is formed when deposits of fibrin collect within the artery and form an insoluble matrix. The fibrin clot eventually is broken down by the naturally occurring enzyme, *plasmin.* Thrombolytic agents work to accelerate this natural process by converting plasminogen to plasmin, which rapidly dissolves the fibrin clot. However, plasmin also breaks down circulating clotting proteins, thus producing excessive fibrin/fibrinogen degradation products (FDPs). The presence of large amounts of FDPs results in significant systemic anticoagulation and can trigger bleeding complications.

First-generation thrombolytics (streptokinase, anistreplase) are nonfibrin selective and activate both fibrin-bound and nonfibrin-bound plasminogen. Alteplase (rt-PA), a second-generation thrombolytic, is fibrin selective or "clot specific" and preferentially activates fibrin-bound plasminogen. Alteplase is also approved for use in management of acute ischemic stroke and massive pulmonary embolism. Retavase (Reteplase) is a deletion mutein of tissue plasminogen activator (t-PA) and is the most recent thrombolytic, with actions that are not as clot specific as t-PA.

Indications that lysis has taken place include decreased chest pain; rapid resolution of ST-segment depression; and a new onset of dysrhythmias. As many as 80% of patients are reported to have had reperfusion dysrhythmias, primarily accelerated idioventricular rhythm and PVCs. Bradycardia and heart block also are seen.

After clot lysis occurs, thrombin is released into the circulation. The thrombin induces platelet clumping and increases the potential for reocclusion. Use of thrombolytic agents results in excessive circulating thrombin and increases the risk of coronary artery reocclusion. Heparin and antiplatelet agents are used as adjuncts to thrombolytic therapy to inhibit the action of free thrombin and prevent reocclusion. GPIIB/IIIA inhibitors (e.g. abciximab [ReoPro]; eptifibatide [Integrilin]; tirofiban [Aggrastat]) are being studied for use with thrombolysis to assist in prevention of reocclusion of clot-lysed vessels.

ASSESSMENT

History and risk factors: Presence of cardiac risk factors (see "Acute Coronary Syndrome," p. 247). Assess patient for absolute and relative contraindications for thrombolytic therapy (Table 4-26). Assess for recent (within 6 mo) streptococcal infection when use of streptokinase or anistreplase is anticipated. Assess for aspirin allergy, since antiplatelet therapy with aspirin usually is initiated.

Subjective findings: Candidates for thrombolytic therapy include patients with clear symptoms of AMI: usually, sudden onset of chest pain/pressure that is unrelieved by sublingual nitrates and lasts >30 min but <6-12 h. The pain may radiate to the neck, jaw, and arms. Intermittent, severe chest pain over hours or days can indicate subtotal occlusion secondary to coronary thrombosis, and these patients also may be considered for thrombolytic therapy. Diaphoresis, nausea, vomiting, anxiety, and other symptoms consistent with the diagnosis of AMI may be present.

Selection of candidates for thrombolytic therapy relies heavily on clinical history and physical examination. The presentation of aortic dissection and acute pericarditis is similar to that of AMI, and these diagnoses must be excluded before proceeding with thrombolytic therapy.

Objective findings: The patient may experience tachycardia, bradycardia, irregular pulse, hypotension, and other findings consistent with AMI (see p. 249). Assess patient for absolute and relative contraindications for thrombolytic therapy (Table 4-26). Assess for and note all venipuncture attempts and superficial injuries that could become active bleeding sites after thrombolysis. Perform a careful baseline neurologic assessment for comparison of subsequent examinations, which are indicated to detect neurologic changes associated with acute stroke.

DIAGNOSTIC TESTS

ECG: 12/15/18-lead ECG is performed to determine presence, location, and extent of myocardial injury. Localized ST-segment elevation of 1 mm in 2 contiguous leads, significant Q waves, and T-wave inversion are findings

**TABLE 4-26   Contraindications and Warnings for Thrombolytic
Therapy**

Contraindications

   Known hypersensitivity to thrombolytic agents
   Active internal bleeding
   History of stroke
   Recent intracranial or intraspinal surgery or trauma
   Known bleeding diathesis
   Severe, uncontrolled hypertension

*Warnings (risks may be increased and should be weighed against
   anticipated benefits)*

   Recent major surgery (e.g., coronary artery bypass graft, obstetrical delivery,
      organ biopsy)
   Previous puncture of noncompressible vessels
   Cerebrovascular disease
   Recent gastrointestinal or genitourinary bleeding
   Recent trauma
   Hypertension (systolic BP ≥180 mm Hg and/or diastolic BP ≥110 mm Hg)
   High likelihood of left heart thrombus (e.g., mitral stenosis with atrial
      fibrillation)
   Acute pericarditis
   Subacute bacterial endocarditis
   Hemostatic defects including those secondary to severe hepatic or renal
      disease
   Severe hepatic or renal dysfunction
   Pregnancy
   Diabetic hemorrhagic retinopathy or other hemorrhagic ophthalmic conditions
   Septic thrombophlebitis or occluded AV cannula at a seriously infected site
   Advanced age
   Currently receiving anticoagulants (e.g., warfarin sodium)
   Any other condition in which bleeding constitutes a significant hazard or
      would be particularly difficult to manage because of its location

---

AV, Arteriovenous.

associated with AMI. ST-segment elevation that decreases after administration
of sublingual NTG suggests coronary artery spasm (Prinzmetal angina), and
thrombolytic therapy is not indicated.

Laboratory studies: Serum enzymes, including cardiac enzymes, troponins,
myoglobin and isoenzymes (e.g., MB bands, MB2:MB1), electrolytes, CBC,
and clotting studies are evaluated before initiating thrombolytic therapy. A
heparin-lock device is used for specimen collection. Do not delay therapy for
confirmation of laboratory values.

COLLABORATIVE MANAGEMENT

Thrombolytics: Prompt identification of candidates for thrombolytic therapy
and rapid initiation of therapy increase the effectiveness of all thrombolytic
agents. Because time is crucial, initiation of thrombolytic therapy may occur in
the prehospital setting or in the emergency department of a smaller hospital
before transfer to a definitive care center. In these settings the thrombolytic
agents are administered peripherally. In other cases thrombolytic agents are
started in the catheterization laboratory, where they are administered via the

intracoronary route while the patient is undergoing fluoroscopic examination. Ideally, thrombolytic therapy is initiated within 30 min of the patient's arrival at the hospital's emergency department. Patients with AMI must be identified expediently and treated rapidly. Table 4-27 compares thrombolytic agents that are in general use.

First-generation thrombolytics

- *Streptokinase:* An enzyme derived from group C β-hemolytic strepto-cocci, it acts as a catalyst for the conversion of plasminogen to plasmin, which lyses the clot. Streptokinase can be administered IV or via the intracoronary route. Because it is an antigen, patients who have had previous exposure to streptococcal organisms may have antibodies against streptokinase. Therefore steroids or antihistamines are adminis-tered before streptokinase therapy to prevent a hypersensitivity reaction. Usual dosage is 1.5 million IU, given IV as a continuous infusion over 60 min.

- *Anistreplase:* A plasminogen activator that induces clot lysis with fewer systemic lytic effects than does streptokinase. Allergic and anaphylactic reactions are possible. Usual dose is 30 IU by IV injection over 2-5 min.

Second-generation thrombolytics

- *Alteplase:* A recombinant tissue plasminogen activator (rt-PA) with the same amino acid sequence as endogenous t-PA. Has clot-specific effects, wherein plasminogen is converted to plasmin only after binding to the fibrin clot. There are no systemic lytic effects, it is non-antigenic, and it has a shorter half-life than do the other agents. Several dosage regimens are approved for coronary thrombolysis:

  ☐ *Accelerated infusions, weight based:* total dose is not to exceed 100 mg. For patients weighing >67 kg, the recommended dose is 100 mg given as a 15-mg IV bolus, followed by a 50-mg infusion over the next 30 min and then 35 mg infused over the next 60 min. For patients weighing <67 kg, a 15-mg IV bolus is given, followed by a 0.75-mg/kg infusion (not to exceed 50 mg) over the next 30 min and then 0.50 mg/kg (not to exceed 35 mg) infused over the next 60 min. The accelerated dosing has been studied only with concomitant use of a heparin infusion (following the drug) and aspirin. The half-life is less than 5 min, and the drug is cleared mainly by the liver.

  ☐ *3-Hour infusion:* 100-mg total dose, administered 60 mg in the first hour (a 6- to 10-mg IV bolus followed by 50- to 54-mg IV infusion); then 20 mg infused over the second hour and 20 mg infused over the third hour. The 3-h infusion is typically followed by a heparin infusion, aspirin, and/or dipyridamole.

- *Reteplase:* a recombinant deletion mutein of tissue plasminogen activator (t-PA), including 355 of the 527 amino acids of native t-PA. Catalyzes cleavage of endogenous plasminogen to generate plasmin. Is not clot specific, so fibrinogen levels fall to lower than seen with rt-PA (alteplase), with a return to baseline value within 48 h after infusion. The half-life is 13-16 min, and the drug is cleared by the liver and kidneys. Dosage: given as two boluses; each over 2 min. An initial 10-mg bolus is given, followed by the second 10-mg bolus 30 min after the initial bolus.

Adjunctive therapy: Standard therapy for AMI is initiated, including oxygen administration, continuous ECG monitoring, nitrates, IV analgesia, β-blockade, and other therapies as indicated. Heparin and antiplatelet agents are given concurrently with thrombolytic therapy to prevent reocclusion.

Coronary angiography: May be performed to assess for patency or reocclusion. Because of the systemic lytic effects of all thrombolytics, it is best to wait 24-48 h after initial thrombolytic therapy. May be used also before "rescue angioplasty" for patients who are given thrombolytics and either reocclude or do not reperfuse after the infusion. See discussion in "Acute Myocardial Infarction," p. 249.

TABLE 4-27   Thrombolytic Dosage Regimens

Name of agent: generic and brands	Streptokinase (Kabikinase, Streptase)	Anistreplase (APSAC, Eminase)	Reteplase (Retavase)	Alteplase (Activase)	Alteplase (Activase)	Alteplase (Activase)
Total time of regimen	Original 30-60 min	Original 2-5 min	Original 30 min	Accelerated 90 min	Accelerated 90 min	Original 180 min
Initial IV bolus		30 units over 2-5 min	10 units over 2 min	15 mg	15 mg	6-10 mg
Second IV bolus at time: 30 min			10 units over 2 min			
Infusion from time 0-≥30 min	1.5 million units IV over 30-60 minutes			Patient weight >67 kg: 50 mg	Patient weight ≤67 kg: 0.75 mg/kg	
Infusion from time 0-60 min						50-54 mg
Infusion from time 30-90 min				35 mg	0.50 mg/kg	
Infusion from time 60-120 min						20 mg
Infusion from time 120-180 min						20 mg
Total dose	1.5 million units	30 units	20 units	100 mg	Varies by weight	100 mg

NURSING DIAGNOSES AND INTERVENTIONS

Pain related to myocardial ischemia; injury; infarction
Desired outcome: Patient's subjective perception of pain decreases within 30 min of onset, as documented by a pain scale.
- Assess location, character, intensity, and duration, using a pain scale. Assess associated symptoms, including SOB, restlessness, diaphoresis, and grimacing.
- Run an ECG rhythm strip and consider obtaining a 12/15/18-lead ECG, per hospital protocol, for episodes of chest discomfort or arm, shoulder, back, or jaw pain.
- Record vital signs during each episode of pain associated with myocardial ischemia.
- Administer prescribed analgesics (e.g., morphine sulfate) and document, compare, and report results of analgesia, as necessary or per protocol.
- Administer oxygen as prescribed, with humidity to reduce the drying effects on oral and nasal mucosa.
- Position the patient in semi-Fowler's position to reduce cardiac workload unless the patient is intolerant of having the head of bed elevated because of hypotension.
- Provide reassurance during episodes of discomfort; stay with the patient to assess for acute changes in assessment or vital signs.

NIC Analgesic Administration; Anxiety Reduction; Calming Technique; Cardiac Care: Acute; Cardiac Precautions; Oxygen Therapy

Knowledge deficit: the atherosclerotic process and the rationale, procedure, and expected outcomes of thrombolytic therapy
Desired outcome: Before initiation of the thrombolytic therapy, patient verbalizes basic knowledge about the atherosclerotic process and thrombolytic therapy.
- Assess patient's knowledge about the atherosclerotic process and the rationale, procedure, and expected outcome of thrombolytic therapy. Explain the goal of therapy: to reduce injury to the heart muscle.
- Explain the need for monitoring and close postprocedural observation.
- Provide emotional support during the procedure, keeping the patient informed about the events that are taking place.
- After the procedure, discuss potential long-term outcomes and the possibility of reocclusion, including interventions the patient can take to prevent it: take prescribed antiplatelet medications; exercise; comply with dietary modifications; and manage or eliminate risk factors such as smoking, hyperlipidemia, hypertension, stress, and obesity.
- Before discharge, instruct patient to report any signs and symptoms of MI that occur after hospitalization: unrelenting chest heaviness or pressure; pain that radiates to the arm, neck, or jaw; accompanying nausea and diaphoresis; and lightheadedness or dizziness.

NIC Teaching: Individual; Teaching: Disease Process

Altered protection related to risk of bleeding/hemorrhage secondary to nonspecific thrombolytic effects of therapy
Desired outcome: Symptoms of bleeding complications are absent as evidenced by BP within patient's normal range; HR ≤100 bpm; blood-free secretions and excretions; natural skin color; baseline or normal LOC; and absence of back and abdominal pain, hematoma, headache, dizziness, and vomiting.
- When patient is admitted, obtain a thorough history, assessing for the following:
  ☐ Risk factors for intracranial hemorrhage: uncontrolled hypertension; cerebrovascular pathology; CNS surgery within previous 6 mo.
  ☐ Bleeding risks: recent or active GI bleeding; recent trauma; recent surgery; bleeding diathesis; advanced liver or kidney disease.

☐ Risk of systemic embolization: suspected left-sided heart thrombus.

☐ History of streptococcal infection or previous streptokinase therapy.

• Monitor clotting studies per agency protocol. Regulate heparin drip to maintain PTT at 1½-2 times control levels or according to protocol. *Never* discontinue heparin without physician's directive.

• Apply pressure dressing over puncture site if cardiac catheterization was performed. Inspect site at frequent intervals for evidence of hematoma formation. Immobilize extremity for 6-8 h after catheterization procedure.

• Avoid unnecessary venipunctures, IM injections, or arterial puncture. Obtain laboratory specimens from heparin-lock device.

• Monitor patient for indicators of internal bleeding: back pain; abdominal pain; decreased BP; pallor; and bloody stool or urine. Report significant findings to physician.

• Monitor patient for signs of intracranial bleeding q2h: change in LOC; headache; dizziness; vomiting; and confusion.

• Test all stools, urine, and emesis for occult blood.

• Use care with oral hygiene and when shaving patient. For more information about safety precautions, see **Altered protection** in "Pulmonary Emboli," p. 238.

NIC Bleeding Reduction; Bleeding Precautions; Surveillance; Hemorrhage Control; Neurologic Monitoring

Decreased cardiac output (or risk for same) related to alterations in rate, rhythm, and conduction secondary to increased irritability of ischemic tissue during reperfusion (usually occurs within 1-2 h after initiation of therapy); reocclusion of thrombolysed vessels; negative inotropic changes secondary to cardiac disease.

Desired outcomes: Within 12 h of initiation of thrombolytic therapy, patient has adequate cardiac output as evidenced by normal sinus rhythm on ECG; peripheral pulses >2+ on a 0-4+ scale; warm and dry skin; and hourly urine output ≥0.5 ml/kg/h. Patient is awake, alert, and oriented without palpitations, chest pain, or dizziness. Within 48 h of initiation of thrombolytic therapy, patient maintains stability as just described.

> **Note:** Reocclusion occurs in as many as 16% of patients within 24-48 h after thrombolysis.

• Monitor ECG continuously during thrombolytic therapy for evidence of dysrhythmias. Consult physician for significant dysrhythmias.

• With any dysrhythmia, check VS and note accompanying signs and symptoms such as dizziness, lightheadedness, syncope, and palpitations.

• Ensure availability of emergency drugs and equipment: atropine; isoproterenol; epinephrine; amiodarone; lidocaine (use cautiously with AMI); defibrillator-cardioverter; external and transvenous pacemaker.

• Evaluate patient's response to medications and emergency treatment.

• Monitor patient for signs of reocclusion: chest pain; nausea; diaphoresis; and dysrhythmias. Consult physician for any signs of reocclusion.

• Obtain 12/15/18-lead ECG if reocclusion is suspected.

• Anticipate and prepare patient for cardiac catheterization, PTCA, PTCA with stent, or repeated thrombolytic therapy.

NIC Hemodynamic Regulation; Circulatory Care; Dysrhythmia Management; Cardiac Care: Acute

Risk for injury related to potential for allergic or anaphylactic reaction to streptokinase or anistreplase secondary to antigen/antibody response

Desired outcome: Patient has no symptoms of allergic response as evidenced by normothermia; RR 12-20 breaths/min with normal pattern and depth (eupnea); HR ≤100 bpm; BP at baseline or within normal limits; natural skin color; and absence of itching, urticaria, headache, muscular and abdominal pain, and nausea.

- Before treatment, question patient about history of previous streptokinase therapy or streptococcal infection. Consult physician for positive findings.
- Administer prophylactic hydrocortisone as prescribed.
- Monitor patient during and for 48-72 h after infusion for indicators of allergy: hypotension (brief or sustained); urticaria; fever; itching; flushing; nausea; headache; muscular pain; bronchospasm; abdominal pain; dyspnea; or tachycardia. These indicators can appear immediately after or as long as several days after streptokinase therapy.
- If hypotension develops, increase rate of IV infusion/administer volume replacement as prescribed. Prepare for vasopressor administration if there is no response to volume replacement.
- Treat allergic response with diphenhydramine or other antihistamine as prescribed.

NIC Shock Management: Vasogenic; Shock Management

Bibliography

Alexander RW, Schlant RC, Fuster V, editors: *Hurst the heart,* ed 9, New York, 1998, McGraw-Hill.

American Heart Association: *Textbook of advanced cardiac life support,* Dallas, Tex, 1994, The Association.

American Heart Association: *1997 Heart and stroke statistical update,* Dallas, Tex, 1997, The Association.

Anderson J: Acute treatment of atrial fibrillation and flutter, *Am J Cardiol* 78(8A):17-21, 1996.

Antman EM, Braunwald E: Acute myocardial infarction. In Braunwald E, editor: *Heart disease: a textbook of cardiovascular medicine,* ed 5, Philadelphia, 1997, Saunders.

Argenziano M, Michler RE, Rose EA: Cardiac transplantation for endstage heart disease, *Heart Vessels* 12:23-27, 1997.

Baas LS: Pericarditis. In *Teaching patients with acute conditions,* Springhouse, Pa, 1992, Springhouse.

Baas LS, Meissner JE: Cardiovascular care. In *Illustrated manual of nursing practice,* ed 2, Springhouse, Pa, 1994, Springhouse.

Barron HV et al: For the NRMI 2 investigators. Regional variation in the treatment of women with acute myocardial infarction in the United States: data from the National Registry of Myocardial Infarction 2 (NRMI 2), *Circulation* 96:3002A, 1997.

Barron HV et al: For the NRMI 2 investigators. Utilization of reperfusion therapy for acute myocardial infarction in the United States: data from the National Registry of Myocardial Infarction 2 (NRMI 2), *Circulation* 97(12):1150-1156, 1998.

Berkowitz SD et al: Incidence and predictors of bleeding after contemporary thrombolytic therapy for myocardial infarction, *Circulation* 95:2508-2516, 1997.

Bittel C: Pre and post cardiac transplantation. In Keen JH, Swearingen PL, editors: *Mosby's critical care nursing consultant,* St Louis, 1997, Mosby.

Boggs R, Woolbridge-King M: *AACN procedure manual for critical care,* ed 3, Philadelphia, 1993, Saunders.

Bonow RO et al: ACC/AHA guidelines for the management of patients with valvular heart disease: executive summary, *Circulation* 98:1949-1984, 1998.

Braunwald E: Pathophysiology of heart failure. In Braunwald E, editor: *Heart disease: a textbook of cardiovascular medicine,* ed 5, Philadelphia, 1997, Saunders.

Bridges MEJ, Woods SL: Cardiovascular chronobiology: implications for critical care nursing, *Crit Care Nurse* 18(4):49-64, 1998.

Burke GW et al: Removal of preformed cytotoxic antibody using Prosorba (Staph Protein-A-Silica) column without immunosuppression, *Transplant Proc* 29:2249-2251, 1997.

Burke L: Securing life through technology acceptance: the first six months after transvenous internal cardioverter defibrillator implantation, *Heart Lung* 25:352-366, 1996.

Casas RE, Marriott HJL, Glancy DL: Value of leads V_7-V_9 in diagnosing posterior wall acute myocardial infarction and other causes of tall R waves in V_1-V_2, *Am J Cardiol* 79:508-509, 1997.

Chase SL: New strategies in the management of patients with heart failure, *Pharmacol Ther,* Feb:84-96, 1999.

Chernecky CC, Berger BJ: *Laboratory tests and diagnostic procedures,* ed 2, Philadelphia, 1997, Saunders.

Cohn JN: The management of chronic heart failure, *N Engl J Med* 335:490-498, 1996.

Collins MA: When your patient has an implantable cardioverter defibrillator, *Am J Nurs* 94(3):34-39, 1994.

Conti CV: Thoracic transplantation in 1998, *Md Med J* 47(5):235-240, 1998.

Copeland JG: Current status and future directions for a total artificial heart with a past, *Artif Organs* 22(11):998-1001, 1998.

Darovic GO: Cardiovascular anatomy and physiology. In Darovic GO: *Hemodynamic monitoring: invasive and non-invasive clinical application,* Philadelphia, 1995, Saunders.

Dracup K, Dunbar SB, Baker DW: Rethinking heart failure, *Am J Nurs* 95(7):22-28, 1995.

Dunnington CS: Sotalol hydrochloride (Betapace): a new antiarrhythmic drug, *Am J Crit Care* 2(5):397-406, 1993.

Eichhorn EJ, Bristow MR: Practical guidelines for initiation of β-adrenergic blockade in patients with chronic heart failure, *Am J Cardiol* 79:794-798, 1997.

Fibrinolytic Therapy Trialists Collaborative Group: Indications for fibrinolytic therapy in suspected acute myocardial infarction: collaborative overview of early mortality and major morbidity results from all randomized trials of more than 1000 patients, *Lancet* 343:311-322, 1994.

Futterman LG, Lemberg L: Radiofrequency catheter ablation for supraventricular tachycardias, *Am J Crit Care* 2(6):500-505, 1993.

Gilbert EM et al: Comparative hemodynamic, left ventricular functional and antiadrenergic effects of chronic treatment with metoprolol versus carvedilol in the failing heart, *Circulation* 94(11):2817-2825, 1996.

Giuliano KK, Warren-Sims T: Transplant issues: infections and immunosuppressant drugs, *Dimens Crit Care Nurs* 18(2):16-19, 1999.

Goldman DS, Hogan TT: Nitrate-tolerance update: mechanism and management, *Pharmacol Ther,* Feb:67-73, 1999.

Grady K, Jalowiec A, White-Williams C: Predictors of quality of life in patients at one year after heart transplantation, *J Heart Lung Transplant* 18(3):202-210, 1999.

Hamm CW et al: Emergency room triage of patients with acute chest pain by means of rapid testing for cardiac troponin T or troponin I, *N Engl J Med* 3337:1648-1653, 1997.

Heidenreich PA, Lee TT, Massie BM: Effects of β-blockade on mortality in patients with heart failure: a meta-analysis of randomized clinical trials, *J Am Coll Cardiol* 30(1):27-34, 1997.

Henning RJ et al: Specific monitoring considerations for patients with cardiac disease. In Darovic GO: *Hemodynamic monitoring: invasive and noninvasive clinical application,* Philadelphia, 1995, Saunders.

Hodgson B, Kizior R: *Saunders' nursing drug handbook,* Philadelphia, 1998, Saunders.

Interqual: *The ISD-A review system with adult ISD criteria,* North Hampton, NH, and Marlboro, Mass, Aug, 1992, Interqual.

Joint National Committee: The fifth report of the Joint National Committee on detection, evaluation, and treatment of high blood pressure (JNC V), *Arch Intern Med* 153:154-183, 1993.

Keen J: *Mosby's critical care and emergency drug reference,* ed 2, St Louis, 1996, Mosby.

Kerber RE: Transthoracic cardioversion of atrial fibrillation and flutter: standard techniques and new advances, *Am J Cardiol* 78(8A):22-26, 1996.

Kim MJ, McFarland GK, McLane AM: *Pocket guide to nursing diagnoses,* ed 7, St Louis, 1997, Mosby.

Kinney MR et al: *AACN's clinical reference for critical-care nursing,* ed 4, St Louis, 1998, Mosby.

Kline-Rogers E, Martin JS, Smith DD: New era of reperfusion in acute myocardial infarction, *Crit Care Nurse* 19(1):21-33, 1999.

Knight L et al: Caring for patients with third generation implantable cardioverter defibrillators: from decision to implant to patient's return home, *Crit Care Nurse* 17(5):46-63, 1997.

Kobashigawa JA: Mycophenolate mofetil in cardiac transplantation, *Curr Opin Cardiol* 13(2):117-121, 1998.

Logston Boggs R, Wooldridge-King M, editors: Organ procurement. In *AACN procedure manual for critical care,* ed 3, Philadelphia, 1993, Saunders.

Mair J et al:. A decision tree for the early diagnosis of acute myocardial infarction in nontraumatic chest pain patients at hospital admission, *Chest* 108:1502-1509, 1995.

Meiser BM et al: Combination therapy with tacrolimus and mycophenolate mofetil following cardiac transplantation: importance of mycophenolic acid therapeutic drug monitoring, *J Heart Lung Transplant* 18(2):143-149, 1999.

Moriguchi JD et al: *Pre-transplant panel reactive antibodies are associated with increased risk of transplant coronary artery disease in cardiac transplant recipients.* Presented at Thoracic Transplantation 1999: In the next millennium, Vail, Colo, March 1999.

Murphy M, Garcia JS, Ramazinski C: Improving the admission process from the emergency department to the critical care areas, *Nurs Clin North Am* 30:31-43, 1995.

Murphy MJ, Berding CB: Use of measurements of myoglobin and cardiac troponins in the diagnosis of acute myocardial infarction, *Crit Care Nurse* 19(1):58-66, 1999.

Myerburg RJ, Castellanos A: Cardiac arrest and sudden cardiac death. In Braunwald E, editor: *Heart disease,* ed 5, Philadelphia, 1997, Saunders.

NASA-JSC Ventricular Assist Device, 1999. website: www.jsc.nasagov

Novacor-Baxter Health Care, Deerfield, Illinois © 1995-2000. website: www.baxtercvg.com/mp/n/n-full.html

O'Connell JB et al: Cardiac transplantation: recipient selection, donor procurement, and medical follow-up, *Circulation* 86(3):1061-1079, 1992.

Olivari MT et al: Treatment of acute vascular rejection with immunoadsorption, *Circulation* 90(5)(part 2):70-73, 1994.

Parnis SM, Conger JL, Fuqua JM: Progress in the development of a transcutaneously powered axial flow blood pump ventricular assist system, *ASAIO J* 43(5):576-580, 1997.

Piano MR et al: The molecular and cellular pathophysiology of heart failure, *Heart Lung* 27:3-19, 1998.

Porterfield LM: The cutting edge in arrhythmias, *Crit Care Nurse* (suppl), June 1993.

Pratt NG: Pathophysiology of heart failure: neuroendocrine response, *Crit Care Nurse Q* 18(1):22-31, 1995.

Rawles J: Should patients with suspected acute myocardial infarction without ST elevation be given thrombolytic therapy? *Eur Heart J* 18:899-906, 1997.

Ross DG: Pacemakers. In Swearingen P, Ross DG: *Manual of medical-surgical nursing care,* ed 4, St Louis, 1998, Mosby.

Ross DG, McDonough MB: Dysrhythmias and conduction disturbances. In Swearingen P, Ross DG: *Manual of medical-surgical nursing care,* ed 4, St Louis, 1998, Mosby.

Ryan TJ, Gunner RM: Improving the odds in acute myocardial infarction, *Hosp Pract,* Sept:97-121, 1997.

Ryan TJ et al: ACC/AHA guidelines for the management of patients with acute myocardial infarction: a report of the American College of Cardiology/American Heart Association Task Force on Practice Guidelines (Committee on Management of Acute Myocardial Infarction), *J Am Coll Cardiol* 28:1328-1428, 1996.

Saint Joseph's Hospital of Atlanta: *Policies, procedures, transplant programs and transplant classes,* 1998-99.

Sayre MR, Gibler WB: New approaches to ruling out acute ischemic coronary syndrome in the emergency department, *Ann Intern Med* 27:75-78, 1996.

Schmid C et al: Cerebral and systemic embolization during left ventricular support with the Novacor N100 device, *Ann Thorac Surg* 65(6):1703-1710, 1998.

Selker HP et al: An evaluation of technologies for identifying acute cardiac ischemia in the emergency department: The National Heart Attack Alert Program Working Group Report, *Ann Emerg Med* 29:59-69, 1997.

Smalling RW: Molecular biology of plasminogen activators: what are the clinical implications of drug design? *Am J Cardiol* 78 (Suppl 12A):2-7, 1996.

Smith TW et al: Management of heart failure. In Braunwald E, editor: *Heart disease: a textbook of cardiovascular medicine,* ed 5, Philadelphia, 1997, Saunders.

Society of Critical Care Medicine: Current concepts in dysrhythmia management. In SCCM: *1998 Educational and scientific symposium highlights,* pp. 5-8, Anaheim, Calif, 1998, The Society.

Starling RC: Radical alternatives to transplantation, *Curr Opin Cardiol* 12:166-171, 1997.

Steward S, Kucia A, Poropat S: Early detection and management of right ventricular infarction: the role of the critical care nurse, *Dimens Crit Care Nurs* 14(6):282-292, 1995.

Tahan HA: Patients waiting for heart transplantation: an analysis of vulnerability, *Crit Care Nurse* 18(24):40-48, 1998.

Thermo Cardiosystems Inc. (TCI): *Heartmate Vented Electric LVAS and Implantable Pneumatic LVAS,* Woburn, Mass, 1999.

United Network of Organ Sharing (UNOS): Policy 3.7, Effective January 20th, 1999. *(See actual policy for detailed criteria and rules.)*

Waldo AL, Pratt CM: Introduction: acute treatment of atrial fibrillation and flutter in perspective, *Am J Cardiol* 78(8A):1-2, 1996.

Wallace CJ: Dual-chamber pacemakers in the management of severe heart failure, *Crit Care Nurse* 18:57-67, 1998.

Young JB: Carvedilol for heart failure: renewed interest in β-blockers, *J Med* 4(8):415-422, 1997.

Zalenski R et al: Value of posterior and right ventricular leads in comparison to the standard 12-lead electrocardiogram in evaluation of ST segment elevation in suspected acute myocardial infarction, *Am J Cardiol* 79:1579-1585, 1997.

Zamora M: *Cytomegalovirus prophylaxis following thoracic transplantation: clinical outcomes and cost-efficacy.* Presented at Thoracic Transplantation 1999: In the next millennium, Vail, Colo, March 1999.

CHAPTER 5

Renal-Urinary Dysfunctions

Acute renal failure

PATHOPHYSIOLOGY

Acute renal failure (ARF) is a syndrome characterized by an abrupt deterioration of renal function, resulting in the accumulation of metabolic wastes, fluids, and electrolytes, usually accompanied by a marked decline in urinary output. If it is undetected or treated inadequately, ARF can lead to parenchymal damage and progress to chronic renal failure. ARF is caused by decreased renal perfusion, parenchymal damage, or obstruction. It is categorized as prerenal, intrarenal, and postrenal (Table 5-1).

Prerenal failure is the result of decreased blood flow to the kidneys. The events leading to prerenal insults cause decreased renal vascular perfusion and usually are associated with systemic hypoperfusion. If renal hypoperfusion exceeds the adaptive mechanisms of autoregulation and renin release, ischemic damage occurs, leading to parenchymal (intrarenal) involvement. Intrarenal involvement usually results from a prolonged mean arterial pressure of <75 mm Hg. Failure of autoregulation enhances the sympathetic response and, coupled with the renin-angiotensin system, causes severe afferent arteriole constriction. This results in a further decrease in glomerular blood flow and glomerular hydrostatic pressure and decreases the glomerular filtration rate. The amount of cellular damage depends on the duration of ischemia. Mild, reversible injury occurs with ≤25 min of ischemia; more severe damage results after 40-60 min of ischemia; and irreversible damage may occur with 60-90 min of ischemia.

The most common cause of ARF is acute tubular necrosis (ATN). ATN is the result of nephrotoxic injury or a prolonged compromise in renal perfusion (ischemic injury). In the acutely ill adult both factors may be operative because renal ischemia tends to potentiate the injury produced by nephrotoxins. Toxic ATN, caused by nephrotoxic agents, is an insult or injury to the tubular cell. Toxic ATN results in tubular cell necrosis, cast formation, and tubular obstruction. The basement membrane usually is not injured, and it often is nonoliguric in nature. Oliguria may occur with both toxic ATN and ischemic ATN. Common nephrotoxic agents are found in Table 5-2.

Fluid, electrolyte, and acid-base disorders that occur with ARF include hypervolemia, hyperkalemia, hyperphosphatemia, hypocalcemia, and metabolic acidosis (Table 5-3). Phosphate levels rise because of impaired excretion of phosphorus by the renal tubules with continued GI absorption. Hypocalcemia results from the lack of active vitamin D, which would otherwise stimulate absorption of calcium from the GI tract. High phosphate levels also inhibit the

TABLE 5-1 Causes of Acute Renal Failure

Prerenal (decreased renal perfusion)	Intrarenal (parenchymal damage; acute tubular necrosis)	Postrenal (obstruction)
Hypovolemia • GI losses • Hemorrhage • Third-space (interstitial) losses (burns, peritonitis) • Dehydration from diuretic use **Hepatorenal syndrome** **Edema-forming conditions** • Right ventricular failure • Cirrhosis • Nephrotic syndrome **Renal vascular disorders** • Renal artery stenosis • Renal artery thrombosis • Renal vein thrombosis	**Nephrotoxic agents** • Antibiotics (aminoglycosides, sulfonamides, methicillin) • Diuretics (e.g., furosemide) • Nonsteroidal antiinflammatory drugs (e.g., ibuprofen) • Contrast media • Heavy metals (lead, gold, mercury) • Organic solvents (carbon tetrachloride, ethylene glycol) **Infection (gram-negative sepsis), pancreatitis, peritonitis** **Transfusion reaction (hemolysis)** **Rhabdomyolysis with myoglobinuria (severe muscle injury)** • Trauma • Exertion • Seizures • Drug related: heroin, barbiturates, IV amphetamines, succinylcholine **Glomerular diseases** • Poststreptococcal glomerulonephritis • IgA nephropathy (e.g., Berger's disease) • Lupus glomerulonephritis • Serum sickness **Ischemic injury**	**Calculi** **Tumor** **Benign prostatic hypertrophy** **Necrotizing papillitis** **Urethral strictures** **Blood clots** **Retroperitoneal fibrosis**

GI, Gastrointestinal; *IV*, intravenous; *IgA*, immunoglobulin A.

TABLE 5-2 Common Nephrotoxic Agents

Drugs	**X-ray contrast media**
Antineoplastics	**Biologic substances**
Methotrexate	Myoglobin
Cisplatin	Tumor products
Antibiotics	**Chemicals**
Cephalosporines	Ethylene glycol
Aminoglycosides	Pesticides
Tetracycline	Organic solvents
Nonsteroidal antiinflammatory drugs	**Heavy metals**
Ibuprofen	Lead
Ketorolac	Mercury
	Gold

absorption of calcium. In turn, hypocalcemia triggers the parathyroid glands to secrete parathyroid hormone (PTH), which mobilizes calcium from the bone.

Generally, there are three identifiable phases or stages of ARF. The first phase usually is characterized by oliguria, a drop in the 24-h urinary output to ≤400 ml. This phase lasts approximately 7-14 days, depending on the underlying pathologic condition. Approximately 30% of patients, however, have a syndrome of nonoliguric renal failure. The diuretic phase is evidenced initially by a doubling of the urinary output from the previous 24-h total. During this phase the patient may produce as much as 3-5 L of urine in 24 h. The recovery phase is marked by a return to a normal 24-h volume (1500-1800 ml). Usually, renal function continues to improve and may take 6 mo-1 yr from the initial insult to return to baseline functional status.

ASSESSMENT

ARF can dramatically affect fluid, electrolyte, and acid-base balances.

History and risk factors: Chronic illness (e.g., hypertension, diabetes), recent infections (e.g., streptococcal), recent episodes of hypotension (major bleeding, major surgery), exposure to nephrotoxins (e.g., carbon tetrachloride, diuretics, aminoglycoside antibiotics, dyes), recent blood transfusion, urinary tract disorder, toxemia of pregnancy or abortion, recent severe muscle damage (rhabdomyolysis with myoglobinuria), burn trauma.

Clinical presentation

Prerenal: Oliguria, urinary sodium (Na^+) <20 mEq/L, elevated specific gravity, increased urine osmolality, normal sediment or presence of hyaline and granular casts, elevated plasma BUN/creatinine ratio (>20:1).

Intrarenal: May have oliguria or be nonoliguric, urinary Na^+ >20 mEq/L, low specific gravity, decreased urinary osmolality, presence of RBC (red blood cell) casts and cellular debris in urine, decreased plasma BUN/creatinine ratio (10:1).

Fluid volume alterations

Excess: Peripheral edema, jugular vein distention, S_3 and S_4 gallops, crackles, increased BP, oliguria.

Deficit: Decreased blood pressure (BP), poor skin turgor, flushed skin, dry mucous membranes, oliguria.

Electrolyte imbalances: Dysrhythmias, altered mental status, GI disturbances, neuromuscular dysfunction.

Metabolic acidosis: Weakness, disorientation, shortness of breath (SOB), Kussmaul respirations, central nervous system (CNS) depression.

Text continued on p. 378

T A B L E 5 - 3   Altered Electrolyte Balance in ARF

Condition/cause	Nursing implications
Hyperkalemia Decreased ability to excrete K$^+$; K$^+$ release with catabolism	• Monitor ECG for tall and peaked T waves, loss of P waves, prolonged PR interval, widened QRS, and cardiac arrest (more likely seen with K$^+$ >6.5 mEq/L). • Monitor serum K$^+$ levels for values ≥5 mEq/L. • Monitor patient for such indicators as paresthesias, muscle weakness or flaccidity, and HR <60 bpm. • Teach patient and significant others the indicators of hyperkalemia and the importance of notifying nurse promptly if they occur. • Provide a list of foods high in potassium (see Table 10-12), and stress the importance of avoiding these foods. • Implement the following to help minimize the cellular release of potassium: □ Ensure that patient consumes only the amount of protein prescribed by physician; enforce sound infection control techniques to minimize risk of infection; and treat fevers promptly. Catabolism of protein, which occurs in these situations, causes potassium to be released from the tissues. □ Ensure that patient consumes the allotted amounts of carbohydrates, and limit strenuous patient activity as prescribed, both of which will spare protein. • Be aware that hyperkalemia can be a fatal complication, especially during the oliguric phase of ARF, because of its adverse effect on cardiac status. Keep emergency supplies (i.e., manual resuscitator, crash cart, emergency drug tray) readily available. • For more information, see "Hyperkalemia," p 651.
Hypokalemia Prolonged, inadequate oral intake; use of potassium-losing diuretics without proper replacement; excessive loss from vomiting, diarrhea, or gastric or intestinal suctioning	• Monitor ECG for prolonged PR interval, flattened or inverted T wave, depressed ST segment, presence of U wave, and ventricular dysrhythmias; ECG changes are more likely to occur at serum K$^+$ levels <3 mEq/L. • Be alert to serum K$^+$ <3.5 mEq/L. • Monitor patient for muscle weakness, soft and flabby muscles, paresthesias, decreased bowel sounds, ileus, weak and irregular pulse, and distant heart sounds. Neuromuscular symptoms are seen at serum levels of approximately 2.5 mEq/L.

K$^+$, Potassium; *ECG,* electrocardiogram; *HR,* heart rate; *ARF,* acute renal failure.

TABLE 5-3 Altered Electrolyte Balance in ARF—cont'd

Condition/cause	Nursing implications
	• Teach patient and significant others the indicators of hypokalemia and the importance of notifying nurse promptly if they occur. • Provide a list of foods high in potassium (see Table 10-12), and assist with planning menus that incorporate them. • Administer potassium-sparing diuretics (e.g., spironolactone, triamterene) as prescribed. • Administer oral or IV potassium supplements as prescribed; for oral route, administer with at least 4 oz water or juice to minimize gastric irritation. • For more information, see "Hypoka-lemia," p. 649.
Hypernatremia Kidney's inability to excrete excess sodium; decreased water intake; increased water losses via osmotic diuresis; excessive parenteral administration of sodium-containing solutions (e.g., sodium bicarbonate, 3% sodium chloride)	• Monitor serum sodium levels for serum Na^+ >147 mEq/L. • Monitor VS and I&O hourly; weigh patient daily. • Be alert to dry mucous membranes, flushed skin, firm and rubbery tissue turgor, hyperthermia, oliguria, or anuria. • Assess sensorium for restlessness and agitation; institute seizure precautions as indicated. • Administer prescribed IV replacement fluids. • Administer diuretics as prescribed. • For more information, see "Hyperna-tremia," p. 647.
Hyponatremia Loss through vomiting, diarrhea, profuse diaphoresis; use of potent diuretics; salt-losing nephropathies; administration of large amount of sodium-free IV fluids (may be associated with fluid volume excess or postobstructive diuresis)	• Monitor for serum Na^+ <137 mEq/L. • Monitor I&O hourly; record weight daily for trend. • Assess patient for abdominal cramps, diarrhea, nausea, dizziness when changing position, postural hypotension, cold and clammy skin, and apprehension. • Provide parenteral replacement therapy as prescribed. • Institute a safe environment for individuals with altered LOC. • For more information, see "Hypona-tremia," p. 644.

IV, Intravenous; *Na+,* sodium; *VS,* vital signs; *I&O,* intake and output; *LOC,* level of consciousness. *Continued*

TABLE 5-3   Altered Electrolyte Balance in ARF—cont'd

Condition/cause	Nursing implications
Hypocalcemia Poor absorption of dietary calcium; precipitation of calcium out of the tissues in the presence of elevated phosphorus level; inadequate absorption and utilization of calcium occurring with lack of conversion of vitamin D to its usable form	• Monitor for serum Ca^{++} <8.5 mg/dl. • Monitor for numbness and tingling around the mouth, muscle twitching, facial twitching, and tonic muscle spasms. Assess for Trousseau sign (carpopedal spasm) and Chvostek sign (spasm of lip and cheek). • Administer calcium and vitamin D supplements as prescribed. Reinforce the necessity of taking these medications as prescribed. • Teach patient and significant others the indicators of hypocalcemia. • Teach the importance of continued medical follow-up to check serum Ca^{++} levels. • For more information, see "Hypocalcemia," p. 654.
Hyperphosphatemia Abnormal retention of phosphates caused by the kidneys' inability to excrete excess phosphorus	• Monitor for serum phosphate >4.5 g/dl. • Although most foods contain generous amounts of phosphate, those especially high in phosphate include beef, pork, dried beans, dried mature peas, and dairy products (see Table 10-13). Monitor patient's diet accordingly. • Administer phosphate binders as prescribed. Assess for constipation, which may result from use of phosphate binders. • Teach patient and significant others the relationship between calcium and phosphate levels in the body. • Emphasize that maintaining good phosphate control and calcium balance may help control itching and prevent future problems with bone disease. • Reinforce the need for follow-up visits to check serum phosphate levels. • For more information, see "Hyperphosphatemia," p. 662.
Hypermagnesemia Administration of magnesium-containing medications to patients with impaired renal function	• Monitor serum Mg^{++} levels >2.5 mEq/L. • Assess for diaphoresis, flushing, hypotension, drowsiness, weak-to-absent DTRs, bradycardia, lethargy, and respiratory impairment. • Teach the above indicators to patient and significant others.

Ca^{++}, Calcium; Mg^{++}, magnesium; *DTR*, deep tendon reflex.

TABLE 5-3   Altered Electrolyte Balance in ARF—cont'd

Condition/cause	Nursing implications
	• Avoid giving medications that contain magnesium (see Table 10-15). Emphasize to patient that such medications should not be taken without physician's approval. • For more information, see "Hypermagnesemia," p. 668.
Metabolic acidosis Kidneys' inability to excrete excess acid produced by normal metabolic processes. Marked tissue trauma, infection, and diarrhea may contribute to a more rapid development of acidosis (often associated with K^+ >5 mEq/L)	• Monitor for HCO_3^- <22 mEq/L and pH <7.35. • Monitor I&O, LOC, and VS. Be alert to Kussmaul respirations, SOB, anorexia, headache, nausea, vomiting, weakness, apathy, fatigue, and coma. • Institute seizure precautions in the presence of altered LOC. • Administer IV fluids and bicarbonate as prescribed. • Teach patient the importance of dietary restrictions, particularly of protein, and of maintaining adequate carbohydrate intake to prevent worsening acidosis. • Stress that patient should report to physician increased temperature and other signs of infection. • Teach patient the importance of taking sodium bicarbonate as prescribed and of maintaining dialysis schedule (both hemodialysis and peritoneal dialysis help correct acidosis). • For more information, see " Chronic Metabolic Acidosis," p. 682.
Uremia Failure of the kidneys to excrete urea, creatinine, uric acid, and other metabolic waste products	• Monitor patient for chronic fatigue, insomnia, anorexia, vomiting, metallic taste in the mouth, pruritus, increased bleeding tendency, muscular twitching, involuntary leg movements, decreasing attention span, anemia, muscle wasting, and weakness. • Teach patient and significant others that the indicators of uremia develop gradually and are very subtle. Explain the importance of notifying nurse of sudden worsening of the symptoms that may be present. • Monitor and record dietary intake of protein, potassium, and sodium. • Use lotions and oils to lubricate patient's skin and relieve drying and cracking.

HCO_3^-, Bicarbonate; *I&O*, intake and output; *LOC*, level of consciousness; *VS*, vital signs; *SOB*, shortness of breath; *IV*, intravenous.   *Continued*

| **T A B L E 5 - 3   Altered Electrolyte Balance in ARF—cont'd** | |
Condition/cause	Nursing implications
	• Provide oral hygiene at frequent intervals, using a soft-bristle toothbrush and mouthwash, to help combat patient's thirst and the metallic taste caused by uremia. Chewing gum and hard candy also may help alleviate thirst and the unpleasant taste.
	• Encourage isometric exercises and short walks, if patient is able, to help maintain patient's muscle strength and tone, especially in the legs.
	• Teach significant others that because of patient's decreasing concentration level, they should communicate with patient by using simple and direct statements.
	• Teach patient to maintain good nutrition by ingesting the allotted amounts of carbohydrates and high–biologic value protein to support cell rebuilding and decrease waste products from protein breakdown.
	• Explain that profuse bleeding can occur with uremia and that knives, scissors, and other sharp instruments should be used with caution.
	• Stress that OTC medications, such as aspirin and ibuprofen, may enhance bleeding tendency.
	• Emphasize the importance of follow-up visits to evaluate the progression of uremia.
	• Stress that dialysis schedule should be maintained to decrease the symptoms of uremia and correct many of the metabolic abnormalities that occur.

OTC, Over-the-counter.

Uremic manifestations: Accumulation of urea, creatinine, uric acid; anemia and bleeding tendencies; fatigue and pallor; increased BP, congestive heart failure, pericarditis with tamponade, pulmonary edema; anorexia, nausea, vomiting, diarrhea; behavioral changes; decreased wound healing ability; increased susceptibility to infection.

Physical assessment

Cardiovascular: S_3 and S_4 gallops, pericardial friction rub, jugular vein distention, tachycardia, dysrhythmias, increased BP, pulsus paradoxus in the presence of fluid volume excess, edema (peripheral, periorbital, sacral), capillary fragility, purpura.

Respiratory: Crackles, hyperventilation.

Neuromuscular: Weakness, lethargy, muscle irritability, muscle tenderness, asterixis.

Cutaneous: Pallor; presence of uremic frost in persons with severe uremia.

DIAGNOSTIC TESTS

Serum blood urea nitrogen (BUN), creatinine, uric acid, and electrolyte levels: Creatinine is the most reliable indicator of renal function. BUN is influenced by hydration, catabolism, GI bleeding, infection, fever, and corticosteroid therapy. BUN, creatinine, and uric acid levels will be elevated in the presence of ARF, as will potassium, phosphorus, and possibly magnesium.

Creatinine clearance test: For clinical purposes this is the most reliable estimation of glomerular filtration rate. Accuracy depends on complete collection. Creatinine clearance decreases with age. Normal creatinine clearance is 95-125 ml/min. In the presence of ARF it usually is <50 ml/min.

Urinalysis: The presence of sediment-containing tubular epithelial cells, cellular debris, and tubular casts supports a diagnosis of ARF. Large amounts of protein and many RBC casts are common in ARF when it is secondary to parenchymal (intrarenal) disease. Sediment is normal when the causes are categorized as prerenal.

Urinary sodium: A prerenal cause is signaled by a sodium count <10 mEq/L.

CBC and coagulation studies (PT, PTT):   Complete blood cell count (CBC), prothrombin time (PT), and partial thromboplastin time (PTT) to evaluate for hematologic complications. Baseline hematocrit (Hct) may be low as a result of ARF, and Hct and hemoglobin (Hgb) will fall steadily if the patient has bleeding or hemodilution from fluid overload.

ABG values: Low $Paco_2$ and plasma pH values reflect the metabolic acidosis associated with ARF.

Ultrasonography: Identifies hydronephrosis, fluid collection, and masses.

Intravenous pyelograms (IVP), both retrograde and antegrade: To diagnose partial or complete obstruction.

Renal scan: Provides information about renal perfusion.

Renal angiography and venography: Assess for the presence or absence of thrombotic or stenotic lesions in the main renal vessels.

COLLABORATIVE MANAGEMENT

Prerenal acute renal failure

Volume replacement: Replacement solutions include free water plus electrolytes lost through the urine, wounds, drainage tubes, diarrhea, and vomiting. Usually losses are replaced on a volume-for-volume basis. Maintenance fluids total approximately 1500 ml/24 h. With a moderate fluid deficit (5% weight loss), at least 2400 ml is given over a 24-h period. A severe deficit (>5% weight loss) requires a replacement of at least 3000 ml/24 h.

Diuretics (furosemide [Lasix], ethacrynic acid [Edecrin]), bumetanide [Bumex], and torsemide [Demadex]):   Decrease filtrate reabsorption and enhance water excretion. They may be used, after adequate hydration, to increase urine output or in an attempt to prevent onset of oliguria. If volume overload is present, diuretics are used to prevent pulmonary edema. Osmotic diuretics, such as mannitol, may be used to increase intravascular volume, promote renal blood flow, increase glomerular filtration rate, and stimulate urinary output. See Table 5-4 for additional information on diuretics.

Dopamine: Low doses, usually ≤2 μg/kg/min, to stimulate dopaminergic receptors, encourage renal vasodilation, and promote renal blood flow. Slightly higher doses (e.g., 3-6 μg/kg/min) are used in mildly hypotensive patients to stimulate dopaminergic and beta $(\beta)_1$-receptors, resulting in improved BP and cardiac output. Doses >7 μg/kg/min lack renal vasodilatory effects and may cause damaging renal vasoconstriction.

Intrarenal acute renal failure

Removal or discontinuation of toxic agent: For example, aminoglycosides, dye load, chemicals.

Dialytic therapy: Maintains homeostasis (see discussion, p. 395).

TABLE 5-4   Diuretic Use in Acute Renal Failure

Types	Mechanisms of action	Potential fluid and electrolyte abnormalities
Osmotic diuretics Mannitol Urea	Increase osmotic pressure of the filtrate, which attracts water and electrolytes and prevents their reabsorption	Hyponatremia Hypokalemia Rebound volume expansion
Loop diuretics Furosemide Ethacrynic acid Bumetanide Torsemide	Inhibit reabsorption of Na^+ and Cl^- at the ascending loop of Henle in the medulla; they produce a vasodilatory effect on the renal vasculature	Hypokalemia Hyperuricemia Hypocalcemia Hypomagnesemia Hyperglycemia and impairment of glucose tolerance Dilutional hyponatremia Hypochloremic acidosis
Thiazides Bendroflumethiazide Benzthiazide Chlorothiazide sodium Hydrochlorothiazide Hydroflumethiazide Polythiazide Trichlormethiazide	Inhibit reabsorption of Na^+ in the ascending loop of Henle at the beginning of the distal loop	Hypokalemia Dilutional hyponatremia Hypercalcemia Metabolic alkalosis Hypochloremia Hyperuricemia Hyperglycemia and impaired glucose tolerance
Thiazide-like diuretics Chlorthalidone Indapamide Metolazone Quinethazone	Action same as thiazides	Same as thiazides
Potassium-sparing diuretics* Amiloride HCl Spironolactone Triamterene	Inhibit aldosterone effect on the distal tubule, causing Na^+ excretion and K^+ reabsorption	Hyperkalemia Hyponatremia Dehydration Acidosis Transient increase in BUN
Carbonic anhydrase-inhibitors Acetazolamide sodium Dichlorphenamide Methazolamide	Block the action of the enzyme carbonic anhydrase, producing excretion of Na^+, K^+, HCO_3^-, and water	Hyperchloremic acidosis Hypokalemia Hyperuricemia

NOTE: Loop or osmotic diuretics (or a combination of both) are used in patients with acute renal failure to prevent hypervolemia and to stimulate urinary output.
NA^+, Sodium; Cl^-, chloride; K^+, potassium; *BUN*, blood urea nitrogen; HCO_3^-, bicarbonate.
*Used with caution in patients with oliguria.

Nutrition therapy: Involves a diet high in carbohydrates to prevent endogenous protein catabolism and muscle breakdown; low in sodium for individuals who retain sodium and water; high in sodium for those who have lost large volumes of sodium and water as a result of diuresis or other body drainage; low in potassium if the patient is retaining potassium; and low in protein to maintain daily requirements while minimizing increases in azotemia. Nutrition is delivered via oral, enteral, or total parenteral nutrition (TPN). (See Table 10-11, p. 642, for a list of foods high in sodium and Table 10-12, p. 650, for a list of foods high in potassium.)

Hematologic problems and blood transfusions: Packed RBCs are given if indicated to maintain a stable Hct. There are two major hematologic complications of renal failure:

Anemia: Caused by decreased erythropoietin, low-grade GI bleeding from mucosal ulceration, blood drawing, and shortened life of the RBCs. Erythropoietin (Epogen) is used for primary prevention and treatment of anemia.

Prolonged bleeding time: Caused by decreased platelet adhesiveness. As renal failure progresses, anemia becomes more profound and platelet adhesiveness decreases further.

Pharmacotherapy

Antihypertensives: See Table 4-21, p. 336.

Phosphate binders (aluminum hydroxide antacids, calcium carbonate antacids, and calcium acetate): Bind phosphorus and control hyperphosphatemia. They are given with meals.

Sodium bicarbonate: Controls metabolic acidosis and promotes shift of potassium back into the cells.

Sodium polystyrene sulfonate (Kayexalate): Oral or rectal preparation that exchanges sodium for potassium in the GI tract to help control hyperkalemia.

Water-soluble vitamin supplements: For patients receiving dialytic therapy. Water-soluble vitamins are diffused across the membrane and are removed during dialysis.

Recombinant erythropoietin (Epogen, Procrit): Intravenous/subcutaneous (IV/SC) preparation given 3×/wk after dialysis in doses of 50-500 U/kg to correct anemia of chronic renal failure. Maintenance doses are given 3×/wk to maintain Hct levels of 33%-38%. Adverse reactions include development or worsening of hypertension; clotting of vascular access; depletion of iron stores; and slight increases in predialysis levels of BUN, creatinine, and potassium in individuals with Hct <30%.

> **Note:** See Table 5-5 for a list of common medications that require dosage modification for patients with ARF. Drugs that require dosage modification in renal failure are those that are excreted primarily by the kidneys. Dosage must be governed by clinical responses, as well as serum levels, if available. Nephrotoxic drugs should be avoided (Table 5-6). Also avoid drugs that are toxic to other organs if they accumulate; those that aggravate uremic symptoms; and those that contribute to metabolic derangements of renal failure.

Postrenal acute renal failure

Relief of obstruction: Achieved via catheterization with indwelling urinary catheter, nephrostomy tube, or ureteral stent to relieve obstruction before surgical intervention, lithotripsy to disintegrate stones, or prostatectomy if benign prostatic hypertrophy is the cause of the obstruction.

Monitoring of fluid and electrolyte balance: Postobstructive diuresis may result in hypovolemia (see p. 638), hyponatremia (see p. 644), hypokalemia (see p. 649), hypocalcemia (see p. 654), and hypomagnesemia (see p. 665). See Table 5-3 for factors leading to altered electrolyte balance in ARF.

Culturing of urine and administration of antibiotics: If indicated.

TABLE 5 - 5   Drugs That Require Dosage Modification in Renal Failure

Antimicrobials	Cardiovascular agents	Analgesics	Sedatives	Miscellaneous
Amikacin	ACE inhibitors	Meperidine	Meprobamate	Cimetidine
Amphotericin B	Digitoxin	Methadone	Phenobarbital	Clofibrate
Chloramphenicol	Digoxin			Glycoprotein IIB, IIIA
Ethambutol	Guanethidine			inhibitors
Gentamicin	Procainamide			Insulin
Kanamycin				Neostigmine
Lincomycin				NSAIDs
Penicillins				Platelet inhibitors
Sulfonamides				
Tobramycin				
Vancomycin				

TABLE 5-6 Drugs to Avoid in Renal Failure

Amiloride
Aspirin
Cisplatin
Lithium carbonate
Magnesium-containing medications (see Table 10-15)
Nitrofurantoin
Nonsteroidal antiinflammatory drugs (e.g., ibuprofen)
Phenylbutazone
Spironolactone
Tetracycline

NURSING DIAGNOSES AND INTERVENTIONS

Fluid volume excess related to compromised regulatory mechanism secondary to acute renal failure

Desired outcome: Within 24-48 h of onset, patient becomes normovolemic as evidenced by balanced intake and output (I&O); urinary output ≥0.5 ml/kg/h; body weight within patient's normal range; BP within patient's normal range; central venous pressure (CVP) 2-6 mm Hg; heart rate (HR) 60-100 beats per minute (bpm); and absence of edema, crackles, gallop, and other clinical indicators of fluid overload.

> **Note:**   Although patient is retaining sodium, his or her serum sodium level may be within normal limits or decreased from baseline because of the dilutional effect of the fluid overload.

- Document I&O hourly. Consult physician if urinary output falls to <0.5 ml/kg/h.
- Weigh patient daily; consult physician regarding significant weight gain (e.g., 0.5-1.5 kg/24 h).
- Assess for and document the presence of basilar crackles, jugular vein distention, tachycardia, pericardial friction rub, gallop, increased BP, increased CVP, or SOB, any of which are indicative of fluid volume overload.
- Assess for and document the presence of peripheral, sacral, or periorbital edema.
- Restrict patient's total fluid intake to 1200-1500 ml/24 h or as prescribed. Measure all output accurately, and replace milliliter for milliliter at intervals of 4-8 h or as prescribed.
- Provide ice chips, chewing gum, or hard candy to help patient quench thirst and moisten mouth.
- Monitor serum osmolality and serum sodium values. These values may be decreased because of the dilutional effect of fluid overload.
- Recognize that if it is delivered, TPN will provide the largest volume of fluid intake for the patient. If total fluid intake is >2000 ml/day, ultrafiltration (UF) with dialysis (see p. 395) or continuous arteriovenous hemofiltration (CAVH) (see p. 395) may be necessary to maintain fluid balance.
- If patient is retaining sodium, restrict sodium-containing foods (see Table 10-11, p. 642) and avoid diluting IV medications with high-sodium diluents. Also avoid sodium-containing medications such as sodium penicillin.

You may also wish to refer to the following interventions from the Nursing Interventions Classification (NIC):

NIC Electrolyte Management: Hyponatremia; Fluid/Electrolyte Management; Fluid Management; Fluid Monitoring; Electrolyte Management: Hypokalemia.

Additional optional interventions include Dysrhythmia Management; Hemodialysis Therapy; Hemodynamic Regulation; Invasive Hemodynamic Monitoring; Medication Management; Positioning; Skin Surveillance; Weight Management

Fluid volume deficit related to active loss secondary to diuresis, vomiting, diarrhea, and hemorrhage; failure of regulatory mechanism with fluid shift to interstitial compartments

Desired outcomes: Within 24 h of this diagnosis, patient becomes normovolemic as evidenced by balanced I&O; urinary output ≥0.5 ml/kg/h; CVP 2-6 mm Hg; HR 60-100 bpm; BP within patient's normal range; and absence of thirst and other indicators of hypovolemia. Patient's weight stabilizes within 2-3 days.

- Weigh patient daily. Consult physician for weight loss of 1-1.5 kg/24 h.
- Monitor and document I&O hourly. Consult physician if patient's output is <0.5 ml/kg/h. With deficit, intake should exceed output by 0.5-1 L (depending on severity of dehydration) q24h.
- Consult physician for increase in losses from vomiting, diarrhea, or wound drainage or sudden onset of diuresis.
- Observe for and document indicators of dehydration and hypovolemia (e.g., poor skin turgor, dry and sticky mucous membranes, thirst, hypotension, tachycardia, decreasing CVP, increasing BUN and creatinine).
- Encourage oral fluids if they are allowed. Ensure that IV fluid rates are maintained as prescribed.
- Approximately 20% of patients with ARF have GI bleeding. Monitor Hgb, Hct, and BUN levels. In the presence of bleeding with ARF, Hgb and Hct values will fall steadily (rapidly if there is massive bleeding).

> **Note:**   A patient with ARF has an Hct in the range of 20%-30% because of the anemia that occurs with renal failure. BUN will increase in the presence of GI bleeding without a concomitant rise in serum creatinine level.

- Test all stools, emesis, and peritoneal dialysate drainage for occult blood. Check urine and dialysate drainage at least q8h.
- To minimize the risk of bleeding, keep side rails up, minimize invasive procedures, use small-gauge needles for injections, minimize blood drawing, and promote the use of electric razors and soft-bristle toothbrushes. If possible, avoid IM/SC injections for 1 h after hemodialysis. Apply gentle pressure to injection sites for at least 2-3 min.
- Inspect gums, mouth, nose, skin, and perianal and vaginal areas q8h for bleeding. Also inspect hemodialysis insertion and peritoneal access sites for evidence of bleeding q8h. Apply a soft, occlusive, sterile dressing to access sites to protect skin from irritation and bleeding caused by catheter movement.

Altered nutrition: less than body requirements, related to catabolic state and excessive metabolic needs secondary to ARF; anorexia and psychologic aversion to dietary restrictions

Desired outcome: Within 72 h of this diagnosis, patient has adequate nutritional intake as evidenced by a caloric intake that ranges from 35-45 calories (cal)/kg normal body weight; a daily protein intake that consists of 50%-75% of high-biologic value proteins; and a nitrogen intake of 4-6 g more than nitrogen loss (calculated from 24-h urinary urea excretion and protein intake).

- Infuse enteral feedings and TPN as prescribed.
- Assess and document patient's intake of nutrients every shift.
- Weigh patient daily. Consult physician for significant findings (e.g., loss of >1.5 kg/24 h).
- As prescribed, use cooling blanket or antipyretic agents to control fever. Fever increases tissue catabolism, which in turn increases metabolic needs.

- The end products of protein metabolism that accumulate in renal failure are reflected by an increase in BUN level. Low-protein diets are used to decrease the nitrogenous load and attempt to control uremia to some extent. Ensure intake of protein with high biologic value (e.g., eggs, meat, fowl, milk, fish), which contains essential amino acids necessary for cell building.
- Be sure that caloric intake ranges from 35-45 cal/kg normal body weight. The exact amount will vary with age, gender, activity, and the degree of preexisting malnutrition. Foods that may be used to increase caloric intake include fats and concentrated carbohydrates.
- Restrict high-potassium foods such as bananas, citrus fruits, fruit juices, nuts, tea, coffee, legumes, and salt substitute. In ARF the kidneys are unable to excrete potassium effectively.
- Sodium requirements will vary greatly. If oliguria is present, sodium intake may be restricted in the diet. If diuresis is present, sodium intake may be increased because of excess sodium loss in the urine. Intervene accordingly.
- Hypocalcemia may be present early in ARF as a result of decreased absorption of calcium from the gut and the presence of hyperphosphatemia. As prescribed, replace calcium orally (e.g., with dairy products) or intravenously and administer phosphate binders as prescribed.
- If patient is anorexic or nauseated, provide small, frequent meals. Present appetizing food in a pleasant atmosphere; eliminate any noxious odors. As indicated, administer medication with prescribed antiemetic ½ h before meals.

NIC Nutrition Management; Nutritional Monitoring; Fluid Management; Fluid Monitoring. Additional optional interventions include Bowel Management; Energy Management; Enteral Tube Feeding; Exercise Promotion; Gastrointestinal Intubation; Hyperglycemia Management; Hypoglycemia Management; Intravenous Insertion; Intravenous Therapy; Medication Management; Mutual Goal Setting; Phlebotomy: Venous Blood Sample; Positioning; Teaching: Individual; Teaching: Prescribed Diet; Total Parenteral Nutrition Administration; Venous Access Devices Maintenance

Risk for infection related to inadequate secondary defenses as a result of immunocompromised state associated with ARF; multiple invasive procedures
Desired outcome: At the time of discharge from ICU, patient is free of infection as evidenced by normothermia; negative culture results of dialysate and body secretions; and WBC count ≤11,000/mm^3. NOTE: After the initial insult, infection is the primary cause of death in ARF.

- Monitor and record patient's temperature q8h. If it is elevated (i.e., >37° C [98.6° F]), monitor temperature q4h. Because ARF may be accompanied by hypothermia, even a slight rise in temperature of 1°-2° may be significant.
- Inspect and record the color, odor, and appearance of all body secretions. Be alert to cloudy or blood-tinged peritoneal dialysate return, cloudy and foul-smelling urine, foul-smelling wound exudate, purulent drainage from any catheter site, foul-smelling and watery stools, foul-smelling vaginal discharge, or purulent sputum. Be aware that uremia retards wound healing, and therefore it is important that all wounds (including scratches resulting from pruritus) be assessed for indicators of infection. Send sample of any suspicious fluid or drainage for culture and sensitivity tests as indicated.
- Monitor WBC count for elevations, and obtain specimens for C&S as prescribed.
- Ensure sound infection control when manipulating central lines, peripheral IV lines, and indwelling catheters. Be aware that catabolism of protein, which occurs with infection, causes potassium to be released from the tissues.
- Avoid use of indwelling urinary catheter in patients with oliguria and anuria. The presence of a catheter in these patients further increases the risk of infection.

- To help maintain the integrity of the oral mucous membranes, provide oral hygiene q2h.
- Reposition patient q2-4h to help maintain the barrier of an intact integumentary system. Provide skin care at least q8h.
- Encourage good pulmonary hygiene by having patient practice deep-breathing exercises (and coughing, if its need is indicated) q2-4h.

NIC Infection Control; Infection Protection. Additional optional interventions include Airway Management; Exercise Promotion and Therapy (all listed); Medication Management; Respiratory Monitoring; Teaching: Disease Process; Tube Care: Urinary; Vital Signs Monitoring

Knowledge deficit: biochemical alterations associated with ARF

Desired outcome: Within 72 h of admission, patient and significant others verbalize accurate information regarding patient's disease state and the measures that can be taken to prevent its occurrence or minimize its effects.

- Determine patient's and significant others' knowledge about patient's disease process and the biochemical alterations (hyperkalemia, hypokalemia, hypernatremia, hyponatremia, hypocalcemia, hyperphosphatemia, hypermagnesemia, metabolic acidosis, and uremia) that can occur.
- Teach patient and significant others the signs and symptoms of the biochemical alterations (see Table 5-3 and **Altered protection,** p. 386).
- Provide lists of foods high in potassium (see Table 10-12), sodium (see Table 10-11), phosphorus (see Table 10-13), and magnesium (see Table 10-14), which patient should add or avoid when planning meals. In addition, provide a list of medications that contain magnesium (see Table 10-15), which should not be taken without physician approval.
- Explain the importance of consuming only the amount of protein prescribed by physician and avoiding exposure to persons with infection or a febrile illness to minimize catabolism of protein, which causes potassium to be released from the tissues. Reinforce that patient should consume the prescribed diet and limit strenuous activity as prescribed, both of which will spare protein and thus minimize potassium release.
- Teach patient to report to physician an increase in temperature or other signs of infection.
- Reinforce the importance of taking vitamin D and calcium supplements as prescribed.
- Teach the relationship between calcium and phosphate levels. Emphasize that maintaining good phosphate control and calcium balance may help control itching and prevent future problems with bone disease.
- Stress the importance of taking phosphate binders (e.g., Amphojel, Alternagel, PhosLo) as prescribed.
- Teach patient not to take over-the-counter (OTC) medications without first consulting physician. Aspirin, for example, exacerbates the bleeding tendency caused by uremia.
- Instruct patient about the importance of maintaining the prescribed dialysis schedule, inasmuch as dialysis will help correct acidosis, uremia, and many of the metabolic abnormalities that occur.
- Teach patient to use lotions and oils to lubricate skin and relieve drying and cracking.
- Stress the importance of follow-up monitoring of serum electrolyte levels.

NIC Teaching: Disease Process; Teaching: Individual; Teaching: Prescribed Medication. Additional optional interventions include Discharge Planning; Medication Management; Weight Management

Altered protection related to neurosensory changes secondary to electrolyte imbalance, metabolic acidosis, and uremia

Desired outcomes: Within 48-72 h of onset, patient verbalizes orientation to time, place, and person and maintains his or her normal mobility.

- Monitor patient for the following mentation and motor dysfunctions associated with ARF:
  - ☐ Hyperkalemia (during oliguric phase): muscle weakness, irritability, paresthesias.
  - ☐ Hypokalemia (during diuretic phase): lethargy; muscle weakness, softness, flabbiness; paresthesias.
  - ☐ Hypernatremia: fatigue, restlessness, agitation.
  - ☐ Hyponatremia: dizziness when changing position, apprehension, personality changes, agitation, confusion.
  - ☐ Hypocalcemia: neuromuscular irritability, tonic muscle spasms, paresthesias.
  - ☐ Hyperphosphatemia: excessive itching, muscle weakness, hyperreflexia.
  - ☐ Hypermagnesemia: drowsiness, lethargy, sensation of heat.
  - ☐ Metabolic acidosis: confusion, weakness.
  - ☐ Uremia: confusion, lethargy, itching, metallic taste, muscle twitching.
- Explain to significant others that patient's decreasing attention level necessitates simple and direct communication efforts.
- To alleviate unpleasant metallic taste caused by uremia, provide frequent oral hygiene. Because patient with uremia is at increased risk for bleeding, ensure use of soft-bristle brushes. If appropriate, provide chewing gum or hard candy, which may help alleviate the unpleasant metallic taste.
- Encourage isometric exercises and short walks, if patient is able, to help maintain muscle strength and tone, especially in the legs.
- Decrease environmental stimuli, and use a calm, reassuring manner in caring for patient.
- Encourage establishment of sleep/rest patterns by scheduling daytime activities appropriately and promoting relaxation method (see **Health-seeking behavior,** p. 302).
- Assess for decreased tactile sensations in the feet and legs, which may occur with peripheral neuropathy. Be alert to the potential for pressure sores and friction burns, which may occur with peripheral neuropathy.
- Use splints and braces to aid in mobility for patients with severe neuropathic effects.

NIC Infection Control; Infection Protection. Additional optional interventions include Nutrition Management; Nutrition Therapy; Nutritional Counseling; Pressure Management; Pressure Ulcer Prevention; Teaching: Individual

Constipation related to immobility; restrictions of fresh fruit and fluids; use of phosphate binders

Desired outcome: Within 48 h of onset, patient has bowel movements of soft consistency.

- Monitor and record the number and quality of patient's bowel movements.
- Administer prescribed stool softeners and bulking agents, such as psyllium husks.
- If these measures fail, administer oil retention or tap water enemas as prescribed. Because excess fluid can be absorbed from the gut, avoid using large-volume water enemas.
- Encourage moderate exercise on a routine basis.
- Establish a regular schedule for fluid intake within patient's prescribed limits.
- Administer metoclopramide as prescribed to increase motility in the presence of autonomic neuropathy.

NIC Constipation/Impaction Management. Additional optional interventions include Exercise Promotion; Medication Administration: Oral; Medication Management; Pain Management; Skin Surveillance

Impaired skin integrity (or risk for same) related to uremia with resulting pruritus and edema

Desired outcome: Patient's skin remains intact.

- Monitor patient for presence of pruritus with resulting frequent and intense scratching.

- Pruritus decreases with reduced BUN level and control of hyperphosphatemia. Monitor laboratory values of BUN and phosphorus, and report levels
  outside the optimal range (BUN >20 mg/dl and phosphorus >4.5 mg/dl or
  2.6 mEq/L).
- Administer phosphate binders (e.g., Alternagel) as prescribed, and if possible,
  reduce patient's dietary intake of phosphorus (see Table 10-13, p. 660).
- Ensure that patient's fingernails are cut short and that the nail tips are smooth.
- Because uremia retards wound healing, monitor scratches for indicators of
  infection.
- Because of reduced oil gland activity in uremia, the patient's skin may be
  quite dry. Use skin emollients liberally, and avoid harsh soaps and excessive
  bathing.
- Advise patient of the potential for bruising because of clotting abnormality
  and capillary fragility.
- Pruritus increases in the presence of secondary hyperparathyroidism. Monitor
  serum calcium and PTH levels, and report elevations (Ca^{++} >10.5 mg/dl and
  PTH >30% above the upper limit of the test used).
- As prescribed, administer oral antihistamine, such as diphenhydramine, to
  relieve itching.

NIC Skin Surveillance; Pressure Ulcer Prevention. Additional optional interventions
include Bathing; Bleeding Reduction; Cutaneous Stimulation; Exercise Promotion and Therapy (all listed); Electrolyte Monitoring; Exercise Promotion:
Stretching; Fluid/Electrolyte Management; Infection Control; Infection Protection; Medication Management; Nail Care; Nutrition Management; Perineal
Care; Surveillance; Vital Signs Monitoring

ADDITIONAL NURSING DIAGNOSES

For patients undergoing dialytic therapy, see nursing diagnoses and interventions in "Renal Replacement Therapies," p. 395. Also see the following as
appropriate: "Nutritional Support," p. 1; "Prolonged Immobility," p. 74;
"Psychosocial Support," p. 83; and "Psychosocial Support for the Patient's
Family and Significant Others," p. 95.

Renal transplantation

Renal transplantation has become an accepted mode of treatment for end-stage
renal disease, to a large extent a result of advances in the development of
immunosuppressive medications in the late 1960s and the 1970s. Approximately 30%-40% of individuals who need transplantation have chronic renal
failure caused by glomerulonephritis; 20%-30% have pyelonephritis or other
interstitial disease; 15%-20% have multisystem disease; and approximately
10% have cystic kidney disease. There are two types of transplant donors—
living and cadaveric. The 1-yr success rate with live donor transplantation
is 90%-95%. The 1-yr success rate with cadaveric transplantation since the
advent of cyclosporine has improved to 80%-90%. The majority of patients
do not have a suitable (medically or psychologically) live donor and therefore
are placed on a cadaveric waiting list. The demand exceeds the supply, with
approximately 40,000 patients awaiting transplantation in the United States
alone.

Rejection and infection remain the major complications after transplantation. Rejection is the phenomenon that represents the recipient's immunologic response to the transplanted kidney. There are two types of lymphocytes
involved in the rejection response, and either or both may participate: B lymphocytes, which form antibodies (humoral immunity), and T lymphocytes,
which produce cell-mediated immunity. The rejection response can be categorized into four distinct types: hyperacute, accelerated acute, acute, and chronic
(Table 5-7).

TABLE 5-7 Types of Renal Rejection

Type	Mechanism	Clinical presentation	Treatment
Hyperacute	Preformed antibodies against donor antigens	Occurs in the operating room. Kidney turns blue and becomes soft and flabby	Removal of kidney
Accelerated acute	May be mediated by humoral antibody or primed lymphocytes (possible presensitization in the recipient)	Occurs 48-72 h after transplantation. Abrupt fall in urine output; leukocytosis or leukopenia; tenderness over kidney; decreased flow on renal scan; profound thrombocytopenia	Bolus IV steroids for 3-4 days; antilymphocyte preparations; poor prognosis for reversal
Acute	Cell-mediated T lymphocytes infiltrate renal tissue; humoral-mediated antigen-antibody complexes, platelets, and fibrin aggregates are present in glomerular and peritubular capillaries; may be a combination of cell-mediated and humoral-mediated	Occurs from 1-2 wk to several months after transplantation. Fever, leukocytosis, and enlarged and tender kidney; drop in urine output, weight gain (1-1.5 kg/24 h), hypertension, elevated BUN and creatinine	Bolus steroids, antilymphocyte preparations, and monoclonal antibody treatments most effective in reversing this type of rejection; good prognosis
Chronic	Probably a combined effect of antibody and cell-mediated components	Occurs months to years after transplantation. Slow, progressive decrease in renal function; hypertension; proteinuria	None known; poor prognosis for graft survival

BUN, Blood urea nitrogen; *IV,* intravenous.

ASSESSMENT FOR REJECTION

Sudden drop in urine output: Oliguria or anuria may develop.

> **Note:**   A sudden drop in output in the first 24 h after surgery, when a Foley catheter is in place, may signal the presence of clot obstruction, which should be ruled out as the first cause of oliguria.

Elevated temperature: Low-grade, persistent fevers of 37.2°-37.8° C (99°-100° F) can occur with rejection. In the presence of accelerated or acute rejection, the patient may have fevers ranging from 37.8°-40° C (100°-104° F).
Edema: May increase in grade from 1+ (slight indentation over bony areas such as the tibia) to 3+ and 4+, with the degree of indentation increasing significantly.
Hypertension: BP that increases ≥10 mm Hg over baseline.
Weight gain: Increase of 2-3 lb over a 24-h period.
BUN and creatinine values: Will increase from previous 24-h levels and continue to rise until rejection is reversed.
24-h urine collection: Will exhibit a change in components (e.g., decreases in creatinine clearance, total amount of creatinine excreted, and urinary sodium excretion; increase in protein excretion).

> **Note:**   In the early postoperative period, the urine may remain bloody for several days, causing urinary protein concentration to be falsely elevated because of Hgb breakdown in the urine.

Renal scan: Will exhibit decreased blood flow.
Kidney assessment: May reveal a firm, large kidney that may be tender on palpation.

DIAGNOSTIC TESTS

Renal scan: Evaluates blood flow to the kidney and rate of excretion of substances into the bladder.
Renal biopsy: Determines presence, type, and severity of rejection.
Renal ultrasound: To rule out possibility of obstruction.

TREATMENT OPTIONS FOR REJECTION

Megadoses of IV methylprednisolone (Solu-Medrol):   Block the production of interleukin-2 (IL-2), thereby barring essential factors for activated T cells; prevent transcription of IL-1. The release of IL-1 and IL-2 is part of the process of helper T-cell and cytotoxic T-cell differentiation, which occurs during the immune response that is triggered when foreign antigens are present in the body. Methylprednisolone also is used for its antiinflammatory properties (Table 5-8).
Antithymocyte or antilymphocyte preparations: See Table 5-8.
Monoclonal antibody (Orthoclone OKT3):   Reacts with and blocks the function of the T3 complex on the surface of the T lymphocytes, causing their entrapment by cells in the spleen and liver and leading to their destruction. The T3 complex is responsible for the ability of the T lymphocyte to identify a transplanted organ as foreign (see Table 5-8).
Graft irradiation: Destroys lymphocytes within the graft. Irradiation is performed with 150 rad for approximately 3 days in succession.

NURSING DIAGNOSES AND INTERVENTIONS

Fear and **Anxiety** related to threat to health status secondary to potential loss of the kidney from rejection
Desired outcomes: Within 48 h after the transplant, patient verbalizes accurate information about the signs and symptoms of rejection. Patient's fear and anxiety are controlled as evidenced by HR ≤100 bpm, BP within patient's

TABLE 5-8 Immunosuppressives (Standard Agents and Prophylaxis)

Drug name	Action	Dosage
Azathioprine (e.g., Imuran)	Blocks proliferation of immunocompetent lymphoid cells; affects the rapidly dividing B and T cells	Ranges from 1.5-2 mg/kg/day; IV or PO
Corticosteroids (prednisone)	Suppress the body's inflammatory and allergic processes	Varies; total dose tapered to 20-30 mg/day by first postoperative month
Cyclophosphamide (e.g., Cytoxan)	See azathioprine	1 mg/kg/day IV or PO
Cyclosporine (e.g., Sandimmune)	Interferes with helper T-lymphocyte function; used in combination with corticosteroids and azathioprine	8-14 mg/kg/day PO; 3-4 mg/kg via continuous IV infusion
Antilymphocyte sera (e.g., ATGAM)	Immunoglobulin preparation that coats the T cells, making them susceptible to phagocytosis	*Prophylaxis:* 10-15 mg/kg IV over 4-6 h for 5-10 days *Rejection:* 10-15 mg/kg IV over 4-6 h for 10-14 days
Monoclonal antibody (Orthoclone OKT3)	Reacts with T3 complex on the surface of the T cells, causing their removal from the circulation	5 mg IV push over 30-60 sec for 10-14 days to treat rejection

NOTE: Each of these agents, when used individually or in combination, leads to an increased incidence of infection and malignancy secondary to their immunosuppressive properties.
IV, Intravenous; *PO,* oral.

normal range, and RR ≤20 breaths/min. Patient demonstrates ability to relax, discusses anxiety related to the rejection, and exhibits increased involvement in his or her own care.
- Provide opportunities for patient to express fears, concerns, and anxieties about kidney rejection.
- Assess patient's knowledge of the signs and symptoms of rejection. Ensure that patient and significant others can verbalize knowledge of the following indicators of rejection:
  ☐ Persistent, low-grade fever of 37.2°-37.8° C (99°-100° F).
  ☐ Increased swelling of feet, ankles, hands, or face.
  ☐ Weight gain >1 kg/24 h.
  ☐ Painful and swollen kidney.
  ☐ Elevated BP.
  ☐ Decreased 24-h urine output.
- Reassure patient that several medication regimens (e.g., corticosteroids,

antilymphocyte preparations, and monoclonal antibody) are available to treat rejection episodes.

- Reassure patient that rejection does not necessarily mean kidney loss. Under most circumstances, rejection can be reversed.
- Reassure patient that retransplantation is a viable option if kidney loss occurs.

NIC Anxiety Reduction; Coping Enhancement. Additional optional interventions include Progressive Muscle Relaxation; Self-Esteem Enhancement; Simple Relaxation Therapy; Support Group

Knowledge deficit: immunosuppressive medications and their side effects

Desired outcome: Within 72 h after initiation of medications, patient and significant others verbalize accurate information regarding the prescribed immunosuppressive agents, the side effects that can occur, and precautions that should be taken.

- Provide patient with verbal and written information for the type of immunosuppressive agent that has been prescribed. Discuss the generic name, trade name, purpose, usual dosage, route, side effects, and precautions (see Table 5-8 for purpose, usual dosage, and route) for each medication. Commonly prescribed medications follow:

Azathioprine (Imuran)

- Major side effects include leukopenia and thrombocytopenia, nausea and vomiting, diarrhea. In addition, it increases the risk of cancer and can contribute to an increased susceptibility to infection and hepatotoxicity.
- Report fever, chills, cough, muscle or joint pain, rapid heartbeat, stomach pain with nausea and vomiting, sores in mouth and on lips.
- Blood should be tested at frequent intervals for evaluation of white blood cells (WBCs) and platelets. Report jaundice promptly to health care provider.
- Hair loss can occur early in the treatment course, but occurs less frequently over time.

Tacrolimus (Prograf)

- Major side effects include nephrotoxicity, hypertension, neurotoxicity, tremors, tingling of the hands and feet, paresthesias, insomnia, headache, tinnitus, hyperglycemia.
- Blood levels of tacrolimus are monitored to ensure maintenance of therapeutic ranges.
- Absorption is increased in a fasting state. Dosing is spaced 12 h apart.
- Because of the tendency to hyperglycemia, monitor blood glucose and follow a diet low in concentrated carbohydrates.
- Report neurologic symptoms immediately. Report nausea and vomiting. Do not repeat dose unless told to do so by the physician.
- Consult the physician before taking any OTC medications.

Corticosteroids

- Major side effects include cushingoid features, edema, hypertension, bone disease, muscle wasting, cataracts, steroid-induced diabetes, acne, GI irritation, capillary fragility.
- Immediately report swelling of ankles, hands, or face; BP >20 mm Hg over baseline; swollen or bleeding gums; night sweats; change in eyesight; muscle weakness.

Cyclosporine (Sandimmune or Neoral)

- Major side effects include nephrotoxicity, hepatotoxicity, leukopenia, thrombocytopenia, hirsutism, muscle pain, fluid retention, edema, tremors, hypertension, nausea, vomiting, diarrhea, gum hyperplasia, anorexia, anaphylaxis (rare but can occur with IV route). Immediately report these symptoms.
- Blood levels of cyclosporine are monitored at frequent intervals to ensure maximal absorption of oral solution. This is particularly important for patients experiencing GI malabsorption.
- To make oral solutions more palatable, mix with orange juice or milk and

drink immediately. Stir the mixture well, and use a glass container because plastic, foam, or paper will absorb the medication. However, most patients now use the capsule form of either Sandimmune or Neoral.
- Rinse syringe and container with milk or orange juice and drink the remaining solution to ensure that all medication has been taken.
- Take medication 1 h before or 2 h after meals, and if taking twice a day, space the doses 12 h apart.
- Tolerance to the medication, with a decrease in side effects, occurs over time.
- Because of gum hyperplasia, brush teeth with soft-bristle toothbrush and nonabrasive toothpaste after meals and snacks.
- Report nausea and vomiting that occur after dose of cyclosporine, and *do not* repeat dose unless told to do so by physician.
- Report headache, breast enlargement, flushing, presence of any skin lesions.
- Protect skin from freezing temperatures (e.g., by wearing a mitten when taking foods out of the freezer).
- Consult physician before taking OTC medications.

Mycophenolate mofetil (CellCept)
- Major side effects include GI distress, neutropenia, anemia, thrombocytopenia, infections.
- Report nausea, vomiting, diarrhea, blood loss in stool, fever, chills, abdominal pain, sores in the mouth and on the lips.
- Blood should be tested to evaluate WBCs and platelets.

Antilymphocyte sera
- Major side effects include local phlebitis, thrombocytopenia, pruritus, serum sickness. Indicators of serum sickness include rashes on the skin or genital area, joint pain and swelling, fever and chills, night sweats. Consult physician for indicators of serum sickness.

Monoclonal antibody
- Major side effects include chills and fever, headache, photophobia, nausea, vomiting, diarrhea, dyspnea, bronchospasm.

> ***Caution:*** Intensive monitoring is required during the first two doses because of the high frequency of side effects just discussed. In addition, risk of pulmonary edema is increased in the presence of fluid volume excess.
> The patient is premedicated with acetaminophen, diphenhydramine, and hydrocortisone to decrease the above symptoms. A chest x-ray must be clear before the first dose is given.

NIC Teaching: Disease Process; Teaching: Individual; Teaching: Prescribed Medication. Additional optional interventions include Discharge Planning; Medication Management; Weight Management

Risk for infection related to inadequate secondary responses as a result of immunosuppression

Desired outcome: Patient is free of infection as evidenced by normothermia; absence of erythema, swelling, and drainage of catheter and wound sites; absence of adventitious breath sounds or cloudy and foul-smelling urine; negative results of urine, wound drainage, and blood cultures; and WBC count 4,500-11,000/mm^3.
- Assess and record patient's temperature q4h; consult physician for elevations ≥37.8° C (100° F).
- Assess and document condition of indwelling IV sites and other catheter sites q8h. Be alert to swelling, erythema, tenderness, and drainage. Consult physician for any of these findings.
- As prescribed, obtain blood, urine, and wound cultures when infection is suspected.
- Be alert to WBC count >11,000/mm^3 or <4,500/mm^3. A below-normal WBC

count with increased band neutrophils on differential (shift to the left) may signal acute infection.

- Inspect graft wound for erythema, swelling, and drainage. Consult physician for significant findings.
- Record volume, appearance, color, and odor of urine. Be alert to foul-smelling or cloudy urine, frequency and urgency of urination, and patient complaints of flank or labial pain, all of which are signs of renal-urinary infection.
- Auscultate lung fields q8h, noting presence of rhonchi, crackles, and decreased breath sounds.
- Use meticulous aseptic technique when dressing and caring for wounds and catheter sites.
- Obtain specimens for urine cultures once a week during patient's hospitalization and once a month after hospital discharge.

NIC Infection Control; Infection Protection. Additional optional interventions include Airway Management; Exercise Promotion and Therapy (all listed); Medication Management; Respiratory Monitoring; Teaching: Disease Process; Tube Care: Urinary; Vital Signs Monitoring

Altered oral mucous membrane related to treatment with immunosuppressive medication

Desired outcomes: Patient's oral mucosa, tongue, and lips are pink, intact, and free of exudate and lesions. Patient states that he or she can swallow without difficulty within 24 h after treatment for altered oral mucous membrane.

- Inspect the mouth daily for signs of exudate and lesions; consult physician if they are present. Teach patient to perform self-inspection of mouth.
- Teach patient to brush with a soft-bristle toothbrush and nonabrasive toothpaste after meals and snacks.
- To help prevent monilial infection, provide patient with mycostatin prophylactic mouthwash for "swish and swallow" after meals and at bedtime.

NIC Oral Health Maintenance; Oral Health Promotion

Impaired skin integrity (or risk for same): herpetic lesions, skin fungal rashes, pruritus, and capillary fragility, related to treatment with immunosuppressive medications

Desired outcome: Patient's skin is intact and free of open lesions or abrasions.

- Assess for and document daily the presence of erythema, excoriation, rashes, or bruises on patient's skin.
- Assess for and document the presence of rashes or lesions in the perineal area, inasmuch as herpetic lesions are common in the immunosuppressed patient.
- Inspect the trunk area daily for the presence of flat, itchy rashes. Skin fungal rashes are common in the immunosuppressed patient.
- Teach patient the importance of daily skin care with water, nondrying soap, and lubricating lotion.
- Use nonallergenic tape when anchoring IV tubing, catheters, and dressings.
- Assist patient with changing position at least q2h; massage areas that are susceptible to breakdown, particularly areas over bony prominences.

NIC Skin Surveillance; Pressure Ulcer Prevention. Additional optional interventions include Bathing; Bleeding Precautions; Cutaneous Stimulation; Exercise Promotion and Therapy (all listed); Electrolyte Monitoring; Exercise Promotion: Stretching; Fluid/Electrolyte Management; Infection Control; Infection Prevention; Medication Management; Nail Care; Nutrition Management; Perineal Care; Surveillance; Vital Signs Monitoring

ADDITIONAL NURSING DIAGNOSES

As indicated, also see "Acute Renal Failure," p. 371. Also see "Organ Rejection" for **Powerlessness** related to actual and perceived inability to control organ rejection episodes, p. 621. For other nursing diagnoses and interventions, see the following sections, as appropriate: "Nutritional Support," p. 1; "Prolonged Immobility," p. 74; "Psychosocial Support," p. 83; and "Psychosocial Support for the Patient's Family and Significant Others," p. 95.

Renal replacement therapies

The patient with renal dysfunction has an increasingly malfunctioning physiologic system. The goal of renal replacement therapy (RRT) is to restore dynamic equilibrium to that system. Indications for RRT in a critical care setting include fluid removal, solute removal, and correction of electrolyte and acid-base abnormalities. RRT uses four principles for solute and water removal: diffusion, osmosis, ultrafiltration, and convection.

Diffusion: Movement of solutes from an area of greater concentration to an area of lesser concentration. Diffusion requires a concentration gradient. During dialysis, high concentrations of waste products and excess electrolytes diffuse into the dialysate, which contains much lower concentrations of these solutes.

Osmosis: Passive movement of water from an area of low solute concentration to an area of high solute concentration. Thus the use of high concentrations of glucose in the peritoneal dialysate causes movement of water from the patient's plasma into the dialysate.

Ultrafiltration: Movement of water from an area of higher pressure to an area of lower pressure. In hemodialysis, negative pressure in the dialysate facilitates the rapid removal of excess water from the blood compartment in which positive pressure exists.

Convection: Removal of a substance with fluid across a semipermeable membrane over time.

INDICATIONS FOR RRT

- Volume excess
- Hyperkalemia and other electrolyte disturbances
- Metabolic acidosis
- Uremic intoxication
    - ☐ Neurologic (encephalopathy)
    - ☐ Hematologic (bleeding caused by platelet dysfunction)
    - ☐ Gastrointestinal (anorexia, nausea, vomiting)
    - ☐ Cardiovascular (pericarditis)
- Need for removal of dialyzable substances (metabolites, drugs, toxins)

DETERMINATION FOR TYPE OF RRT USED

- Availability in the institution of hemodialysis (HD), peritoneal dialysis (PD), continuous arteriovenous hemofiltration (CAVH), or continuous venovenous hemofiltration (CVVH).
- Type best suited for patient's clinical status. Catabolism, for example, causes rapid rises in BUN, creatinine, and potassium values. The patient needs rapid removal of metabolic wastes (i.e., hemodialysis) (Table 5-9). Advantages and disadvantages of RRT methods are found in Table 5-10. Complications of RRT are found in Table 5-11.
- Blood or peritoneal access route availability.
- Ability to effect safe anticoagulation.

PERITONEAL DIALYSIS

The semipermeable membrane used during peritoneal dialysis is the patient's peritoneum. A special catheter is placed in the peritoneal cavity, and dialysate solution is instilled. Water, electrolytes, and waste products cross between the capillary bed of the peritoneum and the dialysate via osmosis and diffusion.

T A B L E 5 - 9   Comparison of Renal Replacement Therapies

	Peritoneal dialysis	Hemodialysis	CAVH	CVVH
Access route	Peritoneal catheter, which may be used immediately	Subclavian or femoral catheter or arteriovenous shunt, which may be used immediately	Arterial and venous catheters or shunt Patient's mean arterial pressure drives flow rate	Double-lumen venous catheter Pump used to achieve flow rate
Semipermeable membrane	Peritoneum; approximately 2.2 m^2 (the total area available for diffusion of solutes)	Cuprophane or cellulose acetate; 1-2 m^2	High-efficiency, high-flux material (polysulfone, polyamide, and polyacrylonitrile)	Same as CAVH
Molecular movement	Diffusion by a concentration gradient	Diffusion by a concentration gradient	Diffusion and convection	Same as CAVH
Water removal	Osmotic pressure, using high glucose concentration	Hydrostatic pressure (pressure gradient across the membrane)	Ultrafiltration—hydrostatic pressure	Same as CAVH

Duration				
6-12 cycles/day, intermittent PD (IPD); 3-4 cycles/day, continuous ambulatory (CAPD); nighttime, continuous cycling (CCPD) machine	3 h, 3/wk; maximum of 3-4 h/day	Continuous	Same as CAVH
Efficiency				
Slow diffusion; less efficient than hemodialysis	High efficiency	High for fluid removal, moderate solute removal	Same as CAVH
Risk of infection				
High	Lower than peritoneal method	High for access infection	Same as CAVH
Major problem				
Development of peritonitis	May not be tolerated by the patient with hemodynamic instability	Dehydration and hypotension	Same as CAVH

CAVH, Continuous arteriovenous hemofiltration; *CVVH*, continuous venovenous hemofiltration.

TABLE 5-10   Advantages and Disadvantages of Methods of Renal Replacement Therapy

Advantages	Disadvantages
Hemodialysis	
Very efficient; requires short, frequent treatments	Special equipment and trained staff
As needed, fluid and chemical balance may be altered rapidly	Heparinization usually required
	Possibility of disequilibrium from too-rapid fluid and biochemical shifts
	Possible difficulty in maintaining vascular access
	Blood loss necessitating transfusion
Peritoneal dialysis	
Simple equipment; rapid initiation of treatment	Time consuming
Systemic anticoagulation not needed	Risk of peritonitis and pneumonia
Slow dialysis; less risk of hypotension and rapid fluid and electrolyte shifts	Desired effects slower to occur
	Protein loss
	Some patient discomfort
Hemofiltration	
Physiologic process	Low-efficiency solute removal
Ideal for the patient who is hemodynamically unstable	Large volume fluid replacement
Allows administration of large volumes (e.g., TPN)	Potential for electrolyte imbalance
Technically simple	Increased responsibilities for ICU nurses
CVVH effective in patients with MAP <70 mm Hg	

TPN, Total parenteral nutrition; *CVVH,* continuous venovenous hemofiltration; *MAP,* mean arterial pressure.

System components
Catheter: Two types are commonly used:
- *Trocar:* A stiff Silastic catheter inserted at the bedside that provides temporary access.
- *Soft Silastic indwelling catheter* (e.g., Tenckhoff): Inserted in the operating room to provide permanent access.

Dialysate: A premixed, sterile electrolyte solution with a composition similar to that of normal plasma. The concentration of ionized calcium is high to maintain a positive calcium balance. Hypocalcemia tends to occur in patients with renal failure, and the goal is to maintain serum calcium levels at 8.5-10 mg/dl. Glucose concentrations are variable inasmuch as hypertonic solutions are used to increase osmotic load for greater filtration. Potassium is added according to patient need.

Methods of peritoneal dialysis
Intermittent peritoneal dialysis (IPD):   Usually involves 3-4 treatments/wk, lasting 8-10 h each session. Hospitalized patients with acute renal failure may undergo dialysis for 24 h every other day.

Continuous ambulatory peritoneal dialysis (CAPD):   Involves extension of the time the fluid remains in the abdomen (dwell time) to 4 h during the day and 8 h during the night, with 4-5 exchanges during a day. Dialysis occurs 7 days a week, 24 h a day. This method is the most physiologic form of dialysis.

TABLE 5-11   Complications of Renal Replacement Therapies

Hemodialysis	Peritoneal dialysis	Hemofiltration
Hypotension	Bowel or bladder	Bleeding
Air embolus	perforation	Infection
Angina and dysrhythmias	Hyperglycemic	Volume depletion
Blood loss (dialyzer	hyperosmolar coma	Blood leakage
rupture)	Hypernatremia	Decreased ultrafiltration
Disequilibrium syndrome	Hypovolemia	Filter clotting
Hemolysis	Metabolic alkalosis	Electrolyte disturbances
Hemorrhage	Peritonitis	Air embolus
Septicemia	**Procedural complications**	with CVVH
Bleeding	Abdominal distention:	
Clotting	failure to drain dialysate	
High-output heart failure	• Catheter obstruction	
Infection	from clots or fibrin	
Phlebitis	• Catheter becoming	
Venous spasm	wrapped in omentum	
	Cuff erosion	
	Catheter malposition	
	Tunnel infection	

CVVH, Continuous venovenous hemofiltration.

Continuous cycling peritoneal dialysis (CCPD): Dialysis treatments are performed continuously throughout the night using a special cycling machine.

HEMODIALYSIS
With hemodialysis an artificial semipermeable membrane is used to diffuse water, electrolytes, and waste products from the blood. The patient's blood is heparinized, passed through the dialyzer, and then returned to the circulation. For acutely ill patients, dialysis may be needed from 3 times/wk to daily.
System components
Dialyzer (artificial kidney): Consists of the blood compartment, dialysate compartment, and the semipermeable membrane. Small molecules, such as electrolytes, water, and waste products, pass through this membrane; RBCs, protein, and bacteria, however, are too large to cross.
Dialysate: Electrolyte solution similar to normal plasma. The potassium concentration varies according to patient need. Glucose may be necessary to prevent changes in the patient's serum glucose and osmolality values. Although glucose is a large molecule, it can cross the semipermeable membrane, resulting in hypoglycemia. Use of a glucose bath reduces the risk of hypoglycemia.
Vascular access: Method used to deliver blood to the dialyzer at a rate of at least 200-300 ml/min.
- *Subclavian or femoral catheter:* Temporary access catheter (usually double lumen) that is placed in a large vein to enhance blood flow (e.g., Tesio, Vascath).
- *Arteriovenous (AV) fistula:* Anastomosis of an artery and vein, resulting in dilated vessels for easy cannulation and increased blood flow.
- *Graft:* Bovine, Gore-Tex, or saphenous vein. The graft connects the artery and vein internally in the arm or thigh.
- *Hemasite:* A T-shaped device inserted into an arterialized vein with a Gore-Tex graft. The "T" projects out of the skin, resulting in an external entry point.

CONTINUOUS ARTERIOVENOUS HEMOFILTRATION OR CONTINUOUS VENOVENOUS HEMOFILTRATION

CAVH and CVVH are two types of renal therapy performed to manage fluid overload in critically ill patients. Their advantage over conventional dialytic therapies is that ultrafiltration occurs gradually, thus avoiding drastic volume changes and rapid fluid shifts. Treatment duration may be 24 h or several days, depending on the total amount of fluid to be removed.

Principles

- Use of a highly permeable, hollow fiber filter (e.g., Amicon Diafilter 20).
- Removal of plasma water and unbound substances, such as urea, calcium, sodium, potassium, chloride, vitamins, and unbound drugs, with a molecular weight between 500 and 10,000 daltons.
- Filtration: Movement of fluid across a semipermeable membrane from an area of greater pressure to one of lesser pressure (pressure gradient).
- Convection: Some elements in plasma water (e.g., urea) conveyed across the membrane as a result of the differences in hydrostatic pressure. The removal of large amounts of plasma water results in the removal of large amounts of filterable solutes.
- For ultrafiltration to occur, there must be a pressure gradient across the membrane that favors filtration. In CAVH or CVVH this is called *transmembrane pressure (TMP)*, and its major determinants are hydrostatic pressure and oncotic pressure. The higher pressure in the blood compartment is a function of the individual's blood pressure. Pressure in the blood compartment is adequate when the systolic pressure is 50-70 mm Hg. Higher pressures enhance ultrafiltration. Negative pressure for ultrafiltration can be achieved by lowering the collection container 20-40 cm below the hemofilter. The differences in hydrostatic pressure also cause the crossing of some elements, such as glucose and some vitamins. The longer it takes for blood to clear the filter, the more likely that intermediate molecules (vitamins, glucose) will be filtered out of the patient's system. Opposing the hydrostatic pressure is oncotic pressure, which is maintained by plasma proteins that do not pass through the membrane. When hydrostatic pressure exceeds oncotic pressure, filtration of water and solutes occurs.

Indications for CAVH or CVVH

- Massive fluid overload: congestive heart failure, acute renal failure, overaggressive fluid resuscitation in multiple trauma.
- Fluid overload in the presence of hemodynamic instability.
- Cardiogenic shock with pulmonary edema.
- Oliguric patient unresponsive to diuretics.
- Patient with anuria who requires large volumes of parenteral fluid: acts as a supplement to hemodialysis to maintain fluid balance.

Method: The hemofilter and lines are primed with normal saline before the treatment is initiated. Blood flows from the arterial (usually femoral or radial) limb of the vascular access through the filter and returns through the venous (usually femoral or cephalic) limb of the access. A continuous infusion of heparin prevents clotting in the lines and filter. Blood is driven through the system by the patient's blood pressure with CAVH, so no pump is used. With CVVH a pump is used to drive the blood flow. As the blood flows through the filter, water, electrolytes, and most drugs not bound to plasma protein diffuse across the membrane and thus become part of the filtrate. If the objective is the removal of large amounts of fluid and solute (urea, potassium, creatinine), it is necessary to infuse large volumes of filtration replacement fluid (FRF) to maintain electrolyte balance. Nursing responsibilities include initiating treatment, monitoring the patient and system, and discontinuing treatment. Tables 5-10 and 5-11 discuss the advantages, disadvantages, and complications of RRTs, including hemofiltration. Table 5-12 discusses troubleshooting major problems with hemofiltration.

TABLE 5-12	**Troubleshooting Major Problems in Hemofiltration**	
Problem	**Cause**	**Intervention**
Hypotension	Cardiac dysfunction Excessive intravascular volume removal	Cardiotonic and pressor support Fluid replacement Recalculate UF rate
Poor ultrafiltration	High hematocrit Decreased MAP Clotted filter	Predilution fluid replacement Pressor support to increase MAP Flush filter; replace if necessary
Clotted hemofilter	Inadequate anticoagulation Poor blood flow rates Kinks in blood tubing	Check ACT or aPPT hourly, and adjust heparin infusion Pressors or fluid replacement to increase MAP Check tubing hourly to guard against kinks Change filter, and restart therapy

UF, Ultrafiltration; *MAP,* mean arterial pressure; *ACT,* activated clotting time; *aPPT,* activated partial thromboplastin time.

COLLABORATIVE MANAGEMENT
For patients undergoing dialysis
Dietary restrictions
Hemodialysis: Between dialysis treatments the main products of protein metabolism and potassium and sodium will accumulate because of the kidneys' inability to excrete excesses of these products. Therefore it is necessary to restrict the intake of protein to decrease the amount of urea generated, to restrict potassium to prevent hyperkalemia, and to restrict sodium to prevent hypernatremia and curb thirst. Recommended guidelines include protein 1-1.2 g/kg/day; sodium 80-100 mEq/day (individualized); and potassium 40-80 mEq/day (individualized).

Peritoneal dialysis: Patients undergoing peritoneal dialysis tend to lose more protein through the peritoneal membrane. Therefore protein restriction is liberalized to 1.2-1.5 g/kg/day to compensate for the extra loss. If peritonitis develops, protein loss can increase from around 10 g/day to 50 g/day. Patients undergoing CAPD may need calorie restrictions because of the added calories they absorb from the glucose contained in the dialysate. If hypertonic solutions are used several times a day, these patients can absorb as much as 600 calories or more from the dialysate. Potassium may be less restricted in these patients because the dialysate is potassium free and allows better diffusion of potassium with less accumulation that would lead to hyperkalemia. Sodium restriction in peritoneal dialysis is approximately 80-100 mEq/day to prevent hypernatremia and control thirst to prevent fluid overload.

Fluid restriction: To prevent fluid overload secondary to the kidneys' inability to excrete excess water. Weight gain between dialysis treatments usually is the result of fluid retention. An attempt is made to limit interdialytic weight gain to 1.5-2 kg by limiting fluid intake to 1500-1800 ml in 24 h. This restriction also is individualized.

Phosphate binders: To prevent or control hyperphosphatemia, which can occur because of the kidneys' inability to excrete excess dietary phosphates.

Vitamin D analogs (dihydrotachysterol—the active form of vitamin D) and calcium replacement: To prevent hypocalcemia and renal osteodystrophy, which may occur because of the body's inability to absorb calcium and maintain serum levels. If hypocalcemia occurs, the parathyroid glands are activated to release parathormone, which releases calcium from the bone to replenish serum levels. Over time, this can lead to bone demineralization and osteodystrophy.

Water-soluble vitamins and folic acid: Are dialyzable and necessitate replacement after dialysis.

For patients undergoing continuous arteriovenous or venovenous hemofiltration
The goal is the removal of excess fluid while maintaining electrolyte balance and adequate fluid intake for homeostasis. In the critically ill adult, catabolic rate is 2-3 times that of normal, and this is balanced with TPN.

TPN: To maintain nutritional requirements.

CAVH: To correct hypervolemic state. A large-bore catheter is used for access.

Predilution fluid replacement: If increased solute removal is required. (See Table 5-13 for differences between predilution and postdilution replacement.)

Filtration replacement fluid: To maintain fluid and electrolyte balance. (See Table 5-14 for calculation of infusion rate of these fluids.) Concentration may vary, depending on the replacement needs of the patient.

Standard fluids infused simultaneously include:
1 L 0.9 NS with 7.5 ml 10% CaCl
1 L 0.9 NS with 1.6 ml 50% $MgSO_4$
1 L 0.9 NS
1 L D_5W with 150 mEq $NaHCO_3^-$
Final composition of fluid for typical patient:
Sodium: 150 mEq/L
Chloride: 114 mEq/L

TABLE 5-13   Approaches to Fluid Replacement

Predilution: replacement fluid infused proximal to the filter	Postdilution: replacement fluid infused distal to the filter
Patient population: Those with poor blood flow and elevated BUN and Hct levels	*Patient population:* All types
Replacement fluid infused into arterial line	Replacement fluid infused into venous line
Used to enhance urea clearance to ≥18%; decreases oncotic pressure, increasing net TMP; moves urea from erythrocytes into plasma	Used to maintain fluid and electrolyte balance
Increases net fluid removal	Less replacement fluid required
Potentially increases filter life	Simplified clearance determination
*Urea clearance 12.5 ml/min	Urea clearance 10.6 ml/min

BUN, Blood urea nitrogen; *Hct,* hematocrit; *TMP,* transmembrane pressure.
*If increased urea clearance is desired, predilution mode of fluid replacement is used.

Bicarbonate: 37 mEq/L
Magnesium: 1.6 mEq/L
Calcium: 2.5 mEq/L
Heparin infusion solution: To prevent clotting in the circuit.
Vasopressors: To maintain arterial pressure, which is necessary for driving the blood through the hemofilter.

NURSING DIAGNOSES AND INTERVENTIONS
For patients undergoing dialysis
Risk for infection related to invasive procedure used to obtain peritoneal or vascular access for dialysis
Desired outcome: Patient is free of infection as evidenced by normothermia; WBC count ≤11,000/mm^3; blood and dialysate free of infective organisms; and absence of erythema, purulent drainage, abdominal or access site pain, and cloudy dialysate.

- Assess and document condition of the access site daily. Be alert to the presence of erythema, purulent drainage, or tenderness.
- Peritonitis accounts for a high incidence of failure with peritoneal dialysis. Use strict aseptic technique when cleansing catheter site and connecting and disconnecting dialysis bags. Use an antiseptic solution such as hydrogen peroxide or povidone-iodine to cleanse the access site. Maintain aseptic technique when cleansing and drying the site. Cover the site with a dry, sterile dressing. Because moist surfaces breed bacteria, change the dressing immediately if it becomes wet.
- Keep all external access devices (shunts, subclavian catheters, femoral catheters, peritoneal catheters) covered with a dry, sterile dressing between treatments.
- Document the appearance of peritoneal dialysis effluent. If peritoneal drainage becomes cloudy or contains flecks of material, send specimen for a culture and obtain a cell count to check for increased white cells in the peritoneal effluent. Consult physician for changes in outflow.
- Report the presence of an elevated temperature, malaise, access site drainage, cloudy dialysate, and abdominal pain.
- Teach patient to notify staff members if symptoms of infection occur.

NIC Infection Control; Infection Protection. Additional optional interventions include Airway Management; Exercise Promotion and Therapy (all listed); Medication Management; Respiratory Monitoring; Teaching: Disease Process; Tube Care: Urinary; Vital Signs Monitoring

---

TABLE 5-14   Calculation of Filtration Replacement Fluid (FRF) Rate

Infusion rate
   Equals ultrafiltrate plus other losses per hour minus all fluid infused minus net removal rate

Example
   Ultrafiltrate = 600 ml/h + Losses (urine, GI) = 100 ml/h – Hyperalimentation 100 ml/h; vasopressors 50 ml/h – Net fluid removal rate 150 ml/h

FRF rate
   = (600 + 100) – (100 + 50 + 150)
        700   –   300

FRF rate
   = 400 ml/h

Altered nutrition: less than body requirements, related to dietary restrictions; protein loss occurring with peritoneal dialysis

Desired outcomes: Patient has adequate nutrition as evidenced by stable weekly body weight. Patient's caloric intake ranges from 35-45 calories/kg body weight/day (may not be appropriate for patient with CAPD, who absorbs calories through the dialysate); high-in-biologic-value protein intake is 50%-75% of patient's daily protein intake. Nitrogen intake is 4-6 g more than nitrogen loss (loss calculated from 24-h urinary urea excretion, and intake estimated from protein intake).

- Document food intake; count calories consumed with each meal. Total caloric intake should be 35-45 calories/kg body weight/24 h.
- Consult with physician and dietitian regarding use of nutritional supplements for maintaining caloric intake.
- For patient undergoing peritoneal dialysis, encourage intake of protein (e.g., milk shakes with protein supplements, custards).
- Weigh patient daily. Be alert to losses ≥10% of patient's normal body weight over a 1-wk period. Daily fluctuations reflect body fluid changes.
- For the patient receiving hemodialysis, encourage the intake of foods that are high in calories (e.g., butter, honey, hard candy, tapioca, sherbet, corn syrup, ginger ale, jellies, jams, marshmallows). Patients undergoing peritoneal dialysis absorb extra calories from the glucose in the peritoneal dialysate.
- Concentrate protein intake on high-in-biologic-value protein foods (e.g., meats, milk, fish, fowl, eggs).
- Minimize the intake of protein from low-in-biologic-value protein foods (e.g., breads, cereals, pastas, grains, fruits, vegetables).
- For patients receiving hemodialysis in particular, suggest the intake of caloric substances that do not contain protein or electrolytes. Commercially available products are Cal-Powder, Controlyte, Hycal, and Polycose.
- As appropriate, refer to dietitian, who can teach the patient and significant others meal-planning techniques that will include restrictions while maintaining a high-calorie intake. Many dialysis patients also are diabetic, and careful meal planning is necessary.
- If patient is anorexic or nauseated, provide small, frequent meals. Present appetizing food in a pleasant atmosphere. As indicated, administer prescribed antiemetic ½ h before meals.

NIC Nutrition Management; Nutritional Monitoring; Fluid Management; Fluid Monitoring. Additional optional interventions include Bowel Management; Energy Management; Enteral Tube Feeding; Exercise Promotion; Gastrointestinal Intubation; Hyperglycemia Management; Hypoglycemia Management; Intravenous Insertion; Intravenous Therapy; Medication Management; Mutual Goal Setting; Phlebotomy: Venous Blood Sample; Positioning; Teaching: Individual; Teaching: Prescribed Diet; Total Parenteral Nutrition Administration; Venous Access Devices Maintenance

Fluid volume excess (or risk for same) related to dietary indiscretions of sodium and fluids; compromised regulatory mechanisms secondary to renal failure

Desired outcome: Within 24-48 h of admission, patient is normovolemic as evidenced by balanced I&O; stable weight; HR ≤100 bpm; BP within patient's normal range; RR 12-20 breaths/min; and absence of edema, crackles, and other physical indicators of hypervolemia.

- Monitor and record I&O q4h, and weight daily; report significant findings to physician. Be alert to weight gain of >0.5-1 kg/24 h.
- Assess and record status of VS, lung sounds, and cardiac rate and rhythm. Be alert to crackles, tachycardia, pericardial friction rub, and pulsus paradoxus.
- Assess for presence of peripheral, periorbital, and sacral edema.
- Maintain fluid restrictions as prescribed.
- Elevate head of bed (HOB) during peritoneal dialysis to relieve pressure of fluid against diaphragm.

- If outflow is poor, change patient's position or irrigate catheter to determine patency.

NIC Electrolyte Management: Hyponatremia; Fluid/Electrolyte Management; Fluid Management; Fluid Monitoring; Electrolyte Management: Hypokalemia. Additional optional interventions include Dysrhythmia Management; Feeding; Gastrointestinal Intubation; Hemodialysis Therapy; Hemodynamic Regulation; Invasive Hemodynamic Monitoring; Medication Management; Phlebotomy: Arterial and Venous Blood Sample; Positioning; Skin Surveillance; Weight Management

Risk for fluid volume deficit related to active loss secondary to excess fluid removal during dialysis; bleeding secondary to heparinization

Desired outcomes: Patient is normovolemic as evidenced by balanced I&O; daily weight within 1-2 lbs of calculated dry weight (true body weight without any excess fluid); BP within patient's normal range; CVP ≥2 mm Hg; and HR ≤100 bpm. Hct is 20%-30% (a range expected for the patient receiving dialysis, inasmuch as anemia is associated with renal failure), and there is no evidence of blood loss caused by line separation or membrane rupture.

- When using hypertonic dialysate for peritoneal dialysis, assess skin turgor, mucous membranes, CVP, BP, and HR for signs of dehydration, which can occur from excessive fluid loss. Be alert to sudden decrease in BP, tachycardia, poor skin turgor, dry mucous membranes, and change in mental status (e.g., restlessness, unresponsiveness).
- When using hypertonic peritoneal dialysate, check finger-stick glucose q4h. Consult physician for blood glucose levels >200 mg/dl.
- Weigh patient daily for trend. Monitor I&O q8h, and consult physician for output >1500 ml over intake.
- Monitor Hct results before each hemodialysis. Notify physician if a >2-point drop occurs.
- If hypotension occurs during peritoneal dialysis, stop the dialysis, consult physician, and encourage oral fluids up to 1000 ml (or per protocol).
- If hypotension occurs during hemodialysis, give normal saline or volume expanders as prescribed and notify physician.
- During hemodialysis, secure lines with tape to prevent disconnection and dislodgment. Consult physician immediately if blood loss occurs because of line separation or dialyzer rupture. As prescribed, send blood sample to laboratory for type and screen.
- Maintain pressure over any venipuncture sites for at least 5 min after needles have been removed.

NIC Electrolyte Management; Fluid Management; Fluid Monitoring; Hypovolemia Management; Intravenous Therapy; Electrolyte Management: Hyperkalemia; Electrolyte Management: Hypermagnesemia; Electrolyte Management: Hypernatremia; Electrolyte Management: Hyperphosphatemia. Additional optional interventions include Dysrhythmia Management; Feeding; Fever Treatment; Gastrointestinal Intubation; Hemodynamic Regulation; Invasive Hemodynamic Monitoring; Medication Management; Nutrition Management; Weight Management; Phlebotomy: Arterial Blood Sample and Venous Blood Sample

Altered peripheral tissue perfusion (or risk for same): Access site, related to interruption of vascular flow secondary to clot formation, pressure, obstruction, or disconnection of vascular access device

Desired outcomes: Patient's access site for dialysis has adequate perfusion as evidenced by palpation of thrill; auscultation of bruit; visualization of blood flow; and warmth of shunt tubing or AV fistula. Warmth and brisk capillary refill (<2 sec) are present in the access extremity.

- Confirm patency of access site by palpating for a thrill (vibratory sensation) and auscultating for presence of bruit (buzzing sound) over shunt or AV fistula. Monitor the access extremity for warmth and brisk capillary refill.
- Notify physician promptly if patency cannot be confirmed. Thrombolytic therapy or embolectomy may be indicated to save the fistula.

- Avoid taking BP, drawing blood, or using restrictive clothing, name bands, or restraints on arm with fistula. Teach patient the importance of these restrictions.
- If using a pressure dressing over the access site, make sure it is snug enough to prevent bleeding but not so tight that it could stop blood flow and promote clot formation. Remove the pressure dressing after it has been on the site for 1-2 h.
- Maintain constant infusion of heparin (e.g., 10 U/ml, or as prescribed, via piggyback) through subclavian or femoral line or flush with heparinized saline and cap as prescribed.
- Flush peritoneal catheter before and after dialysis with 30-50 ml normal saline to ensure patency.
- Always check fistula, graft, or shunt for patency after any hypotensive episode.
- If it is suspected that air has entered the vascular access, clamp the line and place the patient in a left side-lying Trendelenburg position, which will trap air at the apex of the right ventricle of the heart, away from the outflow tract. Call physician *stat,* administer oxygen, and monitor VS carefully.
- For more information, see "Pulmonary Emboli," p. 232.

NIC Circulatory Care. Additional optional interventions include Embolus Precautions; Exercise Promotion; Exercise Therapy (all listed); Surveillance

Altered protection (or risk for same) related to neurosensory alterations secondary to endogenous chemical alteration (dialysis disequilibrium syndrome) occurring with rapid removal of metabolic wastes and changes in serum osmolality

Desired outcome: Patient verbalizes orientation to time, place, and person and does not exhibit signs and symptoms of disequilibrium syndrome: headache, nausea, vomiting, restlessness, asterixis, stupor, coma, or seizures.

- Monitor patient for indicators of disequilibrium syndrome.
- Consult physician for changing LOC and other marked signs of disequilibrium.
- Recognize predisposing factors: BUN >150 mg/dl; hypernatremia (serum sodium >147 mEq/L); severe metabolic acidosis; and history of neurologic problems (e.g., seizures). The syndrome often is prevented by short, frequent dialysis exchanges and by increasing the osmolality of dialysate by adding glucose, glycerol, urea, or mannitol or by giving IV mannitol during treatment.
- Monitor BUN levels before and after dialysis to evaluate for changes occurring along with signs and symptoms of disequilibrium.
- Raise and pad side rails, and keep an appropriate-size airway at the bedside as indicated.

NIC Infection Control; Infection Protection. Additional optional interventions include Nutrition Management; Nutrition Therapy; Nutritional Counseling; Pressure Management; Pressure Ulcer Prevention; Teaching: Individual

Ineffective breathing pattern related to decreased lung expansion secondary to impaired respiratory mechanics occurring with dialysate in the peritoneal cavity

Desired outcome: Patient becomes eupneic within 24 h of this diagnosis.

- Monitor patient's respiratory rate, depth, and pattern and assess breath sounds when dialysate is dwelling in the peritoneal cavity.
- Elevate the HOB to reduce pressure of fluid against the diaphragm and increase vital capacity.
- Schedule deep-breathing exercises and incentive spirometry q2-4h.
- Get patient up in a chair 3-4 times/day if possible.

NIC Airway Management. Additional optional interventions include Acid-Base Monitoring; Analgesic Administration; Aspiration Precautions; Chest Physiotherapy

For patients undergoing continuous arteriovenous or venovenous hemofiltration
Decreased cardiac output (or risk for same) related to decreased preload and electrical changes secondary to fluid and electrolyte shifts occurring with hemofiltration
Desired outcomes: Patient's cardiac output is adequate as evidenced by systolic BP ≥100 mm Hg (or within patient's normal range); HR 60-100 bpm; RR 12-20 breaths/min; peripheral pulses >2+ on a 0-4+ scale; brisk capillary refill (<2 sec); and normal sinus rhythm on ECG.

- Assess and document BP, HR, and RR hourly for the first 4 h of hemofiltration, and then q2h. Be alert to indicators of fluid volume deficit, manifested by a drop in systolic BP to <100 mm Hg, tachycardia, and tachypnea.
- Assess and document peripheral pulses and color, temperature, and capillary refill in the extremities q2h. Be alert to decreased amplitude of peripheral pulses and to coolness, pallor, and delayed capillary refill in the extremities as indicators of decreased perfusion.
- Measure and record I&O hourly. Consult physician for a loss of ≥200 ml/h over desired loss.
- Monitor cardiac rhythm continuously; notify physician of decrease in BP of 20 mm Hg from baseline, tachycardia, depressed T waves and ST segments, and dysrhythmias, which can occur with hypovolemia, potassium changes, or calcium changes.
- Ensure prescribed rates of ultrafiltration and replacement fluid infusion (see Table 5-14), and adjust if ultrafiltration rate changes. Use an infusion pump for replacement fluids to ensure precise rate of infusion. Also maintain TPN and IV rates, as well as oral intake, within 50 ml of the values used to calculate the filtration fluid replacement rate. If any parameters change more than 50 ml, recalculate filtration fluid replacement rate and adjust accordingly.
- Monitor serum electrolyte values, being alert to changes in potassium, calcium, phosphorus, and bicarbonate. Compare patient's values with the following normal ranges: potassium 3.5-5 mEq/L; calcium 8.5-10.5 mg/dl; phosphorus 2.5-4.5 mg/dl; and bicarbonate 22-26 mEq/L. (See "Fluid and Electrolyte Disturbances," p. 636, and "Acid-Base Imbalances," p. 670.)

Risk for fluid volume deficit related to active loss secondary to excessive ultrafiltration during CAVH or CVVH
Desired outcomes: Patient is normovolemic as evidenced by gradual weight loss (<2.5 kg/day) and urinary output ≥0.5 ml/kg/h in nonoliguric patients. Ultrafiltration rate remains within 50 ml of the desired hourly rate.

- Measure and record I&O q30min for the first 2 h and then hourly. Ensure that it is within desired limits.
- Weigh patient q8h. Be alert to daily loss ≥2.5 kg.
- Record cumulative ultrafiltrate loss hourly. Measure amount in the ultrafiltrate container. The difference between this value and total hourly intake is the cumulative loss per hour.
- Check replacement fluid rate hourly to ensure that it is within prescribed limits—usually 25 ml of the calculated rate.
- Consult physician for unanticipated fluid loss from vomiting, diarrhea, fever, and wound drainage.
- Consult physician for increased filtration rate, which may occur because of increased BP; or for increased negative pressure, which may be caused by lowering the ultrafiltration collection device.
- Monitor VS hourly; consult physician for increased arterial pressure (≥10 mm Hg above baseline), which would increase flow through the hemofilter, thereby increasing the rate of ultrafiltration.
- Adjust the filtration replacement fluid rate as prescribed when ultrafiltration rate increases.

- Maintain intake (oral, IV, TPN) within 25-50 ml of the value used to calculate fluid replacement rate.

NIC Electrolyte Management; Fluid Management; Fluid Monitoring; Hypovolemia Management; Intravenous Therapy; Electrolyte Management: Hyperkalemia; Electrolyte Management: Hypermagnesemia; Electrolyte Management: Hypernatremia; Electrolyte Management: Hyperphosphatemia. Additional optional interventions include Dysrhythmia Management, Feeding; Fever Treatment; Gastrointestinal Intubation; Hemodynamic Regulation; Invasive Hemodynamic Monitoring; Medication Management; Nutrition Management; Weight Management; Phlebotomy: Arterial Blood Sample and Venous Blood Sample

Fluid volume excess (or risk for same) related to excessive fluid intake associated with decreased ultrafiltration secondary to hypotension, clogged or clotted filter, or kinked lines

Desired outcome: Patient experiences a gradual fluid loss and becomes normovolemic as evidenced by BP remaining at baseline range; activated clotting time (ACT) 2-3 times that of the baseline value; CVP 2-6 mm Hg; HR 60-100 bpm; RR 12-20 breaths/min; and absence of edema, crackles, and other physical indicators of hypervolemia.

- Monitor BP q30min for the first 2 h and then hourly. Consult physician for a 10 mm Hg drop in BP, which would decrease the rate of ultrafiltration significantly.
- If ultrafiltration rate is decreased to 50% of the baseline, consult physician and decrease FRF rate as prescribed.
- Check tubes hourly for kinks.
- Maintain constant heparin infusion per infusion pump to maintain ACT at 2-3 times that of the baseline value.
- Monitor clotting time q2h. Use of an activated clotting time device is advisable.
- Inspect vascular access filter and lines for patency hourly. If clotting or clogging with protein is suspected, flush the system with 50 ml normal saline to check patency.
- If clots are present, consult physician. As prescribed, change the filter and recheck ACT to ensure necessary adjustment in heparin infusion rate.
- On an hourly basis, assess for and document the presence of physical indicators of hypervolemia: CVP >6 mm Hg; BP elevated ≥20 mm Hg over baseline; tachycardia; jugular venous distention; basilar crackles; increasing edema (peripheral, sacral, periorbital); and tachypnea.

NIC Electrolyte Management: Hyponatremia; Fluid/Electrolyte Management; Fluid Management; Fluid Monitoring; Electrolyte Management: Hypokalemia. Additional optional interventions include Dysrhythmia Management; Feeding; Gastrointestinal Intubation; Hemodialysis Therapy; Hemodynamic Regulation; Invasive Hemodynamic Monitoring; Medication Management; Phlebotomy: Arterial and Venous Blood Samples; Positioning; Skin Surveillance; Weight Management

Knowledge deficit: hemofiltration procedure

Desired outcome: Patient or significant other verbalizes accurate information about the hemofiltration procedure within 24-48 h of the instruction.

- Assess patient's knowledge of the procedure, and intervene accordingly.
- Explain the necessity of vascular access and the sensations that can be anticipated during cannula insertion.
- Explain the importance of and rationale for limited movement of the involved extremity after cannula placement.
- Describe the equipment that will be used for the procedure (e.g., filter, lines, infusion pump).
- Explain that VS will be assessed and blood tests will be performed at frequent intervals to monitor patient's status during the procedure.
- Explain to patient that his or her blood will be visible in the filter and lines.

- Reinforce that a staff member will be close to patient at all times during the procedure and will explain each step as it occurs.
- Explain that the procedure may take 24 h or longer until fluid balance is attained.
- Teach patient that the typical access sites are the femoral artery and femoral vein or the radial artery and cephalic vein.

NIC Teaching: Disease Process; Teaching: Individual; Teaching: Prescribed Medication. Additional optional interventions include Discharge Planning; Medication Management; Weight Management

Impaired physical mobility related to movement restrictions because of access and equipment for hemofiltration

Desired outcomes: Patient exhibits ability to move about in bed with assistance without evidence of disruption of hemofiltration equipment. Patient's skin remains intact, and there is no evidence of muscle atrophy or contracture formation caused by imposed immobility.

- Secure access catheters with gauze wraps (elastic wrap may compress access site and cause clotting) and tape to ensure safe movement of the involved limb without disruption of access cannula.
- Explain to patient the need for care and assistance when moving the involved limb.
- Use soft restraints if movement must be restrained markedly.
- Turn and reposition patient at least q2h, maintaining good body alignment.
- Massage bony prominences during every position change to promote comfort and circulation.
- Support involved extremities with pillows.
- Teach patient assisted ROM exercises on uninvolved extremities. Encourage isometric, isotonic, and quadriceps-setting exercises on uninvolved extremities, especially for patients whose CAVH or CVVH lasts >24 h.

NIC Exercise Therapy: Ambulation; Exercise Therapy: Joint Mobility. Additional optional interventions include Activity Therapy; Body Mechanics Promotion; Circulatory Care; Circulatory Precautions; Fall Prevention; Pain Management; Progressive Muscle Relaxation; Skin Surveillance; Weight Management

Risk for fluid volume deficit related to potential for blood loss secondary to line disconnection or membrane rupture

Desired outcome: Patient's membrane and line connections remain intact, and ultrafiltrate test results are negative for blood.

- Tape and secure all connections within the system.
- Check connections hourly to ensure that they are secure.
- Avoid concealing lines, filter, or connections with linen.
- Position filter and lines close to the access extremity; secure them with gauze wraps and tape to prevent traction on the connections.
- Inspect ultrafiltrate hourly for any signs of blood. If unsure whether ultrafiltrate contains blood, check the solution for occult blood.
- If the test is positive for blood, clamp the ultrafiltrate port and consult physician for further interventions.

NIC Electrolyte Management; Fluid Management; Fluid Monitoring; Hypovolemia Management; Intravenous Therapy; Electrolyte Management: Hyperkalemia; Electrolyte Management: Hypermagnesemia; Electrolyte Management: Hypernatremia; Electrolyte Management: Hyperphosphatemia. Additional optional interventions include Dysrhythmia Management; Feeding; Fever Treatment; Gastrointestinal Intubation; Hemodynamic Regulation; Invasive Hemodynamic Monitoring; Medication Management; Nutrition Management; Weight Management; Phlebotomy: Arterial Blood Sample and Venous Blood Sample

Research Brief 5-1   Continuous renal venovenous dialysis is a treatment option for critically ill patients whose condition is too hemodynamically unstable to tolerate the rapid fluid and electrolyte shifts associated with intermittent hemodialysis. The authors describe establishing a venovenous dialysis program, focusing on initial training, annual competency assessment, and the difficulties that they encountered. Because of the large time commitment and need to maintain competency through frequent exposure, not all of the unit nurses were trained to perform venovenous dialysis.

Giuliano K, Pysznik E: Renal replacement therapy in critical care: implementation of a unit-based continuous venovenous hemodialysis program, *Crit Care Nurse* 18(1):40-51, 1998.

ADDITIONAL NURSING DIAGNOSES

See "Pulmonary Emboli" for **Altered protection,** p. 238. For more information about fluid and electrolytes, see "Fluid and Electrolyte Disturbances," p. 636. Also see "Prolonged Immobility," p. 74.

Bibliography

Dipiro J et al: *Pharmacotherapy: a pathophysiologic approach,* Norwalk, Conn, 1997, Appleton & Lange.

Giuliano KK, Pysznik EE: Renal replacement therapy in critical care: implementation of a unit-based continuous venovenous hemodialysis program, *Crit Care Nurse* 18(1):40-51 1998.

Horne MM, Heitz UE, Swearingen PL: *Pocket guide to fluids and electrolytes,* ed 3, St Louis, 1997, Mosby.

Horne MM, Jansen PR: Renal-urinary disorders. In Swearingen PL, editor: *Manual of medical-surgical nursing care: nursing interventions and collaborative management,* ed 4, St Louis, 1999, Mosby.

Interqual: *The ISD-A review system with adult ISD criteria,* North Hampton, NH, and Marlboro, Mass, Aug, 1992, Interqual.

Kim MJ, McFarland GK, McLane AM: *Pocket guide to nursing diagnoses,* ed 7, St Louis, 1997, Mosby.

Lancaster L, editor: *Core curriculum for nephrology nursing,* ed 2, Pitman, NJ, 1995, Anthony J. Janetti.

Norman DJ, Suki WN, editors: *Primer on transplantation,* Thorofare, NJ, 1998, American Society Of Transplant Physicians.

Parker J, editor: *Contemporary nephrology nursing,* Pitman, NJ, 1998, Anthony J. Janetti.

Rodriguez D, Lewis Sl: Nutritional management of patients with acute renal failure, *Am Nephrol Nurs Assoc J* 24(2):232-241, 1997.

Neurologic Dysfunctions

Myasthenia gravis

PATHOPHYSIOLOGY

Myasthenia gravis (MG) is a chronic, progressive autoimmune disorder that manifests as weakness and abnormal fatigability of the voluntary striated skeletal muscles. The abnormality occurs at the neuromuscular junction on the postsynaptic membrane, where persons with MG exhibit changes of the structural integrity of the membrane and a marked reduction in the number of acetylcholine receptors (AChR). Acetylcholine (ACh), a neurotransmitter, is synthesized and stored in the terminal expansion of motor nerve axons. Neurotransmission involves the release of ACh into the synaptic cleft and the attachment of ACh to AChR on the postsynaptic membrane. In turn, this interaction activates the muscle action potential, which is responsible for muscle contraction. This process takes only milliseconds and is terminated by the removal of ACh from the neuromuscular junction, in part by the action of acetylcholinesterase, which catalyzes the breakdown of ACh, deactivating it. In approximately 85%-90% of patients with MG, an anti-AChR antibody is present, which is believed to cause structural damage to the postsynaptic AChR, inhibit receptor site synthesis, and cause receptor site blockade. If production of new receptor sites is insufficient, neuromuscular transmission eventually fails.

MG is associated with an increased rate of occurrence of other autoimmune disorders, including rheumatoid arthritis, thyrotoxicosis, systemic lupus erythematosus, Sjögren syndrome, polymyositis, ulcerative colitis, and pernicious anemia. Studies have shown that the thymus gland, which plays a role in the development of the immune system, undergoes pathologic changes in 80% of persons with MG. MG usually affects women between 20 and 40 years of age and men after age 40. The peak incidence for women is during the second and third decades and for men in the sixth decade. The overall ratio of women to men is 3:2. The course of the disease depends on the muscle groups involved and the degree of their involvement. Remissions and exacerbations can occur.

ASSESSMENT

Clinical presentation: Weakness and abnormal fatigability of skeletal muscles that worsen as effort is sustained and the day progresses.

Symptom progression
Ocular muscle group: First muscle group to be affected in 65% of patients. During course of disease, 90% will have ocular involvement. Eye signs include ptosis, diplopia, inability to maintain upward gaze.
Muscles of face and neck, bulbar signs: The next area of involvement. *Bulbar signs:* difficulty chewing, dysphagia, dysarthria, inability to close mouth, nasal regurgitation of fluids, mushy and nasal tone to voice, neck-muscle weakness with head bob, inability to raise chin off chest, loss of facial expression, risk of aspiration.
Muscles of limbs and trunk: The last area of involvement. Decreased strength in all extremities; inability to maintain position without support. Weakness greater in proximal muscles than distal. Diaphragmatic and intercostal weakness, dyspnea, ineffective cough, accumulation of secretions, potential for respiratory arrest.
Myasthenic and cholinergic crises: Patients with any of the generalized forms of MG may experience crisis, either myasthenic or cholinergic. Crisis may occur rapidly or incipiently, ultimately resulting in respiratory failure, which necessitates intubation or tracheostomy with mechanical ventilation. Crisis is a dramatic and frightening occurrence for the patient with MG. This individual is acutely aware of how she or he feels and tends to be knowledgeable about the disease. It is important for the nurse to listen to and observe the patient closely, because a subjective complaint of increasing anxiety, apprehension, or insomnia may herald the onset of crisis.

Although respiratory rate (RR) and arterial blood gas (ABG) values can be normal, the patient may be experiencing subtle decreases in chest expansion and air movement as a result of muscle weakness. These changes may be accompanied by increasing dysphagia, dysarthria, and dysphonia and an accumulation of oropharyngeal secretions, which increases the risk of aspiration.
Myasthenic crisis: Results from the need for more medication because of either tolerance to the medication or an exacerbation of the disease caused by infection, trauma, surgery, temperature extremes, stress, endocrine imbalance, or intake of medications with neuromuscular-blocking properties, such as sedatives, tranquilizers, opiates, or antibiotics (e.g., neomycin, kanamycin, gentamicin, streptomycin, tetracycline).
- *Signs and symptoms:* Increasing muscle weakness in spite of normal or increasing drug dosage, increasing anxiety and apprehension, severe ocular and bulbar weakness, and respiratory muscle weakness that occurs rapidly and can lead to respiratory arrest.

Cholinergic crisis: Results from an overdose of anticholinesterase medication, which blocks the AChR sites, causing a neuromuscular depolarizing block.
- *Signs and symptoms:* Increasing muscle weakness, increasing anxiety and apprehension, fasciculations (twitching) around the eyes and mouth, diarrhea and cramping, sweating, pupillary constriction, sialorrhea (excessive salivation), and difficulty breathing and swallowing.

DIAGNOSTIC TESTS

Tensilon test: Edrophonium chloride (Tensilon) is a short-acting anticholinesterase agent that delays hydrolysis of ACh, permitting the ACh released by the nerve to act repeatedly over a longer period. In the patient with MG, weakness and muscle fatigue will improve within 30-60 sec of IV Tensilon injection (2-10 mg) and improvement will last up to 5 min.

This test also identifies the type of crisis. In myasthenic crisis the weakness improves with Tensilon, whereas in cholinergic crisis the symptoms worsen.

> *Caution:* Have atropine sulfate at the bedside during Tensilon test to reverse the effects of Tensilon if the patient is in cholinergic crisis.

Serum antibody titer: Elevated serum antibodies against acetylcholine receptors are present in 80%-90% of cases of generalized MG.

Electromyography (EMG): Muscle action potentials are recorded from selected skeletal muscles. The amplitude of the evoked muscle action potentials falls rapidly in persons with MG.

Mediastinal magnetic resonance imaging (MRI) of the thymus gland: To evaluate for the presence of thymic abnormalities, which are present in 80% of patients with MG. Of this group, 65%-90% have thymic hyperplasia, whereas 10%-15% have gross or microscopic thymomas.

Mediastinoscopy: To evaluate for the presence of thymic abnormalities (see "Mediastinal MRI," above).

Thyroid studies: To evaluate for hyperthyroidism. Frequently, thyroid abnormalities are present in young women with MG. MG also is associated with a condition known as *Hashimoto thyroiditis*, an autoimmune disorder.

Other laboratory studies: Serum creatine phosphokinase (CPK), erythrocyte sedimentation rate (ESR), and antinuclear antibody levels are studied because of the frequent occurrence of other immunologic disorders with MG.

COLLABORATIVE MANAGEMENT

Emergency interventions for myasthenic or cholinergic crisis: Once supportive emergency therapy in an intensive care setting has been instituted, the patient is stabilized, the type of crisis is identified, and specific treatment is begun. Anticholinesterase medications may be withheld or reduced temporarily. A "drug holiday" will improve subsequent patient responsiveness to medication. With the resumption of anticholinesterase medications, dosage, timing, and combinations of medications will need readjustment. In severe MG, plasmapheresis (see p. 414) may hasten improvement in signs and symptoms.

Pharmacotherapy during noncrisis periods: Medications must be given on time to maintain therapeutic effects. Pharmacologic management is patient specific.

Cholinesterase inhibitors: Such as pyridostigmine bromide (Mestinon), neostigmine bromide (Prostigmin), and ambenonium chloride (Mytelase). These drugs inhibit the hydrolysis of ACh by acetylcholinesterase at the neuromuscular junction. Generally pyridostigmine is the choice agent because it is longer acting and has fewer side effects. The patient usually is started on one tablet q3h during the day, and the dose is adjusted as required. Sustained-release preparations usually are given at bedtime to maintain the patient's strength throughout the night and early morning hours.

Immunosuppression: glucocorticosteroids (e.g., ACTH and prednisone) and other immunosuppressive agents: With their use, clinical improvement has been shown in 70%-100% of patients with MG. Although the mechanism of action of steroids has not been established, studies have shown that they exert certain direct influences on neuromuscular transmission. In addition, they suppress the action of the immune system at many levels by decreasing the size of the thymus gland and lymphatic tissue, decreasing circulating lymphocyte population, and decreasing antireceptor reactivity of peripheral lymphocytes. Treatment must be continued indefinitely. Indications for their use include weakness that is uncontrolled by anticholinesterase drugs or surgery and patients who refuse surgery. Glucocorticosteroids produce favorable results in patients with all degrees of muscle involvement, from ocular to severe respiratory impairment. Glucocorticosteroids are used alone or in conjunction with anticholinesterase drugs.

Azathioprine (Imuran) may be used alone or in combination with other therapies in situations in which response to steroids is poor. Side effects can be serious and include toxic hepatitis, thrombocytopenia, leukopenia, leukemia, lymphoma, infections, vomiting, and teratogenic effects.

Immune globulin: Human immune globulin in high doses is reported to provide rapid but temporary relief of symptoms in some individuals with MG.

Plasmapheresis: Involves a complete exchange of plasma with the removal of abnormal circulating antibodies that interfere with the acetylcholine receptors. Table 6-1 describes potential complications with corresponding nursing assessments and interventions. (For additional information about fluid and electrolyte disturbances, see p. 636.)

Thymectomy: Removal of the thymus gland may lead to clinical improvement, especially in patients with hyperplasia of thymic tissue. Two approaches are used: the suprasternal approach or the transsternal approach with sternal splitting. Usually, best results are seen with a combination of surgery and medication in patients <50-60 yr with recent onset of moderate, generalized MG. The suprasternal approach may be less successful because of the presence of residual thymic tissue, which may lead to reactivation of the MG. Plasmapheresis sometimes is used before surgery to increase strength and allow for a decrease in medication dosage.

Respiratory support: Endotrachel (ET) tube or tracheostomy with mechanical ventilation may be necessary, depending on the degree of involvement of the respiratory muscles. (See "Mechanical Ventilation," p. 17.)

Nutritional support: If patient has dysphagia, enteral or parenteral feedings may be needed. (See "Nutritional Support," p. 1.)

NURSING DIAGNOSES AND INTERVENTIONS

Impaired gas exchange related to altered oxygen supply associated with decreases in chest expansion and air movement secondary to weakness and abnormal fatigability of pharyngeal, diaphragmatic, intercostal, and accessory muscles of respiration

Desired outcome: Within 12-24 h of initiation of treatment, patient has adequate gas exchange as evidenced by orientation to time, place, and person; RR ≤20 breaths/min with normal depth and pattern (eupnea); Pao_2 ≥80 mm Hg; $Paco_2$ ≤45 mm Hg; and oxygen saturation ≥94%.

- Assess patient for indicators of altered respiratory function: diminished or adventitious breath sounds; changes in rate, rhythm, and depth of respirations; changes in skin color; nasal flaring or intercostal or suprasternal retractions; and restlessness, irritability, confusion, or somnolence.

- Monitor ventilatory capability via pulmonary function tests. Vital capacity <75% of predicted value, tidal volume <1000 ml (or <patient's normal/ baseline volume), and RR >34 breaths/min are signals of the need for assisted ventilation.

- Monitor ABG and pulse oximetry results. Falling Pao_2 (<60 mm Hg), rising $Paco_2$ (>50 mm Hg), and falling oxygen saturation, coupled with changes in vital capacity, tidal volume, and increasing RR, indicate the need for additional respiratory support.

> **Note:**   If mechanical ventilation already is in place, ventilator settings will vary, depending on patient's size and ABG results. Check ventilator settings at set intervals. Consult with anesthesia and/or respiratory therapy staff members regarding setting changes as patient's needs change.

- Provide pulmonary toilet q2h when patient is awake and prn. In addition, turn patient after each physiotherapy session to facilitate lung expansion, decrease risk of atelectasis, and prevent consolidation of secretions.

You may also wish to refer to the following interventions from the Nursing Interventions Classification (NIC):

NIC Respiratory Monitoring; Airway Management; Coping Enhancement; Acid-Base Monitoring; Oxygen Therapy

Ineffective airway clearance related to ineffective cough; decreased energy; abnormal fatigability of diaphragmatic, intercostal, pharyngeal, and accessory muscles of respiration

Hypovolemia

Can result from rapid removal of up to 3 L of body fluid during plasmapheresis with volume replacement that is too slow during the procedure

- Perform a baseline assessment of patient's weight, skin turgor, and VS before the procedure is begun. During plasmapheresis, monitor patient for thirst, poor skin turgor, dizziness, confusion, nausea, and flattened neck veins. Assess VS continuously for evidence of hypovolemia, including decreased BP and increased HR. Monitor Hct for elevation, which occurs with hypovolemia. Weigh patient after procedure. Remember that 1 L of fluid equals 1 kg; thus hypovolemia can be reflected readily in weight changes.
- Provide fluids during plasmapheresis as prescribed, via oral, enteral, or IV access.
- Monitor and record I&O throughout the procedure. Be alert to oliguria (urinary output <30 ml/h for 2 consecutive hours).
- Protect patients who are dizzy or confused by keeping side rails up and the bed in its lowest position.

Clotting abnormalities

Can result from removal of clotting factors during plasmapheresis

- Assess PT, PTT, and platelet count before and after procedure. Be alert to PT and PTT greater than those of control values and to increased platelet count. Normal ranges are as follows: PT 11-15 sec, PTT 30-40 sec, and platelet count 150,000-400,000/mm^3.
- Be alert to signs of impaired clotting, such as oozing from arterial puncture, venous access, or IV sites. Monitor patient for epistaxis or other signs of hemorrhage, such as elevated pulse rate, decreasing BP, or changes in patient's mental status.
- Apply firm, continuous (e.g., 10 min) pressure to the arterial puncture site once the catheter or needle is removed. A pressure dressing is recommended.
- Check gastric aspirate and stools for occult blood.
- Instruct patient to alert staff to the presence of bleeding from puncture and other sites.

Hypokalemia

Can result from removal of potassium during the plasma exchange

- Assess serum potassium before, during, and after plasma exchange. Be alert to decreasing levels (<3.5 mEq/L).
- Monitor for physical signs of hypokalemia, including bradycardia, fatigue, leg cramps, nausea, and paresthesias.
- Observe cardiac monitor for signs of cardiac dysrhythmias: ST-segment depression, flattened T wave, presence of U wave, and ventricular dysrhythmias. Report abnormal cardiac rhythms to physician.
- During reinfusion of blood, administer potassium as prescribed to prevent hypokalemia and dangerous dysrhythmias. If prescribed, administer antidysrhythmic agents.

CAUTION: Patients on prednisone or digitalis therapy are at increased risk for hypokalemia and should be monitored closely for its occurrence.

L, Liter; *VS,* vital signs; *BP,* blood pressure; *HR,* heart rate; *Hct,* hematocrit; *kg,* kilogram; *IV,* intravenous; *I&O,* intake and output; *PT,* prothrombin time; *PTT,* partial thromboplastin time.

Continued

TABLE 6-1   Nursing Interventions for Complications of Plasmapheresis—cont'd

Hypocalcemia

Can result from binding of calcium to ACD, the anticoagulant used during plasmapheresis

- Assess serum calcium levels before, during, and after plasmapheresis. Be alert to decreasing levels (<8.5 mg/dl).
- Monitor patient for signs of hypocalcemia, such as numbness with tingling of fingers and circumoral area, hyperactive reflexes, muscle cramps, tetany, paresthesia, Chvostek sign (see p. 654), diffuse irritability, emotional instability, impaired memory, and confusion.
- Observe cardiac monitor for evidence of hypocalcemia: prolonged QT interval caused by elongation of ST segment.
- Encourage patient to drink milk before and during the plasma exchange.
- As prescribed, administer calcium gluconate during plasmapheresis if indicators of hypocalcemia occur.

Myasthenic crisis

Can result from removal of circulating anticholinesterase drugs during plasmapheresis

Cholinergic crisis

Can result from removal of antibodies and decreased need for anticholinesterase drugs after plasmapheresis

- In the event of either crisis, have the following available: IV infusion apparatus, medications (edrophonium chloride [Tensilon], neostigmine bromide, atropine, and pralidoxime chloride [Protopam Chloride]), manual resuscitator, oxygen, suction equipment, and intubation tray if intubation is not already in place.
- Monitor patient for evidence of crisis, such as decreased vital capacity (<1 L), inability to swallow, ptosis, diplopia, dysarthria, dysphonia, dyspnea, muscle weakness, and nasal flaring. Stay with patient if these signs appear, and notify physician promptly.

ACD, Acid-citrate-dextrose; *IV,* intravenous; *L,* liter.

Desired outcome: Within 24-48 h of intervention/treatment, patient's airway is clear as evidenced by absence of adventitious breath sounds.

- Assess breath sounds, effectiveness of patient's cough, and the quality, amount, and color of sputum. Consult physician for significant findings, including patient's inability to raise secretions; for secretions that are tenacious, thick, or voluminous.
- Suction secretions as indicated, using hyperoxygenation before and after procedure.

Note: To prevent aspiration of secretions, always suction the trachea and mouth before deflating endotracheal or tracheostomy cuff. Consider use of endotracheal tube (ETT) with continuous supraglottic suction, if available. This is especially important in patients with MG because of their increase in saliva.

- Place patient in semi-Fowler's to high Fowler's position at all times to facilitate chest excursion and decrease risk of aspiration. Fully elevate head of bed (HOB) during feedings to prevent aspiration of food.

- Assess VS for indicators of atelectasis and upper respiratory infection (see **Risk for infection,** which follows). Consult physician for significant findings.
- Increase activity as allowed and tolerated to minimize stasis of secretions and to facilitate expansion of the lung.
- If prescribed, administer or assist with intermittent positive pressure breathing (IPPB) treatments.
- Keep another tracheostomy tube of the same size and an obturator at the bedside in the event of inadvertent extubation.

NIC Airway Management; Artificial Airway Management; Cough Enhancement: Oxygen Therapy; Ventilation Assistance

Risk for infection related to inadequate primary defenses (stasis of secretions); inadequate secondary defenses (suppressed inflammatory response); invasive procedures (e.g., insertion of ET tube); chronic disease

Desired outcome: Patient is free of infection as evidenced by normothermia; HR 60-100 bpm; pulmonary secretions that are clear, thin in consistency, and odorless; and WBC count ≤11,000/mm^3.

- Monitor patient for signs of infection, including temperature ≥37.7° (100° F), tachycardia, and diaphoresis.
- Assess color, consistency, amount, and odor of pulmonary secretions. Consult physician for a change in sputum color (i.e., to green, tan, brown, bloody). Obtain sputum specimens for culture as indicated.
- Monitor CBC results for elevation of WBC count (>11,000/mm^3).
- Administer antibiotics as prescribed.
- Use meticulous hand washing before caring for patient and use sterile technique when performing suctioning and other invasive procedures.
- Protect patient from exposure to persons with infection, particularly upper respiratory infection (URI).
- Turn and reposition patient at least q2h to prevent stasis of secretions.
- See Appendix 8 for more information.

NIC Cough Enhancement; Infection Protection; Surveillance

Impaired swallowing related to decreased or absent gag reflex; decreased strength or excursion of muscles involved in mastication; facial paralysis; mechanical obstruction (tracheostomy tube)

Desired outcome: Before oral foods and fluids are given or reintroduced, patient demonstrates capability for safe and effective swallowing as evidenced by presence of gag reflex and adequate strength and excursion of muscles involved in mastication.

- Assess patient for the presence of the gag reflex, ability to swallow, and strength and excursion of muscles involved in mastication. As indicated, consult with a speech therapist to determine patient's ability to swallow.
- If patient cannot swallow, confer with physician regarding alternate method of nutritional support, such as enteral or parenteral nutrition (see "Nutritional Support," p. 1).

> **Note:** If the patient has an artificial airway, add a few drops of blue food coloring to tube feedings to facilitate assessment of aspiration.

- After patient's gag reflex and ability to swallow return, begin oral feedings cautiously.
  - ☐ When reinstating oral intake, begin with a small quantity of ice chips, which may help stimulate the swallowing reflex, and progress to semisolid foods (e.g., textured food, applesauce) and then to solid foods.
  - ☐ Elevate HOB ≥70 degrees to facilitate gravity flow through the pylorus and to minimize the potential for regurgitation and aspiration.
  - ☐ Provide small feedings at frequent intervals (e.g., q4h while patient is awake).

☐ Avoid cold foods and beverages, which cause bloating and upward pressure on the diaphragm and may impede respiratory excursion.

☐ Keep suction equipment at the bedside; suction excess secretions as necessary after each feeding. Inspect the buccal surface for residual food particles after each meal. Provide materials for oral hygiene after every meal.

- If patient begins oral feedings with a tracheostomy tube in place, elevate HOB ≥70 degrees to facilitate movement of food through the pylorus and to minimize the potential for regurgitation and aspiration. Inflate tracheostomy tube cuff for 30 min before and after feeding to prevent aspiration in the event that the patient vomits or regurgitates. Progress the diet slowly, as described in the previous intervention.

- If patient is unable to communicate verbally, be alert to signs of respiratory distress that can occur in response to aspiration: dyspnea, tachypnea, restlessness, agitation, pallor, and presence of adventitious breath sounds. If these signs occur, discontinue feeding immediately; ensure that HOB is elevated; and provide oxygen via nasal cannula, mask, or ET tube. If a tracheostomy tube is in place, suction through the tube to remove food or secretions that may be obstructing the airway. As prescribed, obtain specimen for ABG analysis or arrange for a chest x-ray.

NIC Aspiration Precautions; Swallowing Therapy; Positioning; Nutrition Management

Sensory/perceptual alterations (visual) related to altered sensory reception associated with diplopia or ptosis

Desired outcome: Within 48-72 h of this diagnosis, patient relates that vision is adequate to perform activities of daily living (ADL).

- Assess for and document signs of weakness of the ocular muscles (i.e., diplopia, ptosis, incomplete closure of the eye).

- Provide an eye patch or frosted lens for the patient with diplopia; alternate the patch or lens to the opposite eye q2-3h during patient's awake hours.

- Provide eyelid crutches for the patient with ptosis, or loosely tape eyelids open but *only* when providing direct care.

- Administer artificial tears in each eye at least q4-6h to lubricate and protect corneal tissue.

- As indicated, provide assistance with ADL and ambulation to protect patient from injury.

- Keep patient's environment consistent to facilitate location of desired objects.

NIC Communication Enhancement: Visual Deficit; Environmental Management; Fall Prevention; Surveillance: Safety

Knowledge deficit: thymectomy procedure, including preoperative and post-operative care

Desired outcome: Before surgery, patient verbalizes understanding of the surgical procedure, including preoperative and postoperative care.

- Assess patient's knowledge of thymectomy and its relationship to myasthenia gravis. Provide explanations as indicated.

- Describe the preoperative routine both verbally and with written material. Discuss preoperative medications, application of antiembolic hose, the potential for postoperative discomfort, and the availability of analgesic agents. Advise patient that the medication regimen may change after surgery, because removal of the thymic tissue may result in improvement in the patient's condition. If the patient will have a thoracotomy approach, explain that chest tubes will be present after surgery; with a transcervical approach, a portable wound drainage system (e.g., Hemovac) will be present to collect wound drainage.

- During the preoperative period, teach coughing and deep-breathing techniques that will be employed after surgery for expanding the lungs and mobilizing secretions into the upper portion of the airway.

- Explain that plasmapheresis may be performed preoperatively to improve the patient's clinical state. (See **Knowledge deficit: purpose and procedure for plasmapheresis,** which follows.)
- Explain that pulmonary function and ABG studies will be performed preoperatively to provide baseline data that will be used to evaluate respiratory status; and again postoperatively to assist in determining the patient's readiness for extubation.
- Prepare patient for the possibility of tracheostomy with assisted ventilation for the preoperative and postoperative periods to prevent respiratory problems that can occur as a result of the stresses of surgery or the risk of myasthenic or cholinergic crisis.
- Before surgery, devise a communication system that uses aids such as a Magic Slate, hand signals, call bell, or word board, inasmuch as patient is likely to require a ventilator postoperatively. (A communication system already may be in place if a ventilator is in use.)
- Explain that the results of a thymectomy are variable and may not be apparent for several months to years.

Knowledge deficit: purpose and procedure for plasmapheresis
Desired outcome: Before the first plasma exchange, patient verbalizes knowledge of the purpose and procedure for plasmapheresis.

- Assess patient's previous experience with and knowledge of plasmapheresis.
- As appropriate, teach patient the following about plasmapheresis: (1) blood is withdrawn via an arterial catheter, anticoagulated, and then passed through a cell separator; (2) the plasma portion of the blood that contains the AChR antibodies is removed; (3) red blood cells (RBCs), white blood cells (WBCs), and platelets are mixed with saline, potassium, and plasma protein fraction and then are returned to the body, minus the plasma, via a venous access.
- Advise patient that plasmapheresis generally is performed to control severe symptoms until other modalities (medications, thymectomy) take effect, when other treatments have failed, or to increase patient's strength and improve general status before surgery.
- Explain that patient should eat before plasmapheresis and that nutrition will be provided during the procedure.
- Advise patient that the nurse will perform several assessment procedures before, during, and after plasmapheresis (see Table 6-1).
- Advise patient that the procedure may take several hours and that it may be performed as often as 3-4 times/wk, depending on patient's condition.
- Explain that the patient's degree of weakness may increase during and after the procedure because of the removal of plasma-bound medications (corticosteroids, anticholinesterase agents). Reassure patient that he or she will be monitored closely during the procedure and will receive appropriate medication after plasmapheresis.

Knowledge deficit: signs and symptoms of myasthenic and cholinergic crises
Desired outcome: Within 24 h of stabilization of respiratory status, patient and significant others verbalize the signs and symptoms of impending myasthenic and cholinergic crises.

- Assess patient's/family's previous experience with and knowledge of myasthenic and cholinergic crises.
- Explain the differences between *myasthenic crisis:* an exacerbation of the myasthenic symptoms, frequently triggered by an infection; and *cholinergic crisis:* an episode triggered by toxic levels of anticholinesterase medication. The crisis, regardless of type, may manifest similar symptoms, including abdominal cramping, diarrhea, generalized weakness, increased pulmonary secretions, and impaired respiratory function.
- Advise patient/family to report immediately indications of crisis.
- Recommend that emergency respiratory support equipment (resuscitator bag and suction apparatus) should be available in the home if patient has a history of crisis events.

- Advise patient to carry an identification card with diagnosis, medications, medication contraindications, and physician's name and phone number.
- Provide address and phone number of Myasthenia Gravis Foundation of America, Inc. Address: 222 South Riverside Plaza, Suite 1540, Chicago, IL 60606; phone: 1-800-541-5454, 1-312-258-0522; fax: 1-312-258-0461; website: www.Myasthenia@myasthenia.org.

ADDITIONAL NURSING DIAGNOSES

See also "Nutritional Support," p. 1; "Mechanical Ventilation," p. 17; "Psychosocial Support," p. 83; and "Psychosocial Support for the Patient's Family and Significant Others," p. 95. Also see "Renal Transplantation" for **Knowledge deficit: immunosuppressive medications and their side effects,** p. 392.

Guillain-Barré syndrome

PATHOPHYSIOLOGY

Guillain-Barré syndrome (GBS) is an acute or subacute postinfectious polyneuritis. The frequency of GBS after an infection, along with its occurrence in conjunction with diseases of lymphoid tissue (e.g., Hodgkin's disease), suggests that it is an autoimmune disorder. Statistically, GBS affects 1.5-2 individuals per 100,000 population.

GBS affects mainly the Schwann cell, which synthesizes and maintains the peripheral nerve myelin sheath. The result is the segmental loss of myelin along the peripheral nerve axon. Cellular inflammatory infiltrates that consist of T and B lymphocytes, macrophages, and neutrophils appear in the areas of myelin loss. Studies suggest that the macrophages penetrate the basement membrane and strip apparently normal myelin from intact axons, causing the characteristic signs and symptoms of GBS. The ventral (motor) root axons of the anterior horn cells, which innervate voluntary skeletal muscles, are primarily involved. Dorsal (sensory) root axons of the posterior horn also are affected but to a lesser degree. Recovery of neurologic function depends on proliferation of Schwann cells and remyelination of axons. Recovery can be expected in 80%-90% of cases, with minor residual deficits occurring in fewer than half of affected patients.

ASSESSMENT

History and risk factors: Respiratory or gastrointestinal (GI) illness 10-14 days before onset of the neurologic symptoms, in which (1) a viral agent such as *parainfluenza 2* virus, measles, mumps, rubella, varicella, or herpes zoster is present (50% of cases); (2) recent vaccination (15% of cases), such as for influenza; (3) recent surgical procedure (5% of cases).

Clinical presentation: Ascending flaccid motor paralysis is the most common presenting sign and is associated with the early loss of deep tendon reflexes (DTRs). Weakness, which usually precedes the paralysis, is symmetric and generally begins in distal muscle groups and ascends to involve more proximal muscles. Muscles of respiration (intercostals and diaphragm) frequently are involved, and approximately half of all patients will require mechanical ventilation. Complaints of distal paresthesias are common. In more serious or prolonged cases, proprioceptive and vibratory dysfunctions are present. In addition, loss of pain and temperature sensations in a glove-and-stocking distribution has been reported. Sensory complaints usually appear first, with muscle weakness developing rapidly over 24-72 h. Approximately 90% of patients reach the peak of dysfunction within 2 weeks.

Autonomic nervous system involvement (a type of autonomic dysreflexia): Occurs in most patients with GBS: sinus tachycardia, bradycardia, orthostatic hypotension, hypertension, excessive diaphoresis, bowel and bladder retention, loss of sphincter control, increased pulmonary secretions, syndrome of inappropriate antidiuretic hormone secretion (SIADH), and cardiac dysrhythmias (a common cause of death).

Cranial nerve involvement: All cranial nerves except I and II may be involved. See Appendix 4.

Physical assessment: Symmetric motor weakness, decreased or absent DTRs, hypotonia or flaccidity of affected muscles, presence of respiratory abnormalities (e.g., nasal flaring, hypoventilation), facial paralysis.

DIAGNOSTIC TESTS

The diagnosis for GBS is based on clinical presentation, history of antecedent illness, and cerebrospinal fluid (CSF) findings.

Lumbar puncture (LP) and CSF analysis: CSF analysis usually shows an elevated protein, without any increase in WBCs. This is referred to as the *albuminocytologic dissociation.* This dissociation usually is noted during the course of GBS and is helpful in differentiating GBS from other central nervous system (CNS) disorders. CSF protein, normally between 15-45 mg/dl, may peak 4-6 wk after onset of GBS to levels of several hundred mg/dl. This elevation may persist for months. CSF pressure, which is normally 0-15 mm Hg, may be elevated in severe cases.

Electrodiagnostic studies: Electromyography (EMG) and nerve conduction velocity (NCV) demonstrate profound slowing of motor conduction velocities and conduction blocks as a result of the demyelination of peripheral nerves. Although these changes may not appear initially, they will become apparent several weeks into the illness.

Pulmonary function studies: May be performed during initial diagnostic evaluation. Vital capacity (VC) of <1 L indicates a possible need for assisted ventilation.

ABG studies: Performed if VC drops below 1 L or if patient demonstrates dyspnea, confusion, restlessness, nasal flaring, use of accessory muscles of respiration, or breathlessness (noted during a count by the patient from 1-10). A decrease in Pao_2 >10-15 mm Hg or increase in $Paco_2$ of 10-15 mm Hg greater than baseline or normal value signals the need for immediate intubation or tracheostomy.

COLLABORATIVE MANAGEMENT

Respiratory support: ET intubation or tracheostomy with assisted mechanical ventilation, as necessary.

Plasmapheresis: Involves a complete exchange of plasma with the removal of abnormal circulating antibodies that affect the peripheral nerve myelin sheath. Removal of these autoantibodies may lessen the duration and severity of GBS. For nursing interventions for complications of plasmapheresis, see Table 6-1.

Maintenance and monitoring of cardiovascular function: As necessary, cardiac monitoring may be initiated for dysrhythmias; arterial pressure monitoring may be used to evaluate hypertension or hypotension; and antihypertensive agents or vasopressors may be administered to maintain BP within normal levels.

Management of bowel and bladder dysfunction: Nasogastric suction and parenteral infusion may be started for patients with paralytic ileus; an indwelling urinary catheter may be inserted in patients with urinary retention.

Nutritional management: Parenteral feedings are given until return of peristalsis. Tube feedings or gastrostomy feedings are used for patients with severe dysphagia. With recovery of gag reflex and swallowing ability, the diet will progress to semisolid and solid foods, which are more readily swallowed than are liquids.

Management of motor dysfunction: Active and passive range-of-motion (ROM) exercises are performed at frequent intervals during all phases of GBS.

Activity must be balanced with caloric intake to prevent muscle wasting. As the patient's condition stabilizes, physical and occupational therapy personnel should be involved in the planning of the rehabilitation process. The primary goal is maintenance of the patient's mobility and independence.

> **Caution:** ROM must not be done strenuously during the acute phase because this may exacerbate weakness and possibly accelerate the demyelinating process.

NURSING DIAGNOSES AND INTERVENTIONS

Impaired gas exchange related to altered oxygen supply associated with decreased lung expansion secondary to weakness or paralysis of intercostal and diaphragmatic muscles

Desired outcome: Within 12-24 h of this diagnosis, patient has adequate gas exchange as evidenced by orientation to time, place, and person; RR 12-20 breaths/min with normal pattern and depth (eupnea); HR ≤100 bpm; BP within patient's normal range; Pao_2 ≥80 mm Hg; $Paco_2$ ≤45 mm Hg; and oxygen saturation ≥94%.

- Assess neurologic function hourly, or as often as needed. Ascending motor and sensory dysfunctions usually occur rapidly (over 24-72 h) and can lead to life-threatening respiratory arrest.
- Monitor patient's respiratory status and results of diagnostic tests for evidence of distress or other abnormalities. Be alert to and consult physician for the following: adventitious (crackles, rhonchi); decreased or absent breath sounds; temperature ≥37.7° C (100° F); increased HR and BP; tidal volume or VC decreased from baseline; decreased Pao_2 or increased $Paco_2$ ≥10-15 mm Hg from baseline or normal values; abnormal respiratory rate or rhythm; increasing restlessness or anxiety; and confusion.
- In the presence of the aforementioned indicators, be prepared to assist with intubation or tracheotomy.
- Prepare patient for the likelihood of these interventions; explain that they will be temporary measures.
- Maintain mechanical ventilation via ET tube or tracheostomy as indicated; check ventilator settings at regular intervals to ensure that they are within prescribed limits. (See "Mechanical Ventilation," p. 17.)
- Continue to monitor ABG results and pulse oximetry. Improvement is indicated by increases in Pao_2 (optimally to ≥80 mm Hg) and oxygen saturation and a decrease in $Paco_2$ (optimally to ≤45 mm Hg). Consult physician for continued abnormalities.

NIC Airway Management; Acid-Base Monitoring; Oxygen Therapy; Respiratory Monitoring

Ineffective airway clearance related to ineffective cough; decreased energy; increasing paralysis of respiratory, pharyngeal, and facial muscles; absence of the gag reflex

Desired outcome: Within 12-24 h of this diagnosis, patient's airway is clear as evidenced by absence of adventitious breath sounds; HR 60-100 bpm; BP within patient's baseline range; RR 12-20 breaths/min with normal depth and pattern (eupnea); tidal volume or VC within baseline parameters; Pao_2 ≥80 mm Hg; $Paco_2$ ≤45 mm Hg; and absence of restlessness.

- Monitor patient for the following: adventitious (crackles, rhonchi), decreased, or absent breath sounds; increased HR and BP; tidal volume or vital capacity decreased from baseline; abnormal respiratory rate or rhythm; decrease in Pao_2 or increase in $Paco_2$; and increasing restlessness or anxiety.
- Suction the airway as determined by auscultation findings. As the paresis or paralysis subsides (usually after 2-4 wk), cranial nerve function will begin to return (i.e., gag, swallowing, coughing). Evaluate patient's ability to cough, whether or not he or she has been placed on mechanical ventilation. Assess

for the presence of adventitious sounds to determine effectiveness of patient's cough.

- Deliver oxygen and humidification as prescribed.
- Maintain mechanical ventilation as prescribed; confirm that ventilator settings are within prescribed limits. (See "Mechanical Ventilation," p. 17.)
- Unless contraindicated, maintain adequate hydration (up to 2-3 L/day) to minimize thickening of pulmonary secretions.
- Turn and reposition patient at least q2h to prevent stasis of secretions.

NIC Positioning; Airway Management; Respiratory Monitoring; Cough Enhancement; Airway Suctioning

Risk for disuse syndrome related to ascending flaccid paralysis and paresthesias

Desired outcomes: Patient maintains baseline/optimal ROM of all joints and baseline muscle size and strength of all muscles.

- Assess neurologic function hourly or as often as indicated. Ascending motor and sensory dysfunction usually occurs rapidly (over 24-72 h). During the stage of GBS crisis when neurologic dysfunction is progressing, assess motor and sensory levels by starting with the lower extremities and working upward to determine level of deficit.
  - ☐ Assess muscle symmetry by using a side-to-side comparison.
  - ☐ Assess muscle strength: *For lower extremities:* have patient pull heel of foot toward the buttocks as you provide resistance by holding onto the foot. *For upper extremities:* have patient extend and flex the wrists and arms against your resistance.
  - ☐ Assess DTRs of the Achilles, patellae, biceps, triceps, and brachioradialis. Normal response is +2; report decreased (+1) or absent (0) response.
  - ☐ Assess for the presence of paresthesia, including the location, degree, and whether it is ascending.
  - ☐ Assess for the presence or absence of position sense by moving patient's big toe or thumb up and down while patient's eyes are closed. Also note presence or absence of vibratory sense by placing a vibrating tuning fork over bony prominences.
  - ☐ Assess for the presence or absence of response to light touch or pinprick by starting at the feet and working upward to determine the level of dysfunction.

> **Note:**   Sensory symptoms usually are milder than are motor complaints, with vibration and position sensations affected most often. However, about 25% of affected patients will experience pain, requiring analgesia. When light touch, pinprick, and temperature sensations are affected, they most often are found in a glove-and-stocking distribution. Patients frequently experience muscle tenderness and sensitivity to pressure.

  - ☐ Assess for cranial nerve dysfunction (see Appendix 4).
- Record and report sensorimotor deficit, including degree of involvement.
- Turn and reposition patient in correct anatomic alignment q2h or more often if requested by patient. Support patient's position with pillows and other positioning aids.
- To maintain patient's muscle function and prevent contractures, ensure that active or passive ROM exercises are performed q2h during all phases of GBS. Involve significant others in exercises, if appropriate.
- Obtain a physical therapy referral, and begin rehabilitation planning process during the early stages of the disorder.
- As indicated, apply splints to hands-arms and feet-legs to help prevent contracture; alternate splints so that they are on for 2 h and off for 2 h.
- Apply antiembolic stockings as prescribed to help promote tissue perfusion and minimize the risk of thrombophlebitis, deep vein thrombosis, and pulmonary emboli.

- Low air loss or fluidized beds may be used to manage the respiratory, autonomic, and musculoskeletal problems that occur with GBS. Use an air mattress to help maintain skin integrity. For interventions related to maintaining skin integrity, see "Wound and Skin Care," p. 55.

NIC Exercise Therapy (all of them); Exercise Promotion; Positioning

Dysreflexia (or risk for same) related to noxious stimulus

Desired outcome: Patient has no symptoms of autonomic dysreflexia (AD) as evidenced by normal T-wave configuration on ECG; HR 60-100 bpm; BP within patient's normal range; cool and dry skin; patient's normal strength; and absence of headache and chest and abdominal tightness.

- Assess for signs of AD: cardiac dysrhythmias; HR <60 bpm or >100 bpm; elevated and sustained BP (e.g., ≥250-300/150 mm Hg); facial flushing; increased sweating, possibly caused by loss of thermal regulation; extreme generalized warmth; profound weakness; and complaints of severe headache or tightening in the chest and abdomen.
- Place patient on cardiac monitor as prescribed.

> **Note:** Because of the risk of fatal cardiac dysrhythmias in GBS, continuous cardiac monitoring is recommended for the first 10-14 days of hospitalization.

- Monitor patient carefully during activities that are known to precipitate AD: position changes, vigorous coughing, straining with bowel movements, and suctioning.
- Be aware of and implement measures to prevent factors that may precipitate AD:
  - ☐ *Bladder stimuli:* urinary tract infection, cystoscopy, urinary catheter insertion, clogged urinary catheter, urinary calculi.
  - ☐ *Bowel stimuli:* fecal impaction, rectal examination, enemas, suppositories.
  - ☐ *Sensory stimuli:* pressure caused by tight clothing, dressings, bed covers, thigh straps on urinary drainage bags; prolonged pressure on skin surface or over bony prominences; temperature changes, such as exposure to a cool breeze or draft.
- If indicators of AD are present, implement the following:
  - ☐ Elevate HOB or place patient in a sitting position to promote decrease in BP.
  - ☐ Monitor BP and HR q3-5min until patient stabilizes.
- Determine and remove offending stimulus:
  - ☐ For example, if patient's bladder is distended, catheterize cautiously, using sufficient lubricant.
  - ☐ If patient has an indwelling urinary catheter, check for obstruction such as granulation in catheter or kinking of tubing. As indicated, irrigate catheter, using no more than 30 ml normal saline.
  - ☐ If urinary tract infection is suspected, obtain a urine specimen for culture and sensitivity once crisis stage has passed.
  - ☐ Check for fecal impaction. Perform the rectal examination gently, using an ointment that contains a local anesthetic (e.g., Nupercainal).
  - ☐ Check for sensory stimuli, and loosen clothing, bed covers, or other constricting fabric as indicated.
- Consult physician if symptoms do not abate within 15-30 min, especially if elevated BP, because the consequences are life threatening: seizures, subarachnoid or intracerebral hemorrhage, fatal cerebrovascular accident.
- As prescribed, administer antihypertensive agents and monitor effectiveness.

NIC Dysreflexia Management; Urinary Elimination Management

Decreased cardiac output (or risk for same) related to decreased afterload secondary to reduced peripheral vascular tone

> **Note:** These patients, while normovolemic, may experience a decreased cardiac output as a result of an enlarged vascular space. This is similar to the vascular response seen in distributive (e.g., anaphylactic, septic) shock.

Desired outcome: Patient has adequate cardiac output as evidenced by BP within patient's normal range; HR 60-100 bpm; urinary output ≥0.5 ml/kg/h; peripheral pulses >2+ on a 0-4+ scale; orientation to time, place, and person; PAWP 6-12 mm Hg; SVR 900-1200 dynes/sec/cm^{-5}; CO 4-7 L/min; and normal sinus rhythm on ECG.

- Monitor patient for indicators of decreased cardiac output: drop in systolic BP >20 mm Hg from baseline, systolic BP <80 mm Hg, or a continuing drop in systolic BP of 5-10 mm Hg with every assessment; HR >100 beats/min; irregular HR; restlessness, confusion, and dizziness; warm and flushed skin; peripheral edema; and decreasing urinary output <0.5 ml/kg/h for 2 consecutive hours. Monitor hemodynamic pressures, particularly PAWP, CO, and SVR.
- Continuously assess cardiac rate and rhythm per cardiac monitor; report changes in rate and rhythm.
- Implement measures to prevent episodes of decreased cardiac output caused by orthostatic hypotension:
  ☐ Change patient's position slowly.
  ☐ Perform ROM exercises q2h to prevent venous pooling.
  ☐ Apply elastic antiembolic hose as prescribed to promote venous return.
  ☐ Avoid placing pillows under patient's knees, "gatching" the bed, or allowing patient to cross the legs or sit with legs in a dependent position.
  ☐ Collaborate with physical therapy personnel in progressing patient from a supine to upright position, with the use of a tilt table.
- As prescribed, administer fluids to treat the hypotension.
- As prescribed, administer vasopressor (e.g., epinephrine) to counteract peripheral vasodilation.

NIC Cardiac Care: Acute; Hemodynamic Regulation; Resuscitation; Shock Prevention

Sensory/perceptual alterations (or risk for same) related to altered sensory transmission secondary to cranial nerve involvement with GBS

Desired outcomes: Patient relates the presence of normal vision and exhibits normal pupillary and gag reflexes, intact corneas, ability to masticate, and full ROM of head and shoulders.

- Assess cranial nerve function (see Appendix 4). Patients with GBS commonly exhibit deficits in cranial nerves III through XII.
- Evaluate cranial nerves III, IV, and V by checking for extraocular eye movements, pupillary light reflex, and degree of ptosis and for the presence of diplopia.
  ☐ If patient experiences a deficit, place objects where patient can see them. Assist patient with ADL as indicated.
  ☐ Cover one eye with a patch or frosted lens if patient is experiencing diplopia; alternate patch or lens q2-3h during patient's waking hours.
  ☐ Use eyelid crutches for patients with ptosis.
- Evaluate cranial nerves V and VII by checking patient's facial sensation and movement, ability to masticate, and the corneal reflex.
  ☐ In the presence of a deficit, assess patient for corneal irritation or abrasion. Apply artificial tear drops or ointments as prescribed. Secure the eyelid in a closed position if corneal reflex is diminished or absent.
- Evaluate cranial nerves IX, X, and XII by checking for pharyngeal sensation and movement (swallowing), the presence or absence of the gag reflex, and control of the tongue.
  ☐ If a deficit is found, suction during oral hygiene. Do not feed patient an oral diet until the gag reflex returns.

- Assess cranial nerve XI by checking patient's ability to shrug the shoulders and turn the head from side to side.
  - ☐ If a deficit is found, position patient's head in a position of comfort and proper anatomic alignment.

NIC Peripheral Sensation Management; Surveillance: Safety

Constipation, colonic related to hypoperistalsis or paralytic ileus associated with neuromuscular impairment

Desired outcome: Within 3-5 days of this diagnosis, patient has a bowel movement or returns to usual pattern of elimination.

- Assess patient's GI status, noting absence or presence and quality of the following: bowel sounds, abdominal distention, nausea, vomiting, and abdominal discomfort. In the presence of hypoperistalsis or paralytic ileus, patient will exhibit (1) high-pitched, tinkling sounds that will be heard early in obstruction or ileus or (2) a decrease or absence of sounds occurring with complete obstruction or paralytic ileus.
- If patient is having bowel movements, determine the amount, consistency, and frequency. Question patient about his or her usual pattern of bowel elimination.
- Begin bowel training program based on patient's needs and status of dietary intake. Examples include the following:
  - ☐ Provide a high-fiber diet if patient is able to chew and swallow without difficulty; give patient prune juice every evening.
  - ☐ Establish a regular time for elimination (e.g., 30 min after meals), and have a bed pan readily available.
  - ☐ Facilitate patient's normal bowel habits: ensure privacy; provide warm oral fluids with each attempt at defecation.
  - ☐ Administer stool softeners (e.g., docusate sodium) or bulk-building additives such as psyllium.
  - ☐ Administer prescribed medicated suppositories.

> ***Caution:*** Care must be taken to avoid stimulation of autonomic dysreflexia by using generous amounts of anesthetic ointment (e.g., Nupercainal) and ensuring gentle insertion when giving suppository or enema.

  - ☐ Provide 2-3 L/day of fluid to prevent dehydration and constipation. This may be contraindicated for patient with impaired renal or cardiac status.

NIC Constipation/Impaction Management; Bowel Management; Nutrition Management

Knowledge deficit: purpose and procedure for plasmapheresis

Desired outcome: Before the first plasma exchange, patient verbalizes knowledge of the purpose and procedure for plasmapheresis.

- Assess patient's previous experience with and knowledge of plasmapheresis.
- As appropriate, teach patient the following about plasmapheresis: blood is withdrawn via an arterial catheter, anticoagulated, and then passed through a cell separator. The plasma portion of the blood that may contain the autoantibody whose target is the peripheral nerve myelin sheath is removed. RBCs, WBCs, and platelets are mixed with saline, potassium, and plasma protein fraction and then are returned to the body, minus the plasma, via a venous access.
- Advise patient that plasmapheresis *may* lessen the duration and severity of the symptoms of GBS.

> **Note:** Benefits of plasmapheresis with GBS have not been determined definitively. Although plasmapheresis is still in the experimental stage with this disorder, some studies have shown a rapid but temporary improvement in symptoms.

- Explain that patient should eat before plasmapheresis and that nutrition will be provided during the procedure.
- Advise patient that the nurse will perform several assessment procedures before, during, and after plasmapheresis. See **Risk for disuse syndrome,** p. 423, for neuroassessment parameters. Also see Table 6-1 for the following complications: hypovolemia, clotting abnormalities, hypokalemia, and hypocalcemia.
- Advise patient that the procedure may take several hours and that it may be performed as often as 3-4 times/wk, depending on the patient's condition.
- Provide address and phone number of Guillain-Barré Syndrome Foundation International. Address: PO Box 262, Wynnewood, PA 19096; phone: 1-610-667-0131; fax: 1-610-667-7036; website: www.gbint@ix.netcom.com.

ADDITIONAL NURSING DIAGNOSES

See also "Acute Spinal Cord Injury" for **Urinary retention,** p. 178. See "Renal Transplantation" for **Knowledge deficit: immunosuppressive medications and their side effects,** p. 392. See "Myasthenia Gravis" for **Risk for infection,** p. 417, and **Impaired swallowing,** p. 417. For other nursing diagnoses and interventions, see the following as appropriate: "Nutritional Support," p. 1; "Mechanical Ventilation," p. 17; "Prolonged Immobility," p. 74; "Psychosocial Support," p. 83; and "Psychosocial Support for the Patient's Family and Significant Others," p. 95.

Cerebral aneurysm and subarachnoid hemorrhage

PATHOPHYSIOLOGY

An aneurysm is a localized dilation of an arterial lumen caused by weakness in the vessel wall; 90% of cerebral aneurysms are berry or saccular. The other 10% comprise fusiform, traumatic, septic, dissecting, and Charcot-Bouchard aneurysms. Recent research suggests that cerebral aneurysms result from degenerative vascular diseases that are complicated by hypertension and atherosclerosis. Aneurysms usually occur at the bifurcation of the blood vessels that compose Willis circle, with 85% in anterior cerebral circulation and 15% in posterior cerebral circulation.

Most aneurysms are silent until they rupture, although nearly half of the affected population experience some warning sign or symptom as a result of expansion of the lesion and compression of cerebral tissue. When rupture occurs, hemorrhage into the subarachnoid space (SAS) and basal cisterns results. If the patient survives the initial effects of subarachnoid hemorrhage (SAH), which include destruction of brain tissue by the force of arterial blood, intracerebral hemorrhage, and sharply increased ICP, he or she also must survive two of the common causes of morbidity and mortality—rebleeding and cerebral arterial vasospasm. Although rebleeding may occur at any time, the greatest incidence is between 3 and 11 days after SAH, with the peak at day 7. Although the mechanisms behind rebleeding are unknown, theories of causation involve the normal process of clot dissolution coupled with fluctuations in arterial pressure. Mortality associated with rebleeding is estimated to be approximately 70%.

Cerebral vasospasm, the constriction of the arterial smooth muscle layer of the major cerebral arteries, causes a dramatic decrease in cerebral blood flow, which in turn leads to cerebral ischemia and progressive neurologic deficit. Vasospasm occurs in as many as 60% of patients with SAH, and its onset is between 4 and 14 days after SAH and peaks between 7 and 10 days. The pathogenesis of cerebral vasospasm is poorly understood but seems to be directly related to the amount of blood in the SAS and basal cisterns. The

TABLE 6-2   Clinical Presentation with Cerebral Salt-Wasting Syndrome and Syndrome of Inappropriate Antidiuretic Hormone (SIADH)

Cerebral salt-wasting syndrome	*SIADH*
Hypotension	Normotension
Postural hypotension	Normal pulse rate or bradycardia
Tachycardia	Normal or low hematocrit
Elevated hematocrit	Increased glomerular filtration rate
Decreased glomerular filtration rate	Normal or decreased BUN and creatinine
Normal or elevated BUN and creatinine	Normal or low urine output
Normal or low urine output	Normovolemia or hypervolemia
Hypovolemia	Normal hydration
Dehydration	Dilutional hyponatremia
True hyponatremia	Hypoosmolality
Hypoosmolality	Increased body weight
Decreased body weight	

BUN, Blood urea nitrogen.

greater the volume of blood, the more pronounced the vasospasm. It is hypothesized that as the clots in the basal cisterns begin to hemolyze, spasmogenic substances are released that precipitate the onset of vasospasm. In addition to rebleeding and vasospasm, the patient with a ruptured cerebral aneurysm and SAH is at risk for communicating hydrocephalus, hypothalamic dysfunction, and hyponatremia.

Communicating hydrocephalus: Communicating hydrocephalus develops in approximately 20% of patients with SAH. This condition occurs as a result of the presence of blood in the SAS and ventricular system. The hydrocephalus may be *acute* (lasting <24 h), *subacute* (lasting >24 h-1 wk), or *delayed* (beginning 10 or more days after SAH). Blood in the SAS and ventricles obstructs flow of CSF, interfering with its circulation and reabsorption and causing a rise in CSF pressure, with concomitant decrease in neurologic status.

Hypothalamic dysfunction: Hypothalamic dysfunction, seen in approximately one third of patients with hydrocephalus after SAH, may result from mechanical pressure on the hypothalamus from a dilated third ventricle. One manifestation of this dysfunction is an increase in serum catecholamines, which leads to overstimulation of the sympathetic nervous system.

Hyponatremia: Hyponatremia may be caused by cerebral salt-wasting syndrome, SIADH, or a combination of factors influencing sodium and water metabolism. Hyponatremia is reported to occur in 10%-50% of patients with SAH. If not identified and corrected early, hyponatremia may lead to intracranial hypertension, cerebral ischemia, seizures, coma, and death. See Table 6-2 for signs and symptoms of cerebral salt wasting and SIADH.

Note: Both hypothalamic dysfunction and hyponatremia are seen more frequently in patients with extensive SAH and are positively correlated with the subsequent development of cerebral vasospasm.

ASSESSMENT

Signs and symptoms before and after rupture depend on the size, site, and amount of bleeding.

TABLE 6-3 Indicators of Increased Intracranial Pressure

Alterations in consciousness: increasing restlessness, confusion, irritability, disorientation, increasing drowsiness, lethargy

Bradycardia

Increasing systolic BP with a widening pulse pressure

Irregular respiratory patterns (e.g., Cheyne-Stokes, ataxic, apneustic, central neurogenic, hyperventilation)

Hemisensory changes and hemiparesis or hemiplegia: caused by involvement of hemispheric sensory and motor pathways

Worsening headache

Pupillary changes

Dysconjugate gaze and inability to move one eye beyond midposition: caused by involvement of cranial nerves III, IV, and VI

Seizures

Involvement of other cranial nerves: depends on the severity of neurologic insult

NOTE: If these indicators of IICP are left untreated, the patient will undergo irreversible brain damage or death. If these indicators occur suddenly, there will be displacement of brain substance (herniation), which will progress rapidly to permanent brain damage or death. For additional information about herniation syndromes, see "Traumatic Brain Injury," p 118.

Warning signs and symptoms (before bleeding): Headaches (possibly localized); occasional ptosis and dilated pupil caused by palsy of cranial nerve III; diplopia, blurred vision, pain above and behind the eye; neck and upper back pain; nausea and vomiting.

Clinical presentation after initial bleeding: Meningeal signs (caused by presence of blood in the SAS) include headache, nuchal rigidity, fever, photophobia, lethargy, nausea, and vomiting. Patients report that the headache is the worst they have ever experienced, a sensation of a "bullet going off in the head."

Increased intracranial pressure (IICP): Caused by SAH or intracerebral hemorrhage and the subsequent cerebral edema (Table 6-3; see also "Traumatic Brain Injury," p. 118).

Indicators of hydrocephalus

Acute: Onset within 24 h; loss of pupillary reflexes; sudden onset of coma or persistent coma after initial SAH.

Subacute: Onset within 1-7 days; gradual changes in level of consciousness (LOC) with confusion, drowsiness, lethargy, and stupor.

Delayed: Onset after 10 days; gradual changes in LOC and orientation with confusion, incontinence, and impaired balance, mobility, and gait; intellectual impairment (slowness, mutism); lack of affect; and presence of frontal lobe reflexes (grasp and sucking), which are abnormal in the adult.

Hyponatremia: Anxiety, confusion, agitation, disorientation, lethargy, stupor, coma, anorexia, nausea, vomiting, abdominal pain, cold and clammy skin, generalized weakness, and lower extremity muscle cramps. See Table 6-2 for signs and symptoms of cerebral salt wasting and SIADH.

Altered hypothalamic regulatory mechanisms: Vomiting, glycosuria, proteinuria, and hyponatremia. Increased circulating catecholamines can cause flushing, diaphoresis, pupillary dilation, decreased gastric motility, increased serum glucose, fever, hypertension, tachycardia, cardiac dysrhythmias, ischemia, and infarction.

Physical assessment: Pathologic reflexes caused by the presence of blood in the SAS.

Kernig sign:　Resistance to full extension of the leg at the knee when the hip is flexed.

Brudzinski sign:　Flexion of the hip and knee with neck flexion.

Fundoscopic assessment:　May reveal retinal hemorrhage(s) at the side of the optic disc. Hemorrhage is caused by blood from the SAS being forced along the optic nerve sheath under high pressure. The patient may complain of blurred vision or blind spots (scotomata).

Hunt-Hess classification system:　Permits objective and continuing evaluation of the patient's initial symptoms and their progression. Grading is performed according to symptom presentation and level of consciousness.

　　Grade I: Asymptomatic, alert, and oriented.

　　Grade II: Alert, oriented, headache, and stiff neck.

　　Grade III: Lethargic or confused; minor focal deficit such as hemiparesis.

　　Grade IV: Stuporous, moderate to severe focal deficits, hemiplegia, possible early decerebrate rigidity, and vegetative disturbances.

　　Grade V: Deep coma, decerebrate rigidity, moribund appearance.

DIAGNOSTIC TESTS

CT:　To identify presence of aneurysm and subarachnoid or intracerebral hemorrhage; and size, site, and amount of bleeding. Scan also may reveal the presence of hydrocephalus caused by blocked CSF reabsorption pathways. If the aneurysm is small, it may not appear on the scan.

Cerebral angiography:　To confirm diagnosis of ruptured aneurysm and SAH. It is used to show the size, location, and vessels involved and the presence of other aneurysms, as well as to determine the accessibility of the aneurysm and the presence of hematoma, vasospasm, and hydrocephalus. Panangiography involving both carotids and vertebrals is recommended because of the 15%-20% chance of multiple aneurysms. Very small aneurysms can be missed on angiogram, as are those that do not fill with contrast material because of the presence of vasospasm or a blood clot within the aneurysm.

LP and CSF analysis:　To confirm presence of blood in the CSF, which signals that SAH has occurred. CSF pressure, which normally is 0-15 mm Hg (75-180 mm H_2O), may be as high as 250 mm H_2O, with the pressure proportionate to the degree of bleeding. Protein may be increased to as much as 80-130 mg/dl (normal is 15-50 mg/dl). WBC count may be greater than the normal of $\leq 10/mm^3$; and CSF glucose may be low (<40 mg/dl) in the presence of SAH.

> **Note:**　Performance of LP in the patient with SAH and IICP carries substantial risk of herniation and rebleeding. It is performed only when results of the CT are nondiagnostic.

Transcranial Doppler (TCD) ultrasonography:　To evaluate the flow of blood through cerebral arteries and permit early detection of cerebral vasospasm.

ABG analysis:　To detect hypoxemia and hypercapnia and to determine appropriate respiratory therapy.

Electrocardiogram (ECG):　To detect cardiac changes and dysrhythmias precipitated by hypothalamic dysfunction.

COLLABORATIVE MANAGEMENT

Respiratory support:　To maintain airway and provide intubation and ventilation as necessary. Serial ABG tests are performed to identify hypoxemia (Pao_2 <80 mm Hg) and hypercapnia ($Paco_2$ >45 mm Hg). Hypercapnia is a potent cerebral vasodilator that can increase ICP in patients who are already at risk.

Bed rest, with aneurysm precautions:　To help prevent stress and strain. An attempt should be made to keep patient in a quiet, calm, and soothing environment with lowered lights and noise level. Active ROM and isometric exercises are restricted during acute and preoperative stages to prevent IICP. Passive ROM is prescribed to prevent formation of thrombi, with subsequent pulmonary emboli. Bowel management program is essential to prevent straining at stool.

Intracranial pressure (ICP) monitoring: See "Collaborative Management" in "Traumatic Brain Injury," p. 125.

HOB elevation: To help facilitate venous outflow from the intracranial cavity and lower ICP. A 30- to 45-degree angle usually is prescribed.

Fluid and electrolyte management: Fluid balance is maintained based on measurement of CVP, weight, pulmonary artery wedge pressure (PAWP), and serum osmolality. Electrolytes are replaced as indicated by patient's clinical data and laboratory values. It is recommended that hyponatremia be treated based on a careful assessment and identification of etiology. If the cause is true hyponatremia (cerebral salt wasting), normal saline, packed RBCs, and colloids are recommended. If the cause is dilutional hyponatremia (SIADH), free water restriction is recommended. Fluid restriction ranges from 500-800 ml/24 h to 1000-1500 ml/24 h. If fluid restriction is not an option, sodium replacement is implemented. All therapies should be administered cautiously with frequent (at least q4h) assessment of fluid and electrolyte status.

Nutrition therapy: Adequate nutritional intake is maintained via parenteral nutrition or lipid emulsions, enteral feedings, and oral intake as indicated by patient's neurologic status. See "Nutritional Support," p. 1.

Pharmacotherapy

Sedatives: Phenobarbital is the drug of choice for reducing restlessness and irritability, which can increase BP and ICP.

Antipyretics: Acetaminophen is used to control fever, which increases cerebral metabolic activity. It may be administered along with using a hypothermia blanket and chlorpromazine to decrease temperature and control shivering. Usually aspirin is avoided because it inhibits clotting.

Analgesics: Acetaminophen and codeine sulfate for mild to moderate pain. Although codeine, when given in usual doses, will not depress neurologic indicators, it can cause constipation and thus should be administered with stool softeners.

Stool softeners: Docusate sodium (Colace) is the drug of choice for preventing straining, which can increase ICP.

Corticosteroids: Dexamethasone (Decadron) is used to relieve cerebral edema and decrease ICP. Its effectiveness is controversial. The patient should be monitored carefully for side effects, including GI tract irritation. Medications that reduce gastric activity reduce the risk of gastritis and ulceration.

Antihypertensives: Hydralazine hydrochloride (Apresoline), reserpine (Serpasil), propranolol (Inderal), labetalol (Normodyne), or sodium nitroprusside (Nipride) is administered to reduce BP in patients with persistent hypertension. They may be used in combination with a thiazide diuretic.

Osmotic diuretics: Mannitol (Osmitrol), urea (Ureaphil), and glycerin (Glycerol) may be used to reduce ICP and treat cerebral edema via diuresis and a slightly hypovolemic state. All must be used with caution because of the risk of electrolyte imbalances and other serious side effects and adverse reactions.

Note: With the rapid movement of extracellular fluid from brain tissue to plasma and the associated decrease in brain volume, potential for rebleeding may be increased after the administration of mannitol. In addition, mannitol may cause a rebound increase in ICP approximately 8-12 h after administration as a result of increased circulating volume. It is suggested that furosemide (Lasix) be used to decrease the rebound effect of mannitol.

TABLE 6-4   Nursing Implications for Administration of Epsilon-Aminocaproic Acid (EACA)

- Be aware that rapid administration may induce hypotension, bradycardia, or cardiac dysrhythmias.
- Monitor for and report the following side effects: nausea, cramps, diarrhea, dizziness, tinnitus, headache, skin rash, malaise, nasal stuffiness, postural hypotension.
- Be alert to clotting or thrombosis, which can be precipitated by this medication. Assess for indicators of thrombophlebitis: calf erythema, warmth, tenderness, or increase in size or positive reaction for Homans sign. Provide pneumatic compression stockings as prescribed.
- Assess for indicators of pulmonary emboli: chest pain, dyspnea, fever, tachycardia, cyanosis, falling BP, restlessness, agitation.
- Monitor and report blood levels of EACA via use of chromatography, which is available in some institutions.
- Consult physician promptly for significant findings.

Loop diuretics: Some physicians use furosemide (Lasix) because it seems to decrease cerebral edema without causing the rise in intracranial blood volume that occurs with mannitol.

Anticonvulsants: Phenytoin and phenobarbital may be used to control or prevent seizures.

Antifibrinolytics: Epsilon (ϵ)-aminocaproic acid (EACA [Amicar]) or tranexamic acid (TEA) may be used to prevent lysis of the aneurysmal clot, which occurs normally between 7 and 14 days postrupture. It delays the spontaneous breakdown of the clot and provides time for further stabilization of the patient in preparation for surgery. EACA usually is administered via continuous infusion for the patient with SAH. The length of therapy is determined by the patient's status and readiness for surgery and the physician's preference (Table 6-4).

Note: Use of antifibrinolytic agents remains controversial. The results of research on these agents have been inconclusive.

Calcium channel blocker: For example, nimodipine (Nimotop), inhibits calcium influx across the cell membrane of vascular smooth muscles, thereby decreasing peripheral vascular resistance and promoting vasodilation. Nimodipine and nicardipine selectively affect cerebral vessels.

Triple H therapy: Each of the following therapies may be used singly or in combination.

Note: Although hypervolemic-hypertensive therapy with hemodilution has been proved to be an effective treatment for vasospasm, it carries great risks, and the patient's BP, ICP, and neurologic status must be monitored closely. If used preoperatively (rare), this therapy may precipitate IICP with rerupture and rebleeding from the aneurysm. When used postoperatively, the patient may experience cerebral edema with cerebral ischemia and subsequent neurologic deficit.

- *Hypervolemia* (saline, whole blood, packed cells, plasma protein fraction [Plasmanate], albumin, and hetastarch [Hespan]): To increase circulating volume to reverse or prevent ischemia caused by vasospasm.

TABLE 6-5   Nursing Interventions After Shunt Placement

- After the shunting, assess patient for indicators of IICP (see Table 6-3) caused by either the disease itself or shunt malfunction.
- Position patient on side opposite the insertion site, either flat or with head elevated slightly (as prescribed) to prevent pressure on shunt mechanism.
- Assess VS; LOC (orientation to time, place, person); pupillary light reflex; and motor function.
- Monitor I&O, and limit fluids as prescribed.
- Avoid severe head and neck rotation, flexion, or hyperextension to prevent kinking, compression, or twisting of the shunt catheter, which would impede CSF flow.
- If the shunt has a valve for controlling drainage or preventing reflux of CSF, pump the valve to ensure proper functioning, according to surgeon's directive. Usually the valve is located behind or above the ear and is the approximate diameter of a fingertip. Pumping involves gentle, serial compressions of the tissue over the shunt. If the valve is working properly, the emptying and refilling of the valve will be felt with palpation.
- Assess for indicators of meningitis (see p. 460), peritonitis (see p. 186), or septicemia (see p. 596) caused by presence of shunt mechanism.

IICP, Increased intracranial pressure; *VS,* vital signs; *LOC,* level of consciousness; *I&O,* intake and output; *CSF,* cerebrospinal fluid.

- *Hemodilution* (albumin and crystalloid fluids): To decrease blood viscosity.
- *Hypertension* (dobutamine [Dobutrex], phenylephrine [Neo-Synephrine], dopamine [Intropin], isoproterenol [Isuprel], norepinephrine [Levophed], metaraminol [Aramine]): To increase BP, thereby increasing cerebral perfusion pressure and preventing ischemia and infarction.

Placement of a shunt for treatment of hydrocephalus: Hydrocephalus develops in 20%-25% of patients with subarachnoid hemorrhage from a ruptured cerebral aneurysm. A shunt is placed to drain CSF and thereby prevent enlargement of the ventricles with compression of cerebral tissue and IICP. The method of CSF drainage depends on the type of hydrocephalus. For acute and subacute types, a ventricular catheter (ventriculostomy) usually is positioned, whereas for chronic hydrocephalus, one end of a small catheter is positioned into a ventricle, with the other end draining into a body cavity or space (e.g., subarachnoid space, cistern, peritoneum, vena cava, pleura). Major complications include infection and malfunction. If the shunt has a valve for the purpose of controlling drainage or preventing reflux of CSF, the surgeon may request that the valve be pumped periodically to ensure proper functioning. For nursing interventions after shunt placement, see Table 6-5.

Surgical interventions: Surgical treatment is based on the patient's clinical status and the neurosurgeon's preference. Surgical timing is a continuing source of controversy. Recent studies demonstrate improved outcome with surgery during the first 24-72 h for patients with grade I or II symptoms. Operating early may prevent rebleeding, an often fatal complication, and allow for initiation of Triple H therapy for vasospasm without risk of rebleeding. Others prefer to wait more than 2 wk, until the peak time for vasospasm (7-10 days after SAH) has passed. Use of antifibrinolytic and antihypertensive agents reduces the risk of rebleeding during the presurgical period. Patients with grades III-V symptoms generally are considered poor surgical risks, especially in the period immediately after SAH. If the condition of these patients is clinically unstable, the trend is to treat them medically until they show improvement and stabilization. Surgery is considered for any patient with a large intracranial clot that causes a life-threatening intracranial shift. It is delayed for patients with cerebral vasospasm until the vasospasm subsides.

Repair of a cerebral aneurysm requires a craniotomy with either clipping or ligation of the neck of the aneurysm, coagulation of the aneurysm, or encasement of the aneurysmal sac in surgical gauze. The method of repair depends on the size, site, and number of perforating arteries, as well as the patient's clinical condition and the surgeon's preference.

Although surgical interventions remain the mainstay of treatment of cerebral aneurysms, new modalities are being used. In selected centers and in selected cases, interventional radiology with use of endovascular balloon therapy is an option. The goal of therapy, achieved either through balloon occlusion of the aneurysm or of the parent vessel, is thrombosis of the aneurysm. Cerebral angioplasty for arterial vasospasm is a new technique used to decrease vascular narrowing and reverse ischemia in patients with new-onset vasospasm, 6-12 h after symptoms presentation. Generally, patient selection is limited to poor surgical candidates with surgically difficult or inaccessible aneurysms.

NURSING DIAGNOSES AND INTERVENTIONS

Decreased adaptive capacity: intracranial, related to compromise of fluid dynamic mechanisms secondary to hemorrhage into the subarachnoid space
Desired outcome: Patient exhibits adequate cerebral perfusion within 24-72 h of treatment as evidenced by orientation to time, place, and person (or consistent with baseline); equal and normoreactive pupils; BP within patient's normal range; HR 60-100 bpm; RR 12-20 breaths/min with normal depth and pattern (eupnea); bilaterally equal motor function, with extremity strength and tone normal for patient; ICP 0-15 mm Hg; cerebral perfusion pressure 60-80 mm Hg; and absence of headache, vomiting, and other indicators of IICP.

- Assess hourly for indicators of IICP (see Table 6-3) and herniation (see "Traumatic Brain Injury," p. 119).
- Calculate cerebral perfusion pressure (CPP) by means of the formula:

$$CPP = MAP - ICP$$

     when

$$MAP = \frac{\text{Systolic BP} + 2(\text{Diastolic BP})}{3}$$

CPP <30 mm Hg is incompatible with life. If ICP monitoring is used, assess for IICP (ICP ≥15 mm Hg or elevated above patient's baseline), and consult physician promptly if it occurs (see discussion in "Traumatic Brain Injury," p. 131).

- Assess for and treat conditions that can cause increasing restlessness with concomitant IICP: distended bladder, constipation, hypoxemia, headache, fear, anxiety.
- Implement measures that help prevent IICP and herniation:
  - ☐ Maintain complete bed rest.
  - ☐ Keep HOB elevated 15-45 degrees or as prescribed to promote cerebral venous outflow.
  - ☐ Avoid hyperflexion, hyperextension, or hyperrotation of the neck to decrease the risk of jugular vein compression, which can impede venous outflow, thereby increasing ICP.
  - ☐ Instruct patient to avoid activities that use isometric muscle contractions

(e.g., pulling or pushing side rails, pushing against the foot board). These activities raise systolic BP, which increases ICP.

☐ Caution patient about straining with bowel movements because this increases intrathoracic pressure, which in turn increases ICP.

☐ Instruct patient to exhale through the mouth when moving in bed or having a bowel movement.

☐ Instruct patient to avoid coughing, because it increases intrathoracic pressure and ICP. Teach patient to open mouth when sneezing to minimize the increase in ICP.

☐ Maintain a quiet, relaxing environment; decrease external stimuli in the room, such as lights or noise. Limit visitors if appropriate, and encourage them to talk quietly with patient and try to keep conversations as nonstressful as possible for the patient.

☐ Minimize vigorous activity by assisting with ADL (feeding, bathing, dressing, toileting).

☐ Maintain a patent airway and adequate ventilation to prevent cerebral hypoxia, which, concomitant with hypoxemia and hypercapnia, can cause dramatic cerebral vasodilation and an increase in cerebral edema and ICP.

☐ Monitor ABG values for evidence of hypoxemia (Pao_2 <80 mm Hg) or hypercapnia ($Paco_2$ >45 mm Hg), which can lead to IICP. Administer oxygen as prescribed.

☐ Avoid vigorous, prolonged suctioning during period of intubation because this can precipitate hypoxemia, hypercapnia, and anxiety, which in turn can increase ICP.

☐ Some sources recommend hyperoxygenation of the patient with 100% oxygen during suctioning to increase Pao_2 and decrease $Paco_2$, which will help prevent cerebral vasodilation. Follow this procedure if it is prescribed.

☐ Limit fluid intake to 1500-1800 ml/24 h as prescribed.

☐ Monitor and record I&O accurately.

• Administer antihypertensive medication as prescribed to keep BP at desired levels.

• Administer stool softeners as prescribed to prevent constipation, which can lead to straining and IICP with herniation.

• As prescribed, administer antitussive agents to prevent coughing and antiemetics to prevent or treat vomiting. Both coughing and vomiting can increase intrathoracic pressure and ICP.

• If IICP occurs suddenly, perform hyperinflation (as prescribed or per agency protocol) with a manual resuscitator at a rate of ≥50 breaths/min to decrease $Paco_2$.

• If prescribed for acutely increased ICP, administer bolus of mannitol (i.e., 1.5-2 g/kg, as a 15%-25% solution infused over 30-60 min). Because of this relatively high dose and rapid infusion rate, monitor renal status before and during administration and evaluate fluid and electrolyte status (see p. 636), body weight, and total output before and after the infusion. Consult physician if cerebrospinal fluid pressure is not reduced within 15 min of starting the infusion.

NIC Cerebral Edema Management; Cerebral Perfusion Promotion; Intracranial Pressure (ICP) Monitoring; Neurologic Monitoring; Positioning: Neurologic

Altered protection related to risk of rebleeding from cerebral aneurysm associated with clotting anomaly secondary to normal fibrinolytic response

Desired outcomes: Patient has no symptoms of rebleeding from ruptured cerebral aneurysm as evidenced by orientation to time, place, and person; equal and normoreactive pupils; BP within patient's normal range; HR 60-100 bpm; RR 12-20 breaths/min with normal depth and pattern (eupnea); bilaterally equal motor function with extremity strength and tone normal for patient; and absence of headache, papilledema, nystagmus, and nausea. ICP is 0-15 mm Hg; CPP is 60-80 mm Hg.

- Assess for signs and symptoms of IICP with herniation, which can signal that rerupture with rebleeding from cerebral aneurysm has occurred. See preceding diagnosis, **Decreased adaptive capacity.**
- Administer antifibrinolytic agent (i.e., EACA) as prescribed to prevent the normal hemolytic response and stabilize the blood clot around the ruptured aneurysm.
- Monitor administration of EACA. Use an infusion controller or pump to ensure accuracy. Initial loading dose of 5 g is followed with 1-1½ g/h, not to exceed 24-36 g in 24 h.
- See Table 6-4 for nursing implications for administering EACA.

▐NIC Surveillance: Safety; Bleeding Precautions

Decreased adaptive capacity: intracranial, related to compromise of fluid dynamic mechanisms secondary to cerebral vasospasm associated with ruptured cerebral aneurysm

Desired outcomes: Patient has baseline or normal neurologic status as evidenced by orientation to time, place, and person; equal and normoreactive pupils; BP within patient's normal range; HR 60-100 bpm; RR 12-20 breaths/min with normal depth and pattern (eupnea); bilaterally equal motor function with extremity strength and tone normal for patient; and absence of headache, papilledema, nystagmus, and nausea. ICP is 0-15 mm Hg or at patient's baseline; CPP is 60-80 mm Hg.

- Assess for indicators of IICP (see Table 6-3) and herniation (see "Traumatic Brain Injury," p. 118), which may occur either abruptly or gradually. Cerebral vasospasm generally affects the major cerebral vessels in the hemisphere or at the site of the ruptured aneurysm and can cause a focal neurologic deficit with or without a major or sudden loss of consciousness. Vasospasm also may be characterized by a gradual onset of confusion and deteriorating LOC associated with focal motor deficits. A headache that worsens over time and increasing BP may precede the onset of more serious neurologic symptoms.
- In the presence of the aforementioned indicators, prepare patient for cerebral angiography or CT with contrast medium, the only methods for confirming the presence of vasospasm and ruling out rebleeding.
- Administer the prescribed medications (i.e., mannitol, nitroprusside sodium, nimodipine) and intravenous fluids (e.g., colloids or whole blood to increase volume, BP, and subsequently cerebral perfusion) for treating cerebral vasospasm.
- If hypervolemic-hemodilution therapy is prescribed, observe for signs and symptoms of fluid overload: imbalanced I&O, tachypnea, adventitious breath sounds (crackles), respiratory distress, decreased Hct, hyponatremia (serum sodium <137 mEq/L), jugular vein distention, peripheral edema, and increased CVP and pulmonary artery pressure (PAP).
- Continue to treat the IICP (see **Decreased adaptive capacity: intracranial,** secondary to hemorrhage into the subarachnoid space, p. 434).

▐NIC Cerebral Edema Management; Cerebral Perfusion Promotion; Intracranial Pressure (ICP) Monitoring; Positioning: Neurologic; Neurologic Monitoring

Constipation related to prolonged immobility; decreased fluid intake; inadequate intake of fiber; restriction against Valsalva maneuver for straining

Desired outcome: Patient has bowel movements within his or her normal pattern (or at least q3-5days) without straining.

- Obtain data regarding patient's normal bowel elimination pattern, including date of most recent bowel movement.
- Assess for indicators of constipation, including abdominal distention, cramping, and complaints of fullness or pressure in the abdomen or rectum. Auscultate for bowel sounds.
- Advise patient to defecate whenever the need arises but to refrain from straining because this can increase ICP dramatically, thus increasing the risk

of rerupturing and rebleeding from the aneurysm. Instruct patient to exhale slowly when defecating, inasmuch as this will help prevent a sudden increase in ICP.

- Assist patient into semi-Fowler's or high Fowler's position to facilitate bowel elimination unless this position is contraindicated. Use of a bedside commode is recommended rather than a bed pan, because the physical and emotional stress of getting on a bed pan may increase ICP more than moving with assistance to a commode.
- Teach patient to select foods high in fiber to facilitate bowel elimination.
- Unless contraindicated, offer patient a warm drink to stimulate peristalsis. Record amount on I&O record.
- Administer stool softeners as prescribed.
- Avoid use of rectal thermometers, suppositories, enemas, or digital evacuation of an impaction. This type of stimulus may cause patient to perform a Valsalva-type maneuver, which in turn may increase intrathoracic and intracranial pressures, resulting in the potential for rerupture and rebleeding from the aneurysm.

NIC Bowel Management; Constipation/Impaction Management

ADDITIONAL NURSING DIAGNOSES

As appropriate, see nursing diagnoses and interventions in "Nutritional Support," p. 1; "Mechanical Ventilation," p. 17; "Alterations in Consciousness," p. 46; "Prolonged Immobility," p. 74; "Psychosocial Support," p. 83; and "Psychosocial Support for the Patient's Family and Significant Others," p. 95. See "Status Epilepticus" for **Risk for trauma** (oral and musculoskeletal), p. 445. See "Meningitis" for **Pain** related to headache, photophobia, and fever, p. 446. Also see "Diabetes Insipidus" for **Risk for fluid volume deficit,** p. 482. See "Syndrome of Inappropriate Antidiuretic Hormone" for **Risk for injury,** p. 485.

Care of the patient after intracranial surgery

Cranial surgery is performed for the following reasons: removal of a space-occupying lesion such as a tumor, hematoma, or abscess; repair of a vascular abnormality such as an aneurysm or arteriovenous malformation (AVM); drainage of cerebrospinal fluid from the ventricular system; correction of skull fractures; biopsy of tissue to confirm a diagnosis and facilitate treatment; control of seizures; and reduction of pain.

The surgical approach selected by the neurosurgeon depends primarily on the location of the pathologic condition. The *supratentorial* approach is used to remove or correct problems in the frontal, temporal, or occipital lobes, as well as in the diencephalic area (pituitary, hypothalamus). Lesions of the cerebellum and brainstem usually require an *infratentorial* (suboccipital) approach. The *transsphenoidal* approach gains access to the pituitary gland to remove a tumor, control bone pain associated with metastatic cancer, or attempt to arrest the progression of diabetic retinopathy in a patient with diabetes mellitus. After intracranial surgery the major goals of treatment are to maintain cerebral function through control of ICP; recognize, prevent, or treat complications; provide supportive care until the patient can resume ADL; and prepare for rehabilitation.

COMPLICATIONS AFTER INTRACRANIAL SURGERY

Increased intracranial pressure with herniation: Cerebral edema, hemorrhage, infection, and surgical trauma can all lead to IICP with herniation (see Table 6-3). Some cerebral edema is expected after intracranial surgery, and it usually peaks about 72 h after surgery (see "Traumatic Brain Injury," p. 118).

Intracranial bleeding: May be intracerebral, intracerebellar, subarachnoid, subdural, epidural, or intraventricular. Bleeding may be caused by the lengthy and extensive surgical procedure, prolonged anesthesia, preexisting medical problems, or medications.

Hypovolemic shock: May occur as a result of general fluid loss associated with use of osmotic diuretics.

Seizures: Generalized or partial seizures can occur as a result of surgical trauma, irritation of cerebral tissue by the presence of blood, cerebral edema, cerebral hypoxia, hypoglycemia, preexisting seizure disorder, or inadequate anticonvulsant levels.

CNS infection: Meningitis, encephalitis, and ventriculitis may occur as a result of bacterial contamination before, during, or after surgery. For example, organisms introduced at the time of injury (e.g., gunshot wound) or a break in sterile technique may lead to CNS infection. (See "Meningitis," p. 460, and "Infection Prevention and Control," Appendix 8.)

Hydrocephalus: May appear preoperatively or occur postoperatively as an acute or chronic complication. Usually it is caused by a slowing or complete stoppage of the flow of CSF through the ventricular system secondary to edema, bleeding, scarring, or obstruction. For a discussion of shunt creation, see "Cerebral Aneurysm and Subarachnoid Hemorrhage," p. 427.

Diabetes insipidus (DI) and SIADH: The result of a disturbance in the hypothalamus or posterior lobe of the pituitary gland. ADH is produced within the supraoptic nuclei of the hypothalamus and stored in the posterior pituitary. DI is the result of a decrease or loss of production of ADH, which leads to excessive urinary output, with a potential for serious fluid and electrolyte problems (see "Diabetes Insipidus," p. 479). This disturbance may result from edema, manipulation, or partial or total removal of the gland. SIADH, a less common problem, is the result of an increase in the release of ADH, which leads to reabsorption of large amounts of water via the renal tubules with concurrent loss of large amounts of sodium. Like DI, SIADH also can cause serious fluid and electrolyte problems (see "Syndrome of Inappropriate Antidiuretic Hormone," p. 484).

Cardiac dysrhythmias: May occur as a result of cerebral hypoxia or ischemia, manipulation of the brainstem, or the irritating effects of blood in the CSF (see "Dysrhythmias and Conduction Disturbances," p. 277).

Tension pneumocephalus: Occurs as a result of air entering the subdural, extradural, subarachnoid, intracerebral, or intraventricular spaces. Is a complication of infratentorial/posterior fossa craniotomy, burr holes for removal of chronic subdural hematoma, and transsphenoidal hypophysectomy.

CSF leakage: Caused by a channel between the subarachnoid space (SAS) and the outside as a result of a tear or rupture of the dura mater. A CSF leak may be present preoperatively after a skull fracture, or it may occur during surgery. CSF leakage from the ear is called *otorrhea*; from the nose it is called *rhinorrhea*. The leakage of CSF indicates an open pathway to the SAS, which carries a serious risk of infection.

Respiratory complications: Respiratory complications after intracranial surgery can be particularly serious because any increase in $Paco_2$ resulting in hypercapnia will lead to cerebral vasodilation with a subsequent increase in intracranial volume, and thus IICP. Respiratory complications include the following:

- Partial or complete airway obstruction caused by accumulation of secretions and improper positioning.
- Neurogenic pulmonary edema caused by a sudden increase in ICP.
- Cerebral edema that causes compression of brainstem respiratory centers.
- Atelectasis and pneumonia.
- Pulmonary embolus.

Gastrointestinal bleeding (Cushing ulcer) and paralytic ileus: The development of GI bleeding is associated with cerebral trauma and the postoperative period after neurosurgery. Although the cause is unclear, it is believed that stress from the trauma or surgery can lead to continued vagal stimulation, which in turn leads to a hyperacidic state that causes gastric erosion, ulceration, and ultimately hemorrhage. Gastric erosion, ulceration, and hemorrhage also can be precipitated by medications, especially the corticosteroids (see "Acute Gastro-intestinal Bleeding," p. 541). Paralytic ileus may occur after neurologic surgery. Decreased or absent peristalsis results from prolonged anesthesia, immobility, trauma, electrolyte deficiencies, and mechanical obstruction (e.g., obstipation). **Thrombophlebitis, deep vein thrombosis (DVT), and pulmonary embolus:** Each of these complications is related to or the result of prolonged bed rest and immobility after intracranial surgery. Other factors, such as a prolonged surgical procedure or preexisting coagulopathies and blood dyscrasias, may influence the postoperative development of these complications.

POSTOPERATIVE NEUROLOGIC DEFICITS

Some neurologic deficit(s) may be present preoperatively and should be noted and documented. Deficits that occur after surgery may be caused by surgical trauma or the presence of cerebral edema, which will interfere with normal brain function. With time, these deficits may improve. The following are some of the neurologic deficits that may be present in the patient after intracranial surgery.

Diminished LOC: The degree of improvement in LOC will depend on the amount of preoperative damage to cerebral tissue. Generally, LOC improves as anesthesia wears off, cerebral edema subsides, and ICP approaches normal.

Communicative and cognitive deficits: The ability to communicate and understand after surgery depends on the degree of preoperative dysfunction, the site of the lesion, the extensiveness of the surgical procedure, and the degree of postoperative cerebral edema.

Broca (expressive, motor, nonfluent) dysphasia: A situation or disorder in which an individual can comprehend the situation and follow commands appropriately but cannot articulate wishes and needs.

Wernicke (receptive, sensory, fluent) dysphasia: A situation or disorder in which an individual does not understand the situation and cannot follow commands appropriately.

Motor and sensory deficits: Motor deficits (weakness or paralysis) are caused by injury or edema to the primary motor cortex and corticospinal (pyramidal) tracts. Generally, improvement will be seen as cerebral edema subsides. Early physical therapy is necessary to prevent long-term disabilities such as foot or wrist drop, contractures, and hip rotation. Sensory deficits are caused by injury or edema to the primary sensory cortex or the sensory association areas of the parietal lobe. In addition, damage to the spinothalamic tracts may cause sensory deficits. Examples of sensory deficits include the inability to distinguish objects according to size, shape, weight, texture, and consistency and the inability to distinguish changes in temperature, touch, pressure, and position. As with motor deficits, improvement in sensory perception generally will occur as cerebral edema subsides.

Cranial nerve impairment: The degree and presence of cranial nerve deficit(s) depend on the site of the lesion, preoperative deficit, the degree of postoperative cerebral edema, and the surgical approach. Infratentorial surgery for lesions in the posterior fossa (brainstem and cerebellum) may involve significant cranial nerve manipulation and trauma, with considerable postoperative cranial nerve deficit. Deficit(s) may improve with decreasing cerebral edema or may be permanent. Assessment of cranial nerve dysfunction is an important nursing function. For more information about the function of all the cranial nerves, see Appendix 4.

Loss of corneal reflex: May be caused by surgical trauma to motor pathways from the frontal lobe or trauma or edema of the brainstem cranial nerve nuclei.

It can result in corneal abrasion, ulceration, and blindness if it is not recognized and treated promptly.

Periocular edema: Can occur after supratentorial surgery with manipulation of the scalp or frontal bones of the cranium or retraction of the frontal lobes.

Hyperthermia: May be caused by injury or irritation of the hypothalamic temperature-regulating centers or the presence of blood in the CSF or may be an indicator of infection. Regardless of the cause, an elevated temperature is detrimental because it increases the metabolic needs of the brain, potentially leading to increased blood flow to the area, with concomitant cerebral edema.

COLLABORATIVE MANAGEMENT AFTER INTRACRANIAL SURGERY

Respiratory support: Oxygen supplements, intubation, and mechanical ventilation are provided as indicated.

Activity restrictions: Will depend on patient's LOC and general condition.

Positioning: For most patients, HOB is elevated 30 degrees to promote venous drainage, thereby reducing ICP.

- In posterior fossa surgery (infratentorial approach), the supporting muscles of the neck are altered. This necessitates turning the patient with the neck in alignment with the head and supporting the head, neck, and shoulders in the process.
- After craniectomy, during which a bone flap is removed, the patient should not be positioned on the side on which bone has been removed. Label patient's head dressing, chart, and bed with this information.
- After procedures in which a large intracranial space has been left because of extensive surgery, patient should not be positioned on operative side immediately after surgery because this may cause a sudden shift in intracranial contents, with subsequent hemorrhage or herniation.

Pharmacotherapy: The following may be prescribed postoperatively:

Corticosteroids (e.g., dexamethasone):   To decrease cerebral edema.

> **Note:**   Current research has not resolved the question of whether steroids are effective in the treatment of cerebral edema.

Osmotic diuretics (e.g., mannitol, urea):   To control cerebral edema causing IICP.

Anticonvulsants (e.g., phenytoin, fosphenytoin, phenobarbital):   To prevent seizures in the immediate postoperative period caused by cerebral edema and irritation as a result of surgical manipulation of the brain. Anticonvulsants may be continued prophylactically for a period of 1-2 yr after surgery.

Antibiotics: To prevent or treat postoperative surgical site infection. Also to treat respiratory or urinary tract infection.

Antipyretics: For prompt treatment of elevated temperature, which, if left untreated, can increase metabolic activity, causing increased use of oxygen and glucose supplies.

Analgesics: To treat or control headache. Drugs of choice are acetaminophen alone or with codeine sulfate.

Antacids (e.g., Maalox):   To prevent the formation of gastric ulceration occurring from steroid use or as a result of surgical stress.

Histamine H_2-receptor antagonists (e.g., ranitidine [Zantac]):   To suppress gastric secretions and thus prevent or facilitate healing of Cushing ulcer.

Fluid and electrolyte management: To prevent or treat increasing cerebral edema. Usually fluids are limited to 1500-1800 ml/day, depending on patient's body size and overall condition.

Nutritional support: The method and type of nutritional support are determined by the patient's condition and may include any of the following: oral feedings, enteral feedings, supplements, or parenteral nutrition (i.e., total parenteral nutrition [TPN], fat emulsion therapy). See "Nutritional Support," p. 1.

Physical medicine consultation:　To evaluate patient for physical, occupational, and speech therapy and to begin planning for rehabilitation.

NURSING DIAGNOSES AND INTERVENTIONS

Risk for injury related to potential for development of gastric ulcer (Cushing) or gastritis secondary to hyperacidic state

Desired outcomes:　Patient's gastric pH is >5, and patient has no symptoms of gastric ulcer and gastritis as evidenced by gastric secretions and stool culture that are negative for blood; HR ≤100 bpm; BP within patient's normal range; and absence of midepigastric discomfort.

- Monitor for indicators of GI bleeding or ulceration: midepigastric discomfort, occult or frank blood in stool or gastric secretions, decreasing BP, increasing HR. If these indicators are present, consult physician and prepare for insertion of a gastric tube.
- Monitor hematocrit (Hct) or hemoglobin (Hgb) results daily; report decreasing values. Normal values are as follows: Hct 37%-47% (female) and 40%-54% (male); Hgb 14-18 g/dl (male) and 12-16 g/dl (female).
- Test gastric drainage pH q4h. Administer H_2-receptor antagonists and/or antacids as prescribed to maintain pH >5.
- Implement measures to prevent ulceration and hemorrhage:
  - ☐ As prescribed, administer sucralfate (Carafate) and histamine H_2-receptor antagonists, antacids to suppress gastric secretions and promote healing.
  - ☐ When administering steroids, aspirin, phenytoin, and other medications that irritate gastric mucosa, administer with a meal or snack.

NIC Surveillance; Bleeding Precautions

ADDITIONAL NURSING DIAGNOSES

See also nursing diagnoses and interventions in "Traumatic Brain Injury," for **Risk for infection (CNS),** p. 130; **Ineffective thermoregulation,** p. 131; **Risk for disuse syndrome,** p. 132; and **Impaired corneal tissue integrity,** p. 132. See also "Cerebral Aneurysm and Subarachnoid Hemorrhage" for **Decreased adaptive capacity** secondary to hemorrhage into the subarachnoid space, p. 434; **Decreased adaptive capacity** secondary to cerebral vasospasm, p. 436; and **Constipation,** p. 436. See "Status Epilepticus" for **Risk for trauma** (oral and musculoskeletal), p. 445. See "Meningitis" for **Pain** related to headache, photophobia, and fever, p. 446. See "Diabetes Insipidus" for **Fluid volume deficit,** p. 482. See "Syndrome of Inappropriate Antidiuretic Hormone" for **Risk for injury,** p. 485. See "Nutritional Support," p. 1; "Prolonged Immobility," p. 74; "Psychosocial Support," p. 83; and "Psychosocial Support for the Patient's Family and Significant Others," p. 95.

Status epilepticus

PATHOPHYSIOLOGY

Status epilepticus is a state of recurring or continuous seizures of at least 20- to 30-min duration, in which the patient does not return to full consciousness from the postictal state before another seizure occurs. If possible, treatment should be initiated immediately to prevent neuronal injury, which is thought to begin within 20-30 min. The two major types of status epilepticus, based on the classification of Gastaut and used by Engel, are generalized status epilepticus and partial status epilepticus. *Generalized status* includes convulsive status (generalized tonic-clonic seizures) and absence status (petit mal seizures). *Partial status* includes simple partial status (focal motor or epilepsia partialis continua) and complex partial status (temporal or nontemporal seizures). The term *nonconvulsive status* also is used to describe absence and complex partial status. Convulsive status (generalized tonic-clonic seizures) is the more common type and is considered a life-threatening medical emergency because of the hypoxia and neuronal metabolic exhaustion that occur. Neuronal death is possible.

A common cause of status epilepticus in persons with epilepsy is noncompliance with medications or a drop in anticonvulsant serum levels caused by alcohol abuse or infection. Other causes for individuals with and without preexisting epilepsy include acute metabolic disturbances (hypoglycemia, hyponatremia, hypocalcemia), cerebrovascular accident, CNS infection (meningitis, encephalitis), CNS trauma or tumors, and alcohol or drug abuse. Prompt treatment is vital in preventing complications such as cardiac dysrhythmias, hyperthermia, aspiration, hypertension, hypotension, anoxia, hyperglycemia, hypoglycemia, dehydration, myoglobinuria, and oral or musculoskeletal injuries. The mortality in status epilepticus is 10%-12%.

ASSESSMENT

History and risk factors:　Epilepsy, drug or alcohol abuse, recent head injury, infection, headaches. If the patient is taking antiepilepsy medications, record the following: drug name, dosage, time last taken, length of time drug has been taken, and any recent medication changes. Determine whether patient is taking any other medications, including name, dose, and time last taken.

Partial status epilepticus

Complex partial status:　Manifested as a prolonged confusional state caused by continuing or recurring seizures. Automatisms (lip smacking, chewing, swallowing) and speech difficulty may be present. Once this period of status passes, postictal confusion and sleepiness may ensue.

Simple partial status:　The second most common form of status epilepticus, it is commonly manifested as focal motor status (epilepsia partialis continua). Usually consciousness remains intact, and motor activity is localized to one area of the body such as the face or hand. It may last for hours or days.

Generalized status epilepticus

Absence status:　Characterized by some alteration in consciousness, ranging from a dreamy state to stupor. Automatisms or mild clonic movements, such as fluttering of the eyelids, may be present. Clinically, absence status is difficult to differentiate from complex partial status.

Convulsive status:　The most common form of status epilepticus, it is characterized by generalized tonic-clonic seizures without return to full consciousness. This is a life-threatening medical emergency requiring immediate intervention.

DIAGNOSTIC TESTS

Serum drug screen:　To rule out drug or alcohol intoxication.

Serum electrolyte, liver enzymes, blood urea nitrogen (BUN), calcium, magnesium, and glucose values; complete blood cell count (CBC):　To rule out electrolyte imbalance or metabolic disturbance as the cause of status epilepticus.

Antiepilepsy serum drug level:　To determine the amount of drug in patient's system.

ABG analysis:　To obtain baseline levels and determine state of oxygenation.

ECG:　To evaluate cardiovascular status, especially during administration of drugs such as phenytoin that may lead to hypotension and dysrhythmias.

Electroencephalogram (EEG):　Performed during the seizure and can differentiate between absence and complex partial status.

CT:　To rule out presence of a brain lesion.

COLLABORATIVE MANAGEMENT

Maintenance of alveolar ventilation and other vital functions: Cardiopulmonary function and VS are assessed closely. Oral airway, oxygen, and if necessary, intubation and respiratory support are initiated.

Prevention of Wernicke-Korsakoff syndrome: 100 mg IV thiamine and 50 ml of 50% glucose are administered if chronic alcohol ingestion or hypoglycemia is suspected.

Pharmacotherapy

Administration of fast-acting anticonvulsant: Given to achieve high serum and brain concentrations. It is not used as a long-acting anticonvulsant.

- Diazepam (Valium):
  - ☐ 0.2 mg/kg up to 20 mg given IV.
  - ☐ Do not infuse faster than 5 mg/min because of respiratory depression that can occur with faster infusion rate.
- Lorazepam (Ativan):
  - ☐ 0.1 mg/kg up to 8 mg given IV.
  - ☐ Do not infuse faster than 2 mg/min.
  - ☐ Monitor respiratory and cardiovascular status continuously during administration of short-acting anticonvulsants.

Administration of long-acting anticonvulsant

- Phenytoin (Dilantin):
  - ☐ Usual loading dose is 18-20 mg/kg given IV.
  - ☐ Do not infuse faster than 50 mg/min, inasmuch as hypotension or dysrhythmias can develop.
  - ☐ Flush line with normal saline only. Microcrystallization, which occurs when phenytoin is used with dextrose, also may occur when it is used in saline as a continuous drip.
  - ☐ Monitor VS closely.
  - ☐ If status persists after 20 mg/kg dose, an additional 5- to 10-mg/kg up to a maximal total dose of 30 mg/kg may be given.

> *Caution:* High doses of phenytoin can cause seizure activity; therefore >30 mg/kg is not recommended.

*OR (if phenytoin is **not** used)*

- Fosphenytoin (Cerebyx) :
  - ☐ Usual loading dose is 20 mg/kg PE (phenytoin equivalents) IV.
  - ☐ Infusion rate is 100-150 PE/min. Hypotension and cardiac dysrhythmias may develop.
  - ☐ Most IV solutions are compatible with fosphenytoin, including dextrose solutions.
  - ☐ Phlebitis and soft tissue damage at IV site are not seen as frequently with fosphenytoin.
  - ☐ Monitor VS closely.
  - ☐ If status persists after 20 mg/kg, an additional 5-10 mg/kg up to a maximal total dose of 30 mg/kg may be given.

Administration of IV phenobarbital: If patient is allergic to phenytoin.
☐ Usual dosage is 20 mg/kg.
☐ Do not infuse faster than 50-75 mg/min.

> *Caution:* If given simultaneously with or after lorazepam or diazepam, respiratory depression and hypotension can occur, possibly necessitating ventilatory support.

For refractory status epilepticus—that continues after administration of benzodiazepines, phenytoin or fosphenytoin, and/or phenobarbital—even more aggressive treatment is required. This is done best with general anesthesia using propofol, midazolam, or pentobarbital.

General anesthesia
- Pentobarbital coma
  - ☐ Given if administration of fast-acting anticonvulsant, long-acting anticonvulsant, or IV phenobarbital is ineffective in stopping the seizure activity.
  - ☐ Loading dose is 5 mg/kg.
  - ☐ Maintenance dose is 0.5-3 mg/kg/h to stop seizure activity or maintain burst suppression on EEG.
  - ☐ Monitor respiratory and cardiovascular activity continuously.
  - ☐ Mechanical ventilation and vasopressors usually are required.
  - ☐ Periodic tapering of pentobarbital is done to see if seizures have remitted.
  - ☐ Patient may be in a coma for days to weeks.
- Propofol
  - ☐ Given for refractory status epilepticus.
  - ☐ Loading dose is 1-2 mg/kg IV.
  - ☐ Initial maintenance dose of 2-10 mg/kg/h to stop seizure activity or maintain burst suppression on EEG. Adjust dose according to EEG findings.
  - ☐ Monitor respiratory and cardiovascular activity continuously.
  - ☐ Mechanical ventilation and vasopressors are required.
  - ☐ Periodic tapering of propofol is done to see if seizures have remitted.
- Midazolam
  - ☐ Given for refractory status epilepticus.
  - ☐ Loading dose is 0.2 mg/kg IV.
  - ☐ Initial maintenance of 0.75-10 µg/kg/min to stop seizure activity or maintain burst suppression on EEG. Maintenance dose is adjusted according to EEG findings.
  - ☐ Monitor respiratory and cardiovascular activity continuously.
  - ☐ Mechanical ventilation and vasopressors are usually required.
  - ☐ Periodic tapering of midazolam is done to see if seizures have remitted.

Intravenous valproic acid (Depacon), paraldehyde, lidocaine, or neuromuscular blockade: Alternative therapies to stop the seizure activity. Neuromuscular blockade will stop the movements but not the electrical activity and is always administered with sedatives.

Nutritional support: Enteral or parenteral nutrition may be necessary, depending on the duration of the status epilepticus and patient's underlying nutritional state.

NURSING DIAGNOSES AND INTERVENTIONS

Impaired gas exchange related to altered oxygen supply associated with hypoventilation and bradypnea secondary to depressant effect of seizures on respiratory center

Desired outcome: Within 1 h of treatment/intervention, patient has adequate gas exchange as evidenced by Pao_2 ≥80 mm Hg; $Paco_2$ 35-45 mm Hg; pH 7.35-7.45; and RR 12-20 breaths/min with normal depth and pattern (eupnea).

- Assess patient's respiratory status, including rate, depth, rhythm, and color. Be alert to use of accessory muscles of respiration, rapid or labored respirations, and cyanosis (a late sign of dysfunction).
- Position an oral airway to help maintain open airway. To prevent injury, avoid forcing airway into mouth.
- Keep patient turned to the side to allow secretions to drain; suction as necessary.
- Monitor ABG values to assess oxygenation. Be alert to hypoxemia (Pao_2 <80 mm Hg) and respiratory acidosis ($Paco_2$ >45 mm Hg; pH <7.35).
- Keep intubation equipment readily available for airway and ventilation assistance.

- Administer oxygen as indicated per nasal cannula, mask, or manual resuscitator.
- Administer antiepilepsy medications within prescribed criteria to avoid further depression of respiratory center.

NIC Airway Management; Oxygen Therapy; Aspirations Precautions

Altered tissue perfusion: cerebral and cardiopulmonary, related to interrupted blood flow secondary to continuous seizure activity or vasodilatory effects of some antiepilepsy medications

Desired outcome: Within 1 h of treatment/intervention, patient has adequate cerebral and cardiopulmonary perfusion as evidenced by orientation to time, place, and person; normal sinus rhythm on ECG; BP within patient's normal range; RR 12-20 breaths/min with normal depth and pattern (eupnea); and absence of headache, papilledema, and other clinical indicators of IICP.

> **Note:** Metabolic demands of the brain and heart are increased greatly during seizure activity; thus adequate perfusion is essential for organ function.

- Maintain airway and ventilation to ensure maximal delivery of oxygen to the brain cells.
- Monitor VS q2-4min. Respiratory depression, decreased BP, and dysrhythmias can occur with rapid infusion of diazepam and phenytoin. BP must be maintained within normal limits for optimal brain perfusion.
- Monitor cardiac status via cardiac monitor. Be alert to dysrhythmias.
- Ensure safe administration of antiepileptic drugs: diazepam at 5 mg/min; lorazepam at 2 mg/min; phenobarbital at 50-100 mg/min; or phenytoin at 50 mg/min. See "Collaborative Management," p. 443, for details.
- Perform baseline and serial neurologic assessments to determine the presence of focal findings that suggest an expanding lesion. (See Table 6-3 for indicators of IICP.)

NIC Cerebral Perfusion Promotion; Neurologic Monitoring; Seizure Management; Cardiac Care: Acute

Risk for trauma (oral and musculoskeletal) related to seizure activity

Desired outcome: Patient's oral cavity and musculoskeletal system do not exhibit evidence of trauma after the seizure.

- Pad the side rails, keep side rails up at all times, maintain bed in its lowest position, and keep an oral airway at the bedside.
- Perform protective measures during the seizures:
  - ☐ Put a soft object such as a flat pillow under patient's head.
  - ☐ Move sharp or potentially dangerous objects away from patient.
  - ☐ Loosen any tight clothing.
  - ☐ Avoid restraining patient, because the force of the tonic-clonic movements could traumatize the patient.
  - ☐ Avoid forcing airway into patient's mouth when jaws are clenched. Force could break teeth, causing patient to swallow or aspirate them.
  - ☐ Avoid use of tongue blade, which could splinter.
  - ☐ Stay with patient; assess and record seizure type and duration. Record any automatic behavior (e.g., lip smacking, chewing movements), motor activity, incontinence, tongue biting, and postictal state.
- After seizure, reorient and reassure patient.

NIC Environmental Management: Safety; Positioning; Seizure Precautions; Seizure Management

Noncompliance with prescribed medication regimen, related to misunderstanding health care recommendations; not understanding importance of following medication schedule; running out of medication; stopping medication intentionally

Desired outcome: Within the 24-h period before discharge from the critical care unit, patient verbalizes understanding of the rationale and importance

of taking the medication as prescribed, as well as the consequence of noncompliance.
- Once a diagnosis of noncompliance with the medication regimen has been established, determine patient's reason for noncompliance.
- Assess patient's understanding of epilepsy and its treatment.
- Ensure that patient is aware that stopping the antiepilepsy medication can result in serious problems, including status epilepticus. Explain that if patient plans to stop the medication for any reason, he or she should do so with physician's guidance so that it can be done as safely as possible, although the risk of status epilepticus would remain.
- Evaluate the effect epilepsy has on patient's life-style.
- Once the problem has been identified, work with the patient to find a solution. For example, if the patient is experiencing a side effect from the medication, such as gastric upset, suggest that patient try taking the medication after meals. If the gastric upset is a result of increasing the medication, advise patient to increase the dose more slowly.
- Refer patient to regional epilepsy support groups and the Epilepsy Foundation of America (EFA), including regional affiliate and national headquarters.
- As appropriate, refer patient to nurse specialist or social worker at regional center for individual counseling.

NIC Teaching: Prescribed Medication; Decision-Making Support; Coping Enhancement; Values Clarification

Knowledge deficit: disease process, treatment, and necessary life-style changes for epilepsy

Desired outcome: Within the 24-h period before discharge from the critical care unit, patient verbalizes understanding of epilepsy, including its etiology, pathophysiology, and seizure classification, as well as its treatment and necessary life-style changes.
- Assess patient's understanding of epilepsy.
- As indicated, teach patient about the disease, its cause, pathophysiology, and seizure classification.
- Ask patient to describe the seizure(s) in detail, including warning signals (aura) that occur at the beginning of the seizure. Explain to patient that this aura or warning is the beginning of the seizure and that patient should lie down or get into a safe position to prevent injury.
- Assess patient's knowledge of the antiepilepsy medication, including its name, purpose, schedule, dosage, precautions, and side effects. Teach patient the importance of maintaining a constant blood level of the medication by taking the medication every day as prescribed. Explain that if the medication is missed or taken erratically, he or she cannot attain the blood level that is necessary for preventing seizure breakthrough. If a dose of medication is missed, instruct patient to notify his or her physician.
- Advise patient that a normal life is possible.
- Teach patient that sleep deprivation can precipitate status epilepticus and that each individual must know his or her own limits. However, having epilepsy does not mean that it is necessary to get more sleep than do persons who do not have epilepsy.
- Teach patient and significant others the safety interventions that should be made during a seizure (see **Risk for trauma** [oral and musculoskeletal] related to seizure activity, p. 445). In addition, explain the importance of easing patient to the floor and turning patient to a side-lying position.
- Inform patient of the state's driving regulations for persons with epilepsy.
- Teach patient the importance of avoiding dangerous machinery and heights if his or her seizures are not being controlled adequately by medications.

NIC Teaching: Individual; Support Group

Ineffective individual coping related to frustration secondary to unpredictable nature of the disease

Desired outcomes: Within 24-48 h of this diagnosis, patient verbalizes feelings, identifies strengths and ineffective coping behaviors, and demonstrates a responsible role in his or her own care.

- Assess patient's knowledge of the disease and its treatment. See preceding diagnosis, **Knowledge deficit.**
- Encourage patient to express feelings of frustration so that you can evaluate areas of major concern.
- Involve patient in decisions regarding care so that he or she has more of a sense of control over the disease (e.g., encourage patient to participate in the decision for scheduling the medications).
- Help patient set realistic goals for employment and living arrangements. Refer patient to regional or local EFA as appropriate.
- To involve patient in self-care, encourage him or her to educate others in what to do should a seizure occur.
- Encourage patient's involvement in support groups in which patient can learn coping strategies from other persons with the same disorder.
- For additional interventions, see the same nursing diagnosis in "Psychosocial Support," p. 83.

NIC Coping Enhancement; Crisis Intervention; Emotional Support; Support System Enhancement

ADDITIONAL NURSING DIAGNOSES

For other nursing diagnoses and interventions, see the following as appropriate: "Mechanical Ventilation," p. 17; "Psychosocial Support," p. 83; and "Psychosocial Support for the Patient's Family and Significant Others," p. 95.

Stroke: acute cerebral infarct and intracerebral hematoma

PATHOPHYSIOLOGY

Stroke is the leading cause of adult disability and the third leading cause of death. Although strokes can occur at any age, the majority occur in individuals over age 55 yr. The term *stroke* refers to an acute vascular injury to the brain. There are two major categories of stroke—ischemic and hemorrhagic. Subcategories of these major stroke types are shown in Figure 6-1. Each stroke type is defined by the pathophysiologic event. This section deals exclusively with acute cerebral infarct and intracerebral hematoma—the clot that remains after the hemorrhage. Subarachnoid hemorrhage (SAH) and arteriovenous malformations (AVM) are discussed on p. 427.

Acute ischemic stroke (AIS) comprises 80% of all strokes. They are caused primarily by thrombi or emboli that interrupt blood flow to the brain and cause an ischemic event that leads to infarction. The ischemic cascade compromises the sodium/potassium (Na^+/K^+) pump, leading to neuronal depolarization and neurotransmitter release. These actions cause a massive flux of ions and water, resulting in brain cell edema. Extracellular K^+ and intracellular calcium (Ca^{++}) rise, and the pH falls. The resulting high concentration of intracellular Ca^{++} and lactic acidosis cause cellular metabolic alterations that ultimately lead to cellular death. The lactic acidosis stimulates the vasomotor center, which causes a marked elevation in arterial pressure. This response is known as the *CNS ischemic response.* Systolic blood pressures <220 mm Hg and diastolic pressures <110 mm Hg should not be treated, since this is the body's natural response to perfuse the ischemic brain. The only exception is if thrombolytic therapy is being considered. Then the blood pressure should be gently lowered to <185/105 mm Hg. Although the CNS ischemic response can be appreciated during the acute phase of stroke, it is most pronounced during a Cushing response just before herniation.

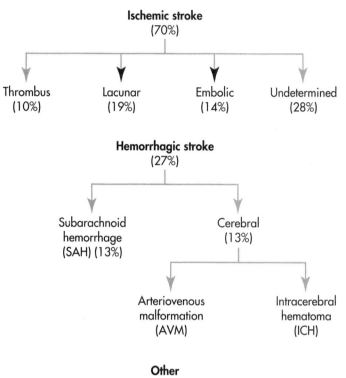

Figure 6-1:   Stroke classification.

The two most common causes of AIS are thrombus and embolic clot formation. A thrombus is a clot formed in the artery, usually occurring in branches of low flow with plaque formation. Cerebral emboli most commonly are formed in the heart and travel to the brain. Some clots are formed in the carotid or other cerebral arteries and break off and migrate to occlude a smaller artery in the brain. Characteristic deficits are produced, depending on the artery involved (Table 6-6).

Intracerebral hematomas (ICHs) can occur in any location of the brain (Table 6-7). Although various pathophysiologic events can result in ICH, the most common cause is hypertension, usually resulting in the rupture of a small penetrating artery in the basal ganglia. Damage occurs as blood destroys and displaces the brain tissue. Because of the lack of blood flow, ischemia develops in the area that surrounds the already injured brain tissue, resulting in even greater injury. Intracerebral blood sometimes ruptures into the lateral ventricle and puts the patient at risk for communicating hydrocephalus. Lobar hemorrhages are less common and, when found in elders, often are caused by cerebral amyloid angiopathy. Other common causes of hemorrhage include vascular malformations, vasculitis, neoplasms, hematologic disorders, and stimulant abuse (cocaine, amphetamines).

T A B L E 6 - 6   Neuroanatomy Related to Neurologic Deficit

Vessel	Area supplied	Deficit
ICA (internal carotid artery)	Right or left hemisphere	Contralateral motor or sensory deficit, aphasia with dominant hemisphere, neglect with nondominant hemisphere, contralateral visual field deficit (hemianopia), contralateral eye deviation
MCA (middle cerebral artery)	Right or left convex surface of the brain, most of the basal ganglia, internal capsule, putamen, and globus pallidus	Contralateral hemiplegia (arm and face > leg), sensory involvement, aphasia of dominant hemisphere, neglect of nondominant hemisphere (denial of weakness), homonymous hemianopia
ACA (anterior cerebral artery)	Right or left frontal lobe, corpus callosum, caudate nucleus, internal capsule	Weakness or sensory loss of contralateral leg and proximal arm; behavior disturbance: abulia, confusion, memory loss, and urinary incontinence
PCA (posterior cerebral artery)	Midbrain, thalamus, choroid plexus, occipital lobe, and medial temporal lobe	Contralateral visual field deficit, color blindness, impaired depth perception, occasional sparing of central vision, memory loss, sensory loss, nystagmus, pupillary abnormalities, ataxia
Vertebral artery	Medulla and/or cerebellum	Face, nose, or eye ipsilateral numbness with contralateral body numbness, facial weakness, vertigo, ataxia, nystagmus, dysphagia, dysarthria
Basilar artery	Pons, midbrain, and/or cerebellum	Quadriplegia or hemiplegia/paresis, locked-in syndrome (pons), dysarthria, dysphagia, ataxia, nystagmus, vertigo, coma

TABLE 6-7 Hemorrhagic Locations and Syndromes

Area	Syndrome
Putamen	Contralateral hemiplegia, hemisensory loss, hemianopia, slurred speech
Thalamic	Contralateral hemiplegia; hemisensory loss; small, poorly reactive pupils; decreased level of consciousness
Pontine	Locked-in syndrome (awake, aware, unable to verbally communicate, quadriplegia), coma
Cerebellar	Occipital headache, ataxia, dizziness, headache, nausea, vomiting
Lobar	Mimics cerebral infarct (e.g., contralateral motor and sensory signs)

ASSESSMENT

Each stroke type has a unique presentation based on the pathophysiology and location of the event. A complete and ongoing physical examination is crucial during the initial phase of stroke to detect further deterioration.

History and risk factors: Hypertension, smoking, aging, and previous history of transient ischemic attack (TIA)/stroke are the strongest risk factors. Risk factors for stroke are classified according to those that can be changed and those that cannot be changed. Risk factors that cannot be changed are age (>55 yr); race (risk for blacks is twice that for whites); gender (risk for males is twice that for females); previous history of stroke, TIA, and acute myocardial infarction (AMI) (increases risk ×10); and family history of stroke or AMI. Risk factors that can be changed include hypertension, heart disease, diabetes mellitus, obesity, hypercholesterolemia, sedentary life-style, and smoking.

Cardiac disease is the most common cause of cerebral embolism. Cardiac disorders such as atrial fibrillation, sick sinus syndrome, dilated cardiac myopathy, ventricular thrombus after AMI, and valvular disease are causes of cardioembolic stroke. Thrombotic strokes usually are caused by local atherosclerosis of large vessels (e.g., internal cerebral artery [ICA] or middle cerebral artery [MCA]) related to occlusion of small, perforating vessels (lacunar infarction).

For acute cerebral infarct/intracerebral hemorrhage
Clinical presentation: Individuals with ischemic strokes caused by MCA occlusion in the dominant hemisphere usually are awake with hemiparesis, aphasia, visual field cut, and sensory loss. Individuals with ICA stroke usually do not experience pain other than a headache, nor do they have altered LOC unless the stroke causes mass effects as a result of swelling or involves the brainstem or thalamic regions bilaterally. Individuals with acute hemispheric infarction have elevated arterial BP and often appear drowsy even in the absence of swelling. Although both thrombotic and embolic strokes can begin abruptly, the former are more likely to evolve over several hours and may fluctuate over several hours or days. In contrast, the deficit caused by embolic strokes usually is maximal at onset and often occurs during activity.

For intracranial hematoma
Clinical presentation: Depends on the size and location of the hematoma. For example, a relatively small hemorrhage into the brainstem may produce quadriplegia and coma, whereas a hematoma of similar size in the basal ganglia may produce hemiparesis without altered LOC. Generally, the larger the

hematoma (as measured by computed tomography [CT]), the worse the prognosis.

Neurologic findings with intracerebral hematoma (ICH) are similar to those with acute ischemic stroke (AIS). However, individuals with ICH are more likely to have altered LOC, vomiting, headache, very high BP, and IICP. Furthermore, the neurologic deficit may evolve over minutes to a few hours, requiring intubation and ICP monitoring. Neurosurgical intervention is often necessary.

For both stroke types

Physical assessment: The Glasgow coma scale (see Appendix 3) is often used to evaluate patients with stroke in critical care. Because this scale primarily measures LOC, it is not an appropriate scale for stroke patients. The National Institutes of Health (NIH) stroke scale (Table 6-8) provides a better measurement of deficits and is easy to use. It also guides the examiner in evaluating cognitive, language, and motor deficits that are unique to stroke. Comprehensive neurologic assessment assists the critical care nurse in detecting declines in neurologic status and responses to interventions.

Complications: The most serious are those that affect the CNS and cardiopulmonary systems.

CNS: IICP associated with extension of the infarct or hematoma and its associated edema, which may cause midline shift and herniation; IICP associated with hydrocephalus after ICH; and seizures, which occur most commonly within the first 24 h but may present at any time.

Cardiopulmonary: ECG changes, including QT prolongation, ST-segment depression, T-wave inversion, and U waves. Ventricular ectopy is also common. Cardiac dysrhythmias after stroke may be caused by release of catecholamin-ergic neurotransmitters into the systemic circulation, causing both hypertension and cardiac muscle damage. Individuals with new ECG changes have a less favorable prognosis. ECG monitoring for the first 24-72 h is recommended, along with evaluation of creatine phosphokinase-myocardial band (CK-MB) isoenzymes.

• • •

The most common causes of death within the first month after stroke are MI, pneumonia, and sepsis. Other complications include pulmonary embolism, deep vein thrombosis, skin breakdown, and depression.

DIAGNOSTIC TESTS

CT: Performed within the first 24 h, primarily as a method of differentiating ischemic from hemorrhagic stroke. Within the first few hours after AIS, the scan appears normal. ICH is easily diagnosed on CT—blood appears as a bright white signal.

CT xenon is a new imaging technique that measures cerebral blood flow (CBF). The measurement provides a regional calculation of actual blood flow. Determination of the CBF guides clinical management of the patient.

MRI and magnetic resonance arteriogram (MRA):   Noninvasive tests that provide detailed information regarding the area of injury or its vascular supply. Diffusion weighted imaging and perfusion weighted imaging are additional tests performed with magnetic resonance. These tests also measure CBF.

Doppler studies: Include transthoracic echocardiogram to evaluate heart structure and function; transesophageal echocardiogram and carotid Doppler or duplex to evaluate blood flow and presence or degree of stenosis in the extracranial carotid arteries; and transcranial Doppler to evaluate the intracra-nial vessels and give information on the velocity of blood flow in the anterior and posterior cerebral circulation. The latter is also used for evaluating vasospasm, determining brain death via detection of cerebral circulatory arrest, intraoperative monitoring, and locating emboli.

TABLE 6-8 National Institutes of Health Stroke Scale

		Baseline	30 min	1 h	2 h	24 h	48 h	7-10 days
1.a. Level of consciousness	Alert 0 Drowsy 1 Stuporous 2 Coma 3							
1.b. LOC questions	Answers both correctly 0 Answers one correctly 1 Incorrect 2							
1.c. LOC commands	Obeys both correctly 0 Obeys one correctly 1 Incorrect 2							
2. Best gaze	Normal 0 Partial gaze palsy 1 Forced deviation 2							
3. Best visual	No visual loss 0 Partial hemianopia 1 Complete hemianopia 2 Bilateral hemianopia 3							
4. Facial palsy	Normal 0 Minor 1 Partial 2 Complete 3							

5. Best motor arm	No drift Drift Can't resist gravity No effort against gravity No movement	0 1 2 3 4						
6. Other arm	For brainstem stroke (Use same scale as above)	0-4						
7. Best motor leg	No drift Drift Can't resist gravity No effort against gravity No movement	0 1 2 3 4						
8. Other leg	For brainstem stroke (Use same scale as above)	0-4						
9. Limb ataxia	Absent Present in upper or lower Present in both	0 1 2						
10. Sensory	Normal Partial loss Dense loss	0 1 2						

From the National High Blood Pressure Education Program, National Institutes of Health, and National Heart, Lung, and Blood Institute: NIH Pub No 93-1088, Jan 1993.

LOC, Level of consciousness.

Continued

T A B L E 6 - 8   National Institutes of Health Stroke Scale—cont'd

		Baseline	30 min	1 h	2 h	24 h	48 h	7-10 days
11. Neglect	No neglect 0 Partial neglect 1 Complete neglect 2							
12. Dysarthria	Normal articulation 0 Mild to moderate dysarthria 1 Near unintelligible or worse 2							
13. Best language	No aphasia 0 Mild to moderate aphasia 1 Severe aphasia 2 Mute 3							
14. Change from previous examination	Same S Better B Worse W							
15. Change from baseline	Same S Better B Worse W							

From the National High Blood Pressure Education Program, National Institutes of Health, and National Heart, Lung, and Blood Institute: NIH Pub No 93-1088, Jan 1993.

> **Research Brief 6-1**   This multicenter national nursing study is collecting data on 800 stroke survivors and the "decision-making partner" to determine the patterns of decision making of obtaining medical care after an acute stroke. This information may help nurses to better educate the public to facilitate more rapid responses to emergent medical care after stroke. Currently, half of the patients who have stroke arrive at the hospital within 24 h. With thrombolytic therapy and other stroke interventions available, the delay to medical care must be reduced.

From O'Donnell L: *Factors related to timing in seeking health care for stroke symptoms,* Grand Rapids, Mich. Manuscript in preparation.

Cerebral angiography: Invasive procedure used to visualize the cerebral blood vessels. It provides more specific information on the cause of stroke by identifying the blood vessel involved. In clinical trials, cerebral angiography is used in conjunction with thrombolytics in patients with AIS to identify the site of acute vessel occlusion, with subsequent injection of a thrombolytic agent to dissolve the clot and restore blood flow to the brain. Cerebral angioplasty is also being investigated.

Laboratory studies: Hematology; chemistry; coagulation profiles; evaluations for syphilis (e.g., via Venereal Disease Research Laboratory [VDRL], rapid plasma reagin [RPR], fluorescent treponemal antibody [FTA]); sedimentation rate to assess for infection or vasculitis; and drug screen (e.g., cocaine, amphetamine).

Less common laboratory tests may include determinations of lupus anticoagulant, anticardiolipin antibody, and hemoglobin electrophoresis (to assess presence of sickle cell disease). In addition, a hypercoagulable profile may be performed to evaluate levels of proteins C and S. These proteins often are deficient in the young (<45 yr) stroke patient, who may have no other risk factors for stroke.

Positron emission tomography (PET) and single photon emission computed tomography (SPECT):   To evaluate brain metabolism and blood flow. These tests are performed more commonly in university-affiliated centers.

LP: To measure CSF pressures and obtain CSF specimen when infection such as meningitis or neurosyphilis is suspected. It also may be performed when SAH is suspected and CT is normal.

Electroencephalogram (EEG):   Although not routinely done, it may show slowing or low voltage over the infarct except in lacunar infarcts, where results are usually normal.

COLLABORATIVE MANAGEMENT

Goals of management are to prevent secondary neurologic damage, prevent secondary complications, and promote optimal functional outcome. Early detection via accurate neurologic examination and immediate medical or surgical intervention help prevent stroke extension, increased brain edema, and hydrocephalus. Medical and nursing interventions are guided by the findings derived from the physical examination.

Prevention of stroke extension: Depends on adequate perfusion of the penumbra, which is the ischemic brain tissue surrounding the initial infarct that is at immediate risk of infarction. Perfusing the penumbra decreases the potential infarct size and optimizes patient outcome. Controlling arterial BP is essential in limiting the infarct size. Close monitoring and use of potent vasoactive medications achieve BP control. A "normal" BP may be too low, causing further ischemia and infarct by decreasing cerebral perfusion. Arterial BP should not be lowered abruptly in patients with AIS. At times, maintenance of a somewhat elevated BP may be warranted, depending on the underlying vascular and brain pathology. In contrast, with ICH many practitioners believe that an elevated BP should be reduced aggressively. The best approach is

TABLE 6-9   Maintenance of Normal Regulatory Functions in Stroke

Function	Intervention/goal	Rationale
Temperature	Normothermia	To decrease metabolic demands and ICP
Respiratory	O₂, positioning, respiratory therapy	To optimize O₂ delivery to the brain and prevent atelectasis and pneumonia
Cardiac	Monitor dysrhythmias, fluid, electrolytes	To optimize CO to promote perfusion to the brain
GI	H₂-blockers, bowel program	To prevent stress ulcers, constipation
Nutrition	NPO, enteral, long-term diet	NPO to prevent aspiration; diet to promote healing, meet caloric needs; long-term diet: low Na⁺, low-fat, weight reduction if needed
GU	Bladder training ASAP	To prevent unnecessary use of Foley catheter, prevent UTI, and avoid embarrassment and possible retention
Musculoskeletal	ROM, positioning, increasing activity as tolerated, sequential compression stockings, mobility beds	To promote proper alignment and prevent contractures and complications of immobility
Skin	Keep clean and dry, pressure relief	To prevent skin breakdown and dependent edema
Communication	Develop appropriate communication techniques; swallow study within 24 h	To prevent aspiration and promote meeting patient's needs

GI, Gastrointestinal; *GU,* genitourinary; *ROM,* range of motion; *ICP,* intracranial pressure; *CO,* cardiac output; *Na⁺,* sodium; *UTI,* urinary tract infection.

unclear, and therefore the treatment of increased BP in ICH necessitates individual consideration.

ICP monitoring and CPP management: Necessary for patients with increased infarct size, increased edema, and hydrocephalus. Patients with IICP may receive mannitol, which draws water osmotically from healthy brain cells. Careful monitoring of ICP for rebound effect is necessary after mannitol infusion. Serum osmolality needs to be monitored to prevent excessive dehydration. Patients with hydrocephalus often require a ventriculostomy. For more information about ICP monitoring and CPP management, see "Traumatic Brain Injury," p. 118.

Optimizing regulatory functions: To prevent secondary complications (Table 6-9). In general, patients with ischemic strokes should be positioned with the HOB flat to increase cerebral perfusion. HOB should be elevated for patients with hemorrhagic strokes to decrease ICP. Patient response determines the best position.

Rehabilitation: Should begin immediately. Consults to physiatrist, physical therapist, occupational therapist, and speech therapist should be made within the first 24 h.

Pharmacotherapy: Thrombolysis with rTPA is initiated for thrombotic stroke, ideally within 60 minutes of onset of symptoms. Although thrombolytic and neuroprotective agents hold great promise, they remain experimental. Other pharmacotherapy is aimed at prevention of secondary neurologic damage and recurrent stroke.

Anticoagulation: IV heparin may be indicated for patients with progressing stroke or unstable signs and symptoms of stroke, such as TIAs, and for cardioembolic stroke. If long-term anticoagulation is planned, the patient is converted to oral warfarin (Coumadin) therapy.

Antiplatelet therapy: To reduce risk of stroke and decrease frequency of TIAs. The most used agent is aspirin, 30 mg to 1300 mg daily. Ticlopidine (Ticlid), an antiplatelet agent, reduces the overall risk for fatal and nonfatal strokes by nearly 25% when compared with aspirin. A third antiplatelet agent, clopidogrel (Plavix), has been approved for patients at risk for ischemic events (myocardial, cerebrovascular, peripheral vascular).

Antihypertensives: Frequently used in the stroke population for control and maintenance of optimal BP. Various agents are used, based on the individual's medical history. Long-term therapy is based on the National Heart, Lung, and Blood Institute (NHLBI) algorithm (see Figure 6-2). In the acute phase, systolic BP is often elevated and requires careful management. Vasoactive IV medications such as sodium nitroprusside (Nipride) or labetalol (Normodyne) are often used. Hypotension is a concern, especially in the patient with IICP, because with hypotension, mean arterial pressure (MAP) is decreased. If MAP is decreased in the presence of a normal or elevated ICP, a decrease in CPP results, further compromising neurologic status. Dopamine or dobutamine may be titrated to keep MAP high enough to maintain CPP >60 mm Hg.

Anticonvulsant therapy: Used for seizures in the acute phase. Generally the patient is given a loading dose of phenytoin (Dilantin) followed by a maintenance dose. Lorazepam (Ativan) or diazepam (Valium) may be used initially, especially if the patient is in status epilepticus (see p. 441).

Sedation: May be necessary for ensuring sleep. A thorough neurologic evaluation to rule out organic causes is indicated for patients who are agitated. Sedation also may be indicated as adjunctive therapy for patients with IICP. Drugs of choice include midazolam (Versed), fentanyl (Sublimaze), or morphine sulfate. Pentobarbital coma is occasionally used for patients who experience high ICP that does not respond to other forms of therapy.

Carotid endarterectomy: Surgical removal of plaque in the obstructed carotid artery to promote blood supply to the brain, which is considered choice treatment for patients with >70% carotid stenosis.

Craniotomy: May be performed for evacuation of a hematoma or for a young ACI patient who has uncontrollable IICP caused by massive edema. When this occurs, a craniotomy with a dural incision or temporal lobectomy is considered. In some institutions hematoma evacuation is performed by aspiration through a burr hole.

NURSING DIAGNOSES AND INTERVENTIONS

Decrease adaptive capacity: intracranial, related to interrupted blood flow secondary to thrombus or emobulus

Desired outcome: Within 72 h of this diagnosis (or optimally on an ongoing basis), patient has adequate cerebral tissue perfusion as evidenced by no decrease in LOC; no evidence of deterioration in motor function on affected side; and no evidence of new or further deterioration of language, cognition, or visual field per NIH Stroke Scale.

Life-style modification: diet, exercise, smoking cessation

Inadequate response

Continue life-style modification, add diuretics or β-blockers
(ACE inhibitors, calcium antagonists, α_1-receptor
blockers, and α-β–blockers have not been tested or
shown to reduce morbidity and mortality)

Inadequate response

Increase dosage *or* substitute drug *or* add a second agent

Inadequate response

Add second or third agent and/or diuretic if not already prescribed

Figure 6-2:   The National Heart, Lung, and Blood Institute treatment algorithm for stroke. β, Beta; α, alpha; *ACE*, angiotensin-converting enzyme. From the National High Blood Pressure Education Program, National Institutes of Health, and National Heart, Lung, and Blood Institute: NIH Pub No 93-1088, Jan 1993.

- Assess for neurologic changes qh in the acute phase. Use NIH Stroke Scale to record and monitor neurologic changes after stroke.
- Maintain ICP ≤15 mm Hg and CPP >60 mm Hg. CPP = MAP − ICP.
- Position patient to maintain adequate cerebral perfusion; avoid extreme hip flexion. When positioning, monitor tolerance to position change. Keep HOB flat as tolerated for patients with ischemic stroke. Keep HOB raised at 30 degrees as tolerated for patients with hemorrhagic stroke.
- Maintain oxygenation by turning as tolerated and suctioning as needed. Assess breath sounds frequently. Avoid activities or conditions that can increase ICP, including excessive coughing, hypercapnia, and hypoxia.
- Maintain adequate systolic blood pressure (SBP). Higher pressures (typically 140-180 mm Hg) necessary to perfuse area of brain at risk of infarction when stroke is ischemic. For patients with hemorrhagic stroke, be sure to maintain adequate BP. Use vasodilators or vasopressors as necessary to optimize BP and maintain CPP >60 mm Hg for all stroke patients.
- Medicate for sedation as prescribed. Monitor response, including effects of sedation and resulting changes in ICP.

NIC Cerebral Perfusion Promotion; Positioning: Neurologic; Neurologic Monitoring
Impaired physical mobility related to decreased motor function of upper and/or lower extremities and trunk after stroke

Desired outcome: At time of discharge from ICU, patient exhibits no evidence of complications of immobility such as skin breakdown, contracture formation, pneumonia, or constipation.

- Turn and position frequently as tolerated.
- Transfer toward unaffected side.
- Teach methods for turning and moving using stronger extremity to move weaker extremity.
- Position weaker extremities when turning to avoid contracture formation, frozen shoulder, or foot drop.
- Begin passive ROM within first 24 h of admission. Monitor response and modify exercises if BP or ICP increases.
- Obtain PT and OT referral as soon as possible to establish appropriate therapy.
- Have patient cough and breathe deeply at scheduled intervals. Provide percussion and postural drainage for patients for whom coughing and deep breathing are ineffective for mobilizing secretions.

NIC Positioning; Exercise Therapy: Joint Mobility; Self-Care Assistance

Impaired verbal communication   related to aphasia secondary to cerebrovascular insult

Desired outcome: At a minimum of 24-h period before discharge from ICU, patient demonstrates improved self-expression and relates decrease in frustration with communication.

- Be aware that aphasia is the partial or complete inability to use or comprehend language and symbols and may occur with dominant (left) hemisphere damage.
  - ☐ *Receptive aphasia* (e.g., Wernicke, sensory) characterized by inability to comprehend spoken words. Patient may respond to nonverbal cues.
  - ☐ *Expressive aphasia* (e.g., Broca, motor) characterized by difficulty expressing words or naming objects. Gesture, groans, swearing, or nonsense words may be used. Use of a picture or word board may be helpful.
- Evaluate nature and severity of the aphasia. Assess ability to point to specific object, follow simple directions, understand yes/no and complex questions, repeat simple and complex words, repeat sentences, name objects, relate purpose or action of the object, fulfill written request, write request, and read.
- Assess for dysarthria, which signals risk for aspiration resulting from ineffective swallowing and gag reflexes. Consult with speech therapist to plan measures to promote independence and facilitate swallowing.
- Decrease environmental distractions, such as television or others' conversations. Fatigue affects ability to communicate; plan adequate sleep/rest.
- Communicate with patient as much as possible. General principles include facing patient and establishing eye contact, speaking slowly and clearly, giving patient time to process communication and give answer, keeping messages short and simple, staying with one clearly defined subject, avoiding questions with multiple choices and instead phrasing questions so that they can be answered "yes" or "no," and using same words each time when repeating a statement or question. If patient does not understand after repetition, try different words. Use gesture, facial expresssions, and pantomime to supplement and reinforce message.
- When helping patients regain use of symbolic language, start with nouns first, and progress to more complex statements. For continuity, keep a record at the bedside of words to be used (e.g., "pill" rather than "medication").
- Treat patient as an adult. It is not necessary to raise the volume of your voice unless patient is hard of hearing. Be respectful.
- When patients have difficulty expressing words or naming objects, encourage them to repeat words after you for practice in verbal expression. Be prepared

> **Research Brief 6-2**   The study was completed at four university settings to determine if the public could be taught to accurately find the radial pulse and determine if that pulse is regular or irregular . Of the participants, 92% were able to find a radial pulse. Of that group, 86% were able to correctly identify a regular pulse and 76% were able to correctly identify an irregular pulse. The aim of the project is to teach the general public to begin to check their pulse monthly and see a health care provider immediately if the pulse is irregular. More than 80,000 new strokes occur each year as a result of undiagnosed atrial fibrillation. This simple technique may promote early identification and treatment of atrial fibrillation and prevent stroke. "Check your Pulse America" is a national campaign resulting from this trial. Nurses in every setting should teach this prevention strategy to patients at risk for heart disease and stroke. More information and free brochures can be obtained by contacting the National Stroke Association @800-STROKES.

From Munschauer R: *Screening for atrial fibrillation in the community: a multicentered validation trial.* Submitted for publication, 1999.

for labile emotions because these patients become frustrated and emotional when faced with their impaired speech.

- Patients who have lost the ability to monitor their verbal output may not produce sensible language but may think they are making sense. Avoid labeling patient "belligerent" or "confused" when the problem is aphasia and frustration.
- Patients with nondominant (right) hemisphere damage often have no difficulty speaking; however, they may use excessive detail, give irrelevant information, and get off on a tangent. Bring patient back to the subject by saying "Let's go back to what we were talking about."
- Provide supportive and relaxed environment for patients unable to form words or sentences or speak clearly or appropriately. If patient makes an error, avoid criticism and use encouragement, e.g., "That was a good try." Acknowledge frustration. To validate patient's message, repeat or rephrase it aloud.
- Ensure that call light is available and patient knows how to use it. If patient is unable to use call light, check frequently and anticipate needs to ensure safety and trust.

NIC Communication Enhancement: Speech, Visual, Hearing Deficits; Active Listening: Anxiety Reduction; Touch

ADDITIONAL NURSING DIAGNOSES

See "Status Epilepticus," p. 441, for **Risk for trauma (oral and musculoskeletal).** See "Traumatic Brain Injury," p. 118, for **Risk for disuse syndrome** and **Impaired corneal tissue integrity.** See "Prolonged Immobility," p. 74.

Meningitis

PATHOPHYSIOLOGY

Meningitis is an inflammation of the brain and spinal cord (CNS), which involves the meninges (dura, arachnoid, pia), invades the brain surface, and damages the cranial nerves. There are several types of meningitis, broadly classified as bacterial (pyogenic), tuberculous, fungal, and aseptic. The first three are discussed here.

Bacterial meningitis: The most common form, it can be community acquired or associated with previous infection, injury (e.g., open/penetrating skull fracture), basilar and facial skull fracture, shunt occlusion/malfunction, craniotomy, otitis media, sinusitis, and bacteremia (e.g., endocarditis, pneumonia).

Streptococcus pneumoniae (S. pneumoniae), a gram-positive coccus, is the leading cause of adult meningitis in the United States. Pneumococcal meningitis is prevalent in crowded conditions and is spread seasonally (late fall and winter). It follows a recent nasopharyngeal colonization of a virulent pneumococcal strain or upper respiratory tract infection (URI), is seen in the presence of pneumococcal disease, is a complication of conditions associated with CSF leaks, and is more prevalent in immunocompromised persons.

Neisseria meningitidis (N. meningitidis), a gram-negative coccus, is the second leading cause of meningitis in adults. Infection is more likely to occur in patients with complement component deficiencies (e.g., congenital or associated with nephrotic syndrome, hepatic failure, systemic lupus erythematosus, multiple myeloma).

Haemophilus influenzae (H. influenzae), the most common cause in children, sometimes affects adults as well. Predisposing factors include URIs, hypogammaglobulinemia, diabetes mellitus, alcoholism, asplenia, and head trauma. With the introduction of *H. influenzae* vaccine type B, bacterial meningitis from this source has diminished substantially in infants and children, making it a disease predominately of adults.

Listeria monocytogenes (L. monocytogenes), a gram-positive rod, is being recognized more frequently as a cause of meningitis, especially in immunocompromised patients and those of extreme ages (very young and very old). Outbreaks have been associated with consumption of contaminated dairy products as well as undercooked chicken, fish, and meats.

Gram-negative species: *Escherichia coli, Klebsiella, Proteus,* and *Pseudomonas spp.* are gaining increasing importance, especially in the elderly, in the immunocompromised, and in head-injured patients.

Borrelia burgdorferi (B. burgdorferi), the tick-borne spirochete and causative agent of Lyme disease may also cause meningitis.

Acute meningitis with negative Gram stain, a community-acquired illness in which the Gram stain is negative, making if difficult to determine the pathogen responsible for the acute disease. Causes of the illness are not often found, but syphilis, bacteremia, and Lyme disease have been identified in some cases. Variables associated with diagnosis of meningitis include presentation in winter months, age older than 60 yr, and co-morbid disease—especially immunodeficiency.

Tuberculous meningitis: *Mycobacterium tuberculosis* meningeal infection tends to occur in elders and children where tuberculous presence is high. Human immunodeficiency virus (HIV)-infected patients are also at high risk.

Fungal meningitis: The most common CNS fungal infection is caused by *Cryptococcus neoformans (C. neoformans),* an opportunistic infection associated with acquired immune deficiency syndrome (AIDS). Less common infections result from other fungi.

ASSESSMENT

History and risk factors: Should include the time symptoms developed, report of traumatic injury, exposures to disease or organisms, and recent surgical procedures.

Clinical presentation

S. pneumoniae: The classic presentation is fever, headache, meningismus, and altered mental status that progresses quickly to coma. Nuchal rigidity and Kernig or Brudzinski sign are present. Nausea, vomiting, profuse sweats, weakness, myalgia, seizures, and cranial nerve palsies also may be present.

N. meningitidis: Fever, early macular erythematous rash progressing rapidly to petechial and purpuric states, conjunctival petechiae, and aggressive

TABLE 6-10 Positive Meningeal Signs	
Test/description	**Positive findings**
Stiff neck sign (nuchal rigidity): Raise patient's head by flexing the neck and attempting to make the patient's chin touch the sternum.	Pain and resistance to neck motion.
Brudzinski sign: Assess for nuchal rigidity.	Flexion of the hips and knees when the examiner flexes the patient's neck.
Kernig sign: Flex the patient's leg at the knee and hip when the patient is supine, and then attempt to straighten the leg.	Pain in the lower back and resistance to straightening the leg.

behavior are typical clinical findings. Dysfunctions of cranial nerves VI, VII, and VIII (see Appendix 4) and aphasia, ventriculitis, subdural empyema, cerebral venous thrombosis, and disseminated intravascular coagulation (DIC) also may occur.

H. influenzae: The most distinguishing sign is early development of deafness, which can occur within 24-36 h after onset. A morbilliform or petechial rash may be present.

L. monocytogenes: Seizures and focal deficits such as ataxia, cranial nerve palsies, and nystagmus are seen early in the course of infection. Conclusive diagnosis may require serology testing.

Gram-negative species: In elders, fever may be absent or low grade and headache may not be reported. Meningeal signs may be subtle, but confusion, severe mental changes, and pneumonia commonly are reported. Nuchal rigidity in elders must be differentiated from degenerative changes of the cervical spine.

B. burgdorferi: The clinical presentation of Lyme disease occurs in stages and is heralded by a "bull's eye" rash that develops within a few days of the tick bite. During stage one, headache, stiff neck, lethargy, irritability, and changes in mental status, especially memory loss, are observed. Stage two occurs over weeks and months after the tick bite and is characterized by persistent headache, nausea, vomiting, malaise, irritability, cranial nerve deficits, mental status changes, peripheral neuropathies, and myalgias. Arthritic-type symptoms and brain parenchymal changes are observed in the third stage of the disease.

Acute meningitis with negative Gram stain: Signs and symptoms are similar to other types of meningitis, with fever and neck stiffness being the most frequent findings. The Gram stain for bacteria is negative, but CSF white blood cell count is elevated.

M. tuberculosis: Has a slow onset, and neurologic damage occurs even before treatment is sought. Symptoms include headache, lethargy, confusion, nuchal rigidity, cranial nerve abnormalities, SIADH, weight loss, and night sweats. Kernig and Brudzinski signs are present; the chest x-ray may be clear, and purified protein derivative (PPD) may be nonreactive.

C. neoformans: Typical symptoms of meningitis occur, but since the infection is subacute, fever and headache may have a subtle pattern lasting weeks. Positive meningeal signs (Table 6-10); alterations in mental status (e.g., hyperactivity, bizarre behavior, emotional lability, poor judgment); and photophobia may be reported. Seizures are uncommon, but focal neurologic deficits such as cranial nerve III and IV dysfunction, nausea, and vomiting may occur.

TABLE 6-11   Meningitis: Typical CSF Finding

Findings	White cell count	Glucose	Protein
Normal	0-5/mm^3 lymphocytes	40-80 mg/dl	15-50 mg/dl
Bacterial	Predominantly polycytes: 1,000-10,000	<40 mg/dl	100-500 mg/dl
Viral	Predominantly lymphocytes (may see polycytes initially)	Normal	Slightly elevated
Tuberculous	Elevated lymphocytes: 100-400; lymphocyte elevation minimal or absent in immunocompromised patients	<40 mg/dl or 50% of blood sugar drawn simultaneously	100-500 mg/dl; may increase gradually with progression of disease
Fungal	Predominantly elevated lymphocytes	Slightly decreased	Elevated
Lyme disease	Mildly elevated lymphocytes	Normal	Mildly elevated
Aseptic (nonbacterial)	Elevated lymphocytes	Normal	50-100 mg/dl

Physical assessment: A complete neurologic examination should be performed to establish patient's baseline neurologic function. One or more tests for meningitis usually are positive (see Table 6-10).

DIAGNOSTIC TESTS

CSF analysis: The single most important laboratory test for diagnosing meningitis; CSF is obtained through intraventricular catheter, ventriculostomy and reservoir via high cisternal or cervical approach, and LP. An LP should not be performed if there is a history of head injury, focal neurologic deficits are present, or papilledema is visualized on funduscopic examination, inasmuch as these signs are associated with IICP (see Table 6-3). Antibiotic therapy should not be delayed if CSF samples cannot be obtained. The CSF is analyzed for cell count with white cell differential, glucose, protein, Gram stain, acid-fast stain, culture, and sensitivity (Table 6-11). Other tests of the CSF include the following:

Counterimmunoelectrophoresis (CIE): Detects bacterial antigens in the cerebrospinal fluid.

Cytokine measurements of CSF: Strong correlation found between bacterial meningitis and early presence of interleukin-6 (IL-6) and tumor necrosis factor in neonates.

Latex agglutination: Detects microbial antigens in the CSF.

Limulus lysate assay: May confirm bacterial infection (gram-negative organisms) even when cultures and Gram stains are negative.

TABLE 6-12 Common Drug Therapy for the Management of Meningitis

Causative agent	Therapy
Bacterial meningitis	
Streptococcus pneumoniae	Vancomycin or rifampin plus ceftriaxone
Haemophilus influenzae	Cefoxitin or ceftriaxone
Neisseria meningitidis	Penicillin G—if inadequate response, change to ceftriaxone or cefotaxime
Listeria monocytogenes	Penicillin, ampicillin, plus gentamicin
Pseudomonas	Ceftazidime
Mycobacterium tuberculosis	Isoniazid, rifampin, ethambutol, pyrazinamide These drugs may be used alone, or together in any combination
Gram-positive cocci	Vancomycin plus penicillin G plus aminoglycosides
Gram-negative cocci	Penicillin G
Gram-positive bacilli	Ampicillin, penicillin, plus aminoglycosides
Gram-negative bacilli	Cephalosporin plus aminoglycosides
Fungal	
Cryptococcus neoformans	Amphotericin B plus flucytosine, or fluconazole or itraconazole

Enzyme-linked immunosorbent assay (ELISA): To detect mycobacterial antigens or antimycobacterial antibodies in CSF.

Blood, urine, and sputum cultures: Help identify the infecting organisms.

Serum WBC count: Assesses for presence of infection.

CT with contrast and MRI: To rule out hydrocephalus and detect exudate, abscesses, and intracranial pathology, including tumors.

COLLABORATIVE MANAGEMENT

Rapid sterilization of the CSF via appropriate pharmacologic therapy (Table 6-12): Prophylaxis, using appropriate drug therapy for individuals exposed to *N. meningitidis* (rifampin or spiramycin) or *H. influenzae* meningitis, is recommended.

Adjunctive pharmacologic therapies: Dexamethasone is believed to decrease inflammation by reducing cytokines produced by bacterial products; however, its use is controversial. If given, dexamethasone should be administered before or with antimicrobial medications and 2 days of dosing is recommended. Monoclonal antibodies also have been investigated as therapy because of their ability to decrease inflammation by deactivating bacterial cell surface components and cytokines produced from leukocyte activation (see box, p. 465).

Nutritional management: Patients who are able should continue oral feeding along with IV therapy. Enteral feeding may be initiated. Parenteral nutrition should be initiated if enteral feeding is contraindicated or not tolerated by the patient.

Anticonvulsant therapy: Initiated if seizures are observed, or it may be administered prophylactically. Seizures increase the metabolic rate, requiring an increase in cerebral blood flow, which may be detrimental in meningitis associated with cerebral edema and intracranial hypertension.

USE OF STEROIDS IN THE TREATMENT OF BACTERIAL MENINGITIS

BIOLOGICAL BASIS FOR EFFECTIVENESS	BIOLOGICAL BASIS FOR POTENTIAL HARM	EFFECT IN ADULTS	EFFECT IN CHILDREN
Reduces inflammation	Suppresses immune mechanisms	Evidence for use of dexamethasone is not convincing	Dexamethasone in *Haemophilus influenzae* B protects against hearing loss
Reduces cerebral and spinal cord edema	Masks other infection	Limit use to those with high bacterial concentrations, elevated intracranial pressure, or edema	Dexamethasone is beneficial in bacterial forms if commenced before antibiotics
Reduces inflammation of small blood vessels and prevents slow flow to brain tissue	Reduces meningeal inflammation and decreases drug penetration into subarachnoid space	Randomized trials are needed before recommendations can be made for future changes	Dexamethasone is not associated with adverse effects if limited to 2 days
	Associated with GI hemorrhage, fungal infections, electrolyte imbalance, and hyperglycemia		More studies are needed to determine the effect of steroids in other forms of meningitis

Modified from Quagliarello V, Scheld M: Drug therapy: treatment of bacterial meningitis, *N Engl J Med* 336(10):708-716, 1997; Quagliarello V, Scheld M: Drug therapy: treatment of bacterial meningitis, *N Engl J Med* 336(10):708-716, 1997; Prasad K, Menon G: Steroids in tuberculosis meningitis (Cochrane Review). In *The Cochrane Library*, Issue 2: Update Software 1998. Updated quarterly.

Maintenance of normothermia and fever treatment: Reduces the risks (increased cerebral blood flow and intracranial pressure) associated with increased metabolic rate. Fever should be controlled by antipyretics such as acetaminophen or use of other cooling measures such as tepid baths.

Infection prevention: According to hospital and Centers for Disease Control and Prevention (CDC) guidelines. Transmission-Based Precautions are initiated as needed until effectiveness of antimicrobial treatment is established. See "Infection Prevention and Control," Appendix 8.

Rehabilitation consults: Include physical therapy (PT), occupational therapy (OT), and speech and should be initiated as soon as patient is stable, to minimize physical and cognitive complications.

Evaluation of need for support services: For patient and significant others, including home health care, support groups, and social services.

NURSING DIAGNOSES AND INTERVENTIONS

Decreased adaptive capacity: intracranial, related to compromised fluid dynamic mechanisms secondary to brain and spinal cord inflammation

Desired outcomes: Within 72 h of initiation of antimicrobial therapy, patient's ICP returns to normal range as evidenced by orientation to time, place, and person; bilaterally equal and normoreactive pupils; bilaterally equal strength and tone of extremities; absence of cranial nerve palsies; RR 12-20 breaths/min with normal depth and pattern (eupnea); HR 60-100 bpm; BP within patient's normal range; and absence of headache, vomiting, papilledema, and other clinical indicators of IICP. After instruction, patient verbalizes knowledge of the importance of avoiding Valsalva-like activities.

- Assess neurologic status at least hourly. Monitor pupils, LOC, and motor activity; perform cranial nerve assessments (see Appendix 4). A decrease in consciousness is an early indicator of IICP and impending herniation. Changes in pupillary size and reaction, a decrease in motor function (i.e., hemiplegia, abnormal posturing), and cranial nerve palsies also may be signs of impending herniation.
- Monitor patient for physical indicators of IICP (see Table 6-3).
- Monitor VS at frequent intervals. Be alert to changes in respiratory pattern, fluctuations in BP and pulse, widening pulse pressure, and slow HR.
- Optimize cerebral oxygenation by maintaining a patent airway and delivering oxygen as prescribed. Be sure patient's neck is free of constricting objects such as tracheostomy ties and oxygen tubing.
- Avoid overhydration, which would add to cerebral edema, by ensuring precise delivery of IV fluids at consistent, prescribed rates.
- Ensure timely delivery of medications that are prescribed for the prevention of sudden increases or decreases in ICP, BP, HR, or RR.
- Teach patient the importance of avoiding activities that increase ICP: coughing, straining, and bending over.
- If patient shows evidence of IICP, implement measures to decrease ICP (see Table 2-5, p. 129).

NIC Cerebral Edema Management; Cerebral Perfusion Promotion; Intracranial Pressure (ICP) Monitoring: Neurologic Monitoring; Positioning: Neurologic

Pain related to headache, photophobia, and fever secondary to meningeal irritation

Desired outcome: Within 2 h of initiation of pain treatment, patient's subjective evaluation of discomfort improves, as documented by a pain scale.

- Monitor patient for the presence of pain and discomfort. Devise a pain scale with patient, rating discomfort from 0 (no pain) to 10.
- Monitor temperature q2h and prn. Administer tepid baths or cooling blanket and prescribed antipyretics/antibiotics to keep temperature within prescribed limits.
- Maintain an environment of comfort for the patient. This should be

approached on an individual basis so that environment can be manipulated to enhance physiologic and psychologic comfort and safety.

- Provide patient care allowing for uninterrupted periods (at least 90 min) of rest. If intracranial pressure is elevated, clustering care is contraindicated. Organize visiting hours so that patient can have uninterrupted periods of rest.
- Darken patient's room to minimize the discomfort of photophobia. Provide blindfolds if darkening the room is not possible.
- Administer analgesics as prescribed. Use the pain scale to document the degree of relief obtained.
- See p. 61 for other pain interventions.

Risk for infection related to potential for cross-contamination secondary to communicable nature of bacterial and aseptic meningitis

Desired outcome: Other patients, staff members, and patient's significant others do not exhibit evidence of having acquired meningitis: diminished LOC, confusion, fever, headache, nuchal rigidity, and other signs (see "Assessment" and "Diagnostic Test" data).

For patients with bacterial meningitis

- Bacterial meningitis is transmitted via droplet contact. Provide patient with a private room.
- Initiate Transmission-Based Precautions: Droplet, upon admission and maintain them for at least 24 h after start of antimicrobial therapy.
  - ☐ Standard Precautions should be instituted to provide safety and protection regardless if infection is bacterial, fungal, or viral. Be alert for airborne pathogens as well as those in stool or oral secretions.

ADDITIONAL NURSING DIAGNOSES

See "Status Epilepticus" for **Risk for trauma** (oral and musculoskeletal), p. 445. Because these patients are at risk for SIADH, see "Syndrome of Inappropriate Antidiuretic Hormone" for **Risk for injury,** p. 485. See also appropriate nursing diagnoses and interventions in "Septic Shock," p. 593, inasmuch as these patients are at risk for septic shock. As indicated, see other nursing diagnoses and interventions in "Nutritional Support," p. 1; "Prolonged Immobility," p. 74; "Psychosocial Support," p. 83; and "Psychosocial Support for the Patient's Family and Significant Others," p. 95.

Bibliography

Bader MK: The complexity of caring for patients with ruptured cerebral aneurysm: case studies, *AACN Clinical Issues: Adv Prac Acute Crit Care* 8(2):182-195, 1997.

Bader MK et al: New neurointerventional therapies for stroke patients, *Dimens Crit Care Nurs* 16(6):301-311, 1997.

Barch C, issue editor: Stroke, *J Cardiovasc Nurs* 13(1):v-96, 1998.

Barch C et al: Common problems and proven solutions to acute stroke management, *Stroke Interven* 1(3):5-10, 1998.

Barnett H et al: *Stroke: pathophysiology, diagnosis, and management,* ed 2, New York, 1992, Churchill Livingstone.

Bell TE et al: Transcranial Doppler: correlation of blood velocity measurement with clinical status in subarachnoid hemorrhage, *J Neurosci Nurs* 24(4):215-219, 1992.

Bolton CF: The changing concepts of Guillain-Barré syndrome, *N Engl J Med* 333(21):1415-1416, 1995.

Brott T et al: Measurements of acute cerebral infarction: a clinical examination scale, *Stroke* 20(7):864-870, 1990.

Calder J: Listeria meningitis in adults, *Lancet* 350:307-308, 1997.

Campbell PJ, Edwards SM: Hyperdynamic therapy: the nurse's role in the treatment of cerebral vasospasm, *J Neurosci Nurs* 29(5):318-324, 1997.

Davenport RJ et al: Gastrointestinal hemorrhage after acute stroke, *Stroke* 27(3):421-424, 1996.

Elmore J et al: Acute meningitis with a negative Gram's stain: clinical and management outcomes in 171 episodes, *Am J Med* 100(1):78-84, 1996.

Evans V, Barr J: Case study: nursing care of the patient with vertebral artery aneurysm treated by endovascular stenting and coil implantation, *J Neurosci Nurs* 30(5):279-282, 1998.

Farkkila M, Pentilla P: Plasma exchange therapy reduces the nursing care needed in Guillain-Barré syndrome, *J Adv Nurs* 17:672-675, 1992.

Fischer P: Acute seizures and status epilepticus: advances in therapy, *Clin Nurs Prac Epilepsy* 4(1):10-12, 1997.

Fowler SB: Neurotrauma family interventions, *J Trauma Nurs* 4(3):68-75, 1997.

Hickey JV: Myasthenic crisis: your assessment counts, *RN* 54(4):54-59, 1991.

Hickey JV: *The clinical practice of neurological and neurosurgical nursing,* ed 4, Philadelphia, 1997, Lippincott.

Huston CJ: Cervical spine injury, *Am J Nurs* 98(6):33, 1998.

Huston CJ, Boelman R: Autonomic dysreflexia, *Am J Nurs* 95(6):55, 1995.

Interqual: *The ISD-A review system with adult ISD criteria,* North Hampton, NH, and Marlboro, Mass, Aug, 1992, Interqual.

Iowa Outcomes Project. Johnson M, Maas M, editors: *Nursing Outcomes Classification (NOC),* St Louis, 1997, Mosby.

Jastremski CA: Head injuries, *RN* 61(12):40-46, 1998.

Kaufman HH: *Intracerebral hematomas,* New York, 1992, Raven.

Kernich CA, Kaminski HJ: Myths & facts ... about myasthenia gravis, *Nursing '96* 26(7):21, 1996

Kim MJ, McFarland GK, McLane AM: *Pocket guide to nursing diagnoses,* ed 7, St Louis, 1997, Mosby.

Klugman K, Koornhof H: Penicillin-resistant pneumococcal meningitis, *Lancet* 350(9085):1176-1177, 1997.

Lammertse DP: Recovery of neurologic function in spinal cord injury: a review of new and experimental therapies, *Top Spinal Cord Inj Rehabil* 2(3):95-100, 1997.

Larsen R: Treatment of cryptococcal meningitis, *N Engl J Med* 337(21):1557-1558, 1997.

Latov N: Immune-mediated neurological diseases: immunology of neurological diseases, *J Care Manage* 3(5):6-7, 16-18, 1997.

Lopate G, Pestronk A: Autoimmune myasthenia gravis, *Hosp Pract* 28(1):109-112, 115-117, 121-122, 1993.

Lowenstein DH, Alldredge BK: Status epilepticus, *N Engl J Med* 338(14):970-976, 1998.

Lucke KT: Pulmonary management following acute spinal cord injury, *J Neurosci Nurs* 30(2):91-104, 1998.

McIntyre P et al.: Dexamethasone as adjunctive therapy in bacterial meningitis: a meta-analysis of randomized clinical trials since 1988, *JAMA* 278(11):925-931, 1997.

McMahon-Parkes K, Cornock MA: Guillain-Barré syndrome: biological basis, treatment and care, *Intensive Crit Care Nurs* 13(1):42-48, 1997.

Miller L, Choi C: Meningitis in older patients: how to diagnose and treat a deadly infection, *Geriatrics* 52(8):43-55, 1997.

Moore K: Spotting vasospasm is vital for these patients, *RN* 60(6):60, 1997.

Murray DP: Impaired mobility: Guillain-Barré syndrome, *J Neurosci Nurs* 25(2):100-104, 1993.

National High Blood Pressure Education Program, National Institutes of Health, and National Heart, Lung, and Blood Institute: NIH Pub No 93-1088, Jan 1993.

NINDS: *Rapid identification and treatment of acute stroke,* NIH Pub No 97-423, Aug 1997.

NINDS Stroke Study Group: rt-PA stroke treatment, *J Neurosci Nurs* 29(6): 349-401, 1997.

O'Donnell L: An elusive weakness: myasthenia gravis, *Med-Surg Nurs* 5(1):44-49, 1996.

O'Donnell LE: Immune-mediated neurological diseases: management of myasthenia gravis—an overview, *J Care Manage* 3(6):4-5, 17-18, 1997.

Pacheco T et al.: Failure of cefotaxime treatment in an adult with streptococcus pneumoniae meningitis, *Am J Med* 102(3):303-305, 1997.

Pieper DR et al: Surgical management of patients with severe head injuries, *AORN J* 63(5):854-870, 1996.

Plum F, Posner J: *Diagnosis of stupor and coma,* ed 3, Philadelphia, 1980, Davis.

Pope W: External ventriculostomy: a practical application for the acute care nurse, *J Neurosci Nurs* 30(3):185-190, 1998.

Prasad K, Menon G: Steroids in tuberculous meningitis (Cochrane Review). In The Cochrane Library, Issue 2: Update Software 1998. Updated quarterly.

Quagliarello V, Scheld M: Drug therapy: treatment of bacterial meningitis, *N Engl J Med* 336(10):708-716, 1997.

Rusy KL: Rebleeding and vasospasm after subarachnoid hemorrhage: a critical care challenge, *Crit Care Nurs* 16(1):41-48, 1996.

Schooley Y: *Recommendations for the nursing management of the hyperacute ischemic stroke patient*, American Association of Neuroscience Nurses Clinical Guideline Series, 1998.

Schuchat A et al.: Bacterial meningitis in the United States in 1995, *N Engl J Med* 337: 970-976, 1997.

Segatore M: Hyponatremia after aneurysmal subarachnoid hemorrhage, *J Neurosci Nurs* 25(2):92-99, 1993.

Segreti J, Harris A: Acute bacterial meningitis, *Infect Dis Clin North Am* 10(4):797-809, 1996.

Seybold ME: Update on myasthenia gravis, *Hosp Med* 27(4):71-72, 77-78, 80, 1991.

Stamatos CA et al: Meeting the challenge of the older trauma patient, *Am J Nurs* 96(5):40-48, 1996.

Stephens A: Systems and diseases: the immune system. I. Myasthenia gravis, *Nurs Times* 93(46):56-59, 1997.

The Italian Guillain-Barré Study Group: The prognosis and main prognostic indicators of Guillain-Barré syndrome: a multicentre prospective study of 297 patients, *Brain* 119:2053-2061, 1996 (Dec, part 6).

Titler M, Bulechek G, McCloskey J: Use of the nursing intervention classification by critical care nurses, *Crit Care Nurs* 16(4):38-54, 1996.

van der Horst et al.: Treatment of cryptococcal meningitis associated with the acquired immunodeficiency syndrome, *N Engl J Med* 337(11):15-21, 1997.

Working Group on Status Epilepticus: Treatment of convulsive status epilepticus: recommendations of the Working Group on Status Epilepticus, *JAMA* 270(7):854-859, 1993.

Zafonte RD, Mann NR: Cerebral salt-wasting syndrome in brain injury patients: a potential cause of hyponatremia, *Arch Phys Med Rehabil* 78(5):540-542, 1997.

CHAPTER 7

Endocrinologic Dysfunctions

Diabetic ketoacidosis

PATHOPHYSIOLOGY

Diabetic ketoacidosis (DKA) is a life-threatening complication of diabetes mellitus that is characterized by hyperglycemia, ketosis, acidosis, dehydration, and electrolyte imbalance. It occurs most commonly in persons with type 1 diabetes mellitus who experience illness, infection, trauma, or surgery but may occur also in the severely stressed individual with type 2 diabetes. A relative or absolute insulin deficiency prevents the normal utilization of serum glucose and results in cellular starvation despite the abundance of glucose in the serum. The unmet energy requirements of the cells stimulate gluconeogenesis and glycogen conversion in the liver through the release of counterregulatory hormones. The body is forced to break down fat and protein stores to meet energy requirements. The rate of breakdown exceeds the body's ability to use these alternate energy sources, however, and ketone bodies accumulate in the blood. Ketones cause the blood pH level to drop, which results in the potential for profound metabolic acidosis. Hyperglycemia results in increased serum osmolality with movement of water out of the cells.

Glucose and ketones not reabsorbed by the renal tubule cause an osmotic diuresis, with losses of sodium, potassium, phosphorus, magnesium, and body water, which can lead to dehydration and, if severe, hypovolemic shock. Increased blood viscosity and platelet aggregation can result in thromboembolism. Despite significant loss of potassium in the urine, the patient initially will present with normal or elevated plasma potassium because of the dramatic shift of potassium out of the cells secondary to insulin deficiency, acidosis, and tissue catabolism. Dehydration also decreases tissue perfusion, and the resulting lactic acid waste products exacerbate the existing acidosis. The lowered pH level stimulates the respiratory center, producing the deep, rapid respirations known as *Kussmaul respirations.* The large amount of plasma ketones lends a fruity or acetone odor to the breath. If not treated promptly, elevated serum osmolality, acidosis, and dehydration depress consciousness to the point of coma. Death can result from hypovolemia or profound central nervous system (CNS) depression.

ASSESSMENT

History and risk factors: Type 1 or type 2 diabetes mellitus, recent physical stressor such as illness, infection, trauma, or surgery (most episodes of DKA are precipitated by infection), insufficient exogenous insulin replacement, severe emotional stress, omission of insulin.

Clinical presentation: Recent polyuria, polydipsia, polyphagia, weight loss, weakness, fatigue, nausea, vomiting, abdominal pain.

Physical assessment: Dry and flushed skin, dry mucous membranes, poor skin turgor, altered level of consciousness (LOC) (irritability, lethargy, coma), fruity odor to the breath, Kussmaul respirations. Because fluid loss is largely intracellular, the presence of hypotension and tachycardia suggests severe volume loss.

Electrocardiogram (ECG) and hemodynamic findings: ECG may show dysrhythmias associated with hyperkalemia: peaked T waves, widened QRS complex, prolonged PR intervals, flattened-to-absent P wave. After insulin therapy is initiated, hypokalemia is possible (see p. 649).

> **Note:**   For additional assessment information, see Table 7-1.

DIAGNOSTIC TESTS

See Table 7-1.

COLLABORATIVE MANAGEMENT

Rehydration: Isotonic saline (0.9%) is administered rapidly (1-2 L during the first hour) to correct the fluid deficit, which is typically 4-6 L but may be even greater. After initial fluid replacement, 0.45% saline is administered to continue the rehydration. Dextrose is added to the IV solution once the blood glucose falls to approximately 250 mg/dl, to prevent hypoglycemia and allow the continued administration of insulin necessary to correct ketoacidosis.

Rapid-acting insulin: A loading dose of regular insulin may be given, followed by continuous IV insulin infusion at approximately 0.1 U/kg/h. It is essential that blood glucose be reduced gradually to reduce the risk of cerebral edema. The dosage is adjusted on the basis of serial glucose measurements. The insulin drip may be discontinued *temporarily* or IV dextrose increased to 10% if the serum glucose drops to <100 mg/dl before correction of acidosis. Follow unit protocol, or consult the physician. Be aware that insulin, when added to IV solutions, adheres to the container and plastic tubing. The tubing should be flushed with 50-100 ml of the insulin solution to saturate the tubing before actual administration.

Restoration of electrolyte balance: Potassium is closely monitored and replaced once insulin is administered and potassium returns to the intracellular compartment. Potassium replacement is essential to correct the existing body deficit and prevent severe hypokalemia. Deficits may range from 300-900 mEq and will require days to replace. Phosphate replacement (usually as potassium phosphate) may be indicated if severe depletion has occurred in the presence of prolonged acidosis. Meticulous monitoring of phosphate *and* calcium levels is essential if phosphate replacement is prescribed, because supplemental phosphate may depress plasma calcium levels secondary to calcium-phosphorus binding (see "Hypophosphatemia," p. 659).

Intravenous (IV) bicarbonate: May be prescribed in the presence of severe acidosis (pH <7.1). It is not routinely given in DKA because of the potential for paradoxic cerebral spinal fluid acidosis and hypokalemia. The acidosis of DKA is best corrected by insulin therapy. Hyperchloremic acidosis, secondary to DKA or aggressive volume replacement with isotonic saline, usually resolves without treatment.

Insertion of gastric tube: May be indicated in comatose or obtunded patients when the risk of vomiting and aspiration from gastric distention or paralytic ileus is high.

TABLE 7-1   Comparison of Diabetic Ketoacidosis (DKA) and Hyperglycemic Hyperosmolar Nonketotic Syndrome (HHNS)

Criterion	DKA	HHNS
Diabetes type	Type 1	Type 2
Typical age-group	Any age	Usually >50 yr
Signs and symptoms	Polyuria, polydipsia, polyphagia, weakness, orthostatic hypotension, lethargy, changes in LOC, fatigue, nausea, vomiting, abdominal pain	Same as DKA, but slower onset and, very commonly, neurologic symptoms predominate
Physical assessment	Dry and flushed skin, poor skin turgor, dry mucous membranes, decreased BP, tachycardia, altered LOC (irritability, lethargy, coma), Kussmaul respirations, fruity odor to the breath	Same as DKA, but no Kussmaul respirations or fruity odor to the breath; instead, occurrence of tachypnea with shallow respirations
History and risk factors	Recent stressors such as surgery, trauma, infection, MI; insufficient exogenous insulin; undiagnosed type 1 diabetes mellitus	Undiagnosed type 2 diabetes mellitus; recent stressors such as surgery, trauma, pancreatitis, MI, infection; high-calorie enteral or parenteral feedings in a compromised patient; use of diabetogenic drugs (e.g., phenytoin, thiazide diuretics, thyroid preparations, mannitol, corticosteroids, sympathomimetics)
Monitoring parameters	*ECG:* Dysrhythmias associated with hyperkalemia: peaked T waves, widened QRS complex, prolonged PR interval, flattened or absent P wave. Hypokalemia (K^+ <3 mEq/L), which may produce depressed ST segments, flat or inverted T waves, or increased ventricular dysrhythmias	ECG evidence of hypokalemia as listed with DKA *Hemodynamic measurements:* CVP >3 mm Hg below patient's baseline; PADP and PAWP >4 mm Hg below patient's baseline

Diagnostic tests		
Serum glucose: 200-800 mg/dl	800-2000 mg/dl
Serum ketones: positive at >1:2	Usually absent
Urine glucose: positive	Positive
Urine acetone: "large"	Negative
Serum osmolality: 300-350 mOsm/L	>350 mOsm/L
Bicarbonate: <15 mEq/L	Normal or slightly decreased if mild acidosis present
Serum pH: <7.2	Normal or mildly acidotic (pH <7.4)
Serum potassium: normal or elevated >5.0 mEq/L initially and then decreased	Normal or <3.5 mEq/L
Serum sodium: elevated, normal, or low	Elevated, normal, or low
Serum Hct: elevated because of osmotic diuresis with hemoconcentration	Elevated because of hemoconcentration
BUN: elevated >20 mg/dl	Elevated
Serum creatinine: >1.5 mg/dl	Elevated
Serum phosphorus, magnesium, chloride: decreased	Decreased
WBC: elevated, even in the absence of infection	Normal unless infection present
Onset	Hours to days	Days to weeks
Mortality	<10%	10%-25% because of age-group and complications such as stroke, thrombosis, renal failure

LOC, Level of consciousness; BP, blood pressure; MI, myocardial infarction; ECG, electrocardiogram; Hct, hematocrit; BUN, blood urea nitrogen; WBC, white blood cell count; CVP, central venous pressure; PADP, pulmonary artery diastolic pressure; PAWP, pulmonary artery wedge pressure.

Research Brief 7-1 This retrospective study of 39 patients admitted for severe diabetic ketoacidosis (DKA) from the emergency care unit of a teaching hospital was designed to assess the efficacy of bicarbonate therapy for management of DKA. Twenty-four patients received intravenous 120 ± 40 mmol of sodium bicarbonate; 15 did not receive sodium bicarbonate. Data from the literature and this study are not in favor of the use of bicarbonate in the treatment of DKA with pH values between 6.90 and 7.10.

From Viallon A et al: Does bicarbonate therapy improve the management of severe diabetic ketoacidosis? *Crit Care Med* 27(12):2690-2693, 1999.

Treatment of underlying cause: For example, infection is treated with appropriate antibiotics.

NURSING DIAGNOSES AND INTERVENTIONS

Fluid volume deficit related to decreased circulating volume secondary to hyperglycemia-induced osmotic diuresis

Desired outcomes: Within 12 h of initiating treatment, patient is euvolemic as evidenced by blood pressure (BP) ≥90/60 mm Hg (or within patient's normal range); mean arterial pressure (MAP) ≥70 mm Hg; heart rate (HR) 60-100 beats per minute (bpm), central venous pressure (CVP) 2-6 mm Hg, pulmonary artery wedge pressure (PAWP) 6-12 mm Hg, balanced intake and output (I&O), urinary output ≥0.5 ml/kg/h, firm skin turgor, and pink and moist mucous membranes. ECG exhibits normal sinus rhythm.

- Monitor vital signs (VS) q15min until patient's condition is stable for 1 h. Monitor hemodynamic status, including CVP, MAP, pulmonary artery pressure (PAP), pulmonary capillary wedge pressure (PCWP), if available. Consult physician promptly for the following: HR >120 bpm or BP <90/60 or decreased ≥20 mm Hg from baseline, MAP decreased ≥10 mm Hg from baseline, CVP <2 mm Hg, and PAWP <6 mm Hg.
- Monitor hydration status (e.g., moist mucous membranes, adequacy of pulses, and orthostatic blood pressure), as appropriate.
- Monitor I&O. Decreasing urinary output may signal diminishing intravascular fluid volume or impending renal failure. Consult physician for urine output <0.5 ml/kg/h for 2 consecutive hours.
- Administer IV therapy, as prescribed. Be alert to indicators of fluid overload, which can occur as a result of rapid infusion of fluids: jugular vein distention, dyspnea, crackles (rales), CVP >6 mm Hg.
- Monitor for abnormal serum electrolyte levels as available. Be alert for the development of hypokalemia, a common complication of treatment. Normal range for serum potassium is 3.5-5 mEq/L and for serum sodium is 137-147 mEq/L.
- Monitor for an increase in anion gap (>14 mEq/L), signaling an increased production or decreased excretion of acid products. Anion gap should decrease steadily to normal with successful treatment of DKA.
- Monitor for cardiac dysrhythmias, including disturbance of both rhythm and conduction. Observe specifically for ECG changes typical of hyperkalemia (p. 652) or hypokalemia (p. 649).
- Observe for clinical manifestations of electrolyte imbalance associated with DKA and its treatment:
  - ☐ *Hypokalemia:* ECG changes, muscle weakness, anorexia, drowsiness, hypoactive bowel sounds.
  - ☐ *Hypophosphatemia:* Muscle weakness, malaise, confusion, respiratory failure, decreased oxygen delivery, decreased cardiac function.

☐ *Hypomagnesemia:* Anorexia, nausea, vomiting, lethargy, weakness, personality changes, tetany, tremor or muscle fasciculations, seizures, confusion.
• Weigh patient daily, and monitor trends.

You may also wish to refer to the following interventions from the Nursing Interventions Classification (NIC):

NIC Hyperglycemia Management; Fluid/Electrolyte Management; Fluid Monitoring; Invasive Hemodynamic Monitoring; Acid-Base Management: Metabolic Acidosis; Electrolyte Management: Hypokalemia

Risk for infection related to inadequate secondary defenses (suppressed inflammatory response) as a result of protein depletion and hyperglycemia

Desired outcome: Patient is free of infection as evidenced by normothermia; HR ≤100 bpm; BP within patient's normal range; white blood cell (WBC) count ≤11,000/mm^3, and negative culture results.

• Monitor for systemic and localized signs and symptoms of infection. Be aware that initially fever may be suppressed secondary to acidosis. Monitor laboratory results for increased WBC count. An initial elevation of WBC count may be a reflection of dehydration and increased adrenocortical secretion.
• Wash hands before and after each patient care activity. Use antimicrobial soap for hand washing, as available.
• Because patient is at increased risk of bacterial infection, use of invasive lines should be limited. Change peripheral and central line sites and dressings according to agency guidelines. Central lines should be removed as soon as feasible. Schedule dressing changes according to agency policy, and inspect the site(s) for signs of local infection, including erythema, swelling, or purulent drainage. Document the presence of any of these indicators, and consult physician accordingly.
• Use meticulous aseptic technique when caring for or inserting indwelling catheters, to minimize the risk of bacterial entry via these sites.
• Because of the increased risk of infection, use of indwelling urethral catheter is indicated only when continuous accurate assessment of urine output is essential.
• Provide good skin care to maintain skin integrity. Assess for areas of decreased sensation on the extremities. Use pressure-relief mattress on the bed to help prevent skin breakdown.

NIC Infection Protection; Skin Surveillance

Risk for injury related to altered cerebral function secondary to hyperosmolality, dehydration, cerebral edema associated with DKA, or hypoglycemia

Desired outcomes: Patient verbalizes orientation to time, place, and person; normal breath sounds are auscultated over patient's airways; and patient's oral cavity and musculoskeletal system remain intact and free of injury.

• Monitor patient's orientation, LOC, and respiratory status, especially airway patency, at frequent intervals. Keep an appropriate-size oral airway, manual resuscitator and mask, and supplemental oxygen at the bedside. Notify physician of change in patient condition.
• Reduce the likelihood of injury caused by falls by maintaining bed in lowest position with side rails up at all times and using soft restraints as necessary.
• Insert gastric tube in comatose patients, as prescribed, to decrease the likelihood of aspiration. Attach to low, intermittent suction, and ensure patency of tube q4h.
• Elevate head of bed (HOB) to 45 degrees to minimize the risk of aspiration.
• Monitor blood glucose qh while on insulin infusion. Consult physician if blood glucose drops faster than 100 mg/dl/h or if it drops to <250-300 mg/dl. Obtain prescription for glucose-containing IV solution to prevent hypoglycemia and allow the continued administration of insulin necessary to correct acidosis.

NIC Neurologic Monitoring; Hyperglycemia Management; Hypoglycemia Management

Knowledge deficit: new-onset diabetes or misunderstanding of the causes and prevention of DKA

Desired outcome: By the time of discharge from ICU, patient verbalizes understanding of the causes, symptoms, and prevention of DKA and available resources.

- Consider referral to diabetes educator if this is a new-onset diabetes or the individual lacks adequate self-management skills. Provide instructions in simple terms, incorporating patient teaching into patient care routines.
- Explain the relationship of DKA to illness and stress. Emphasize the importance of adhering to the entire diabetes regimen, including meal planning, medication, exercise, and monitoring.
- Review sick-day guidelines for individuals with diabetes (i.e., need for increased fluid and insulin with illness) with patient and significant others.
- Alert patient and significant others to hospital and community resources (e.g., certified diabetes educator, dietitian, social worker, local American Diabetes Association [ADA], consumer health library, and support groups).
- Provide address for ADA for educational material related to the disease, its complications, and appropriate treatment: American Diabetes Association, Inc., 18 East 48th St, New York, NY 10017.

NIC Teaching: Disease Process; Teaching: Prescribed Diet; Teaching: Prescribed Medication; Teaching: Prescribed Activity/Exercise; Emotional Support

ADDITIONAL NURSING DIAGNOSES

See "Hyperglycemic Hyperosmolar Nonketotic Syndrome," p. 478, for **Altered peripheral tissue perfusion.** See also nursing diagnoses and interventions in "Prolonged Immobility," p. 74; "Psychosocial Support," p. 83; and "Psychosocial Support for the Patient's Family and Significant Others," p. 95.

Hyperglycemic hyperosmolar nonketotic syndrome

PATHOPHYSIOLOGY

Hyperglycemic hyperosmolar nonketotic syndrome (HHNS) is a life-threatening emergency resulting from a relative insulin deficiency that causes severe hyperglycemia and dehydration. It occurs most commonly in older patients with type 2 diabetes, especially if previously undiagnosed. Usually HHNS is precipitated by an acute exacerbation of a chronic disease or a stimulus, such as trauma or infection, that provokes a stress response. The stressor combines with a decreased insulin reserve to initiate the pathophysiologic sequence. Although the body's available insulin is insufficient to control the blood glucose, it usually is adequate to prevent lipolysis and the formation of ketone bodies, thereby avoiding metabolic acidosis. The hyperglycemia of HHNS is more severe than that in DKA, and it results in significant serum hyperosmolality and pronounced osmotic diuresis. Severe dehydration and electrolyte loss occur, and individuals may lose from 15%-25% of their body water. Fluids are pulled from the body cells in response to the hyperosmolality, and significant intracellular dehydration may result. Neurologic deficits frequently occur in response to the severe dehydration and hyperosmolality. The blood becomes more viscous and flow is impeded, increasing the risk of thromboemboli. Increased cardiac workload and decreased renal and cerebral blood flow may result in myocardial infarction, renal failure, and stroke.

The dramatic osmotic diuresis that occurs with HHNS results in significant electrolyte depletion. Sodium and potassium levels are variable at diagnosis, although total body deficiencies of both always are present. Phosphorus and magnesium deficiencies also are common.

Unlike DKA, in which acidosis produces severe symptoms that require prompt hospitalization, symptoms of HHNS develop slowly and frequently are nonspecific. The cardinal symptoms of polyuria and polydipsia are the first to appear, but they may be ignored by older adults or their families. Neurologic deficits may be mistaken for senility. Because of the similarity of these symptoms to other disease processes common to this age-group, proper diagnosis and treatment may be delayed, allowing progression of pathophysiologic processes.

ASSESSMENT

History and risk factors: Type 2 diabetes mellitus; acute exacerbation of a chronic illness, particularly renal or cardiovascular; ingestion of high-caloric enteral or parenteral feedings; stressors, such as trauma or infection, which increase insulin need; use of diabetogenic drugs (e.g., glucocorticoids, some diuretics, phenytoin, thyroid preparations).

Clinical presentation: Polyuria, polydipsia, weight loss, weakness, orthostatic hypotension, lethargy, confusion progressing to coma. Neurologic symptoms are common, ranging from focal findings to frank coma. Although almost all patients present with altered mental status, only 50% are comatose. Seizures may be present in as many as 25% of all patients.

Physical assessment: Poor skin turgor, dry mucous membranes, tachycardia, tachypnea with shallow respirations.

ECG and hemodynamic findings: Evidence of hypokalemia (increased premature ventricular complexes [PVCs], depressed T waves), CVP >3 mm Hg below patient's baseline, pulmonary artery diastolic (PAD) pressure >4 mm Hg below patient's baseline, and PAWP >4 mm Hg below patient's baseline.

> **Note:**   Because these patients usually are >50 yr old and have preexisting cardiac or pulmonary disorders, hemodynamic factors often cannot be evaluated on the basis of normal values but rather on what is normal or optimal for each individual patient. CVP, PAWP, and PAD pressures therefore should be evaluated in terms of deviations from patient's baseline and concurrent clinical status. See Table 7-1 for a comparison of DKA and HHNS.

DIAGNOSTIC TESTS

See Table 7-1.

COLLABORATIVE MANAGEMENT

Replacement of electrolytes and extracellular fluid volume: Most often, 0.45% saline or isotonic saline is used; potassium phosphate and magnesium supplements are added on the basis of laboratory values. Usually half of the estimated fluid deficit is replaced during the first 12 h and the remainder over the next 24 h. To prevent hypoglycemia, dextrose will be added to the IV solution once the blood glucose falls to 250-300 mg/dl.

Rapid-acting insulin: Usually administered in low doses. Because of poor tissue perfusion in these patients, the IV route is preferred. In the majority of cases, continuous drips are used and titrated on the basis of blood glucose levels. In HHNS, some insulin secretion occurs and patients may be extremely sensitive to supplemental doses. Despite severe hyperglycemia, HHNS often requires less insulin to correct than does DKA. The condition sometimes can be treated with fluid alone.

Insertion of pulmonary artery flow-directed catheter: To assess fluid status on a continuous basis.

Treatment of underlying cause: The most frequent cause is infection, which is treated with appropriate antibiotics.

NURSING DIAGNOSES AND INTERVENTIONS

Altered tissue perfusion: peripheral, related to interruption of blood flow (thromboembolism) secondary to increased viscosity of blood, increased platelet aggregation and adhesiveness, and patient immobility

Desired outcome: By the time of hospital discharge, patient has adequate perfusion as evidenced by peripheral pulses >2+ on a 0-4+ scale; brisk capillary refill (<2 sec); warm skin; and absence of swelling, bluish discoloration, erythema, and discomfort in the calves and thighs.

- Maintain adequate hydration to prevent increased blood viscosity. Monitor hematocrit (Hct) results. With proper fluid replacement, values should return to normal (40%-54% [male] or 37%-47% [female]) within 24-48 h. Assess for falling blood urea nitrogen (BUN) and creatinine as an indicators of improved renal perfusion.
- Perform a comprehensive appraisal of peripheral circulation (e.g., check peripheral pulses, edema, capillary refill, color, and temperature of extremity). Consult physician immediately for any decrease in amplitude or absence of pulse(s).
- Be alert to indicators of deep vein thrombosis such as erythema, pain, tenderness, warmth, swelling, bluish discoloration, or prominence of superficial veins in the extremities, especially the lower extremities. Arterial thrombosis may produce cyanosis with delayed capillary refill, mottling, and coolness of the extremity. Report significant findings to physician immediately.
- Assist with or perform range-of-motion (ROM) exercises to all extremities q4h to increase blood flow to the tissues.
- Change the patient's position at least q2h as appropriate.
- Apply pneumatic sequential compression stockings or similar devices to the lower extremities as prescribed to help prevent thrombosis.
- Administer antiplatelet or anticoagulant medication as appropriate.
- Instruct the patient on the importance of prevention of venous stasis (e.g., not crossing legs, elevating feet without bending knees, exercise).

NIC Hyperglycemia Management; Neurologic Monitoring; Fluid/Electrolyte Management; Fluid Monitoring; Intravenous (IV) Therapy; Invasive Hemodynamic Monitoring; Circulatory Care; Hypoglycemia Management

Knowledge deficit: new-onset diabetes or causes of HHNS

Desired outcome: Before discharge from ICU, patient verbalizes understanding of the basics of diabetes management and prevention of HHNS.

- Teach patient the causes, prevention, and treatment of HHNS. Allow patient to verbalize fears and feelings about the diagnosis; correct any misconceptions. As needed, explain the disease process of diabetes mellitus and HHNS and the common early symptoms of worsening diabetes, including polyuria, polydipsia, polyphagia, dry and flushed skin, and increased irritability.
- Stress the importance of daily testing of blood glucose levels, or as prescribed, before meals and at bedtime. Explain that blood glucose >250 mg/dl should be reported to physician. As indicated, review testing procedure with patient.
- Explain the importance of taking diabetes medication as prescribed. In addition, explain that increased medication may be required during periods of physical and emotional stress and that blood glucose levels should be monitored closely during these times, as well as during illness or injury.
- Describe specific components of the diabetic regimen as appropriate. Review the importance of regular exercise, consistent dietary intake, preventive measures for avoiding infection, and prompt management of minor injuries.
- Describe procedures for obtaining medical-alert bracelet or card identifying patient's diagnosis.
- Stress the necessity for continued medical follow-up.
- In addition, provide booklets or pamphlets from the ADA or pharmaceutical companies about diabetes and appropriate treatment. Refer patient and significant others to a diabetes education program, if needed.

NIC Teaching: Disease Process; Teaching: Prescribed Diet; Teaching: Prescribed Medication; Teaching: Prescribed Activity/Exercise; Emotional Support

ADDITIONAL NURSING DIAGNOSES

See also "Diabetic Ketoacidosis" for **Fluid volume deficit,** p. 474; **Risk for infection,** p. 475; and **Risk for injury,** p. 475. For other nursing diagnoses and interventions, see the following as appropriate: "Psychosocial Support," p. 83; and "Psychosocial Support for the Patient's Family and Significant Others," p. 95.

Diabetes insipidus

PATHOPHYSIOLOGY

Diabetes insipidus (DI) results from a profound deficiency of the antidiuretic hormone (ADH) or decreased renal responsiveness to ADH. It may be caused by a neurogenic dysfunction involving either a deficiency in the synthesis of ADH in the posterior pituitary gland or damage to the hypothalamus, which stimulates its release (central DI [CDI]). DI also may be nephrogenic (NDI) in origin secondary to decreased water permeability of the collecting tubules caused by decreased ADH effect. DI is frequently temporary, occurring suddenly in response to head injury, major trauma, tumor, or inflammation. In some situations, however, the condition may become permanent. Transient DI typically resolves after approximately 5-7 days. If resolution of the problem does not occur within that time frame, the patient usually progresses to permanent polyuria and polydipsia.

Regardless of the cause, the characteristic feature of DI is the excretion of large quantities of hypotonic urine, frequently 10-12 L/day or more. As a result of the loss of free water, the extracellular fluid volume decreases dramatically, causing plasma osmolality and serum sodium to rise. If individuals are unable to respond adequately to the stimulus of thirst, they face significant risks from extracellular and intracellular dehydration, hypotension, and hypovolemic shock. The increased blood viscosity increases the risk of thromboemboli. Dehydration, decreased cerebral perfusion, and electrolyte imbalance frequently produce neurologic symptoms ranging from confusion, restlessness, and irritability to seizures and coma.

ASSESSMENT

History and risk factors
Central DI: Brain tumors, especially in the hypothalamus or pituitary region; neoplasms such as leukemia or breast cancer; surgery in the area of the pituitary gland; intracranial hemorrhage; head injury, especially to the base of the brain; meningitis or encephalitis; any disorder that causes increased intracranial pressure (IICP); cerebral hypoxia.
Nephrogenic DI: Medications (lithium, demeclocycline HCl [Declomycin]); hypercalcemia; hypokalemia; osmotic diuresis; congenital disorder.
Clinical presentation: Polyuria with dilute urine; extreme thirst.

Note: As much as 5-12 L/day of urine may be excreted, with specific gravity of 1.000-1.005.

Physical assessment: Unremarkable in the individual who experiences and can safely satisfy thirst. If fluid intake is inadequate, patients may show signs of dehydration, such as poor skin turgor, dry mucous membranes, orthostatic hypotension, hypotension, and tachycardia. Altered LOC may be present if serum hyperosmolality and hypernatremia develop. Altered LOC and neurologic changes also may be related to the precipitating event.

Monitoring parameters
Urine output: >200 ml/h for 2 consecutive hours or >500 ml/h in the presence of any of the aforementioned risk factors.
CVP: <2 mm Hg.
PAWP: <6 mm Hg.

DIAGNOSTIC TESTS

Urine osmolality: Decreased to <200 mOsm/kg in the presence of disease; may be higher if volume depletion is present.
Specific gravity: <1.007.
Serum osmolality: Increased to >300 mOsm/kg.
Serum sodium: Increased to >147 mEq/L.
Plasma ADH: Decreased in central DI.
Water deprivation test: Preliminary measurements of weight, serum and urine osmolality, and urine specific gravity are obtained. Fluid intake is prohibited, and the aforementioned values are measured hourly until urine specific gravity exceeds 1.020 and urine osmolality exceeds 800 mOsm/kg (a negative result) or when 5% of body weight is lost or urine specific gravity does not increase for 3 consecutive hours (a positive result). Less dramatic results may indicate partial DI. To establish a definite diagnosis of DI, it is necessary also to perform the vasopressin test (see next entry).

> *Caution:*   The water deprivation test can take up to 16 h to complete and may produce hypernatremia, severe dehydration, and hypovolemic shock. Patients must be monitored continuously throughout the test. This test may not be necessary for temporary DI in the critical care setting.

Vasopressin test: Vasopressin (exogenous ADH) is administered subcutaneously. Urine specimens are collected q30min for 2 h and evaluated for quantity and osmolality. Urine osmolality generally will rise significantly in response to the ADH unless the DI has a nephrogenic origin, in which case the response may be minimal.

> *Caution:*   This test can induce congestive heart failure secondary to fluid overload in susceptible persons.

COLLABORATIVE MANAGEMENT

Rehydration: Hypotonic IV solutions frequently are used to replace free water lost in the urine. Fluid replacement is very rapid until hemodynamic status becomes stabilized, at which time it is then based on urine output. Hypernatremia, if present, should be corrected slowly, especially if it is chronic. Symptomatic hypernatremia should be corrected more rapidly than asymptomatic hypernatremia.
Exogenous ADH (vasopressin):   Several preparations are available, and dosage is adjusted to patient response. Potential side effects include hypertension, angina, or myocardial infarction (MI) related to its vasoconstrictive effects on blood vessels; abdominal cramping and increased peristalsis from smooth muscle excitation; and water intoxication. Use of desmopressin has become increasingly popular because it produces fewer side effects (Table 7-2).
Thiazide diuretics in combination with a low-sodium diet: Major form of therapy for nephrogenic DI. This approach reduces the loss of free water in the urine. Amiloride hydrochloride (a potassium-sparing diuretic) is the medication of choice for the treatment of lithium-induced NDI. Nonsteroidal antiinflammatory drugs (NSAIDs) may be used as adjunctive therapy in NDI.
Transsphenoidal hypophysectomy: Although not an appropriate treatment for transient DI that occurs after injury or surgery, this surgical approach to the pituitary gland is the treatment of choice for pituitary tumors of all types, whether or not the pituitary gland itself is removed. It produces immediate

TABLE 7-2 Vasopressin Preparations

Generic name	Trade name	Route	Onset	Duration	Total daily dose	Comments
Desmopressin acetate	DDAVP	Intranasal	1-2 h	8-12 h	0.1-0.4 ml (10-40 µg) qd in 1-2 doses	Administered by nasal spray or rhinal tube applicator. Action decreased by nasal congestion/discharge or atrophy of nasal mucosa. Stored in refrigerator. Drug of choice for chronic CDI.
		Subcutaneous	Within ½ h	1½-4 h	0.5-1 ml (2-4 µg) qd in 2 divided doses	Keep refrigerated. More potent than intranasal route.
		Intravenous	Within ½ h	1½-4 h	0.5-1 ml (2-4 µg) qd in 2 divided doses	Keep refrigerated. More potent than intranasal route.
		Oral tablets	1-2 h	8-12 h	0.1-0.8 mg in 2-3 divided doses	Simple to use. More consistent absorption and few side effects.
Vasopressin	Pitressin	Subcutaneous	1-2 h	2-6 h	5-10 units (20 units/ml); given q2-4h	Used primarily to confirm the diagnosis, differentiate between CDI and NDI, and treat acute situations.
Lysine vasopressin	Diapid	Intranasal	Within 1 h	3-8 h	7-14 µg in 4 doses (q6h)	Lower cost than DDAVP for patients with partial CDI who require 1-2 daily doses.

CDI, Central diabetes insipidus; *NDI,* nephrogenic diabetes insipidus.

results, has a low mortality, and can be effective in the treatment of tumors that are resistant to radiation therapy.

To enter the sella turcica through the sphenoid process, the upper lip is elevated and an incision is made in the gingiva above the maxilla. Because of the site of the incision, patients are at high risk for postoperative infection, particularly of the brain. To minimize this possibility, antibiotic nasal sprays are used preoperatively, and nasal packing impregnated with an antibiotic ointment is kept in place for 24-72 h after surgery. Complications include pituitary hemorrhage, frontal lobe damage, and hormonal deficiencies after removal of the gland. Tumors occur most often in the anterior pituitary gland; therefore most postoperative hormone deficiencies are caused by a lack of anterior pituitary hormones. In addition, the patient may have IICP caused by edema or bleeding in the sella turcica and will return from surgery with bilateral periorbital ecchymosis.

NURSING DIAGNOSES AND INTERVENTIONS

Fluid volume deficit related to failure of regulatory mechanisms (resulting in polyuria) secondary to ADH deficiency or altered ADH action
Desired outcome: Within 12 h of initiating therapy, patient is normovolemic as evidenced by BP 110-120/70-80 mm Hg (or within patient's normal value); CVP $\geq$2 mm Hg; PAWP $\geq$6 mm Hg; HR 60-100 bpm; intake equal to output plus insensible losses; and stable weight.
- Keep careful I&O records. Urine output >200 ml/h for 2 consecutive hours, or 500 ml/h, in the presence of risk factors (see p. 479), should be reported to physician promptly.
- Give fluids as appropriate. Keep water pitcher full and within easy reach of patient. Administer hyperosmolar tube feedings or solutions with extreme caution. They can worsen fluid losses through the gastrointestinal (GI) tract by inducing osmotic diarrhea.
- Administer hypotonic solutions (e.g., D_5W, $D_5$0.225 or 0.45 NaCl) for intracellular rehydration. Usually, fluids are administered as follows: 1 ml IV fluid for each 1 ml of urine output. In patients with brain injury, moderate diuresis may be permitted to avoid the need for administering osmotic diuretics. Hypernatremia, if present, must be corrected slowly (at a rate no greater than 0.5 mEq/L/h or 12 mEq/L/day) to prevent cerebral edema, seizures, permanent neurologic damage, or death.
- Administer vasopressin as ordered. Observe for and document effects. Also be alert to side effects of therapy: hypertension, cardiac ischemia, hyponatremia.
- Weigh patient daily, at the same time and using the same scale and garments to prevent error. Consult physician for weight loss >1 kg/day.
- Observe for indications of dehydration (e.g., poor skin turgor, delayed capillary refill, weak/thready pulse, dry mucous membranes, hypotension).
- Monitor hemodynamic status, including CVP, MAP, PAP, and PCWP, if available.
- Monitor laboratory studies, including serum sodium, serum and urine osmolality, and urine specific gravity; report significant findings to physician. Normal values are as follows: serum sodium 137-147 mEq/L, serum osmolality 275-300 mOsm/kg, urine osmolality 300-900 mOsm/24 h, and urine specific gravity 1.010-1.030. Monitor urine specific gravity qh to evaluate response to therapy. Patients may be allowed to develop hypotonic polyuria between doses of vasopressin to demonstrate persistence of DI when transient or triphasic DI is suspected.
- Instruct patients with permanent DI to wear a medical-alert bracelet with diabetes *insipidus* noted. Immediate family members should be familiar with the patient's current treatment plan in case they are contacted in an emergency.

NIC Fluid/Electrolyte Management; Fluid Monitoring; Hypovolemia Management;

Intravenous (IV) Therapy; Invasive Hemodynamic Monitoring; Electrolyte Management: Hypernatremia

Decreased adaptive capacity: intracranial, related to interruption of blood flow secondary to cerebral edema or intracranial bleeding after transsphenoidal hypophysectomy

Desired outcomes: Within 24 h after initiating treatment, patient has adequate intracranial adaptive capacity as evidenced by ability to verbalize orientation to time, place, and person; respiratory rate (RR) 12-20 breaths/min with a normal pattern and depth (eupnea); equal and normoreactive pupils; and bilaterally equal motor strength and tone that are normal for patient. Patient verbalizes understanding of the importance of avoiding Valsalva-type activities.

- Elevate HOB 30 degrees to minimize intracranial pressure (ICP).
- Perform checks of neurostatus at frequent intervals to assess for signs of IICP, including changes in LOC, respiratory rate or rhythm, and pupillary reflexes (see Table 6-3, p. 429).
- Teach patient to avoid coughing, sneezing, straining, bending, or other Valsalva-type activities because they can increase stress on the operative site, increase ICP, and cause cerebrospinal fluid (CSF) leak. Explain to patient that if coughing or sneezing becomes necessary, it should be done with the mouth open to minimize the increase in ICP. As appropriate, administer cathartics, stool softeners, or antiemetics to minimize straining and nausea.
- If IICP develops, implement the interventions described in Table 2-5, p. 131; see also "Care of the Patient After Intracranial Surgery," p. 437.

NIC Neurologic Monitoring; Cerebral Edema Management; Intracranial Pressure (ICP) Monitoring

Risk for infection related to inadequate primary defenses secondary to incisional opening into sella turcica

Desired outcomes: Patient is free of infection as evidenced by normothermia; verbalization of orientation to time, place, and person; and absence of the indicators of CSF leakage or nuchal rigidity.

- Inspect nasal packing at frequent intervals for frank bleeding or evidence of CSF (nonsanguineous) leak. Using a glucose reagent stick, test all clear drainage for the presence of glucose to determine if it is CSF. Because a CSF leak would signal a serious breach in cranial integrity, elevate the HOB to minimize the chance of bacterial migration into the brain. Consult physician promptly for suspected CSF leaks.
- Be alert to indicators of infection, including elevated temperature, nuchal rigidity, and altered LOC.
- To prevent injury to operative site, which could lead to infection, teach patient to avoid brushing teeth until instructed to do so by physician. Provide mouthwash and sponge-tipped applicators for oral hygiene.
- For additional information, see "Care of the Patient After Intracranial Surgery," p. 437.

NIC Incision Site Care; Infection protection; Neurologic Monitoring

Knowledge deficit: management of permanent DI; care after transsphenoidal hypophysectomy

Desired outcome: Before discharge from ICU, patient verbalizes understanding of the basics of DI management and care after transsphenoidal hypophysectomy, if appropriate.

- Teach patient appropriate administration of exogenous vasopressin and its side effects.
- Explain the importance of weighing daily at the same time of day and in the same clothing and reporting weight gains or losses to physician.
- Demonstrate the method for accurate measurement of urine specific gravity and the importance of keeping accurate records of test results.
- Teach the indicators that necessitate medical attention, including signs and symptoms of dehydration and water intoxication.

- Explain the importance of obtaining a medical-alert bracelet and identification (ID) card.
- Stress the importance of continued medical follow-up.

Care after transsphenoidal hypophysectomy
- Explain the necessity for lifetime exogenous hormone replacement if the anterior pituitary gland was removed or damaged.
- If the entire pituitary gland was removed, teach the indicators of hormone replacement excess or deficiency.
  - ☐ *Adrenal hormone excess:* weight gain, moon face, easy bruising, fatigue, polyuria, polydipsia.
  - ☐ *Adrenal hormone deficiency:* weight loss, easy fatigability, abdominal pain, excess pigmentation.
  - ☐ *Thyroid hormone excess:* heat intolerance, irritability, tachycardia, weight loss, diaphoresis.
  - ☐ *Thyroid hormone deficiency:* bradycardia, cold intolerance, weight gain, slowed mentation.
  - ☐ *Androgen replacement deficiency:* some degree of sexual dysfunction, ranging from menstrual irregularities to infertility and impotence.
- For patients with permanent need for hormone replacement, explain the method for obtaining a medical-alert bracelet and ID card outlining diagnosis and appropriate treatment in the event of an emergency.

NIC Teaching: Disease Process; Teaching: Prescribed Medication; Emotional Support

ADDITIONAL NURSING DIAGNOSES

Also see "Diabetic Ketoacidosis" for **Risk for injury,** p. 475. Also see "Hyperglycemic Hyperosmolar Nonketotic Syndrome," p. 478, for **Altered peripheral tissue perfusion.** As appropriate, see "Psychosocial Support," p. 83, and "Psychosocial Support for the Patient's Family and Significant Others," p. 95.

Syndrome of inappropriate antidiuretic hormone

PATHOPHYSIOLOGY

Syndrome of inappropriate antidiuretic hormone (SIADH) develops as a result of excessive levels of circulating ADH. The causes of SIADH typically fall into one of three categories: (1) excessive production or release of ADH secondary to CNS disorders or increased intracranial pressure; (2) respiratory disorders, which increase the release of ADH by an unknown mechanism; or (3) ectopic ADH secretion by malignant tumors, particularly tumors of the lung. In addition, it can occur with the general stress of surgery, positive pressure ventilation, or from a wide variety of medications.

In the presence of increased ADH, water that normally would be excreted in the urine is inappropriately reabsorbed and returned to the circulation, diluting the serum sodium and decreasing serum osmolality. Fluid volume expansion increases glomerular filtration and decreases the release of aldosterone, both of which act to increase urinary excretion of sodium, further reducing the serum sodium level. As the sodium level decreases, an osmotic gradient is created that causes water to move into the cells. Increased intracellular fluid in the brain can result in cerebral edema with altered neurologic function and, ultimately, death if the condition is not treated.

ASSESSMENT

History and risk factors: Cancer of the lung, pancreas, duodenum, and prostate can secrete a biologically active form of ADH. Other common causes include head trauma, brain tumor, hemorrhage, and infection. Positive pressure ventilation, physiologic stress, chronic metabolic illness, pulmonary infections (e.g., tuberculosis, pneumonia, pulmonary abscess), and medications (e.g., thiazide and thiazide-like diuretics, chlorpropamide, carbamazepine, antipsychotics, antidepressants, NSAIDs) have been linked with SIADH.

Clinical presentation: Decreased urine output with inappropriately concentrated urine. Signs of water intoxication may appear, including lethargy, headache, declining LOC, seizures, nausea, vomiting, and eventually coma.

Despite retention of excess water, edema rarely develops. A reduction in the stimulus to the release of aldosterone minimizes fluid volume expansion and edema formation. In addition, retained water expands both the extracellular and intracellular fluid compartments. The primary symptoms of SIADH are neurologic secondary to water movement into the brain cells. The severity of symptoms depends on the degree of cerebral overhydration and how quickly hyponatremia develops. Hyponatremia that develops quickly (<48 h) is more likely to be associated with symptoms than hyponatremia that develops chronically.

Physical assessment: Weight gain without edema; slightly elevated BP.

Monitoring parameters: CVP >6 mm Hg; PAWP >12 mm Hg in the absence of underlying cardiac or pulmonary disease; and urine output <0.5 ml/kg/h with specific gravity >1.030 in the presence of adequate fluid intake.

DIAGNOSTIC TESTS

Serum sodium level: Decreased to <130 mEq/L.

Plasma osmolality: Decreased to <275 mOsm/kg.

Urine osmolality: Elevated disproportionately in relation to plasma osmolality.

Urine sodium level: Increased to >40 mEq/L.

Urine specific gravity: >1.030.

Plasma ADH level: Elevated.

COLLABORATIVE MANAGEMENT

Fluid restriction: Based on urine output. Usually fluids are limited to 1000 ml/day. Once the serum sodium level is normal, fluids may be increased to urine output plus estimated insensible losses.

Isotonic (0.9%) or hypertonic (3%) sodium chloride: May be given if the patient has severe hyponatremia. Supplemental sodium solutions may be administered with IV furosemide (Lasix) or osmotic diuretics, such as mannitol, to promote water excretion.

Demeclocycline (Declomycin) or lithium: Inhibits action of ADH on the distal renal tubules to promote water excretion.

Treatment of underlying cause: SIADH associated with surgery, trauma, or drugs usually is temporary and self-limiting. In chronic situations the focus will be on treating the underlying cause, which may include cancer, surgery, radiation, or chemotherapy.

NURSING DIAGNOSES AND INTERVENTIONS

Risk for injury related to hyponatremia; induced alteration in neurologic function; too-rapid correction of hyponatremia

Desired outcomes: Within 48 h of initiating treatment, patient verbalizes orientation to time, place, and person. CVP, PAWP, and BP are within patient's normal range. Patient remains free of signs of injury.

- Assess LOC, VS, hemodynamic measurements, and I&O hourly; weigh patient daily. Be alert to decreasing LOC; elevated BP, CVP, and PAWP; urine output <0.5 ml/kg/h; and weight gain. Promptly consult physician for significant findings or changes.
- Obtain laboratory specimens for analysis of altered sodium levels (e.g., serum and urine sodium, serum and urine osmolality, urine specific gravity)

as appropriate. Be alert to decreased serum sodium and plasma osmolality, urine osmolality elevated disproportionately in relation to plasma osmolality, and increased urine sodium. Normal values are as follows: urine specific gravity 1.010-1.030, serum sodium 137-147 mEq/L, urine osmolality 300-1090 mOsm/kg, and serum osmolality 275-300 mOsm/kg. Consult physician for significant findings.

- Maintain fluid restriction as appropriate. Explain necessity of this treatment to patient and significant others. Do not keep water or ice chips at the bedside. Ensure precise delivery of fluid administered intravenously by using a monitoring device.

- Elevate HOB no more than 10-20 degrees to promote venous return and thus reduce ADH release. Decreased venous return is a stimulus to the release of ADH.

- Administer demeclocycline, lithium, and furosemide as prescribed; carefully observe and document patient's response.

- Administer hypertonic sodium chloride as prescribed. Rate of administration usually is based on serial serum sodium levels. To minimize the risk of too-rapid correction of hyponatremia, ensure that laboratory specimens are drawn on time. *Serum sodium should not increase more than 12 mEq/L in 24 h because of the risk of neurologic damage (central pontine myelinolysis), particularly if the hyponatremia developed chronically.* Monitor for indications of fluid overload (e.g., crackles, elevated CVP or PCWP, edema) as appropriate. Consult physician promptly for significant findings.

- Institute seizure precautions. These include padded side rails, supplemental oxygen, bite block, and oral airway at the bedside, as well as side rails up at all times when staff member is not present.

- Provide bedside care in a calm, unhurried manner to help minimize stress and pain, both of which will increase ADH release.

NIC Fluid/Electrolyte Management; Neurologic Monitoring; Electrolyte Management: Hyponatremia; Seizure Precautions

ADDITIONAL NURSING DIAGNOSES
See also "Hyponatremia" for **Altered protection,** p. 644.

Acute adrenal insufficiency

PATHOPHYSIOLOGY
Adrenal insufficiency (decreased production of adrenocortical hormones) occurs as a result of either dysfunction of the adrenal glands (primary) or inadequate stimulation of the adrenal glands by the anterior pituitary (secondary). Conditions associated with primary adrenal insufficiency include autoimmune disease, infection, bilateral adrenal hemorrhage, bilateral adrenalectomy, tumor invasion, and enzymatic deficiencies. A decrease in the production of adrenocortical hormones (both glucocorticoids and mineralocorticoids) caused by a reduction in functioning adrenal tissue is also termed *Addison disease.* Secondary adrenal insufficiency is associated with exogenous steroid administration and destruction of the pituitary gland by tumors, infarcts, trauma, surgery, or infection. Mineralocorticoid release is maintained in secondary adrenal insufficiency, since it depends on the action of angiotensin II rather than pituitary release of adrenocorticotropic hormone (ACTH).

Acute adrenal insufficiency (addisonian crisis) is a life-threatening condition characterized by severe fluid and electrolyte imbalances related to both mineralocorticoid and glucocorticoid deficiencies. Mineralocorticoid (aldosterone) deficiency results in large urinary losses of sodium and water with the development of hyponatremia and hypovolemia. In addition, hyperkalemia and metabolic acidosis can develop because of decreased urinary excretion of potassium and hydrogen. Glucocorticoid (cortisol) deficiency intensifies the clinical effects of hypovolemia by causing a decrease in vascular tone and decreased vascular response to catecholamines (epinephrine and norepinephrine). Cortisol depletion also may cause hypoglycemia as a result of the body's inability to maintain blood glucose levels in the fasting state. Severe hypotension, shock, and eventually death will occur without adequate parenteral adrenocortical hormone and fluid replacement. In patients with chronic insufficiency, acute crises may be prevented by tripling replacement hormone doses during periods of stress.

ASSESSMENT

History and risk factors: Addisonian crisis may be precipitated by any extreme emotional or physiologic stressor, at which time the need for adrenal hormones is increased dramatically. Patients who take exogenous steroids are also at risk if physiologic demands increase or doses are withdrawn abruptly. Addisonian crisis is also a potential complication of adrenalectomy or hypophysectomy. It also may develop with sepsis and human immunodeficiency virus (HIV) disease.

Clinical presentation: Hypotension (particularly postural), tachycardia, confusion, weakness, nausea, abdominal pain, hyperthermia (in some individuals).

Physical assessment: Orthostatic hypotension, poor skin turgor, sunken and soft eyeballs, muscle weakness, weight loss. Patients with primary adrenal insufficiency may have a bronze hue to the skin secondary to excess production of ACTH.

ECG findings: Signs of hyperkalemia: peaked T waves, widening QRS complex, lengthened PR interval, and flattened to absent P wave. As hyperkalemia worsens, these signs progress and may result in asystole.

DIAGNOSTIC TESTS

Random serum cortisol levels: Decreased.

Corticotropin stimulation test: Adrenal function is considered abnormal if the plasma cortisol level is <18 µg/dl after an injection of synthetic ACTH (cosyntropin).

Serum sodium levels: Decreased to <137 mEq/L.

Serum aldosterone levels: Depressed in primary Addison disease.

Serum potassium levels: Increased to >5 mEq/L initially; may decrease dramatically with treatment.

Fasting blood glucose levels: Decreased to <80 mg/dl.

BUN and serum creatinine: Often increased secondary to renal hypoperfusion.

COLLABORATIVE MANAGEMENT

Glucocorticoid replacement: The crisis state requires supraphysiologic doses. An immediate IV bolus of hydrocortisone usually is administered, followed by repeat doses as needed q6-8h or by continuous infusion. Emergency mineralocorticoid replacement (fludrocortisone) usually is unnecessary because of the mineralocorticoid effects of hydrocortisone.

IV fluids: Rapid volume restoration is essential. Initially, D_5NS is the fluid of choice. Typically, 1 L of fluid is given in 1 h, followed by an additional 1-2 L over the next 6-8 h as needed. Volume expanders may be used if hypotension persists.

IV glucose: Supplemental glucose usually is included in the IV fluids to correct the hypoglycemia.

Supplemental sodium: Usually provided in the form of normal saline during volume replacement.

Insertion of flow-directed pulmonary artery catheter: To assess volume status on a continuous basis.

Vasopressors: May be used if the patient does not respond to the initial therapy (see Appendix 7). Because these patients have decreased response to catecholamines, vasopressors and inotropic agents will be less effective than they would be in normal individuals.

Treatment of underlying cause.

NURSING DIAGNOSES AND INTERVENTIONS

Fluid volume deficit related to failure of regulatory mechanisms secondary to impaired secretion of aldosterone, causing increased sodium excretion with resultant diuresis

Desired outcome: Within 8 h of initiating treatment, patient is normovolemic as evidenced by BP within patient's normal range; HR 60-100 bpm; RR 12-20 breaths/min with normal pattern and depth (eupnea); CVP 2-6 mm Hg; PAWP 6-12 mm Hg; normal sinus rhythm on ECG; and orientation to time, place, and person.

- Monitor VS and hemodynamic measurements q15min until they have been stable for 1 h. Consult physician promptly for BP <90/60 mm Hg, HR >120 bpm, CVP <2 mm Hg, and PAWP <6 mm Hg.
- Monitor patient at frequent intervals for evidence of hypotension. Measure BP and HR with patient reclining and then sitting. A drop of ≥20 mm Hg or an increase in HR >20 bpm and lasting for more than 3 min after changing position indicates mild to moderate dehydration.
- Administer IV fluids as prescribed to replace extracellular fluid volume. Initially, rapid fluid replacement is essential.
- Maintain accurate I&O record. Weigh patient daily at the same time of day with the patient wearing the same clothing and using the same scale.
- Monitor for manifestations of electrolyte imbalance. Imbalances associated with adrenal insufficiency include:
  ☐ *Hyponatremia:* headache, malaise, muscle weakness, abdominal cramps.
  ☐ *Hyperkalemia:* lethargy, nausea, hyperactive bowel sounds with diarrhea, numbness or tingling in extremities, muscle weakness.
- Monitor patient continuously on cardiac monitor; observe for ECG changes typical of hyperkalemia (see "ECG Findings," p. 652).
- Monitor laboratory test results for abnormalities. With appropriate treatment, serum sodium levels should rise to normal and serum potassium levels should fall to normal. Normal values are: serum sodium 137-147 mEq/L; serum potassium 3.5-5.0 mEq/L. Prevent rapid correction or overcorrection of hyponatremia. Serum sodium levels should not increase more than 12 mEq/L during the first 24 h of treatment because of the risk of neurologic damage.
- Assess patient's LOC and respiratory status at frequent intervals. Institute safety measures as indicated. Reorient and reassure patient as needed.
- Encourage oral fluid intake as patient's condition stabilizes. Add sodium-rich foods (see Table 10-11, p. 642) as tolerated. Begin oral glucocorticoid replacement therapy as prescribed.
- Consult physician if sign and symptoms of fluid and/or electrolyte imbalance persist or worsen.

NIC Fluid Monitoring; Neurologic Monitoring; Hypovolemia Management; Electrolyte Management: Hyponatremia; Electrolyte Management: Hyperkalemia

Risk for injury related to potential for acute regulatory dysfunction (cortisol and aldosterone deficiency) secondary to increased psychologic, emotional, or physical stressors with increased hormonal demand and inadequate adrenal reserves

Desired outcomes: Patient verbalizes orientation to time, place, and person and has stable weight, urine output <80-125 ml/h, HR 60-100 bpm, BP within patient's normal range, and normothermia.

- Monitor for signs of increasing crisis: urinary output increased from usual amount, changes in LOC, orthostatic hypotension, nausea, vomiting, and tachycardia. Consult physician promptly for any of these findings.
- Provide a quiet environment to reduce external stimuli and stress. Transfer patient to private room if possible.

- Adjust lighting to meet needs of individual activities, avoiding direct light in the eyes.
- Control or prevent undesirable or excessive noise when possible.
- Monitor patient for hyperthermia. Maintain a cool environmental temperature. As prescribed, use tepid baths, antipyretics, and cooling blankets as needed to reduce body temperature.
- Prevent unnecessary interruptions, and allow for rest periods. Assist patient with care, and provide 90-min periods of uninterrupted rest as often as possible. Speak softly and reassuringly to patient.
- Limit the number of visitors and the length of time they spend with patient. Caution visitors not to discuss stress-provoking topics with patient but, rather, to speak softly and reassuringly.
- Maintain strict environmental asepsis, and monitor patient carefully for signs of infection. Avoid exposing patient to staff members or visitors who have colds or infections.

NIC Fluid Monitoring; Environmental Management; Infection Protection

Knowledge deficit: prevention of acute adrenal insufficiency in patients with chronic adrenal insufficiency or steroid therapy

Desired outcome: Before discharge from ICU, patient verbalizes understanding of factors that increase the risk of adrenal crisis, how to avoid adrenal crisis, precautions that must be taken, and when to notify physician.

- Teach patient about prescribed medications, including purpose, dosage, route of administration, and potential side effects (Table 7-3). Medication

---

T A B L E 7 - 3   Patient and Family Education Concerning Glucocorticoid and Mineralocorticoid Replacement

Glucocorticoids (e.g., cortisone acetate, prednisone)
- Take medication in a diurnal pattern to mimic normal secretion (i.e., two thirds of dose in the morning and one third of dose in the afternoon).
- Take steroids with food to decrease gastric irritation.
- Weigh self regularly, and report to physician gains of >2 lb/wk.
- Avoid exposure to infection, and be alert to indicators of infection (e.g., fever, nausea, diarrhea, malaise).
- Contact physician promptly during periods of physical or emotional stress; dosages will require adjustment at these times.
- Indicators of overreplacement: weight gain (moon face, truncal obesity); edema; thin, fragile skin (striae, easy bruising); slow wound healing; chronic fatigue; emotional lability.
- Indicators of underreplacement: weight loss; hyperpigmentation; skin creases; anorexia; nausea; abdominal discomfort; chronic fatigue; depression; irritability.

Mineralocorticoids (e.g., fludrocortisone, desoxycorticosterone acetate)
- As prescribed, modify diet with liberal amounts of sodium (see Table 10-11, p. 642), protein, and carbohydrates.
- Weigh self regularly, and report to physician sudden gains or losses >2 lb/wk.
- Contact physician promptly during periods of physical or emotional stress; dosages will require adjustment at these times.
- Indicators of overreplacement: edema, muscle weakness, hypertension.
- Indicators of underreplacement: excessive urination, weight loss, decreased skin turgor.

administration should mimic normal diurnal pattern of plasma cortisol levels (e.g., two thirds in the morning and one third in late afternoon).

- Provide dietary instruction: dietary sodium and potassium may need to be adjusted on the basis of the patient's clinical condition and drug therapy (see discussions of sodium and potassium in "Fluid and Electrolyte Disturbances," p. 636).
- Explain the importance of controlling stress, both emotional and physiologic, which increases adrenal demand. Teach patient to seek medical intervention during times of increased stress (e.g., fever, infection), inasmuch as medication dosages may need to be increased.
- Teach indicators of overreplacement and underreplacement of steroids, which require prompt medical attention (see Table 7-3).
- Stress the importance of never abruptly discontinuing use of any steroid preparation. Use must be tapered to avoid precipitation of crisis.
- Remind patient of the importance of continued medical follow-up.
- Explain the procedure for obtaining a medical-alert bracelet or card identifying patient's diagnosis.

NIC Teaching: Disease Process; Teaching: Prescribed Medication; Emotional Support

ADDITIONAL NURSING DIAGNOSES

See also "Diabetic Ketoacidosis" for **Risk for infection,** p. 475, and **Risk for injury,** p. 475. See "Hyperglycemic Hyperosmolar Nonketotic Syndrome" for **Altered peripheral tissue perfusion,** p. 478. For other nursing diagnoses and interventions, see "Psychosocial Support," p. 83, and "Psychosocial Support for the Patient's Family and Significant Others," p. 95.

Bibliography

Bell DS, Alele J: Diabetic ketoacidosis: why early detection and aggressive treatment are crucial, *Postgrad Med* 101(4):193-198, 203-204, 1997.

Bianco CM: Diabetes insipidus, *Am J Nurs* 96(8):30-31, 1996.

Chan TYK: Drug-induced syndrome of inappropriate antidiuretic hormone secretion: causes, diagnosis and management, *Drugs Aging* 11(1):27-44, 1997.

Fried LF, Palevsky PM: Hyponatremia and hypernatremia, *Med Clin North Am* 81(3):585-609, 1997.

Goldberg RB, Machado R: Atypical ketoacidosis in type 2 diabetes, *Hosp Pract* 33(3):105-108, 111-112, 117-118, 1998.

Gross P et al: The treatment of severe hyponatremia, *Kidney Int* 53(64):S6-S11, 1998.

Gonzalez-Campoy JM, Robertson RP: Diabetic ketoacidosis and hyperosmolar nonketotic state: gaining control over extreme hyperglycemic complications, *Postgrad Med* 99(6):143-152, 1996.

Halperin ML, Goldstein MB: *Fluid, electrolyte and acid-base physiology*, ed 3, Philadelphia, 1999, Saunders.

Horne MM, Heitz UE, Swearingen PL: *Pocket guide to fluids and electrolytes,* ed 3, St Louis, 1997, Mosby.

Kokko JP, Tannen RL: *Fluids and electrolytes,* ed 3, Philadelphia, 1996, Saunders.

Lauro R, Karp BI: Myelinolysis after correction of hyponatremia, *Ann Intern Med* 126(1):57-62, 1997.

Malcoff CD, Carey RM: Adrenal insufficiency, *Curr Ther Endocrinol Metab* 6:142-147, 1997.

Matz R: Managing fluid abnormalities in uncontrolled diabetes mellitus, *J Crit Ill* 12(5):278-282, 1997.

Olkers W: Adrenal insufficiency, *N Engl J Med* 335(16):1206-1212, 1996.

Schrier RW, editor: *Renal and electrolyte disorders*, ed 5, Philadelphia, 1997, Lippincott-Raven.

Singer I, Oster JR, Fishman LM: The management of diabetes insipidus in adults, *Arch Intern Med* 157(12):1293-1301, 1997.

Umpierrez GE, Khajavi M, Kitabchi AE: Review: diabetic ketoacidosis and hyperglycemic hyperosmolar nonketotic syndrome, *Am J Med Sci* 311(5): 225-233, 1996.

Verbalis JG: Adaption to acute and chronic hyponatremia: implications for symptomatology, diagnosis, and therapy, *Semin Nephrol* 18(1):3-19, 1998.

CHAPTER 8

Gastrointestinal Dysfunctions

Gastroesophageal varices

PATHOPHYSIOLOGY

Liver disease (e.g., cirrhosis) or anatomic problems within the hepatic portal system increase portal pressure, causing gastroesophageal veins to become tortuous, dilated, and engorged with blood. As resistance to blood flow in the portal venous system increases, portosystemic collateral channels open and divert portal blood into the systemic circulation. These collaterals manifest as varicosities at the lower end of the esophagus, rectum, umbilicus, and ovaries, and sometimes in the small bowel or stomal sites. As hepatic portal pressure increases, veins dilate beneath the vascular mucosa. Eventually, the overlying submucosa retreats, leaving the veins unprotected. Further pressure increases and/or reflux of digestive juices from the stomach causes erosion into the venous walls with subsequent rupture, hemorrhage, and hematemesis. Blood loss is influenced by severity of rupture in addition to exacerbating factors such as clotting disorders and thrombocytopenia. The risk of bleeding from varices increases with hepatic venous pressure gradients (HVPG) greater than 12 mm Hg. High morbidity and mortality are associated with variceal hemorrhage. As many as 50% of patients die from the first bleeding episode.

In Western countries the most common cause of portal hypertension is cirrhosis. Cirrhosis itself causes loss of hepatocytes, degeneration of the parenchyma, and swelling and eventually shrinkage of the liver into a hard, fibrotic mass. Life-supporting functions of the liver (detoxification, hormonal metabolism, vitamin absorption, and bilirubin metabolism) gradually decline as blood flow to the liver is shunted by collateral vessels and obstructed by increasing fibrosis.

Large portosystemic shunts result in complications, including hepatic encephalopathy, septicemia, and metabolic abnormalities. In addition, acute blood loss from variceal bleeding results in hypoxic damage to liver cells and may precipitate complications of hepatic insufficiency such as jaundice, ascites, and encephalopathy. Childs-Pugh classification scores assist in determining the mortality rate from esophageal varices. Respectively, Childs class A= 5%, class B= 25%, and class C= 50%. Variceal hemorrhage with subsequent liver failure is a leading cause of death in patients with liver cirrhosis and portal hypertension.

ASSESSMENT

History and risk factors: Excessive ethanol ingestion (averaging >60 g/day); previously diagnosed cirrhosis, hepatitis, parasitic infection, schistosomiasis, intraabdominal or biliary infection, biliary disease, traumatic portal vein injury, congenital liver disease, and tumor invasion. The following events may precipitate bleeding in patients with gastroesophageal varices: (1) insertion of a gastric tube, (2) coagulopathy and/or heparin therapy, (3) mechanical irritants (e.g., rough or unchewed food), (4) Valsalva maneuver, (5) vigorous coughing, (6) erosion of mucosa (e.g., erosive gastritis, esophagitis).

Clinical presentation: Massive, painless bleeding, possibly with signs of shock, is usually the first and most common presentation. The average amount of blood lost during a single bleeding episode is 10 units. Melena, with or without hematemesis, is another frequent occurrence. Acute gastritis, peptic ulcer disease, and Mallory-Weiss syndrome (see "Acute Gastrointestinal Bleeding," p. 541) may contribute to the usually massive blood loss. Rapid blood loss leads initially to thirst, dizziness, disorientation, and hypovolemic shock, and eventually to coma and death as the hemorrhage continues. High portal venous pressures with massive bleeding (40% of blood volume) result in death within 10-30 min.

Physical assessment: Hematemesis of frank red blood and/or old swallowed blood that resembles coffee grounds, along with cool, pale skin, syncope, vertigo, altered mental status, and restlessness, are readily apparent. Pale, dry oral mucosa, cracked lips, poor skin turgor, and "sunken-looking" eyeballs are further evidence of hemorrhage. Yellowing of the skin and sclera is associated with jaundice, which is frequently present. Mild to marked edema generally develops within hours of bleeding onset. This is the result of stimulation of the sympathetic nervous system and baroreceptors, which causes release of antidiuretic hormone (ADH) and results in sodium and water retention. Splenomegaly is commonly associated with portal hypertension. In persons with cirrhosis, the liver usually is small and firm. An enlarged and tender liver is associated with hepatic inflammation. Large hemorrhoids may be present on rectal examination, along with stool that contains occult or frank blood. If aspiration of gastric contents has occurred, coarse crackles and rhonchi may be auscultated.

Vital signs and hemodynamic measurements: Vital signs usually reflect a hypovolemic state: tachycardia, tachypnea, decreased BP with orthostasis. Hemodynamics reflect a hypovolemic or hyperdynamic state. In the presence of a hypovolemic state, central venous pressure (CVP), pulmonary artery pressure (PAP), and pulmonary artery wedge pressure (PAWP) are decreased. Cardiac output (CO) is variable, depending on adequacy of stroke volume and the presence of tachycardia. Systemic vascular resistance (SVR) is increased if sympathetic stimulation predominates, or it is decreased in association with a hyperdynamic state similar to systemic inflammatory response syndrome (SIRS). If hypovolemia is corrected, a hyperdynamic cardiovascular state is present. The CO is elevated, peripheral vascular resistance is lowered, pulses are bounding, and the extremities are warm and flushed.

DIAGNOSTIC TESTS

Hematologic tests: Hematocrit (Hct), hemoglobin (Hgb), and red blood cells (RBCs) will be decreased because of acute large blood volume loss and mild anemia associated with hypersplenism. If a slow bleed is present and equal amounts of plasma and cells are being lost, the Hct and Hgb may not show a decrease for 24 h. If bleeding continues without fluid replacement, lost volume is compensated for by shifting fluid from the intracellular space.

Reticulocyte counts increase as bone marrow increases production of immature RBCs to replace those lost. Initially, platelets increase as the body attempts to form clots. As platelets are depleted by continued bleeding, counts fall. Liver disease and alcoholism cause increases in mean corpuscular volume (MCV). When the MCV is increased, the RBC is said to be macrocytic and thus anemia may be termed *macrocytic* and *normochromic* (normal Hgb). Platelet and white blood cell (WBC) counts may be decreased initially because of splenic enlargement. Prothrombin time (PT) is prolonged as a result of coagulopathies in patients with hepatocellular disease. The clotting deficiency is usually unresponsive to vitamin K therapy.

Biochemical tests: An elevated blood urea nitrogen (BUN) is caused by elevated blood proteins from the digestion of blood in the gastrointestinal (GI) tract. Hypernatremia is the result of hypovolemia. Urine osmolality is increased because of ADH secretion, increased protein intake (from hemorrhaged blood in the gut), and cirrhosis. The severity of liver damage can be estimated by elevations of values in serum total bilirubin, decreases in albumin (see "Hepatic Failure", p. 503), and prolongation of PT.

Ammonia is an end product of protein metabolism and is formed from the action of bacteria on proteins in the intestines and from hydrolysis of glutamine in the kidneys. The liver normally removes most of the ammonia from the portal vein flow and converts it to urea for excretion by the kidneys. When the liver is not functioning properly and blood is shunted from the liver by collateral vessels, ammonia levels build. Large protein loads from gastrointestinal bleeding may result in greatly increased ammonia levels.

Note: A fasting venous blood sample for serum ammonia is obtained, placed on ice, and transported immediately to the laboratory to ensure accuracy of the test.

Blood alcohol: Ethyl alcohol levels may be tested on admission to distinguish acute intoxication from encephalopathy.

T A B L E 8 - 1   Nursing Care of the Patient Undergoing Esophagoscopy

Before procedure
- Explain procedure to patient and significant others.
- Maintain NPO status for 8 h before procedure.
- Administer premedication as prescribed, usually at a reduced dose if cirrhosis or hepatitis is present, and monitor for side-effects.
- Clear stomach of blood and gastric contents immediately before endoscope is passed.
- Verify patency of 2 large-bore (>16-gauge) IV catheters.

During procedure
- Keep patient in side-lying position to reduce the likelihood of aspiration.
- Have nasopharyngeal suction equipment as well as a crash cart readily available.

After procedure
- Maintain side-lying position until patient is fully alert to reduce the likelihood of aspiration.
- Ensure that 2-4 h after the procedure the gag reflex has returned.
- Note evidence of change in rate of hemorrhage.
- Monitor for: aspiration pneumonia (evidenced by difficulty breathing, diminished breath sounds, coarse crackles and rhonchi); cardiac dysrhythmias; perforation (evidenced by retrosternal pain, bleeding, fever, dysphagia); and cervical neck perforation (evidenced by crepitus, neck throat pain).

Occult blood tests: To test for blood in stool or gastric secretions. Occult blood may persist in the stool for as long as 3 wk after a significant GI bleed.
Esophagoscopy: Visualizes the esophagus and stomach directly via a fiberoptic esophagoscope. Varices in the esophagus and upper portion of the stomach are identified, and attempts are made to identify the exact source of bleeding. Variceal bleeding may be treated by endoscopic sclerotherapy during the endoscopic procedure (see "Collaborative Management," p, 497). Aspiration, cardiac dysrhythmias, and severe hemorrhage are serious complications of the procedure. Endotracheal intubation may be performed before the procedure to protect the airway. See Table 8-1 for nursing implications of esophagoscopy. If bleeding is more than 0.5 ml/min, visualization of the origin of the bleeding may be impossible. This is when selective angiography may be useful.
Angiographic studies: Angiographic studies (arteriography/radionuclide scanning) may localize acute bleeding rates as low as 0.1-0.2 ml/min. The most common procedure is portal venography by indirect angiography. The femoral artery is catheterized, and contrast material is injected into the splenic artery. Contrast material flows through the spleen into the splenic and portal veins. The procedure establishes patency of the portal vein and visualizes the portosystemic collateral vessels to determine cause and effective treatment for variceal bleeding. This procedure is used to establish portal venous anatomy before operations such as portal systemic shunt or hepatic transplantation. In patients with previously constructed surgical shunts, patency may be confirmed. See Table 8-2 for nursing implications of angiographic studies.

Hepatic vein wedge pressure (HVWP) is measured by introducing a double-lumen balloon catheter into the femoral vein and threading it into one

---

T A B L E 8 - 2   Nursing Care of the Patient Undergoing Angiographic Studies

Before procedure
- Explain procedure to patient and significant others.
- Maintain NPO status for 8 h before procedures.
- Verify patency of IV catheter.
- Note allergies to seafood, iodine, and contrast material.
- Administer sedative as prescribed, usually at a reduced dose if cirrhosis or hepatitis is present.

During procedure
- Assist radiology personnel with positioning and draping patient.
- Monitor vital signs q15min or more often for evidence of anaphylaxis or hemorrhagic shock.

After procedure
- Check vital signs q15min initially and q1-2h once patient's condition has stabilized.
- Maintain patient in supine position with affected leg straight.
- Check dressing often for signs of continued bleeding from puncture site.
- Keep pressure dressing and sandbag over puncture site for 6-8 h.
- Evaluate distal pulses and perfusion in affected extremity q1-2h for 8 h. Arterial thrombosis and large hematomas that compromise femoral blood flow may develop as a result of manipulation of the artery and clotting abnormalities associated with liver disease.
- Monitor urine output q1-2h and report volume <0.5 ml/kg/h.

of the hepatic veins. This is an accurate measurement of the liver's contribution to resistance in the portal system. Normal HVWP is 5-6 mm Hg; values of about 20 mm Hg are typical for patients with cirrhosis.

Direct access to the portal vein may be achieved through transhepatic portography. During this procedure varices may be obliterated by injection of thrombin or Gelfoam into veins that supply the varices. NOTE: Transhepatic portography involves a direct puncture through the liver and has many of the same risks as does liver biopsy. Patients returning from this procedure should be positioned on their right side and monitored closely. (See Table 8-7, p. 513).

Liver biopsy: See "Hepatic Failure," p. 512.

COLLABORATIVE MANAGEMENT

Stabilization of the bleeding varices is the immediate concern. The two priorities are restoring blood volume and assessing and monitoring the degree of vascular compromise. Once stabilized, short-term and long-term management of gastroesophageal variceal bleeding depends on the underlying cause of portal hypertension, the severity of the bleeding episode, previous bleeding episodes, and previous response to therapy. Preserving and optimizing liver function are especially important for patients with cirrhosis and underlying hepatocellular disease to reduce the risk of disabling encephalopathy.

Fluid resuscitation: Large-bore intravenous (IV) lines are necessary to infuse isotonic fluids until albumin, packed red cells, and fresh-frozen plasma are available. To monitor the progress of the resuscitation, a Foley catheter and central venous catheter (preferably a pulmonary artery catheter) should be placed. The central venous catheter will provide hemodynamic monitoring of vital signs (VS), CVP, PAWP, and other parameters essential to prevent hypovolemic shock while avoiding overtransfusion and associated cardiopulmonary problems. In addition, overtransfusion increases variceal pressure and triggers rebleeding.

D_5W, sodium chloride, and Ringer's lactate (RL) are used for initial resuscitation and volume replacement. Excessive use of saline infusions is avoided because sodium is retained and contributes to ascites. Ringer's lactate is not recommended for patients with significant liver dysfunction because the damaged liver may not be able to convert the lactate to bicarbonate. Serum lactate accumulates and contributes to metabolic acidosis. Packed red cells are transfused as soon as they are available to maintain an Hct of 28%-30%. This Hct should be higher in patients with an underlying cardiac condition to prevent the complications associated with cardiac ischemia. Platelets are given if the platelet count is markedly reduced or if spontaneous bleeding from sites other than varices occurs. Albumin is administered if the patient continues to be hypovolemic despite an Hct above 28% or if the patient is hypoalbuminemic. Serial Hct evaluations are necessary to estimate ongoing blood loss and need for RBC replacement.

Vasopressin (Pitressin):   Vasopressin is a naturally occurring, potent vasoconstrictor that is given IV at 0.1-0.4 U/min. Generally it is used until bleeding has been under control for at least 12 h. Vasopressin constricts the mesenteric, splenic, and hepatic arteriolar beds, causing a reduction of blood flow to the portal vein, which lowers portal venous pressure. Blood flow reduction is dose dependent. Vasopressin has systemic vasoconstrictive and cardiotoxic side effects. Nitroglycerin should be coadministered to potentiate the reduction in portal pressure while reducing the cardiac side effects (Table 8-3).

β-Adrenergic blocking agents: Propranolol (Inderal) and other beta (β)-adrenergic receptor blockers are used to decrease portal venous pressure by decreasing cardiac output, inhibiting renin release by the kidneys, and reducing sympathetic stimulation.

T A B L E   8 - 3   Adverse Effects of Vasopressin

Cardiovascular

    Increased cardiac afterload

    Baroreceptor-mediated bradycardia

    Reduced cardiac output

    Impaired cardiac contractility

    Dysrhythmias, including premature ventricular complex (PVC) and ventricular tachycardia

    Myocardial ischemia and infarction

    Potentially fatal dysrhythmias

Gastrointestinal

    Splanchnic vasoconstriction resulting in bowel ischemia, mesenteric infarction, and necrosis

    Increased gut motility resulting in abdominal cramps and diarrhea

Other

    Increased water reabsorption by the kidneys, resulting in antidiuresis, fluid overload, hyponatremia, and increasing ascites

    Stimulation of release of plasminogen activator and factor VIII

    Respiratory arrest

    Cerebral hemorrhage

    Limb ischemia

Somatostatin: A natural hormone that decreases splanchnic blood flow. It has been shown to be as effective as vasopressin with fewer and less serious side effects.

Gastric intubation: A nasogastric (NG) tube is placed in patients with GI bleeding to rule out a rapid bleed. This procedure may cause additional bleeding; therefore some practitioners will avoid NG tube insertion if the source of bleeding is known to be variceal. Lavage with iced water or saline is considered controversial. If lavage is used to clear blood from the stomach or to prepare for endoscopy/sclerotherapy, room temperature water/saline is recommended.

Endoscopic sclerotherapy: Works by injecting a sclerosing solution of sodium tetradecyl sulfate, morrhuate sodium, polidocanol, ethanolamine oleate, or ethanol into the varices. The solution causes inflammation with fibrosis and then obliteration of the varices. The risk of rebleeding is reduced in patients who undergo sclerotherapy, because of scar tissue formation. Sclerotherapy can be repeated if not initially successful. Varices at the same level of the esophagus cannot be injected at the same time because of circumferential scarring leading to esophageal stricture. This treatment is used both to control acute bleeding and to manage long-term bleeding via chronic, serial injections. Complications of varying degrees may occur (Table 8-4). Ulcer prophylaxis with antacids, H_2-receptor blockers, or sucralfate may be initiated.

Esophageal balloon tamponade: Used for severe upper GI bleeding if sclerotherapy or ligation plus intravenous vasopressin fail or if death is imminent from massive hemorrhage. The multilumen/multiballoon Sengstaken-Blakemore (S-B), Minnesota tube, or single-balloon Linton tube is inserted through a nostril or the mouth. It is passed into the stomach, where the gastric balloon is inflated with 250-300 cc of air. It is then pulled snug against the gastroesophageal junction. The esophageal balloon is inflated to 20-40 mm Hg. Esophageal balloon tamponade is useful for control of acute bleeding because

TABLE 8-4   Side-Effects and Complications of Esophageal Sclerotherapy

Anticipated mild side-effects
   Mild retrosternal pain
   Transient fever
   Diminished breath sounds
   Transient dysphagia
   Local ulceration

Serious side-effects/complications
   Bleeding from remaining varices, ulcers, gastric varix, or portal hypertensive gastropathy
   Stricture formation evidenced by prolonged dysphagia
   Perforation evidenced by bleeding, severe substernal pain, or fever
   Pulmonary problems including aspiration pneumonia, pleural effusion, mediastinitis, empyema, atelectasis
   Bronchoesophageal fistula
   Bacteremia/septicemia evidenced by fever, tachycardia, positive blood culture results
   Anaphylaxis
   Gastric wall necrosis
   Chylothorax, pneumothorax, or subcutaneous emphysema

---

direct, constant pressure is applied to the varices. Traction on the tubes is essential for effective tamponading by constant pressure on the varices. The balloon is not to be inflated more than 24 h. Esophageal necrosis, esophageal rupture, and tissue necrosis are some side-effects from tamponade. If bleeding resumes after deflation, surgery is indicated. See Table 8-5.

Transjugular intrahepatic portal-systemic shunts (TIPS/TIPSS):   This nonsurgical procedure is useful for patients with little hepatic function left, such as pretransplant patients. Ninety percent of TIPS procedures are successful. Variceal rebleeding rates are approximately 20%. One to three vascular stents are placed within the liver to connect the portal and hepatic vein. Blood from the spleen and bowels bypasses the diseased liver on its way back to the heart.

Surgical management: Emergency surgery for variceal bleeding is associated with a higher mortality than elective procedures, particularly in patients of Childs-Pugh class C. Ideally, it is best to stabilize the patient and control acute bleeding medically. Surgery can then be performed at a later date with less risk to the patient. Numerous surgical procedures exist that directly control bleeding or indirectly reduce variceal pressure, which will stop bleeding.

Surgeries that are a direct interruption of portosystemic blood flow are as follows: transabdominal, transthoracic, or transthoracoabdominal esophageal transection; gastric devascularization with splenectomy (Suguira procedure); gastric transection; or selective shunts (distal splenorenal and gastric venocaval). Nondecompressive surgery and portocaval shunts may reduce the risk of first bleed. Surgical procedures in many of these high-risk patients is not advisable because of the increased mortality. Many of these procedures bypass the liver completely, which allows for encephalopathy. Combination therapy may be a better option, particularly in those patients in Child-Pugh class C (see "Hepatic Failure," p. 503, for additional information on portal hypertension).

Other: Similar to sclerotherapy in its role in treatment of varices, cyanoacrylate is injected into a varix. The major concern of this treatment is the potential for toxicity.

T A B L E 8 - 5	**Nursing Implications for the Patient Undergoing Esophageal Balloon Tamponade**

Before insertion
- Check all lumens for patency.
- Inflate all balloons, and check for leaks.
- Label each lumen to prevent confusion and accidental deflation of gastric balloon after insertion.
- Have water-soluble lubricant, manometer, wall suction, large syringe, and traction pad or helmet readily available.
- Assist physician with emptying stomach of blood.
- Have Yankauer and endotracheal suction equipment at bedside for use in the event of vomiting.
- Schedule chest x-ray to confirm tube placement immediately after insertion.

After insertion
- Elevate head of bed 30-45 degrees to prevent esophageal reflux.
- Check tube traction and esophageal balloon pressure q2-4h.
- Ensure patency and low, intermittent suction of gastric and nasopharyngeal lumens.
- Perform oral care q2-4h.
- Ensure that scissors are readily available to transect the tube if respiratory distress occurs.

Banding of the varices is an alternative to sclerotherapy. Elastic O rings are used. Because of the large overtube needed to introduce the rings, patients require heavy sedation. This procedure is beneficial, particularly if the varices are large. Some surgeons prefer to use both sclerotherapy and banding together, thereby reducing the chance of rebleeding.

Orthotopic liver transplant has dramatically changed the 5-year survival rate from 20%-30% to 60%-70% for those patients in Childs-Pugh class C. Liver transplant is a last resort, and many patients undergo numerous other procedures first.

NURSING DIAGNOSIS AND INTERVENTIONS

Fluid volume deficit related to active loss of circulating blood volume secondary to variceal bleeding

Desired outcomes: Within 12 hours of this diagnosis, patient becomes normovolemic as evidenced by mean arterial pressure (MAP) >70 mm Hg; HR 60-100 beats per minute (bpm); brisk capillary refill (<2 sec); CVP 2-6 mm Hg; PAWP 6-12 mm Hg; cardiac index (CI) >3 $L/min/m^2$; urinary output >0.5 ml/kg/h; and is oriented to time, place, and person.

- Administer prescribed fluids at rapid rate (wide open for active, massive bleeding). See "Fluid Resuscitation," p. 496, for types of fluids indicated. Minimize IV infusion of sodium-containing solutions, which can contribute to fluid sequestration (ascites) and precipitate hepatorenal syndrome in susceptible patients (see "Hepatic Failure," p. 503).
- Monitor for distended neck veins, crackles in the lungs, peripheral edema, and weight gain. All of these symptoms signal fluid overload.
- Monitor BP q15min, or more frequently in the presence of brisk bleeding. Be alert to decreases in MAP >10 mm Hg less than baseline.
- Monitor HR, electrocardiogram (ECG), capillary refill, respiratory rate (RR), and cardiovascular status q15min, or more frequently in the presence of

active bleeding or if using vasopressin or similar agents. Be alert to increases in HR, delayed capillary refill, and changes in level of consciousness (LOC), which reflect hypovolemia. Be aware that an altered LOC can be caused by encephalopathy as well as by hypovolemia. Anticipate vasopressin-induced reflex bradycardia; consult physician if bradycardia is severe (HR <60 bpm) or compromises tissue perfusion.

- Measure central pressures and thermodilution CO/Cl q1-2h, or more frequently if the patient is unstable or receiving vasoactive agents. Be alert to low or decreasing CVP and PAWP. Assess for signs of overaggressive fluid resuscitation, including elevated CVP, PAP, and PAWP and aggravation of variceal bleeding in some patients. Anticipate compensatory increases in CO/Cl, with Cl usually >3. Monitor Svo_2 as available to evaluate adequacy of tissue oxygenation. Evaluate volume status by noting increases or decreases in PAWP values and urinary output.

- Measure urinary output hourly, as well as urine osmolality levels, color, quantity, and specific gravity of urine. Be alert to output <0.5 ml/kg/h for 2 consecutive hours. Anticipate decreased urinary output after initial dose of vasopressin. Expect diuresis after vasopressin has been discontinued.

- Monitor for physical indicators of hypovolemia, including cool extremities, capillary refill >2 sec, absent or decreased amplitude of distal pulses, and change in LOC.

- Measure and record all GI blood losses from hematemesis, hematochezia (red blood through rectum), and melena. Test all stools and gastric contents for occult blood.

- Administer vasopressin as prescribed. Ensure patency of IV catheter. Monitor for serious side effects such as bradycardia, ventricular irritability, chest pain, abdominal cramping, hyponatremia, water intoxication, and oliguria (see Table 8-3). Administer vasopressin concurrently with IV nitroglycerin to reduce adverse cardiovascular effects and improve efficacy. Consult physician and reduce rate of infusion in the presence of serious adverse effects.

- Be alert to adverse side effects of esophageal sclerotherapy: infection, pulmonary complications (i.e., Pao_2 <80 mm Hg, basilar crackles, diminished breath sounds), and esophageal ulceration (i.e., difficulty swallowing, pain, continued bleeding). Anticipate mild retrosternal pain and transient fever after the procedure.

- Avoid use of indwelling gastric tubes for routine gastric drainage because they irritate varices and may prolong or renew bleeding.

You may also wish to refer to the following interventions from the Nursing Interventions Classification (NIC):

NIC Bleeding Precautions; Blood Product Administration; Fluid/Electrolyte Management; Hypovolemia Management; Shock Management

Decreased cardiac output   related to altered rate or rhythm secondary to myocardial ischemia from prolonged, massive bleeding or vasopressin-induced coronary vasoconstriction; decreased preload secondary to acute blood loss; increased afterload secondary to vasoconstrictive effects of shock or vasopressin therapy

Desired outcome: Within 24 h of this diagnosis, patient's cardiac output is adequate as evidenced by normal sinus rhythm on ECG; CI within normal limits or increased (>3 L/min/m^2); MAP >70 mm Hg; and Svo_2 60%-80%.

- Monitor BP, HR, ECG, and PAP (see first four entries under preceding nursing diagnosis, **Fluid volume deficit**).

- Monitor arterial blood gas (ABG) values for evidence of hypoxemia. Be alert to and consult physician for Pao_2 <80 mm Hg. Administer oxygen if its need is indicated by ABG values. Place patient in semi-Fowler's position to optimize oxygenation; keep pulse oximeter on.

- Monitor Hct; consult physician for values <28%-30% (for each unit of packed RBCs transfused, Hct increases approximately 3%).
- Monitor patient for evidence of myocardial ischemia if Hgb is greatly decreased or if the patient is receiving vasopressin (see ninth entry in preceding nursing diagnosis). Observe ECG for ventricular dysrhythmias and ST-segment changes. Instruct patient to report chest discomfort promptly. Administer PRN nitrites as prescribed.
- Minimize patient's activity during acute bleeding episode to reduce myocardial oxygen demands. Explain and encourage adherence to total bed rest regimen. As available, monitor Svo_2 to evaluate adequacy of tissue oxygenation (see Table 1-16, p 36). Patients with baseline cardiopulmonary disease may need to be transfused to an Hct of 30% to prevent cardiac ischemia.
- Measure thermodilution CO q1-2h. Be aware that a "normal" CO may be a low value for the patient with a hyperdynamic circulatory state associated with cirrhosis. Maintain CI >3 L/min/m^2.
- Maintain MAP >70-80 mm Hg (see preceding nursing diagnosis, **Fluid volume deficit**) to promote adequate tissue perfusion. Avoid excessive fluids and hypervolemia, which could increase variceal bleeding. Supplemental O_2 via nasal cannula may be necessary to decrease or prevent ischemia in those patients with poor oxygenation.

NIC Cardiac Care: Acute; Hemodynamic Regulation; Oxygen Therapy; Shock Management; Invasive Hemodynamic Monitoring

Ineffective airway clearance related to tracheobronchial obstruction by esophageal balloon device; tracheobronchial obstruction by pharyngeal secretions above the inflated esophageal balloon device; perceptual/cognitive impairment secondary to encephalopathy

Desired outcome: Within 4 h of this diagnosis, patient's airway becomes clear as evidenced by auscultation of normal breath sounds, absence of adventitious sounds, and RR 12-20 breaths/min with normal depth and pattern (eupnea).

- Position patient in a side-lying position during vomiting episodes unless he or she is fully alert and is more comfortable in an upright position.
- As necessary, suction oropharynx with Yankauer or similar suction device to remove blood and secretions.
- Auscultate lung fields during and after vomiting episodes for presence of rhonchi, which can signal aspiration of gastric contents. Auscultation at frequent intervals is necessary while inflated esophageal balloon device is in place to ensure device is not partially occluding the airway.
- Provide oral care at frequent intervals to assist in mobilizing oropharyngeal secretions. A dilute solution of hydrogen peroxide and normal saline may be helpful in removing dried blood from the teeth and oral mucosa. Use saline to rinse hydrogen peroxide solution from patient's mouth.
- Monitor for early signs of respiratory failure: increasing RR, work of breathing (WOB), and $Paco_2$ and decreasing Spo_2 via continuous pulse oximetry and decreasing Pao_2.
- Implement the following interventions for patients with an S-B or similar tube:
  ☐ Consult physician regarding possibility of endotracheal (ET) intubation (before S-B tube insertion), particularly if decreased mental status, massive variceal bleed, or massive hematemesis is present.
  ☐ Verify proper tube placement by immediate chest x-ray.
  ☐ Be certain that oral secretions are suctioned from above the inflated esophageal balloon via a proximal tube or an additional lumen in the tube for this purpose. Label proximal tube or lumen with the warning "Do Not Irrigate."
  ☐ Ensure patency of gastric and esophageal drainage lumens. Irrigate gastric lumen q1-2h and as necessary to ensure patency.

☐ Be aware that proximal migration of the esophageal balloon or rupture of the gastric balloon may result in total airway obstruction. Auscultate breath sounds q1-2h. Keep a pair of scissors in an obvious place near the patient at all times to cut and immediately deflate all lumens of the S-B tube should respiratory distress occur.

☐ Check security of tape, tube connections, and traction initially and q2h. Firm traction is established by taping the tube to a helmet or a firm, padded retainer. The traction device should be designed so that it minimizes pressure to facial tissue and prevents tissue necrosis.

☐ Document quantity and characteristics of gastric drainage q4h.

NIC Aspiration Precautions; Artificial Airway Management; Oxygen Therapy; Respiratory Monitoring

Altered tissue perfusion (or risk for same):   gastrointestinal, related to interruption of venous and arterial blood flow secondary to pressure on esophageal tissue from balloon tamponade; hypovolemia secondary to variceal hemorrhage

Desired outcomes: Esophageal balloon pressure is maintained within pre-scribed range (usually 20-45 mm Hg). Patient has no symptoms of esophageal perforation as evidenced by BP within patient's normal range; HR 60-100 bpm; PAP >20/6; PAWP >6 mm Hg; SVR <1200 dynes/sec/cm^{-5}; CI >3 L/min/m^2; and absence of sudden substernal chest or back pain.

* Check and record the esophageal balloon pressure q2-4h. Maintain within prescribed range (usually 20-45 mm Hg). Release pressure at prescribed intervals.

* Carefully document date and time of balloon inflation and deflation. Tissue necrosis is likely to occur if balloons are left inflated for >24 h.

* After 24 h, assist physician in relieving traction and deflating the esopha-geal balloon. The tube remains in place with the gastric balloon inflated for the next 24 h, and the patient is closely monitored for rebleeding. If no further rebleeding occurs, the gastric balloon is deflated and the tube removed.

* Promptly consult physician for signs of esophageal perforation: sudden epigastric or substernal pain, back pain, shock state.

NIC Gastrointestinal Intubation; Shock Management

Impaired swallowing (or risk for same) related to mechanical obstruction secondary to edema or stricture formation after sclerotherapy; irritated esophageal tissue secondary to sclerotherapy or balloon tamponade

Desired outcome: By the time of discharge from ICU or hospital, patient swallows food and demonstrates ability to pass food through the lower esophagus into the stomach.

* After sclerotherapy treatments, evaluate patient for subjective complaints of difficulty in swallowing or pain during swallowing. Consult physician for significant findings.

* Plan a soft and bland diet, as tolerated by patient, which can be initiated 24 h after sclerotherapy.

* Instruct patient to avoid mechanically or chemically irritating foods. Initially, foods that are too hot, too cold, or too spicy should be avoided.

* Caution patient that certain foods or substances (e.g., alcohol) may cause a burning sensation during the swallowing process because of esophageal mucosal erosion. Instruct patient to avoid mechanical or chemical irritants.

NIC Swallowing Therapy; Nutrition Management

Ineffective thermoregulation (or risk for same) related to infusions of non-warmed blood, blood products, and intravenous fluids; too rapid fluid loss secondary to esophageal variceal bleeding

Desired outcomes: Patient will not drop body temperature more than 2° F per hour while fluid resuscitation is ongoing nor develop shock from body temperature being too low.

> **RESEARCH BRIEF 8-1** Since its introduction in 1988, transjugular
> intrahepatic portosystemic shunt (TIPS) has become the standard of care for
> many patients with variceal bleeding and refractory ascites. It also is used as a
> prophylactic treatment against rebleeding, a palliative treatment in liver cancer,
> and as a bridge to transplantation. It works by decompressing the portal system
> through creation of a side-to-side portosystemic anastomosis. Over the 11-year
> period since the introduction of TIPS, nine studies have been conducted using
> endoscopic procedures versus TIPS along with endoscopic treatment and rescue
> TIPS. Because of advanced stages of illness in patients, TIPS may be used to
> improve short-term quality of life versus long-term survival.

From Rossle M et al: The first decade of the transjugular intrahepatic portosystemic shunt
(TIPS): state of the art, *Liver* 18(2):73-89, 1998.

- Use blood warmer for all infusions, particularly blood and blood products,
  thus allowing body temperature to stay closer to normal.
- Institute active external rewarming measures: provide warm blankets, cover
  patient's head to decrease heat loss. Do not rewarm faster than 1° C per hour;
  otherwise rewarming shock may ensue.
- Monitor temperature q1-2h.

Knowledge deficit: lack of exposure to health care information or cognitive
limitation secondary to hepatic encephalopathy

Desired outcome: Within the 24-h period before hospital discharge, patient
states the signs and symptoms of variceal hemorrhage, the importance of
medical follow-ups, and the necessity of avoiding activities that increase the
risk of variceal bleeding.

- Teach patient the signs and symptoms of actual or impending hemorrhage,
  including nausea, dark stools, lightheadedness, vomiting of blood, or passing
  of frank blood in stools. Stress importance of seeking medical attention
  promptly if indicators of hemorrhage appear.
- Stress the importance of medical follow-up for management of variceal
  bleeding—either chronic sclerotherapy or shunt surgery.
- Teach patient about prescribed medications, including drug name, purpose,
  dosage, schedule, precautions, and potential side effects.
- Caution about the necessity of avoiding heavy lifting, straining, and other
  activities associated with the Valsalva maneuver. Stool softeners, increased
  oral fluids, and a bulking agent may be necessary daily to prevent straining
  at stool.
- Teach the importance of avoiding mechanically irritating foods, such as nuts,
  corn chips, and improperly chewed food. Stress importance of avoiding
  nonsteroidal antiinflammatory drugs (NSAIDs) and alcohol, which irritate
  the esophageal and gastric mucosa.

ADDITIONAL NURSING DIAGNOSES

If portal hypertension is caused by cirrhosis, refer to "Hepatic Failure" for
additional nursing diagnoses. For other nursing diagnoses and interventions, see
"Psychosocial Support," p. 83, and "Psychosocial Support for the Patient's
Family and Significant Others," p. 95.

Hepatic failure

PATHOPHYSIOLOGY

No matter its cause or duration of onset, hepatic failure causes necrosis of liver
parenchyma with accompanying sequelae. Worldwide, hepatitis B virus (with
or without accompanying hepatitis D) is still the most common cause of hepatic

failure, accounting for as many as 60% of all cases. Damage to the hepatocytes and liver structure can be acute or chronic. The amount of destruction to the liver varies with duration of illness, underlying etiology, preexisting conditions, treatment, and life-style changes (e.g., eliminating alcohol).

Fulminant hepatic failure: Fulminant hepatic failure (FHF) is divided into three types, based on length between appearance of jaundice to development of encephalopathy. The three types are *hyperacute, acute,* and *subacute.* Patients with hyperacute liver failure develop encephalopathy within 7-8 days from onset of jaundice. Most of these cases are caused by acetaminophen overdose, *Amanita* mushroom poisoning, or acute hepatitis A, B, or B with D. Progression from jaundice to encephalopathy occurs within 8-29 days in patients with acute liver failure. Causes of acute liver failure include hepatitis A or B and chronic excessive alcohol consumption. Hepatitis A infection is very hepatotoxic, and a large inoculation, especially in an immunocompromised host, leads to a higher mortality. Patients presenting with history of jaundice to encephalopathy of 5- to 26-wk duration frequently have hepatitis C as the major cause of liver failure. Many of them present to physicians or emergency departments when damage to the liver parenchyma is extensive, necessitating immediate orthotopic liver transplantation as the only life-saving treatment. In the absence of preexisting liver disease, FHF is generally reversible when the condition is treated promptly.

Chronic hepatic failure: Loss of hepatocytes, parenchyma, and impaired function of 6-mo or longer duration are hallmarks of chronic liver failure. Chronic liver disease is associated with widespread tissue necrosis, fibrosis, nodule formation in the liver, and eventual cirrhosis, ultimately resulting in hepatic failure. The usual causes of chronic liver failure are long-term alcohol ingestion, chronic viral hepatitis, prolonged cholestasis, and metabolic disorders.

Jaundice associated with hepatic failure occurs when the failing liver is unable to metabolize bilirubin. Metabolic encephalopathy, with varying degrees of consciousness and mental function, is attributed to ammonia toxicity and other metabolic derangements. Increased intracranial pressure (ICP) and cerebral edema are present with acute hepatic failure but usually are not seen in chronic hepatic failure. Cerebral edema is present in as many as 80% of patients with fulminant hepatic failure and is a frequent cause of death. In patients with cirrhosis, diversion of portal blood flow via large collateral vessels contributes to encephalopathy. Bleeding tendencies are caused by inadequate vitamin K absorption, failure of the liver to synthesize clotting factors or clear activated clotting factors, and thrombocytopenia. Infections, including sepsis, are common as a result of a generalized state of debilitation and failure of the liver to produce immune-related proteins and filter blood from the intestines.

Circulatory abnormalities often are present and include a hyperdynamic systemic circulation, with increased cardiac output and decreased vasomotor tone. Circulatory changes in the pulmonary system include dilation of the pulmonary vasculature and pulmonary arteriovenous shunting with ventilation-perfusion mismatch. Increased preglomerular vascular resistance reduces glomerular filtration and may result in functional renal failure (hepatorenal syndrome). Fluid retention and ascites are attributed to several factors, including (1) intrahepatic vascular obstruction with transudation of fluid into the peritoneum; (2) defective albumin synthesis, resulting in decreased colloid osmotic pressure with failure to retain intravascular fluid; and (3) disturbances of various hormones, including renin, aldosterone, and renal prostaglandins, resulting in sodium and water retention. Ascites and edema are associated with chronic and acute hepatic failure, although massive ascites usually is the result of cirrhosis.

Metabolic abnormalities include severe hypoglycemia because of a loss of hepatic glycogen stores and impaired degradation of insulin. Dilutional hyponatremia is caused by secondary hyperaldosteronism. Hypokalemia occurs frequently because of hyperaldosteronism, excessive renal losses prompted by alkalosis, and use of loop diuretics. Hypokalemia increases renal production of ammonia, which contributes to hepatic encephalopathy.

King's College Hospital criteria are widely used to assess prognosis of patients with fulminant hepatic failure. *For patients with FHF from acetaminophen:* predictors of a poor prognosis are a pH <7.30 (independent of encephalopathy grade) or a PT >100 sec (INR >6.5) with a serum creatinine >3.4 mg/dl in stage 3 or 4 of encephalopathy. *For patients with FHF from other causes:* accurate predictors of a poor outcome are a PT >100 sec (INR >6.5) regardless of the stage of encephalopathy or any three of the following regardless of encephalopathy grade: (1) age <10 or >40 years, (2) non-A, non-B hepatitis, (3) duration of jaundice before onset of encephalopathy of more than 7 days, (4) PT >50 sec (INR >3.5), or (5) serum bilirubin >17.5 mg/dl.

ASSESSMENT

History and risk factors: Worldwide, viral hepatitis accounts for the most cases of fulminant hepatic failure. Other causes include previous chronic hepatic or biliary diseases (including cirrhosis, hepatitis, cholecystitis) and metabolic liver diseases (Wilson disease, alpha$_1$-antitrypsin deficiency). History of chronic alcohol ingestion or history of taking alcohol with other medications (e.g., acetaminophen), previous blood transfusion, and exposure to hepatotoxic agents such as halothane, MAO inhibitors, herbal preparations, isoniazid, acetaminophen (>10 g), carbon tetrachloride, "ecstasy," and bacterial agents are additional factors. Underlying conditions such as heart disease (which may slowly be causing ischemic liver injury), chronic renal failure (possibly from chronic chemical exposure), and history of cancer elsewhere in the body (particularly breast, lymphoma) are contributing factors.

Clinical presentation: One or more of the following are present: cerebral dysfunction, jaundice, portal hypertension, variceal bleeding, elevated aminotransferases, elevated bilirubin, and increased prothrombin time. Ascites and edema are also common findings. In the later stages of hepatic failure, deep coma, seizures, and decerebrate posturing are possible. In the absence of jaundice, laboratory evaluation of PT and liver function tests are necessary to prevent a misdiagnosis of septicemia, drug overdose, or a psychotic episode.

Physical assessment: An element of hepatic encephalopathy must be present for the diagnosis of fulminant hepatic failure. Grade I encephalopathy includes lethargy, depression, slurred speech, subtle personality changes, euphoria, and sleep disturbances. In grade II, the patient experiences inappropriate behavior, disorientation, and restlessness and is more drowsy than in grade I. In grade III, patients experience somnolence but are arousable by gentle stimulation. They respond inappropriately to questions and may stare blankly as if catatonic. In grade IV, the patient is in a coma and may be able to respond to pain with deep stimulus. It is during grade III that patients are sedated, intubated, and placed on a ventilator to protect the airway and reduce the risk of cerebral edema.

Jaundice is usually present first in the sclera and, as bilirubin increases in the serum, generalized yellowing of the skin occurs. Persons with jaundice may have abdominal pain, nausea, vomiting, and change in stool and urine color. Fluid sequestration (noted as edema, ascites, and weight gain), weight loss, and muscle wasting are also seen in patients with chronic hepatic failure. Small, bright-red vascular spider veins (spider telangiectasis, spider angioma) are frequently found on the abdomen, face, neck, and arms of a patient with cirrhosis. In fulminant hepatic failure, they are usually absent. In chronic hepatic failure, asterixis, a flapping tremor of the hands when the arms are extended, may be present.

Fetor hepaticus is a foul-smelling, fecal-type odor detectable on a patient's breath with severe liver disease. Coagulopathies are responsible for multiple ecchymotic areas, purpura, and bleeding of the oral and nasal mucosa. Hyperdynamic circulatory changes are manifested by tachycardia, warm extremities, an active precordial impulse, and frequently a soft systolic ejection murmur. Fine crackles may be auscultated if pleural effusion, ascites, or pulmonary edema is present. Cyanosis and nail clubbing are seen in liver disease. These findings are consistent with pulmonary arteriovenous shunting and ventilation-perfusion mismatch. Dyspnea, decreased breath sounds, and dullness to percussion are associated with pulmonary edema or hydrothorax (excess fluid in the pleural cavity). In chronic liver disease, the liver is usually small and hard. Individuals with fulminant hepatic failure often have an enlarged, firm liver. Patients with chronic failure usually have an enlarged spleen. Distended abdomen with shifting dullness to percussion and positive fluid wave are present because of ascites. With severe ascites, hernias are common and the umbilicus frequently is everted. Usually, jugular vein distention is the result of increased right atrial pressure (RAP) caused by increased intrapleural pressures from diaphragmatic elevation. Hormonal changes that result in gynecomastia, testicular atrophy, and scant body hair are common in men with chronic hepatic disease.

Vital signs and hemodynamic monitoring: Elevated temperature caused by infection; normal to bounding pulses; low to normal BP; elevated cardiac output associated with decreased peripheral vascular resistance and expanded total blood volume. In the presence of tense ascites, which increases intraabdominal pressure, patient will exhibit impaired right ventricular filling with decreased stroke volume and decreased cardiac output. With massive variceal hemorrhage or late septic shock, pulses will be diminished and BP will be low, reflecting circulatory collapse.

DIAGNOSTIC TESTS

Virologic markers: See Table 8-6.

Liver-related serum biochemical tests

Alanine aminotransferase (ALT/serum glutamic pyruvic transaminase [SGPT]):   This enzyme is found primarily in the liver, and its measurement is used to monitor potentially hepatotoxic drugs, treatment for hepatitis, and progression of postnecrotic cirrhosis. It is useful in determining whether jaundice is caused by liver disease or has a hemolytic cause. Increased levels are found in hepatocellular injury, hepatitis, pancreatitis, obstructive jaundice/biliary obstruction, cirrhosis, metastatic liver tumor, liver congestion, and liver injury in myocardial infarction. Values over 300 IU/L are present with acute hepatic failure.

Aspartate aminotransferase (aspartate aminotransferase [AST]/serum glutamic-oxaloacetic acid transaminase [SGOT]):   This enzyme is present in organs with high metabolic activity such as the heart, liver, skeletal muscle, kidney, brain, pancreas, spleen, and lungs. Damage to the cells of these organs will cause a rise in the AST approximately 12 h after injury, and levels remain elevated for 4-6 days. In liver disease, elevations 10-100 times normal are not unusual, especially in acute hepatitis, active cirrhosis, and hepatic necrosis.

Alkaline phosphatase (ALP):   ALP is found in the liver, bone, placenta, plasma, intestine, and teeth. ALP is elevated to varying degrees in liver diseases such as obstructive jaundice, hepatocellular carcinoma, biliary cirrhosis, hepatitis, and cirrhosis of the liver.

Gamma-glutamyl transpeptidase (GGT/GGTP):   An enzyme present in liver, kidney, prostate, and spleen tissue. Elevations occur in metastasis to the liver, cirrhosis of the liver, and alcoholic liver disease.

Bilirubin: Total bilirubin is a by-product of hemolysis. Elevations occur with excessive RBC destruction or when the liver is unable to process normal amounts of bilirubin. Elevations occur in viral hepatitis and cirrhosis. Conjugated (direct) bilirubin circulates until it reaches the liver, joins glucuronide, and is excreted into the bile. Unconjugated (indirect) bilirubin is protein-bound. An elevation of both occurs in hepatitis, cirrhosis, and hepatic metastasis. A persistently elevated level of bilirubin is a poor prognostic sign.

Text continued on p. 512

TABLE 8-6 Types and Characteristics of Viral Hepatitis

	Hepatitis A	Hepatitis B	Hepatitis C	Hepatitis D	Hepatitis E	Hepatitis G
Likely modes of transmission	Enteric; fecal-oral. Usually through food or drinking contaminated water.	Contact with blood, body fluids (seminal fluid, vaginal secretions, saliva, open sores; found also in tears, urine, breast milk).	Contact with blood, serum, or body fluids, perinatal transmission, blood transfusions, sexual contact.	Similar to HBV; but an incomplete virus that can cause infection only in the presence of HBV.	Enteric; fecal-oral. Is foodborne or waterborne.	Contact with blood, body fluids, serum; possibly vectorborne.
Population most often affected	Varies, based on hygienic and sanitary conditions. Children, employees in daycare centers, international travelers, household contacts, sexual and possibly injection drug users.	Sexually active young adults, injection drug users, hemophiliacs, hemodialysis patients, prisoners or prison personnel, international travelers, those with multiple sexual partners.	Injection drug users, health care workers, transfusion recipients before 1991.	Infects individuals only with HBV infection, so risk factors same as HB.	After flooding in countries with poor sanitation. In 20% of pregnant women, infection is fatal. Countries with the most outbreaks: Nepal, North Africa, Mexico, and the former Soviet Union.	As for HBV and HCV.

Continued

HBV, Hepatitis B virus; *HCV,* hepatitis C virus.

TABLE 8-6 Types and Characteristics of Viral Hepatitis—cont'd

	Hepatitis A	Hepatitis B	Hepatitis C	Hepatitis D	Hepatitis E	Hepatitis G
Incubation	2-6 wk.	1-6 mo.	18-180 days (45-55 days average).	Variable; not well established.	Range is 15-65 days; average is 40 days.	Believed to be 2-6 wk.
Serum markers	Antibody to HAV (anti-HAV) of the IgM class in the acute state. When recovered, anti-HAV of the IgG class. If vaccinated, anti-HAV IgG is present in serum.	In the acute stage, anti-HB$_c$IgM, HB$_s$Ag, and HB$_e$Ag. In the chronic stage, anti-HB$_c$ Total HB$_s$Ag, HB$_e$Ag (during increased replication), HB$_e$Ab (during low replication). When recovered, anti-HB$_c$ Total will be present along with anti-HB$_s$Ag. If vaccinated, anti-HB$_s$Ag is present.	HCV antibody indicates exposure but does not differentiate between acute and chronic exposure. HCV quantitative RNA measures virus circulating in the serum and is a measure of treatment effectiveness.	RIA test for total antibody (anti-HD) to delta antigen. With this test, both IgG and IgM antibodies are measured. Delta antigen (HDAg), IgM antibody to HDAg (IgM anti-HD), and HDV-RNA.	Immune electron microscopy (IEM) identifies HEV antigen and antibody. IgG anti-HEV is detectable over years. IgM antibodies are usually detectable only up to 7 mo. HEV-RNA can be used to diagnose non-A, non-B, non-C cases.	HGV antibody.

	HAV	HBV	HCV	HDV	HEV	HGV
Measures for reducing exposure	Hand washing, good personal hygiene, sanitation, Standard Precautions (see Appendix 8).	Standard Precautions (see Appendix 8), hand washing, good personal hygiene, condom use, sterilization of nondisposable items, avoiding used needles, carefully handling needles and sharps, use of safety engineered devices.	As for HBV.	As for HBV.	As for HAV.	As for HBV.
Prophylaxis	Immunization with HAV vaccine, especially if traveling outside of the United States or already infected with HCV.	Immunization of all health care workers with blood and body fluid exposure, as well as high-risk groups. Routine immunization of children, screening of all blood and blood products, barrier precautions during sexual activity.	Screening all donated blood/blood products, protective devices for health care workers, use of Standard Precautions. No vaccine or cure.	Immunization against HBV.	Gamma-globulin manufactured from sources in endemic countries has shown little protective effect against HEV. The best prophylaxis to date is sanitary measures.	Screening of donated blood; protective devices for health care workers, Standard Precautions. No vaccine or cure available.

HAV, Hepatitis A virus; *IgM*, immunoglobulin M; *IgG*, immunoglobulin G; HB_c, hepatitis B core (antigen); HB_sAg, hepatitis B surface (antigen); HB_eAg, hepatitis B early antigen; *RNA*, ribonucleic acid; *HDV*, hepatitis D virus; *RIA*, radioimmunoassay; *HGV*, hepatitis G virus; *HEV*, hepatitis E virus. *Continued*

TABLE 8-6 Types and Characteristics of Viral Hepatitis—cont'd

	Hepatitis A	Hepatitis B	Hepatitis C	Hepatitis D	Hepatitis E	Hepatitis G
Treatment	Symptomatic.	Supportive measures and monitoring for progression towards chronic disease or fulminant hepatitis (rare). For chronic cases, Lamivudine 100 mg PO daily, or interferon 5 micro units subcutaneously injected daily for 6 mo.	When acute, patient should be monitored for progression to chronic or fulminant state. Most patients are diagnosed in the chronic state, years after contracting the virus. For chronic disease: interferon injected subcutaneously three times a week; or, combination of interferon three times weekly with daily PO ribavirin.	Interferon products may be tried.	Supportive.	Chronic liver disease not associated with this virus. No treatment is recommended at this time.

| Comments | Can cause FHF if superimposed on chronic HCV. | Chronic hepatitis may develop. FHF may ensue, especially if coinfected with HDV. | Chronic hepatitis develops in 85% of those infected. HAV and HBV vaccination is important. HAV or HBV superimposed on HCV can cause FHF. 50% of all liver transplants in the United States are the result of hepatitis C infection. | Fulminant hepatitis occurs ten times more often in HDV and HBV *coinfection*. HDV acquired after chronic HBV infection is termed *superinfection*. Superinfection of HDV with chronic HBV infection can cause acute hepatitis. | During epidemics, the case fatality rate for HEV is 1%-2%. Coinfection with HAV and HEV, is possible. Not endemic to the United States, Canada, or Western Europe. | Many with HCV also have HGV. May not cause a disease state. More HGV is detectable in serum versus the liver. As many as 4% of U.S. blood donors are HGV positive. |

FHF, Fulminant hepatic failure.

Albumin: Maintains blood oncotic pressure and coagulation proteins needed to form a fibrin clot. Decreased levels seen with ascites and severe liver disease. Persistently low levels suggest a poor prognosis.

Other serum biochemical tests

Sodium: Fluid is retained in greater quantity than sodium, resulting in hyponatremia. Patients with cirrhosis, tense ascites, hepatorenal syndrome, and end-stage liver disease are often hyponatremic.

Potassium: Hypokalemia is observed in those with liver disease accompanied by ascites and those with chronic alcoholic liver disease. If the patient has hepatorenal syndrome, hyperkalemia is observed.

Glucose: Hypoglycemia is usually present in severe or terminal liver dysfunction, causing altered mentation and lethargy. This is the result of impaired gluconeogenesis and glycogen depletion in the cirrhotic liver.

BUN: In liver failure the BUN is decreased. If the patient is bleeding and has renal insufficiency, the BUN may be elevated.

Ammonia: Increased because of the failing liver's inability to clear nitrogenous and other waste products. GI bleeding or an increase in intestinal protein from dietary intake will also increase ammonia levels (see Gastroesophageal Varices, p. 492).

Hematologic tests: As many as 70% of patients have platelet counts <100,000/mm^3 because of platelet destruction and malfunctioning hepatic synthesis of platelets. An increase in mean corpuscular volume (MCV) may be present, causing the RBCs to be macrocytic. The anemia present in hepatic failure is then termed *macrocytic* and *normochromic* (normal Hgb). Elevated thrombin-antithrombin III complex is present, which can cause intravascular coagulation. On rare occasions disseminated intravascular coagulation (DIC) results. If GI bleeding is present, a decreased Hgb and Hct are evident. Leukocytes usually are normal unless sepsis is present, causing an elevation. The PT measures factors I, II, V, VII, and X. PT prolongation indicates disease progression and a worsening prognosis. Vitamin K does not cause a response when administered unless the prolongation of the PT is the result of a vitamin K deficiency.

Liver biopsy: After local anesthetic agent is administered, a special needle is inserted into the eighth or ninth intercostal space in the midaxillary line to obtain a specimen (percutaneous liver biopsy). If a percutaneous biopsy is not feasible because of prolonged PT or a platelet count <50,000/mm^3, a transvenous biopsy may be performed via the jugular and hepatic vein. Before biopsy, laboratory tests should include a complete blood cell count (CBC), platelet count, a PT/partial thromboplastin time (PTT), and a type and cross-match. Patients are instructed to exhale and stop breathing while the needle is inserted during the biopsy. Patient movement during the procedure may cause puncture of an abdominal organ or a lung. (See Table 8-7 for nursing care of the patient undergoing liver biopsy.)

Electroencephalogram (EEG):   Often abnormal in hepatic encephalopathy. None of the findings are specific since many metabolic disorders produce abnormal EEGs.

Brain flow studies: If patient is in a hepatic coma, brain death cannot be confirmed by EEG. Therefore brain blood-flow study (technetium scan) is required if an assessment of brain function is needed.

Psychometric testing: Evaluates for hepatic encephalopathy. A common test is the Reitan number-connection (trail-making) test. The patient's speed and accuracy at connecting a series of numbered circles are evaluated at intervals. A daily handwriting test is an easy check of intellectual deterioration or improvement.

Abdominal paracentesis: An incision is made into the skin of the abdomen. A cannula, catheter, or hollow trocar is inserted through the incision into the abdominal cavity, and fluid is removed for analysis of protein, electrolytes, WBCs, and culture. Ascites fluid may also be drained but can result in

---

TABLE 8-7 Nursing Care of the Patient Undergoing Liver Biopsy

Before biopsy
- Explain the procedure to patient and significant others.
- Explain to patient that he or she may feel pushing on the right side during the procedure.
- Explain to patient that a "sharp" right shoulder pain may be felt during the biopsy.

During biopsy
- Assist patient with remaining motionless.
- Coach patient in sustaining exhalation during puncture (or manually ventilate intubated patient to prevent lung inflation during puncture) to avoid pneumothorax.

After biopsy
- Position patient on the right side for several hours after the biopsy to tamponade the puncture site.
- Auscultate breath sounds immediately after the procedure and at 1-2 h intervals for 6-8 h after the procedure to detect pneumothorax or hemothorax (unlikely but serious complications). Diminished sounds on the right side and tachypnea suggest one of these conditions.
- Enforce bed rest for 6-8 h after biopsy to minimize the risk of hemorrhage from the puncture site.
- Monitor patient for indicators of peritonitis or intraperitoneal bleeding, which can occur as a result of puncture of blood vessels or major bile duct: severe abdominal pain, abdominal distention and rigidity, rebound tenderness, nausea, vomiting, tachycardia, tachypnea, pallor, decreased BP, rising temperature.
- If bleeding is suspected, contact physician and obtain an ultrasound of the abdomen, to include the liver.
- Right shoulder pain may persist for 24-48 h after biopsy of the liver.

---

hypovolemic shock because of rapid intravascular fluid shifts. Vital signs including temperature should be checked often, along with intake and output (I&O). Peritonitis is a complication.

See **Fluid volume deficit,** p. 518, for nursing implications.

Urinalysis: Urine sodium excretion (<10 mEq/day) with normal urinary sediment is a sign of hepatorenal syndrome, which may observed in fulminant hepatic failure. Another disorder, acute tubular necrosis, is usually diagnosed if urine sodium excretion is >20 mEq/day and urinary sediment shows cellular casts. Gross inspection may reveal dark urine that produces a yellow foam when shaken. Increased urobilinogen and bilirubin will be present. In the presence of ascites, the 24-h urine volume will be decreased and the 24-h sodium value will be reduced (<5 mEq/day in severe cases).

Liver scan: A radioactive labeled compound that is easily absorbed by the Kupffer cells of the liver is injected into the patient. The radiation that is emitted can be photographed with a scintillation camera or x-ray. This test is best used to determine the presence of three-dimensional lesions. Computed tomography (CT) or ultrasound can aid in determining the size of the liver and abnormal tissue. Ultrasound is also useful for biopsy when "blind" methods have been attempted without success.

ECG: Factors such as hypokalemia, acidosis, or hypoxia may cause cardiac dysrhythmias. The heart should be monitored continuously, as should oximetry.

COLLABORATIVE MANAGEMENT

Correction of precipitating factors: Hepatic failure may develop suddenly in a patient with compensated liver disease. Sustained hypoxia or hypotension from any cause can aggravate hepatocellular failure and must be corrected promptly. Ethanol, hepatotoxic drugs, and hepatotoxic alternative therapies are eliminated. Sedatives and tranquilizers may contribute to hepatic encephalopathy and should be discontinued.

Fluid and electrolyte management: Free water clearance is affected in FHF, causing hyponatremia even though increased total body sodium is present. If hyponatremia is profound, sodium-containing fluids are avoided because they contribute to ascites and peripheral edema and may potentiate renal insufficiency. D_5W generally is used for fluid resuscitation to prevent hypernatremia. Mannitol or albumin is given to increase intravascular oncotic pressure and maintain intravascular volume. Potassium is decreased with the use of mannitol. Hypokalemic alkalosis can worsen encephalopathy and precipitate dysrhythmias. Fresh frozen plasma may be used if clotting factors are deficient, but infusions of large amounts can lead to hypernatremia. Packed RBCs are given if there is brisk bleeding or a low Hct. CVP or PAP monitoring along with ICP monitoring should be initiated to ensure adequate tissue perfusion without fluid overload. A hyperdynamic circulatory state is supported by fluid administration and sympathomimetic agents (e.g., dopamine) as necessary. NOTE: Accurate measurements and careful interpretation of hemodynamic parameters are essential because fluid balance is delicate in critically ill patients with hepatic failure; also, hemodynamic measurements can be difficult to interpret because of the hyperdynamic circulatory state. Svo_2 monitoring is helpful in evaluating the adequacy of tissue oxygenation.

Bed rest: Necessary to reduce metabolic demands placed on the liver during normal daily activity.

Nutritional therapy: The catabolic rate in FHF increases four times over normal. Therefore, to ensure tissue repair, a high-calorie, 80- to 100-g protein diet of high biologic value is indicated for patients without evidence of encephalopathy, inasmuch as the liver is capable of significant regeneration under optimal circumstances. Sodium is moderately restricted unless significant ascites and peripheral edema are present. Then a 500-mg or less sodium-restricted diet is prescribed. If GI function is impaired and the patient is unable to tolerate enteral feedings, parenteral nutrition is initiated. Total caloric intake should be 2500-3000/day.

For the patient with acute hepatic encephalopathy, protein is eliminated totally from the diet until recovery. During recovery, vegetable protein (preferred vs. animal protein) is gradually reintroduced at 10-20 g every 48-72 h. It is gradually increased to 40 g/day. This dose at this rate prevents tissue catabolism. Use of enteral or parenteral branched-chain amino acid supplements in an attempt to correct the amino acid imbalance that is common among patients with an encephalopathic condition is advocated by some, but their effectiveness is controversial. Potassium loss must be replaced by potassium-rich foods or supplements.

Pharmacotherapy: Some commonly used drugs that are hepatotoxic. See Table 8-8.

Sedatives: Avoided if at all possible because they can precipitate or contribute to encephalopathy. If sedative use is necessary, oxazepam (Serax) is the best choice because it can be eliminated safely by patients with hepatic disease. Other sedatives may be used cautiously and in reduced dosages.

Histamine H_2-receptor antagonists: Prophylactic H_2-receptor antagonists are prescribed to block acid secretion and prevent gastric erosions, which are common in patients with chronic or severe hepatic failure. Ranitidine or famotidine is the preferred agent because of the hepatic side effects of cimetidine.

TABLE 8-8 Drugs With Hepatotoxic Potential

Acetaminophen	Ketoconazole
Ampicillin	Methotrexate
Carbamazepine	Methyldopa
Carbenicillin	Monoamine oxidase (MAO) inhibitors
Carbon tetrachloride	Nonsteroidal antiinflammatory drugs (NSAIDs)
Chloramphenicol	Oral contraceptives
Chlorpromazine	Penicillin
Clindamycin	Phenytoin
Cocaine	Propylthiouracil
Dantrolene	Rifampin
Ethanol	Salicylates
FUDR (intraarterial)	Sulfonamides
Halothane	Tetracyclines (especially parenteral)
Hydrochlorothiazide	Valproic acid
Isoniazid	

Sucralfate (Carafate): Binds to gastric erosions and coats the gastric/duodenal mucosa.

Dextrose: Moderate to severe hypoglycemia can occur because of impaired gluconeogenesis and impaired insulin degradation. Checks of blood sugar levels q6-8h are necessary to detect hypoglycemia. In the event of hypoglycemia, a bolus of 50% dextrose or continual infusion of a 10% solution is indicated.

Protection of health care workers: Health care workers whose jobs involve potential exposure to blood or other body fluids should be vaccinated with the hepatitis B vaccine. Health care workers must protect themselves from potential infection by consistent use of appropriate infection control measures (see Appendix 8).

Management of bleeding complications: Fresh-frozen plasma and platelets are administered to correct defects in clotting factors and thrombocytopenia. Vitamin K may be prescribed to help correct bleeding tendencies. Serious coagulopathies that require specialized component therapy may develop (see "Disseminated Intravascular Coagulation," p. 579).

Management of respiratory failure: Intubation or mechanical ventilation may be indicated in the following instances: impaired gag reflex caused by advanced encephalopathy; aspiration of gastric contents; or impairment of ventilation secondary to ascites. Continuous pulse oximetry is used for patients with respiratory failure or those at high risk for same. The need for adequate tissue oxygenation is crucial inasmuch as hepatic hypoxia significantly contributes to hepatic failure.

Management of ascites
Restriction of fluid intake
Restriction of physical activity
Sodium: If ascites causes discomfort, pain, or dyspnea, sodium is limited to <500 mg/day.

Diuretics: If more conservative measures are ineffective in controlling ascites, spironolactone (Aldactone), an aldosterone antagonist with weak diuretic action and potassium conservation, may be used. Another potassium-sparing diuretic, amiloride, may be used as well. If these are ineffective, more potent diuretics such as furosemide (Lasix) or thiazides are added with concurrent use of potassium supplement. For severe ascites, mannitol may be added to the regimen. The goal with diuresis is 1 L/day, as estimated by a weight loss of 0.5 kg/day. Too-rapid diuresis may lead to acute hypovolemia, shock, and hepatorenal syndrome. Hypokalemia should be prevented to reduce the chance of encephalopathy or worsening encephalopathy.

Paracentesis: Repeated daily removal of 4-6 L/day of ascitic fluid may be attempted as a temporary measure for refractory ascites. Concurrent administration of salt-poor albumin aids in maintaining intravascular volume.

Peritoneal-venous shunt: A shunt system (e.g., LeVeen, Denver) may be placed surgically in patients with refractory or life-threatening ascites. The peritoneal cavity is drained by a long, perforated catheter, which is connected to a pressure-sensitive valve. The valve attaches to a subcutaneous catheter that drains into the intrathoracic superior vena cava. The device is designed so that fluid can flow in only one direction—from the peritoneum into the bloodstream. The many complications include fluid overload, infection, DIC, peritonitis, and shunt occlusion. A rapid increase in intravascular volume may precipitate variceal hemorrhage in susceptible persons. See Table 8-9 and **Fluid volume excess,** p. 519, for nursing implications.

Management of hepatorenal syndrome: Hepatorenal syndrome (HRS) is directly related to liver disease. It is thought to result from the renal vasoconstrictor response to systemic vasodilation of liver failure. The resultant renal failure is not related to a malfunction of any structure in the kidney but, rather, to altered blood flow into the cortex of the kidney. This decrease in blood flow allows the kidneys to be vulnerable to insults. Eventually HRS may progress to acute tubular necrosis (ATN) from hypotension or the toxic effects of drugs. Once HRS is present, it is difficult to manage. If possible, eliminating precipitating factors (nephrotoxic drugs, overzealous paracentesis) is encouraged. Sodium-containing solutions are avoided, even in the presence of significant hyponatremia. Renal dialysis seldom is employed because it does not improve survival and can lead to complications such as GI hemorrhage and shock.

Management of encephalopathy

Elimination or correction of precipitating factors: As many as 80% of patients with cirrhosis and liver failure have some degree of cerebral dysfunction or encephalopathy as a result of metabolic causes or hepatic decompensation. The causes and precipitating factors are now known to be many: changes in the permeability of the blood-brain barrier, an increase in endogenous benzodiazepines, impairment of neuronal membrane sodium-potassium adenosinetriphosphatase (ATPase), abnormal neurotransmitter balance, GI bleed, increased dietary protein, and electrolyte disturbance.

Restriction of physical activity: Less stress on all the organs of the body, including those that may be affected by chronic liver disease. Less activity reduces the number of metabolites that must be processed by the liver.

Restriction or elimination of dietary protein: Can be reintroduced if symptoms improve.

Early and thorough catharsis by magnesium citrate or tap water enema: Very helpful to eliminate blood in intestines from GI bleeding. Also useful in eliminating protein if it is lingering in the bowel from ileus, constipation, or other causes.

Administration of neomycin: Broad-spectrum antibiotic used with caution and for short periods of time because of the possibility of ototoxicity, nephrotoxicity (especially in those with renal impairment), lethargy, and yeast superinfection. BUN and creatinine must be monitored q6h. This antibiotic works against the bacteria that break down protein into ammonia.

Administration of lactulose: A nonabsorbable, synthetic disaccharide that decreases the pH of the colon by its conversion into lactic, acetic, and formic acids. The unmetabolized lactulose left in the colon produces osmotic diarrhea. Ideally, the dose is adjusted to produce 2-3 semiformed stools/day.

TABLE 8-9   Nursing Care After Peritoneal-Venous Shunt Surgery

- Measure urinary output hourly and CVP or PAP q1-2h.
  - □ Anticipate rapid fluid mobilization, as evidenced by increased CVP and increased urinary output.
  - □ Notify physician of abnormal CVP, PAP, or lack of diuresis. Failure to mobilize ascitic fluid may signal shunt occlusion or failure.
  - □ Report lessening of urinary output since renal function may diminish after this procedure.
- Administer IV diuretics as prescribed; monitor K^+ levels; and administer K^+ supplements as prescribed.
  - □ Anticipate prescribed K^+ supplements during the first 24 h after surgery.
  - □ Be aware that furosemide (Lasix), which frequently is prescribed, may cause K^+ depletion. Likewise, the anticipated diuresis depletes K^+.
- Instruct and coach patient in the use of the incentive spirometer or similar hyperinflation device.
  - □ Devices that create inspiratory resistance and encourage deep inspiration promote negative inspiratory pressure and facilitate flow of ascitic fluid.
  - □ Encourage patient to cough hourly.
- Apply elastic abdominal binder.
  - □ This intervention facilitates the flow of ascitic fluid by increasing the pressure gradient externally.
- Monitor for evidence of variceal bleeding; report evidence of bleeding to physician.
  - □ Expanded blood volume may increase variceal pressure, resulting in bleeding. Bleeding is evidenced by a sudden decrease in Hct (a mild dilutional decrease is anticipated in the immediate postoperative period), unexplained nausea, lightheadedness, dark stools, or hematemesis. (See "Gastroesophageal Varices," p. 492.)
- Monitor for evidence of peritonitis, endocarditis, or other infection.
  - □ Infection occurs frequently. Anticipate antibiotic coverage during the immediate postsurgical period. Assess abdominal incision for leakage of peritoneal fluid, which is a common occurrence. Change the dressing immediately if leakage is detected.
- Monitor for evidence of postshunt coagulopathy.
  - □ See Altered protection, p. 523, for details.
- Monitor for other postshunt complications.
  - □ Assess for lower extremity edema. After some shunting procedures, none of the venous blood passes through the liver and protein end products are not completely detoxified. These patients are usually placed on a low-protein diet.

CVP, Central venous pressure; *PAP*, pulmonary artery pressure; *IV*, intravenous; K^+, potassium; *Hct*, hematocrit.

Caution: Lactulose may worsen hypernatremia and promote cerebral edema. It should be used with caution.

ICP monitoring: Brain damage may occur when ICP is about 25 mm Hg. This can occur quickly and without obvious accompanying signs/symptoms. It is advisable to use an ICP monitor to detect cerebral edema and guide pharmacologic management (e.g., mannitol, furosemide) and other therapeutic measures. See discussion in "Traumatic Brain Injury," p. 118.

Hepatic transplantation: The orthotopic liver transplant survival rate is more than 80% for the first year after transplant. In cases of chronic progressive or acute hepatocyte damage, it is the only treatment available. Because organs are in such limited supply, new methods are being sought to extend the life of the native liver until a donor liver becomes available. Hepatocyte transplantation, bioartificial liver support, extracorporeal whole-organ perfusion, and xenotransplantation are ways in which waiting time to transplantation is bridged.

NURSING DIAGNOSES AND INTERVENTIONS

Fluid volume deficit related to decreased intake secondary to medically prescribed restrictions; decreased circulating volume secondary to hypoalbuminemia, altered hemodynamics, fluid sequestration, diuretic therapy, diarrhea from lactulose, bleeding varices

Desired outcomes: Within 24 h of this diagnosis, patient becomes normovolemic as evidenced by MAP >70 mm Hg; HR 60-100 bpm; brisk capillary refill (<2 sec); distal pulses >2+ on a 0-4+ scale; CVP 2-6 mm Hg; PAP 20-30/8-15 mm Hg; PAWP 6-12 mm Hg; CI >3 L/min/m^2; SVR 900-1200 dynes/sec/cm^{-5}; urinary output >0.5 ml/kg/h; and patient oriented to person, place, and time.

- Monitor and document BP hourly, or q15min in the presence of unstable VS. Be alert to MAP decreases >10 mm Hg from previous measurement.
- Monitor and document HR, ECG, and cardiovascular status hourly, or more frequently in the presence of unstable VS. Be alert to increases in HR suggestive of hypovolemia or circulatory decompensation. Be aware that HR increases also may be caused by fever related to infection or cerebral edema, and monitor for dyrhythmias from electrolyte imbalances secondary to diarrhea, gastric suctioning, or diuretic therapy.
- Measure central pressures and thermodilution CO q1-4h. Be alert to low or decreasing CVP, PAWP, and CO. Calculate SVR q4-8h, or more frequently in unstable patients. An elevated HR, decreased PAWP, CO less than baseline, or CI <3, along with decreased urinary output, suggest hypovolemia. Because of altered vascular responsiveness, the SVR may not be increased in patients with hypovolemic hepatic failure. Be aware that a "normal" CO value actually may be too low for these patients. A hyperdynamic circulatory state should be supported. Monitor Svo$_2$ as available to evaluate the adequacy of tissue oxygenation.
- Measure and record urinary output hourly. Be alert to output <0.5 ml/kg/hr for 2 consecutive hours. Estimate volume status and adequacy of cardiovascular function by evaluating BP, HR, CVP, PAP, PAWP, urinary output, distal pulse amplitude, capillary refill, and level of consciousness. Consider cautious increases in fluid intake (e.g., 50-100 ml/h), and then reevaluate volume status as already described. Use extreme caution in administering potent diuretics, inasmuch as they may precipitate encephalopathy or renal disease by causing rapid diuresis and electrolyte changes.
- Estimate ongoing fluid losses. Weigh patient daily. Measure all drainage from peritoneal or other catheters q2-4h. Compare 24-h intake with output, and record the difference. Weight loss should not exceed 0.5 kg/day because more rapid diuresis can lead to intravascular volume depletion and impair renal function.
- Monitor serum albumin and total protein, and consult physician if levels are reduced. Administer albumin replacements as prescribed.
- If fluid volume deficit is related to variceal hemorrhage, see this nursing diagnosis in "Esophageal Varices," p. 492.

NIC Electrolyte Management; Fluid Management; Cerebral Edema Management; Electrolyte Management: Hypokalemia

Fluid volume excess: interstitial or intracellular, related to compromised regulatory mechanisms secondary to acute or chronic hepatic failure

Desired outcomes: Within 48 h of this diagnosis, patient becomes normovolemic as evidenced by CVP 2-6 mm Hg; PAWP 6-12 mm Hg; HR 60-100 bpm; RR 12-20 breaths/min with normal depth and pattern (eupnea); decreasing or stable abdominal girth; and absence of crackles, edema, uncomfortable ascites, and other clinical indicators of fluid volume excess.

- Monitor VS, hemodynamic parameters, and cardiovascular status q1-2h, more frequently if patient is undergoing ultrafiltration therapy, and immediately after peritoneal-venous shunt surgery. Be alert to CVP values >6 mm Hg or PAWP >12 mm Hg. Consult physician for elevated values.
- Monitor for peripheral edema. Note severity and location. Jugular vein distention at a 45-degree head-of-bed (HOB) elevation may indicate fluid overload or decreased cardiac output.
- Monitor patient for evidence of fluid overload. Note presence of dyspnea, tachypnea, rhonchi, orthopnea, basilar crackles that do not clear with coughing, labored and/or shallow breathing, elevated BP, S_3 heart sound. Consult physician if these signs develop.
- Use minimal amounts of fluids necessary to administer IV medications and maintain IV catheter patency.
- If fluids are restricted, offer mouth care and/or ice chips (included as part of oral fluid measurement).
- Measure and record abdominal girth daily. Be aware that abdominal girth measurements are subject to error and great care is necessary to ensure accuracy. Measure at the widest point, and mark this level for subsequent measurements. If tolerated by the patient, measure him or her in the supine position. If the supine position is not possible, measure patient in the same position each time. Weigh daily at the same time, in the same clothing, using the same scale and method.
- Monitor serum electrolyte levels, especially sodium and potassium, and consult physician for significant deviations from normal. Normal values are serum sodium 137-147 mEq/L and serum potassium 3.5-5.0 mEq/L.
- Ensure proper functioning of peritoneal-venous shunt in patients after surgery (see Table 8-9).

NIC Electrolyte Management: Hypernatremia; Fluid Management; Invasive Hemodynamic Monitoring

Altered nutrition: less than body requirements, related to inability to digest food secondary to anorexia, nausea, and medically prescribed dietary restriction; decreased absorption of nutrients secondary to decreased intestinal motility, altered portal blood flow, decreased intestinal absorption of vitamins and minerals, altered protein metabolism; the diseased liver's inability to utilize nutrients

Desired outcomes: Within 3-4 days of this diagnosis, patient has adequate nutrition as evidenced by a state of nitrogen balance as shown by daily fecal excretion of 2-3 g of nitrogen and 13-20 g of urinary nitrogen, thyroxine-binding prealbumin 200-300 mcg/ml, and retinol-binding protein 40-50 mcg/ml. Blood glucose levels remain within an acceptable range of 100-160 mg/dl.

- Confer with physician, dietitian, and pharmacist (if parenteral feedings are necessary) to estimate patient's current nutritional and metabolic needs, based on anthropometric data, creatinine excretion, albumin, and transferrin, as well as presence of encephalopathy, chronic hepatic disease, infection, and nutritional status before hospitalization. For general information, see "Nutritional Support," p. 1.

- In the absence of adequate bowel functioning or with poor oral intake, consult physician regarding administration of parenteral (preferred) or enteral nutrients. If insertion of a feeding tube becomes necessary, use caution to minimize the risk of rupturing gastroesophageal varices. If parenteral feedings are being administered, monitor IV site for infection and other complications.
- Note, monitor, and record food/fluid ingested and daily caloric intake. Note all sources of food (including meals not prepared in the hospital), paying particular attention to foods that contain sodium and significant amounts of protein.
- Administer vitamin supplements as prescribed, particularly the fat-soluble ones.
- Encourage food brought from home if desired by patient, and make sure it meets prescribed dietary restrictions.
- Encourage bed rest to reduce metabolic demands on the liver and to promote hepatic regeneration. Increase patient's activity levels gradually as condition improves.
- Monitor blood glucose levels q8h or as prescribed. Monitor patient for clinical indicators of hypoglycemia: altered mentation, irritability, diaphoresis, anxiety, weakness, and tachycardia. Consult physician for blood glucose levels <65 mg/dl. Administer D_{10} or D_{50} as prescribed for hypoglycemia. Clinical signs of hypoglycemia can be confused with hepatic encephalopathy. Be sure to validate clinical signs with blood glucose levels. Be aware that mild elevations in blood sugar are anticipated in some patients with chronic liver disease. Administer hypoglycemic agents as prescribed for blood glucose levels >160 mg/dl.

NIC Nutrition Management; Hypoglycemia Management; Energy Management

Impaired gas exchange related to altered oxygen supply secondary to arteriovenous shunting, ventilation-perfusion mismatch, and diaphragmatic limitation associated with ascites, hydrothorax, or central respiratory depression occurring with encephalopathy

Desired outcomes: Within 4 h of this diagnosis, patient has adequate gas exchange as evidenced by Pao_2 >80 mm Hg; $Paco_2$ <45 mm Hg; RR 12-20 breaths/min with normal depth and pattern (eupnea); oxygen saturation >92% with or without oxygen supplementation or mechanical ventilation; and orientation to person, place, and time.

> **Note:** Level of consciousness is difficult to evaluate in the presence of moderate to severe hepatic encephalopathy, and obtaining a baseline level of consciousness is imperative.

- Monitor and document respiratory rate q1-4h. Note pattern, excursion, depth, and effort.
- Administer supplemental oxygen as prescribed to enhance cerebral and hepatic oxygenation.
- Maintain body positions that optimize ventilation. Elevate HOB 30 degrees or higher, depending on patient comfort and hemodynamic status. If patient has increased ICP, the HOB should not be elevated above 20 degrees. If patient has unilateral lung problem, position him or her with the unaffected lung dependent. Correlate body position with blood gas and oximetry results.
- Monitor Pao_2, $Paco_2$, and oxygen saturation; consult physician for abnormalities. Continuous pulse oximetry should be in use. Monitor ABGs and electrolytes as available.
- Assess patient q4-8h for indicators of atelectasis (e.g., diminished breath sounds, basilar crackles, difficulty breathing), hydrothorax (e.g., diminished breath sounds, dullness to percussion), and pulmonary infection (e.g., yellow, green, or thick sputum, rhonchi, fever). Consult physician if physical assessment findings suggest respiratory complications.

- Evaluate obtunded patient for presence of gag reflex. Consult physician regarding need for ET intubation if the gag reflex is depressed. Suction mouth frequently; offer/assist with frequent mouth care.

NIC Oxygen Therapy; Aspiration Precautions

Altered thought processes related to endogenous chemical alteration (accumulation of ammonia or other central nervous system [CNS] toxins occurring with hepatic dysfunction), therapeutically restricted environment, sleep deprivation, hypoxia, sensory overload (noise, personnel) in ICU, and medication (side effects, toxic levels from liver's inability to detoxify appropriately)

Desired outcomes: By the time of hospital discharge, patient exhibits stable personality pattern, age-appropriate behavior, intact intellect appropriate for level of education, distinct speech, and coordinated gross and fine motor movements. Handwriting is legible, and psychometric test scores are improved from baseline range.

- Avoid or minimize precipitating factors (Table 8-10).
  - ☐ Help patient keep circadian rhythms in sync (e.g., keep lighting in room appropriate for the time of day, activities of daily living [ADL] to the correct time of day).
  - ☐ Check gastric secretions, vomitus, and stools for occult blood. Consult physician promptly if test results are positive for blood or if GI bleeding is obvious.
  - ☐ Evaluate Hct and Hgb for evidence of bleeding. Consult physician for very low values or values that deviate from baseline. Anticipate mild to moderate anemia.
  - ☐ Consult physician promptly for indicators of infection (see **Risk for Infection,** p. 522).

TABLE 8-10   Factors That Contribute to Hepatic Encephalopathy

Chronic factors

Portal-systemic shunting (entry of portal blood into systemic veins without being metabolized by the liver): may occur via damaged liver, collateral vessels, or surgically created portacaval anastomosis

Dietary protein intake

Intestinal bacteria

Acid-base imbalance

Progressive hepatic insufficiency

Precipitating factors

Dehydration/electrolyte imbalance: may occur with overdiuresis, diarrhea, vomiting, or other factors

Excessive paracentesis

Surgery in a cirrhotic patient

Excessive alcohol ingestion

Sedatives/hypnotics

Infection

Constipation

Extrahepatic bile duct obstruction

Acute hepatocellular damage

Viral hepatitis

Alcoholic hepatitis

Drug/chemical reactions (see Table 8-8)

Drug overdose

☐ Evaluate serum ammonia levels (normal levels are 40-110 mg/dl). Report significant elevations from baseline. Ammonia values and their measurement vary greatly and do not always correlate directly with encephalopathy. To help ensure accurate results, place specimens for ammonia analysis on ice and transport immediately to laboratory.

☐ Be alert to potential sources of electrolyte imbalance (e.g., diarrhea, vomiting, occult bleeding).

☐ Avoid use of sedative or tranquilizing agents. If sedatives are necessary, oxazepam (Serax) and antihistamines (e.g., Benadryl) are the safest.

☐ If patient is pulling out tubes, apply mitts rather than restraints.

☐ Avoid use of conventional and alternative drugs that are hepatotoxic (see Table 8-8).

☐ Correct hypoxemia; administer supplemental oxygen as necessary (see **Impaired gas exchange,** p. 520).

• Evaluate patient for CNS effects such as personality changes, childish behavior, intellectual impairment, slurred speech, ataxia, and asterixis.

• Administer daily handwriting or psychometric tests (if appropriate for patient's level of consciousness) to evaluate mild or subclinical encephalopathy. Report significant deterioration in handwriting or in test scores.

• Consult physician for abnormal EEG reports.

• Eliminate dietary protein for patients with severe encephalopathy. As prescribed, reintroduce protein gradually as tolerated after patient's clinical symptoms improve (i.e., patient becomes more alert; neuromuscular coordination improves).

• Administer enemas as prescribed to clear the colon of intestinal contents that contribute to encephalopathy. Repeat enemas as necessary to ensure thorough cleansing of the colon.

• Administer neomycin as prescribed to reduce intestinal bacteria, which contribute to the production of cerebral intoxicants. Monitor patient for evidence of ototoxic (i.e., decreased hearing) and nephrotoxic (e.g., urinary output <0.5 ml/kg/h, increased creatinine levels) effects caused by neomycin. Avoid neomycin administration for patients with renal insufficiency.

• Administer lactulose as prescribed to reduce ammonia formation in the intestine. Consult physician to adjust dose to produce 2-3 semiformed stools daily. Avoid lactulose-related diarrhea because it may cause dangerous dehydration and electrolyte imbalance.

• Protect confused or unconscious patient from injury.

☐ Enlist the aid of family or friends to watch patient during confused or restless periods.

☐ Have call light within patient's reach at all times.

☐ Tape all catheters and tubes securely to prevent dislodgment.

• Consider possibility of seizures in the patient with severe encephalopathy; have airway management equipment readily available.

• Minimize unnecessary noise, lights, and other environmental stimuli. For more information, see "Psychosocial Support" for **Sensory/perceptual alterations,** p. 86, and **Sleep pattern disturbance,** p. 86.

• Monitor ICP and cerebral perfusion pressure (CPP). For patients with increased intracranial pressure (IICP), position carefully (HOB <20 degrees) and avoid fluid overload, hypercarbia, and hypoxemia. Administer mannitol and furosemide (Lasix) as prescribed. Sedation or coma induction may be indicated if cerebral edema does not respond to the measures just mentioned.

NIC Environmental Management; Delirium Management; Intracranial Pressure Monitoring

Risk for infection related to inadequate secondary defenses (impaired reticuloendothelial system phagocytic activity and portal-systemic shunting); multiple invasive procedures; chronic malnutrition in the individual with cirrhosis

Desired outcome: Patient is free of infection as evidenced by normothermia; HR <100 bpm; RR <20 breaths/min; negative culture results; WBC count <11,000/mm^3; clear urine; and clear, thin sputum.

- Monitor VS for evidence of infection (e.g., increases in heart and respiratory rates). Check rectal or core temperature q4h for increases. Avoid measuring temperatures rectally in the patient with rectal varices.
- If temperature elevation is sudden, obtain specimens for blood, sputum, and urine cultures or from other sites as prescribed. Consult physician for positive culture results.
- Monitor CBC, and consult physician for significant increases in WBCs. Be aware that a normal or mildly elevated leukocyte count may signify infection in patients with hepatic failure inasmuch as patients with chronic liver disease often have leukopenia, with WBC counts <3000/mm^3.
- Evaluate secretions and drainage for evidence of infection (e.g., sputum changes, cloudy urine).
- Evaluate IV, central line, and paracentesis site(s) for evidence of infection (erythema, warmth, unusual drainage). It is normal for a paracentesis puncture site to have a small amount of drainage immediately after the procedure. Prolonged or foul-smelling drainage can signal infection.
- Prevent transmission of infectious agents by washing hands well before and after caring for patient and by wearing gloves when contact with blood or other body substances is possible. Dispose of all needles and other sharp instruments in puncture-resistant, rigid containers. Keep containers in each patient room and in other convenient locations. Avoid recapping and manipulating needles before disposal. Teach significant others and visitors proper hand-washing technique. Restrict visitors with evidence of communicable disease.
- Administer antibiotics as prescribed. Use caution and reduced dosage when administering antibiotics (especially aminoglycosides) to patients with low urinary output or renal insufficiency.

NIC Infection Protection; Surveillance

Altered protection related to clotting anomaly; thrombocytopenia; itching; disorientation

Desired outcomes: Patient's bleeding, if it occurs, is not prolonged. Patient's skin is not damaged from scratching. Patient's confusion (if present) and level of consciousness will not lead to injury (see **"Altered thought processes,** p. 521).

- Avoid giving intramuscular (IM) injections. If they are necessary, use small-gauge needles and maintain firm pressure over injection sites for several minutes. Avoid massaging IM injection sites.
- Maintain pressure for several minutes over venipuncture sites. Inform laboratory personnel of patient's bleeding tendencies.
- Avoid arterial punctures. If it is necessary to obtain ABG values, consult physician regarding use of an indwelling arterial line. If this is not possible, be certain to maintain pressure over the arterial puncture site and elevation for at least 10 min.
- Monitor PT levels and platelet counts daily. Consult physician for significant prolongation of the PT or for significant reduction in the platelet count.
- Assess patient for signs of bleeding. Note oral and nasal mucosal bleeding and ecchymotic areas, and test stools, emesis, urine, and gastric drainage for occult blood. Be alert to prolonged bleeding or oozing of blood from venipuncture sites and incisions. Consult physician for positive findings.
- Use electric rather than safety razor for patient shaving. Provide soft-bristle toothbrush or sponge-tipped applicator and mouthwash for oral hygiene.
- Avoid indwelling gastric drainage tubes if possible, because they may irritate gastric mucosa or varices, causing bleeding to occur.

- Administer fresh-frozen plasma and platelets as prescribed. Monitor carefully for fluid volume overload (see **Fluid volume excess,** p. 519).
- Administer vitamin K as prescribed.
- A postshunt coagulopathy may develop in some patients after peritoneal-venous shunt surgery. Monitor these patients closely (see fifth intervention of this diagnosis).
- If fibrin split products (FSP) are present in the blood and thrombocytopenia is significant, the patient may have DIC (see "Disseminated Intravascular Coagulation," p. 579).
- When moving patient, avoid shearing forces to skin.
- Keep sheets free of wrinkles. Keep clothing from bunching against patient's skin.
- Dry skin well after AM care. Provide adequate lotion to skin, avoid massaging it in deeply, and rub gently.
- Use paper tape if it is necessary to place tape directly on skin. If possible, use gauze to secure a dressing or IV and tape over the gauze to prevent it from unwrapping.

Altered tissue perfusion: renal, related to risk of diminished arterial flow secondary to increased preglomerular vascular resistance (see Table 8-11 for other contributing factors)

Desired outcome: By the time of transfer from ICU, patient has adequate renal perfusion as evidenced by urinary output >0.5 ml/kg/h.

- Monitor CVP, PAWP, and SVR q1-4h to ensure optimal filling pressures (see **Fluid volume deficit,** p. 518). Monitor filling pressures hourly immediately after paracentesis or if patient is dehydrated or hemorrhaging.
- Monitor serum and urine sodium levels. Serum sodium <120 mEq/L and urine sodium <10 mEq/L are associated with the development of hepatorenal syndrome. Consult physician for significant alterations in serum and urine sodium levels. Normal values are 135-147 mEq/L for serum and >10 mEq/L for urine.
- Monitor creatinine and potassium values, and consult physician for significant increases. Be aware that BUN level is not an accurate indicator of renal function, especially in the patient with hepatic failure, because alterations in hepatic function can cause decreased BUN values and GI bleeding results in increased BUN values. Normal serum creatinine is 0.7-1.5 mg/dl, and normal serum potassium is 3.5-5 mEq/L.
- Minimize infusion of sodium-containing fluids because they contribute to ascites and peripheral edema and may potentiate functional renal failure.
- Monitor for hypophosphatemia (normal values 2.5-4.8 mg/dl) as evidenced by mental confusion, metabolic acidosis, anorexia, cardiac dysrhythmias, hemolytic anemia, lethargy, and bone pain. Administer replacement therapy as ordered.

T A B L E 8 - 1 1   Factors That May Reduce Renal Perfusion in Persons With Chronic Liver Disease

Dehydration: Diuresis, vomiting, diarrhea, or inadequate intake

Lactulose therapy: Results in frequent, loose stools (>3-4/day) with dehydration

NSAIDs: Results in renal prostaglandin inhibition and a reduced glomerular filtration rate

Hemorrhage: Results in reduced effective plasma volume/intravascular volume depletion

Paracentesis: Causes fluid shifts with a new reduction in effective plasma volume

---

NSAIDs, Nonsteroidal antiinflammatory drugs.

- Monitor for hypomagnesemia (1.8-3.0 mg/dl) as evidenced by muscle weakness, nausea, vomiting, tremors, tetany, and lethargy. Administer replacement therapy as ordered.
- For patients receiving lactulose, adjust dosage so that patient has 2-3 soft stools/day.
- For additional information, see nursing diagnoses and interventions in "Acute Renal Failure," p. 371.

Impaired tissue integrity related to chemical irritants (bile salts), impaired mobility, and fluid excess (tissue edema)

Desired outcomes: Patient's tissue remains intact; pruritus is relieved or reduced within 12 h of this diagnosis.

- Bathe patient with a nonsoap cleanser such as Cetaphil. Follow baths with unscented lotion, which should be applied while the skin is still moist.
- Use a low-pressure mattress to minimize pressure on fragile tissues.
- Turn, reposition (at least q2h), and provide appropriate support to body and over bony prominences to prevent pressure sores.
- If patient is confused or obtunded, place his or her hands in soft gloves or mitts to minimize damage from scratching and keep nails short.
- Administer cholestyramine (e.g., Questran, LoCholest, Cholestid) as prescribed to reduce bile acids in the serum and skin and thereby relieve itching. Avoid administration of other oral medications within 2 h of cholestyramine administration because they may bind with it in the intestine and reduce its absorption.
- Also see last four interventions under "**Altered protection,**" p. 523.

Knowledge deficit: lack of exposure to health care information; cognitive limitation secondary to hepatic encephalopathy

Desired outcome: Within the 24-h period before hospital discharge, patient states signs and symptoms of early hepatic encephalopathy; the importance of medical follow-up; need to adhere to the prescribed diet; importance of rest; infection control measures; availability of alcohol and drug treatment programs; medication instructions; and signs and symptoms of other complications.

- Stress importance of sufficient rest and adherence to prescribed diet.
- Infection control: If hepatic failure is related to hepatitis B virus (HBV) infection, HBV prophylaxis should be considered for sexual partners and household contacts with possible exposure to HBV (e.g., those who share toothbrushes, razors). Teach patient and exposure contacts practices that reduce the risk of exposure (e.g., condom use). Prescreening for the presence of HB antibodies is encouraged if it does not delay treatment for more than 14 days after last exposure. A dose of hepatitis B immune globulin (HBIG) is recommended immediately for sexual contacts and household contacts with possible blood and body fluid exposure. A second HBIG vaccine is to follow 1 mo later. The HB vaccine series should be initiated for sexual and household contacts at risk. The first and second vaccines can be given at the same time the two HBIG vaccines are given. Make sure both vaccines are given in separate areas. The HB vaccines are to be given deltoid IM only.
- If hepatic failure is related to hepatitis C virus (HCV), no prophylaxis is available to exposed persons. Therefore baseline HC antibodies should be drawn and 1 mo later a second should be drawn. Based on results, an infectious disease consult may be indicated, along with possible treatment. It is important to note, however, that those with sexual exposure have only a 5%-8% chance of seroconversion. Those with exposure to blood, particularly through hollow-bore needles, have the greatest chance of seroconversion.
- Inform patient about the availability of alcohol-treatment and drug-treatment programs if alcohol- and drug-related hepatic failure has occurred.
- Explain the availability of support groups (i.e., Alcoholics Anonymous, Al-Anon) for patients and family members when hepatic failure is related to chronic alcohol ingestion.

> **RESEARCH BRIEF 8-2** Patients with subclinical hepatic encephalopathy (SHE) are assumed to have impaired functioning in their work performance or daily lives. Results of psychometric testing using Number Connection Test Part A (NCT-A), Digit Symbol Test (DST), and automated analysis of the electroencephalogram (EEG), along with "Health-related Quality of Life" and the "Sickness Impact Profile" (SIP) questionnaires, demonstrated that patients with SHE do have impaired functioning in daily lives. The study also found that reproducibility of the tests is high, even when several months elapse between testing. Treatment of patients with stable liver disease who have SHE is warranted.

From Groeneweg M et al: *Hepatology* 28(1):45-49, 1998.

- Caution about the importance of avoiding over-the-counter (OTC) medications without first consulting physician. Advise patient to confer with physician regarding use of acetaminophen, NSAIDs, and aspirin (ASA) for minor aches and pains after hospital discharge.
- Provide a list of patient's prescribed medications, including drug name, dosage, purpose, schedule, precautions, and potential side effects.
- Teach the signs and symptoms of infection: fever; unusual drainage from paracentesis or other invasive procedure sites; warmth and erythema surrounding the invasive sites; or abdominal pain. Have patient demonstrate technique for measuring oral temperature with type of thermometer used at home.
- Teach the signs and symptoms of unusual bleeding, including prolonged mucosal bleeding, very large or painful bruises, and dark stools. Caution patient that, if possible, major dental procedures should be postponed until bleeding times normalize.
- Inform patient about sodium restriction if ascites developed during the course of the illness.
- Advise protein restriction if the patient has residual or chronic encephalopathy. Instruct patient to avoid constipation by increasing bulk in the diet or by using agents prescribed by physician.
- Caution about the necessity of alcohol cessation for at least several months after complete recovery from the acute episode. After full recovery, one or two glasses of beer or wine a day usually are allowed if hepatic failure was not related to alcohol ingestion.
- Instruct patient to weigh daily and to report weight loss or gain of >5 lb.

ADDITIONAL NURSING DIAGNOSES

As appropriate, see the following for additional nursing diagnoses and interventions: "Nutritional Support," p. 1; "Mechanical Ventilation," p. 17; "Prolonged Immobility," p. 74; "Psychosocial Support," p. 83; and "Psychosocial Support for the Patient's Family and Significant Others," p. 95.

Acute pancreatitis

PATHOPHYSIOLOGY

Pancreatitis is an autodigestive process of pancreatic tissue by its own enzymes. Chronic pancreatitis is an ongoing inflammatory disorder characterized by irreversible damage, causing pain and ultimately loss of function. With acute pancreatitis, elevated pancreatic enzymes and inflammation result in sudden abdominal pain and pancreatic dysfunction. Episodes may recur, but the gland remains normal before and after the attack. Initially, pancreatic ductal flow becomes obstructed because of biliary stones, reflux, sludge, sphincter spasm, or structural weakness, resulting in injury to the adjacent acinar cells, where pancreatic enzymes are stored in their inactive form. Once acinar cell damage has occurred, enzymes are released and activated, resulting in necrosis or autodigestion of the organ. Autodigestion remains the most accepted of several pathogenic theories. Although alcohol and gallstone disease account for the majority of cases, several other factors are believed to prematurely activate pancreatic enzyme secretions, such as endotoxins, ischemia, anoxia, tumors, trauma, and certain drugs (Table 8-12).

Acute pancreatitis may be clinically classified as mild or severe. In cases of mild acute pancreatitis, there is minimal interstitial edema with sporadic acinar cell damage with no organ system failure. Patients usually improve in 48-72 h with supportive care. Severe acute pancreatitis is a life-threatening condition that is accompanied by necrosis, infection, organ failure, and increased mortality. It is characterized by edema and vascular insult frequently leading to rupture of the pancreatic ducts and spillage of pancreatic enzymes into the peritoneum, which results in a chemical peritonitis and systemic inflammation. Vascular damage causes leakage of fluid from the capillaries. Vasoactive amines, including bradykinin and kallikrein, contribute to capillary leakage and depress myocardial function. The net effect is hypovolemia and cardiovascular failure. Necrosis and hemorrhage are precursors of complete pancreatic dysfunction. Ranson's criteria is a scale of severity for acute pancreatitis based on age and laboratory studies. Pancreatitis is classified as severe when three or more of Ranson's criteria are met (Table 8-13).

Complications: Marked depletion of intravascular plasma volume is the result of fluid sequestration into the interstitium and retroperitoneum. Massive,

---

TABLE 8-12 Precipitating Factors for Acute Pancreatitis

Mechanical blockage of pancreatic ducts
- Biliary tract disease (e.g., gallstones)
- Structural abnormalities (e.g., pancreas divisum)

Toxic/metabolic factors
- Alcohol
- Hypertriglyceridemia
- Hypercalcemia (e.g., hyperparathyroidism)

Infection

Trauma
- External
- Surgical
- Iatrogenic

Ischemia
- Prolonged/severe shock
- Vasculitis

Tumors

Drugs
- NSAIDs
- Estrogens
- Corticosteroids
- Thiazides
- Tetracycline
- Sulfonamides

NSAIDs, Nonsteroidal antiinflammatory drugs.

TABLE 8-13   Ranson's Criteria for Classifying the Severity of Pancreatitis

At presentation
   Age >55 yr
   WBC >16,000
   Glucose >2000
   AST >250
   LDH >350

During initial 48 hours
   Base deficit >4 mEq/L
   BUN increased >5 mg/dl
   Fluid sequestration >6 L
   Serum Ca^{++} <8
   Hematocrit decrease >10%
   pO2 (from ABG) <60 mm HG

WBC, White blood count; *AST*, aspartate aminotransferase; *LDH*, lactate dehydrogenase; *BUN*, blood urea nitrogen; Ca^{++}, calcium; pO_2, partial pressure of oxygen.

life-threatening hemorrhage from rupture of necrotic tissue results in serious blood volume depletion. Hypoalbuminemia frequently is present and contributes to hypovolemia. Hypotension persists in some patients despite volume repletion. These patients are likely to have decreased vascular tone and other findings associated with a hyperdynamic circulatory state. Edema and increased vascular permeability are additional consequences attributed to vasoactive amines. If hypovolemia is not detected and treated promptly, acute renal failure becomes likely. Mild to severe respiratory failure with hypoxemia is common. Respiratory insufficiency is related to right-to-left vascular shunting within the lung and alveolocapillary leakage caused by circulating proteolytic enzymes and vasoactive amines. In addition, elevation of the diaphragm, atelectasis, and pleural effusion caused by subdiaphragmatic inflammation can compromise ventilation further. Intravascular coagulopathy develops in some patients, which can lead to life-threatening complications such as pulmonary emboli. Hypocalcemia, which is common, is attributed to calcium binding in areas of fat necrosis within the pancreas and small intestine. The formation of pancreatic pseudocysts or abscesses as a result of necrosis and the collection of purulent material within the tissue can lead to rupture, which in turn can cause sepsis. The ensuing circulatory and respiratory failure often leads to death.

ASSESSMENT

History and risk factors: Excessive alcohol ingestion; biliary tract disease; high cholesterol levels; use of drugs such as steroids, furosemide, thiazides, NSAIDs; viral infections (especially mumps and hepatitis); penetrating and blunt injuries to the pancreas. Pregnancy, primary hyperparathyroidism, uremia, and renal transplantation have been implicated as causes because they can lead to ductal stone formation and, as a result, pancreatitis.

Clinical presentation: Sudden onset of pain (often after excessive food or alcohol ingestion) lasting 12-48 h, described as mild discomfort to severe distress, and located from the midepigastrium to the right upper quadrant (RUQ). The pain may radiate to the back. Nausea, vomiting, and restlessness typically accompany the pain; diarrhea, melena, and hematemesis also may be present. Abdominal tenderness is common. Dyspnea and cyanosis, which are signs of ARDS (see p. 243), may occur as serious complications of acute pancreatitis. With biliary tract disease, jaundice may be present. Grey Turner sign (a blue-red-purple or green-brown discoloration of the flank) and Cullen sign (faint blue-tinged discoloration around the umbilicus) are associated with pancreatitis; however, both signs are uncommon. Urine output decreases as the body attempts to conserve intravascular volume. Hypocalcemia manifests as numbness or tingling in the extremities that can progress to tetany if calcium is severely depleted.

Physical assessment: Diminished or absent bowel sounds reflective of GI dysfunction and ileus. Palpation will reveal localized tenderness in the RUQ or diffuse discomfort over the upper portion of the abdomen. Mild to moderate ascites is present. Breath sounds may be decreased or absent, suggesting focal atelectasis or pleural effusion. Effusions usually are left sided but can be bilateral. Auscultation of crackles reflects hypoventilation caused by pain, early ARDS, or microemboli. In the presence of hemorrhage or severe hypovolemia, the hands will be cool and sweaty, capillary refill will be delayed, and peripheral pulses will be diminished. With severe hypocalcemia, Chvostek sign (facial twitching after a tap over the facial nerve) or Trousseau sign (spasm of the hand that occurs when the arm is constricted with a BP cuff) may be elicited.

Vital signs and hemodynamic measurements: Increased temperature associated with tachycardia and increased BP. Tachycardia, decreased BP, decreased PAP, and decreased CO are present with hemorrhage, shock, or dehydration. Increase in pulmonary vascular resistance (PVR) suggests the presence of ARDS or pulmonary emboli. If systemic inflammation or sepsis is present, CO may be elevated and SVR decreased.

DIAGNOSTIC TESTS

Hematologic studies: Leukocytosis with a WBC count of 11,000-20,000/mm^3 is reflective of the inflammatory process. Hct and Hgb levels vary, depending on the presence of hemorrhage (decreased) or dehydration (increased).

Chemistry studies: Serum amylase level usually is elevated 3-5 times that of normal for the first several days. As damage subsides, the level decreases. Amylase may be normal or even decreased in patients with necrotizing acute pancreatitis because of severe pancreatic damage and decreased amylase secretion. Serum lipase levels parallel amylase levels and are more specific for pancreatitis. Serum lipase may remain elevated for up to 14 days. Generally, urine amylase is elevated for 1-2 wk. The amylase/creatinine clearance ratio usually is elevated with obvious pancreatitis. Hypocalcemia is a frequent finding, and values <8 mg/dl are not uncommon. Because part of the calcium is protein bound, serum levels depend on albumin levels. As serum albumin levels decrease, reductions in serum calcium levels are anticipated. Hyperglycemia and glycosuria are consequences of glucagon release. Blood glucose values are commonly >200 mg/dl. Persistent elevation of liver enzymes suggests hepatic inflammation caused by alcohol ingestion or viral hepatitis. Increased serum bicarbonate and hypokalemia values reflect metabolic alkalosis, usually the result of vomiting or gastric suctioning.

Coagulation studies: Decreases in platelets and fibrinogen will be present. Elevations in circulating levels of fibrin are associated with microthrombi in the pancreas and other tissues.

ABG values: Decreased arterial oxygen tension is a common finding and may be present without other symptoms of pulmonary insufficiency. Early hypoxia produces a mild respiratory alkalosis. Arterial oxygen saturation may be diminished.

ECG: ST-segment depression and T-wave inversion may be seen as a result of the shock state, the severe pain that causes coronary artery spasm, or the effect of trypsin and bradykinins on the myocardium. Hypocalcemia results in widening of the ST segment.

Radiologic procedures: Abdominal x-ray may show dilation of the bowel and ileus. Chest x-ray findings are helpful in distinguishing effusions from atelectasis and in diagnosing ARDS. Endoscopic retrograde cholangiopancreatography (ERCP) sometimes is helpful after the acute episode in identifying stones or stenosis. However, endoscopic pancreatography (see below) is generally more valuable in detecting abnormalities and is less likely to worsen the course of the disease. Barium studies may reveal displacement of the stomach or duodenum caused by edema or pseudocysts.

CT: Estimates size of the pancreas; identifies fluid collection, cystic lesions, abscesses, and masses; visualizes biliary tract abnormalities; and monitors inflammatory swelling of the pancreas.

Endoscopic pancreatography: Employed to visualize the opening to the pancreas directly and to observe for swelling, ductal abnormalities, and presence of tumors or stones.

COLLABORATIVE MANAGEMENT

Treatment is more palliative than curative. Efforts are directed at pain relief and resting the pancreas until the autodigestive process subsides.

Analgesia: Opioid analgesics are administered for relief of severe pain. Continuous or intermittent IV routes are used, depending on the severity of the pain. Patient-controlled analgesia (PCA) is a helpful mode of delivery. Many opioid analgesics, including morphine, fentanyl, and meperidine (Demerol), cause spasm of pancreatic and biliary ducts and may impede ductal flow. Some authorities believe that meperidine is less likely to cause ductal spasm and therefore recommend it for analgesia in patients with pancreatitis. Epidural blockage may be employed for severe pain.

Fluid and electrolyte management: The inflammatory process results in fluid sequestration and extensive intravascular volume loss. Nausea, vomiting, gastric suctioning, and hemorrhage contribute to the hypovolemic state. Colloids and crystalloids are administered to replace volume losses and minimize interstitial edema. Crystalloids alone may be used initially if serum protein levels are adequate. Fluid sequestration in the peritoneum and interstitium continues until the acute phase is arrested; therefore continual volume replacement is essential. If serum potassium and calcium levels are decreased, replacement therapy is necessary. Because hypercalcemia has been implicated in the genesis of pancreatitis, calcium replacement is prescribed cautiously.

Suppression of pancreatic secretions: Accomplished by withholding oral feedings, including water; aspirating gastric secretions via gastric suction; reducing gastric acidity by administering histamine H_2-receptor antagonists and antacids; and reducing physical activity. Gastric suction has not been shown to offer any clear advantage and should be used only for patients with severe nausea and vomiting, abdominal distention, or pain not relieved by analgesia.

Respiratory support: Pulmonary congestion, pleural effusion, and atelectasis result in respiratory insufficiency. Abdominal distention and retroperitoneal fluid sequestration cause diaphragmatic elevation and ventilatory restriction. Early respiratory failure is detected by a decrease in oxygen tension or oxygen saturation. Frequent or continuous pulse oximetry is performed during the first 2-3 days of therapy to detect early hypoxemia. Oxygen is initiated if hypoxemia is present. If severe pulmonary insufficiency develops, patient requires ET intubation and positive pressure ventilation. IV fluids are given cautiously to prevent cardiopulmonary compromise.

Nutritional support: Parenteral feedings that provide nutrients necessary for tissue healing are initiated for patients with severe pancreatitis. High-glucose parenteral regimens compound the hyperglycemia that is commonly present in pancreatitis. For this reason a higher percentage of calories given as fats may be preferable. Use of long-chain fatty acids for patients with acute pancreatitis is controversial because there is concern that fatty-acid administration may exacerbate the pancreatitis. Oral feedings are not indicated during the acute episode because they result in pancreatic inflammation by stimulating glandular secretions. A feeding jejunostomy tube may be inserted to provide enteral feedings for some patients and may become the preferred feeding route because it has been found safe and without adverse effects, as well as extremely cost effective. Jejunal feeding tubes are placed orally, percutaneously, or surgically. Low-fat oral feedings are begun after the initial episode subsides and bowel function returns.

Peritoneal lavage: Removes toxic factors present in peritoneal exudate and can result in immediate clinical improvement in many patients with severe pancreatitis. The procedure is similar to peritoneal dialysis. A soft lavage catheter is positioned in the peritoneum, and continual lavage is instituted for 2-7 days, depending on the patient's clinical response. Generally, 2 L of an isotonic, balanced electrolyte solution is infused into the peritoneum over a 15-min period. The solution dwells in the peritoneum for 20-30 min and then is drained into a bedside collection container for 15-20 min. The cycle is repeated hourly. Common lavage additives include potassium, heparin, and a broad-spectrum antibiotic.

Surgical management: In general, nonsurgical management of acute pancreatitis is most effective. Because acute pancreatitis is easily confused with acute abdominal emergencies that require urgent surgery, exploratory laparotomy is necessary for some patients. More aggressive surgical procedures, such as early pancreatic drainage or débridement, remain controversial.

Antibiotic coverage: Prophylactic antibiotic use is necessary in severe, acute pancreatitis to reduce the chances of septic complications and improve the chances for survival.

NURSING DIAGNOSES AND INTERVENTIONS

Fluid volume deficit related to active loss secondary to fluid sequestration within the peritoneum and hemorrhage associated with tissue necrosis; insufficient oral intake

Desired outcome: Within 24 h of this diagnosis, patient becomes normovolemic as evidenced by MAP >70 mm Hg; HR 60-100 bpm; normal sinus rhythm on ECG; CVP 2-6 mm Hg; PAWP 6-12 mm Hg; CO $\geq$4-6 L/min; CI $\geq$3 L/min/m^2; SVR 900-1200 dynes/sec/cm^{-5}; PVR 60-100 dynes/sec/cm^{-5}; brisk capillary refill (<2 sec); peripheral pulses >2+ on a 0-4+ scale; urinary output $\geq$0.5 ml/kg/h; and stable weight.

- Administer crystalloids, colloids, or a combination of both as prescribed.
- Monitor BP q1-4h if losses are caused by fluid sequestration, inadequate intake, or slow bleeding. Monitor BP q15min if patient has active blood loss or unstable VS. Be alert to MAP decreases of $\geq$10 mm Hg from previous BP.
- Monitor HR, ECG, and cardiovascular status hourly. Monitor these parameters q15min, or more frequently in the presence of active bleeding or unstable VS. Be alert to increases in HR, which suggest hypovolemia.

Note: Increases in HR also may be caused by fever or hypermetabolic state.

- Measure hemodynamic parameters (i.e., CVP, PAWP, CO) and thermodilution CO q1-4h. Be alert to low or decreasing CVP, PAWP, and CO. Calculate SVR and PVR q4-8h, or more frequently in unstable patients. An elevated HR, decreased PAWP, decreased CO (CI <3 L/min/m^2), and increased SVR suggest hypovolemia. As available, monitor Svo$_2$ to evaluate adequacy of tissue oxygenation. Pulmonary hypertension is anticipated in patients with ARDS. Assess for signs of overaggressive fluid resuscitation (see **Fluid volume excess** p. 532).

- Measure urinary output hourly. Be alert to output <0.5 ml/kg/h for 2 consecutive hours. Evaluate intravascular volume and cardiovascular function, and increase fluid intake promptly if decreased urinary output is caused by hypovolemia and hypoperfusion.
- Monitor for physical indicators of hypovolemia, including cool extremities, delayed capillary refill (>2 sec), and decreased amplitude of or absent distal pulses.
- Estimate ongoing fluid losses. Measure all drainage from tubes, catheters, and drains. Note the frequency of dressing changes because of saturation with fluid or blood. Weigh patient daily, using the same scales and method. Compare 24-h urine output with 24-h fluid intake, and record the difference.
- Evaluate character of all fluid losses. Note color and odor. Be alert to the presence of particulate matter, fibrin, and clots. Test GI aspirate, drainage, and excretions (including stool) for the presence of occult blood.

NIC Fluid/Electrolyte Management; Fluid Monitoring; Hemodynamic Regulation; Hypovolemia Management; Invasive Hemodynamic Monitoring; Shock Prevention; Bleeding Precautions; Bleeding Reduction; Hypervolemia Management

Decreased cardiac output related to myocardial depression secondary to circulating vasoactive amines or hypocalcemia; decreased preload secondary to hypovolemia

Desired outcome: Within 12 h of this diagnosis, cardiac output becomes adequate as evidenced by CI $\geq$2.5 L/min/m^2; brisk capillary refill (<2 sec); peripheral pulses >2+ on a 0-4+ scale; urinary output $\geq$0.5 ml/kg/h; and warm skin.

- Restore acceptable preload by correcting hypovolemia (see preceding nursing diagnosis, **Fluid volume deficit**).
- Administer inotropic agents as prescribed. Monitor hemodynamic parameters carefully to minimize adverse affects of inotropic therapy (see Appendix 7).
- Provide patient with frequent rest periods. Space out procedures and treatments to allow long periods (at least 90 min) of uninterrupted rest.
- Minimize anxiety-producing situations, and assist patient with reducing anxiety (see **Health-seeking behavior,** p. 302, and **Anxiety,** p. 84).

NIC Cardiac Care: Acute; Hemodynamic Regulation; Shock Management: Cardiac; Dysrhythmia Management; Anxiety Reduction; Energy Management

Fluid volume excess related to excessive intake secondary to overaggressive fluid resuscitation and peritoneal lavage

Desired outcome: Within 24 h of this diagnosis, patient becomes normovolemic as evidenced by MAP 70-105 mm Hg; HR 60-100 bpm; RR 12-20 breaths/min with normal pattern and depth (eupnea); CVP 2-6 mm Hg; PAWP 6-12 mm Hg; CI $\geq$2.5 L/min/m^2; and absence of adventitious breath sounds and S$_3$ gallop.

- Evaluate patient q1-4h for clinical indicators of fluid volume excess: dyspnea, orthopnea, increased respiratory rate and effort, S$_3$ gallop, or crackles. Document and report changes and new findings.
- Measure hemodynamic parameters (BP, HR, CVP, PAWP) hourly in patients undergoing peritoneal lavage or in patients with evidence of hypervolemia (i.e., CVP or PAWP increased from baseline or above normal or presence of clinical indicators of fluid volume excess).
- As prescribed, administer inotropic agents to augment myocardial contractility. Evaluate effectiveness by measuring CO and calculating CI q1-2h and by measuring urine output q1-2h. Document and report CI <2.5 L/min/m^2 and urine output <0.5 ml/kg/h for 2 consecutive hours.
- Administer furosemide (Lasix) or other diuretic as prescribed to promote diuresis. Document response to diuretic therapy by noting onset and amount of diuresis.

T A B L E   8 - 1 4   Nursing Interventions for the Patient Undergoing Peritoneal Lavage for Acute Pancreatitis

- Ensure sterile technique throughout all phases of lavage to prevent serious complications caused by infection.
- Warm lavage fluid to patient's body temperature to prevent cramping, hypothermia, and discomfort.
- Measure lavage infusion fluid loss/retention. Document input and output throughout entire procedure. Document and report daily fluid balance—either excess or deficit.
- Turn patient gently from side to side as needed to promote drainage.
- Monitor patient carefully for decrease in ventilatory excursion caused by pressure from lavage fluid. Drain fluid and consult physician promptly if signs and symptoms of respiratory distress develop.
- Maintain head of bed at 30 degrees or higher.
- Check urine for glucose, and monitor blood glucose levels. Glucose in the lavage fluids can contribute to the glucose intolerance that frequently occurs in patients with pancreatitis. Insulin administration may be required in some instances.
- Note and document characteristics (color, odor, clairity, amount) of lavage return. Document and report changes.

- Carefully implement peritoneal lavage as prescribed (see "Collaborative Management," p. 531, and Table 8-14).

Pain related to chemical injury to the peritoneum and surrounding tissue secondary to release of pancreatic enzymes

Desired outcomes: Within 2-4 h of this diagnosis, patient's subjective evaluation of discomfort improves, as documented by a pain scale. Ventilation and hemodynamic status are uncompromised as evidenced by MAP 70-105 mm Hg; HR 60-100 bpm; and RR 12-20 breaths/min with normal depth and pattern (eupnea).

- As prescribed, administer IV opiate analgesic before pain becomes severe. Be aware that fentanyl, morphine, meperidine, and other opioid analgesics have been linked with biliary spasm and symptoms of biliary colic.

Note: Opioid analgesics decrease intestinal motility and delay return to normal bowel function.

- Pancreatitis can be very painful. Prepare significant others for personality changes and behavioral alterations associated with extreme pain and opiate analgesia. Family members sometimes misinterpret patient's lethargy or unpleasant disposition and may even blame themselves. Reassure them that these are normal responses.
- Supplement analgesics with nonpharmacologic maneuvers to aid in pain reduction. Modify patient's body position to optimize comfort. Many patients with abdominal pain find a dorsal recumbent or lateral decubitus bent-knee position most comfortable.
- Because anxiety reduction contributes to pain relief, ensure consistency and promptness in delivering analgesic.
- Patients and family members sometimes are distressed at the health team members' inability to relieve pain. Provide continual reassurance that all possible measures are being implemented.

- Monitor respiratory pattern and LOC closely because both may be depressed by the large amounts of opiate analgesics usually required to control pain.
- Monitor HR and BP q1-4h. Monitor CVP and PAWP q4h, or more frequently in unstable patients. Consult physician for significant deviations from baseline. Be aware that opiates cause vasodilation and can result in serious hypotension, especially in patients with volume depletion.
- Evaluate effectiveness of medication, and consult physician for dose and drug manipulation. If medications are not effective, prepare patient for splanchnic block or other pain-relieving procedure.

NIC Analgesic Administration; Pain Management; Patient-Controlled Analgesia (PCA) Assistance; Environmental Management: Comfort; Coping Enhancement; Teaching: Prescribed Medication; Simple Guided Imagery; Respiratory Monitoring

- For additional interventions for pain, see p. 61.

Impaired gas exchange related to alveolar-capillary membrane changes secondary to microatelectasis and pulmonary fluid accumulation

Desired outcome: Within 4 h of this diagnosis, patient has adequate gas exchange as evidenced by Sao_2 $\geq$92%; Pao_2 $\geq$80 mm Hg; $Paco_2$ 35-45 mm Hg; RR 12-20 breaths/min with normal depth and pattern (eupnea); patient oriented to time, place, and person; and clear and audible breath sounds.

- Monitor and document respiratory rate q1-4h as indicated. Note pattern, degree of excursion, and whether patient uses accessory muscles of respiration. Consult physician for significant deviations from baseline.
- Auscultate both lung fields q4-8h. Note presence of abnormal (crackles, rhonchi, wheezes) or diminished sounds.
- Be alert to early signs of hypoxia, such as restlessness, agitation, and alterations in mentation.
- Monitor Sao_2 via continuous pulse oximetry or ABG values frequently during the first 48 h. Many patients with pancreatitis do not have obvious clinical symptoms of respiratory failure, and a decreased arterial oxygen tension may be the first sign of failure. Consult physician if Pao_2 is <60-70 mm Hg or if oxygen saturation falls below 92%.
- Administer oxygen as prescribed. Check oxygen delivery system at frequent intervals to ensure proper delivery because oxygen is critical to these patients.
- Maintain body position that optimizes ventilation and oxygenation. Elevate HOB 30 degrees or higher, depending on patient's comfort. If pleural effusion or other defect is present on one side, position patient with the unaffected lung dependent to maximize the ventilation-perfusion relationship.
- Avoid overaggressive fluid resuscitation (see **Fluid volume excess,** p. 532).

NIC Acid-Base Management; Airway Management; Oxygen Therapy; Respiratory Monitoring; Positioning; Fluid Monitoring; Hypervolemia Management

- See "Acute Respiratory Distress Syndrome," p. 243, for additional information.

Risk for infection related to tissue destruction with resulting necrosis secondary to release of pancreatic enzymes

Desired outcome: Patient remains free of infection as evidenced by core or rectal temperature $\leq$37.8° C ($\leq$100° F); negative culture results; HR 60-100 bpm; RR 12-20 breaths/min; BP within patient's normal range; CI $\leq$4 L/min/m^2; SVR 900-1200 dynes/sec/cm^{-5}; and orientation to time, place, and person.

- Check rectal or core temperature q4h for increases. Be aware that hypothermia may precede hyperthermia in some patients.
- If temperature suddenly rises, obtain specimens for culture of blood, sputum, urine, and other sites as prescribed. Monitor culture reports, and report positive findings promptly.

- Evaluate orientation and LOC q2-4h. Document and report significant deviations from baseline.
- Monitor BP, HR, RR, CO, and SVR q1-4h. Be alert to increases in HR and RR associated with temperature elevations. An elevated CO (CI >4 L/min/m^2) and decreased SVR (<900 dynes/sec/cm^{-5}) suggest systemic inflammatory response or sepsis.
- Administer parenteral antibiotics in a timely fashion. Reschedule antibiotics if a dose is delayed for more than 1 h. Recognize that failure to administer antibiotics on schedule can result in inadequate blood levels and treatment failure. Monitor peak and trough levels for patients receiving aminoglycoside antibiotics. Aminoglycosides are used frequently; therefore monitor patient for hearing loss. Older adults are especially susceptible to the ototoxic and nephrotoxic effects of aminoglycosides. Monitor levels of BUN, creatinine, and urinary output, which are indicators of renal function.

NIC Medication Management; Vital Signs Monitoring; Temperature Regulation; Intravenous (IV) Therapy

Impaired tissue integrity: GI tract, related to release of chemical irritants into the pancreatic parenchyma and surrounding tissue, including the peritoneum

Desired outcomes: By the time of hospital discharge, patient exhibits no further GI tissue destruction as evidenced by reduction in pain; GI aspirate, stools, drainage, and vomitus negative for blood; and return of bowel sounds and bowel function. Gastric pH value remains >5.

- Withhold oral feedings to avoid stimulation of pancreatic enzymes.
- Ensure patency of gastric sump tube to provide continual gastric drainage and prevent pancreatic stimulation. Do not occlude the air vent of double-lumen tube because this may result in vacuum occlusion. Check placement of gastric tube at least q8h, and reposition as necessary.
- Administer antacids and histamine H$_2$-receptor antagonists as prescribed to decrease gastric and pancreatic secretions and to reduce gastric pH. Monitor gastric pH, and administer antacids to maintain pH value >5.
- Because increased activity can stimulate gastric secretions, limit patient's physical activity during the acute phase.
- Test GI aspirate, drainage, and excretions for the presence of occult blood q12-24h.
- Initiate peritoneal lavage as prescribed (see Table 8-14) to remove irritants from the peritoneum.

NIC Oral Health Maintenance; Acid-Base Management; Gastrointestinal Intubation; Bleeding Precautions

Altered nutrition: less than body requirements, related to decreased oral intake secondary to nausea, vomiting, and NPO status; increased need secondary to tissue destruction or infection

Desired outcomes: Patient maintains baseline body weight and demonstrates a state of nitrogen balance on nitrogen studies.

- Collaborate with physician, dietitian, and pharmacist to estimate patient's individual metabolic needs, based on activity level, presence of infection or other stressor, and nutritional status before hospitalization. Develop a plan of care accordingly.
- As prescribed, provide parenteral nutrition during acute phase of pancreatitis. Monitor closely for evidence of hyperglycemia (e.g., Kussmaul respirations; rapid respirations; fruity acetone breath odor; flushed, dry skin; deteriorating LOC), which commonly is associated with pancreatitis. Administer insulin as prescribed.
- Administer enteral feedings via feeding jejunostomy as prescribed for patients with intestinal peristalsis.
- Monitor bowel sounds q4h. Document and report deviations from baseline. Withhold oral or jejunostomy feedings if bowel sounds are absent.

- Monitor blood or urine glucose levels q4-8h or as prescribed. Consult physician for blood levels >200 mg/dl.
- Begin low-fat oral feedings when acute episode has subsided and bowel function has returned. This may take several weeks in some patients.

NIC Nutrition Management; Nutritional Monitoring; Enteral Tube Feeding; Aspiration Precautions; Total Parenteral Nutrition (TPN) Administration; Venous Access Devices (VAD) Maintenance; Hyperglycemia Management; Hypoglycemia Management

- For additional detail, see "Nutritional Support," p. 1.

Knowledge deficit: lack of exposure to health care information

Desired outcome: Within the 24-h period before hospital discharge, patient verbalizes knowledge regarding availability of alcohol rehabilitation programs, prescribed medications, importance of a low-fat diet, indicators of actual or impending GI hemorrhage, indicators of infection, and the importance of seeking medical attention promptly if signs of recurring pancreatitis appear.

- Inform patients whose pancreatitis is caused by excessive alcohol intake about the availability of alcohol rehabilitation programs.
- Teach patient about prescribed medications, including drug name, dosage, purpose, schedule, precautions, and side effects.
- Advise patient about the importance of adhering to a low-fat diet if prescribed.
- Instruct patient about the indicators of actual or impending GI hemorrhage: nausea, vomiting blood, dark stools, lightheadedness, passing frank blood in stools.
- Teach the indicators of infection: fever, unusual drainage from surgical incisions or peritoneal lavage site, warmth or erythema surrounding surgical sites, and abdominal pain. Have patient demonstrate oral temperature-taking technique using glass thermometer or type of thermometer that will be used at home.
- Stress the importance of seeking medical attention promptly if signs of recurrent pancreatitis (i.e., pain, change in bowel habits, passing blood in the stools, or vomiting blood) or infection (see **Risk for infection,** p. 534) appear.

NIC Teaching: Disease Process, Individual, Prescribed Activity Exercise, Prescribed Diet, Prescribed Procedure/Treatment, Prescribed Medication; Behavior Modification

ADDITIONAL NURSING DIAGNOSES

As appropriate, see nursing diagnoses and interventions in the following: "Acute Respiratory Distress Syndrome," p. 243; "Acute Renal Failure," p. 371; "Enterocutaneous Fistulas," p. 549; "Disseminated Intravascular Coagulation," p. 579; and "Septic Shock," p. 593. Also see "Prolonged Immobility," p. 74; "Psychosocial Support," p. 83; and "Psychosocial Support for the Patient's Family and Significant Others," p. 95.

Peritonitis

PATHOPHYSIOLOGY

Peritonitis can be classified as either *primary* or *secondary*. Primary peritonitis occurs spontaneously without any apparent source of contamination. It occurs most commonly in conjunction with cirrhosis of the liver. Secondary peritonitis is an inflammation of all or part of the peritoneal cavity and is caused by diffuse microbial proliferation or chemical irritation from leakage of corrosive gastric or intestinal contents into the peritoneum. Ruptured appendix, perforated peptic ulcer, bowel rupture related to ulcerative colitis or Crohn disease, pancreatitis, abdominal trauma, and ruptured abdominal abscesses are among the many etiologic factors associated with peritonitis. Indwelling tubes and catheters, such as those used for postoperative drainage and continuous ambulatory peritoneal dialysis (CAPD), are foreign bodies that compromise peritoneal integrity and permit the entry of infective organisms that can trigger peritonitis.

Regardless of the initiating factor, the inflammatory process is similar in every case. The initial reactions, which usually are triggered by histamine release, include hyperemia, edema, and vascular congestion. Fluid shifts from intravascular to interstitial spaces as a result of increased vascular permeability. The circulating blood volume is depleted, and hypovolemic shock may ensue. The transudated fluid contains high levels of fibrinogen and thromboplastin. The fibrinogen is converted to fibrin by the thromboplastin. Under normal conditions the peritoneum has fibrinolytic abilities to stop the fibrin formation. When the peritoneum is weakened or injured, however, this ability is hampered and fibrin adhesions form around the damaged area. The fibrin deposits form a barrier that harbors and protects bacteria from the body's defenses, resulting in multiple pockets of infection, which can lead to recurrent infection or septicemia. In most cases the fibrin deposits dissolve, but prolonged or severe inflammation can result in the continuing presence of fibrin, leading to adhesions and potential bowel obstruction.

ASSESSMENT

History and risk factors: Inflammatory processes such as diverticulitis, appendicitis, or Crohn disease; obstructive events in the small bowel and colon; vascular events such as ischemic colitis, mesenteric thrombosis, or embolic phenomena; blunt or penetrating trauma, especially to hollow viscera; severe hepatobiliary disease; and CAPD. General risk factors include those related to poor tissue healing and infection (e.g., advanced age, diabetes, vascular disease, advanced liver disease, malignancy, malnutrition, and debilitation).

Clinical presentation: The primary symptom is pain, which may be quite severe, causing the patient to maintain a fetal position and resist any movement that aggravates the pain. Its onset can be sudden or insidious, with the location varying according to the underlying pathology. Fever and restlessness are common findings in many patients. Nausea, vomiting, anorexia, and changes in bowel habits also may be present and are reflective of GI dysfunction.

Physical assessment: Auscultation of all four quadrants usually reveals diminished or absent bowel sounds. The complete absence of bowel sounds suggests an ileus—a frequent complication of peritonitis. Palpation of the abdomen elicits tenderness that can be generalized or localized, depending on the nature and extent of infection. Rebound tenderness, guarding, and involuntary rigidity also may be present. Occasionally, mild to moderate ascites is observed, depending on the cause of peritonitis. RR is rapid, and the patient usually has a shallow ventilatory pattern to minimize abdominal movement and pain; as a consequence, breath sounds may be diminished. Fluid shifts and hypovolemia can cause restlessness and confusion because of impaired cerebral perfusion.

Vital signs and hemodynamic measurements: Usually, fever is present, accompanied by tachypnea and tachycardia as a result of increased metabolic demands. During the acute phase the cardiovascular system may be compromised by large fluid shifts from the intravascular space into the abdominal interstitium and peritoneum. This disruption of intravascular volume can lead to hypovolemia with marked tachycardia, hypotension, low CO, decreased PA pressures, and decreased urine output. Depending on disease progression, the patient may exhibit signs of septic shock. Endotoxemic vasodilation is manifested by a low SVR, with an initial increase in HR and CO. This state complicates the initial hypovolemia and may result in a dangerously low MAP, thus impairing renal, cardiac, and cerebral perfusion. See Table 4-17 for a comparison of the hemodynamic profiles for persons with hypovolemic and septic shock.

DIAGNOSTIC TESTS

Hematologic studies: Leukocytosis will be present, with the WBC count usually >20,000/mm^3. Initially, the Hgb and Hct values may be increased because of hemoconcentration, but they will decrease to baseline levels as normal intravascular volume is restored.

Blood chemistry studies: Depending on the severity of the patient's condition, blood electrolyte levels may be abnormal. If nausea and vomiting are persistent, metabolic alkalosis is expected. This state is reflected by high CO_2 and low Cl^- values. Serum albumin levels often are decreased, especially with bacterial peritonitis. The underlying disease process affects chemistry studies (e.g., patients with pancreatitis usually have elevated amylase levels).

Radiologic procedures: The abdominal x-ray usually reveals dilation of the large and small bowel, with edema of the small bowel wall. Free air in the abdomen suggests visceral perforation. With CT, abscesses can be visualized and sometimes drained during the procedure, thus avoiding surgery.

Ultrasonography: Useful in locating small amounts of loculated fluid, as well as in differentiating fluid collections in the abdomen.

Diagnostic paracentesis: Abdominal paracentesis involves the insertion of a catheter or trocar into the abdomen to obtain specimens. Sterile saline is infused through the catheter, and the return fluid is analyzed for RBC, WBC, amylase, and bacteria content. If ascites is present, it may not be necessary to infuse saline because fluid can be removed directly for analysis.

COLLABORATIVE MANAGEMENT

Because peritonitis usually is a complication of another condition, the aim of therapy is to treat the underlying disease process. Following are some of the general therapies that apply to the management of peritonitis.

Antimicrobial therapy: Most commonly, both aerobic and anaerobic organisms are found within the abdomen. Usually a combination of an aminoglycoside, such as gentamicin (Garamycin), with a third-generation cephalosporin, such as cephazolin, or penicillin/beta-lactamase inhibitor is utilized to provide full antimicrobial coverage. For patients undergoing CAPD, vancomycin (Vancocin) may be added if indicated by culture growth. Therapeutic levels are drawn to guide therapy. Refer to Table 8-19 for nursing implications for aminoglycoside therapy.

Pain management: The degree of discomfort caused by peritonitis varies greatly. Opiate analgesics are used to ensure patient comfort but are given cautiously to avoid compromise of abdominal and respiratory function. These analgesics usually require frequent administration, with the dose titrated for each individual.

Fluid and electrolyte management: With bacterial peritonitis a significant intravascular volume depletion may occur. In most cases crystalloids are used initially unless there is evidence of decreased intravascular proteins, in which event colloids such as albumin are indicated. If peritonitis is complicated by hemorrhage, packed RBCs may be given. Electrolyte replacement, typically potassium, is implemented according to laboratory findings. See "Septic Shock," p. 593, for additional information.

Nutritional therapy: Because of the inflammatory process, GI function is compromised and motility is minimal or absent. An enteric tube is inserted to reduce or prevent distention and promote function. Initially, the patient is placed on NPO status until some GI function is regained. When resumption of bowel sounds or passage of flatus signals the return of GI motility, enteral nutrition is begun. If the return of gastric motility is delayed for several days, parenteral nutrition may be necessary.

Surgical management: Surgery is often necessary, depending on the cause of peritonitis. All intraabdominal foreign material is removed, and nonviable tissue is débrided. Leaky anastomoses are identified and repaired. If present, bowel perforations and obstructions are corrected and abscesses are drained.

NURSING DIAGNOSES AND INTERVENTIONS

Fluid volume deficit related to active loss secondary to fluid sequestration within the peritoneum

Desired outcome: Within 8 h of this diagnosis, patient becomes normovolemic as evidenced by the following parameters: MAP 70-105 mm Hg; HR 60-100 bpm; normal sinus rhythm on ECG; CVP 2-6 mm Hg; PAWP 6-12 mm Hg; CI 2.5-4 L/min/m^2; urinary output ≥0.5 ml/kg/h; warm extremities; peripheral pulses >2+ on a 0-4+ scale; brisk capillary refill (<2 sec); patient oriented to time, place, and person; and stable weight.

- Monitor BP q1-4h, depending on patient stability. Be alert to MAP decreases of ≥10 mm Hg from previous BP reading.
- Monitor HR and ECG q1-4h, or more often if VS are unstable. Be alert to increases in HR, which suggest hypovolemia. Usually the ECG will show sinus tachycardia. In the presence of hypokalemia caused by prolonged vomiting or gastric suction, ECG may show ventricular ectopy, prominent U wave, and depression of the ST segment.

> **Note:** HR increases also may be caused by fever.

- Measure CVP, PAWP, and thermodilution CO q1-4h, depending on patient stability. Be alert to low or decreasing CVP, PAWP, and CO. Calculate SVR q4-8h, or more frequently in unstable patients. A decreased CVP and PAWP, decreased CO (CI <2.5 L/min/m^2), and increased SVR (>1200 dynes/sec/cm^{-5}) suggest hypovolemia.
- Measure urinary output hourly. Be alert to output <0.5 ml/kg/h for 2 consecutive hours, which may signal intravascular volume depletion. Consult physician and increase fluid intake promptly if decreased urinary output is caused by hypovolemia and hypoperfusion.
- Monitor patient for physical indicators of hypovolemia, including cool extremities, capillary refill >2 sec, decreased amplitude of peripheral pulses, and neurologic changes such as restlessness and confusion.
- Estimate ongoing fluid losses. Measure all drainage from tubes, catheters, and drains. Note the frequency of dressing changes as a result of saturation with fluid or blood. Weigh the patient daily, using the same scales and method. Compare 24-h body fluid output with 24-h fluid intake, and record the difference.

NIC Fluid/Electrolyte Management; Fluid Monitoring; Hemodynamic Regulation; Hypovolemia Management; Invasive Hemodynamic Monitoring; Shock prevention; Dysrhythmia Management

Pain related to biologic or chemical agents causing injury to the peritoneum and intraperitoneal organs

Desired outcomes: Within 2 h of this diagnosis, patient's subjective evaluation of discomfort improves, as documented by a pain scale. Nonverbal indicators of discomfort, such as grimacing, are absent.

- Monitor patient for the presence of discomfort. Devise a pain scale with the patient, such as rating discomfort from 0 (no pain) to 10. Administer analgesics promptly, before pain becomes severe. Consistency and promptness in delivering analgesics also may help to decrease patient's anxiety, which can contribute to the severity of the pain. Rate the degree of pain relief obtained by using the pain scale. Be aware that opiate analgesics decrease GI motility and may delay the return of normal bowel function.
- Modify patient's body position to optimize comfort. Many patients with severe abdominal pain find a dorsal recumbent or lateral decubitus bent-knee position more comfortable than other positions.

- Monitor respiratory pattern and LOC hourly, because both may be depressed if large amounts of opiates are required to control the pain.
- Monitor HR and BP q1-4h. Monitor CVP and PAWP q4h, or more frequently in unstable patients. Consult physician for significant deviations. Be aware that many opiates cause vasodilation and can result in serious hypotension, especially in patients with volume depletion.
- Evaluate effectiveness of the medication on an ongoing basis. On the basis of the patient's clinical response, discuss dose and drug manipulation with physician.
- Avoid administration of analgesics to newly admitted patients until they have been fully evaluated by a surgeon, because analgesics can mask important diagnostic clues.

NIC Analgesic Administration; Pain Management; Environmental Management: Comfort; Coping Enhancement; Simple Guided Imagery; Respiratory Monitoring

- See p. 61 for additional interventions for patients with pain.

Altered nutrition: less than body requirements, related to decreased intake secondary to impaired GI function

Desired outcomes: Patient maintains baseline body weight, and nitrogen studies show a state of nitrogen balance within 5-7 days of this diagnosis.

- Monitor bowel sounds q1-8h; report significant changes (i.e., sudden absence or return).
- Maintain NPO status during the acute phase of peritonitis. Gradually increase oral or enteral intake when gastric motility returns.
- If patient has abdominal distention, measure and document abdominal girth q8h. Distention can signal complications such as ileus or ascites.
- Administer histamine H_2-receptor antagonists, antacids, and sucralfate as prescribed to reduce corrosiveness of gastric acid and prevent complications such as stress ulcers.
- Administer prescribed antiemetic medications as indicated.
- Ensure that gastric, intestinal, and other GI drainage tubes are functioning properly. Evaluate character of the drainage (see Table 2-14, p. 191). Irrigate or reposition tubes as necessary. Patency and proper position of decompression tubes, such as the Miller-Abbott type, are essential for proper function.

NIC Nutrition Management; Nutritional Monitoring; Gastrointestinal Intubation; Enteral Tube Feeding; Aspiration Precautions; Tube Care: Gastrointestinal

- For additional information, see "Nutritional Support," p. 1.

Risk for infection related to inadequate primary defenses (traumatized tissue, altered perfusion); tissue destruction; environmental exposure to pathogens

Desired outcome: Septicemia does not develop as evidenced by HR 160-100 bpm; RR 12-20 breaths/min; SVR 900-1200 dynes/sec/cm^{-5}; CI 2.5-4 L/min/m^2; normothermia; negative culture results; and orientation to time, place, and person.

- Monitor VS and hemodynamic measurements for evidence of septicemia: increases in HR, RR, and CO (CI >4 L/min/m^2) and a decrease in SVR (<900 dynes/sec/cm^{-5}). Check rectal or core temperature q4h for increases. Be aware that hypothermia may precede hyperthermia in some patients. Also note that older adults and those who are immunocompromised may not demonstrate a fever, even with severe sepsis.
- If the patient has a sudden temperature elevation, obtain culture specimens of blood, sputum, urine, and other sites as prescribed. Monitor culture reports, and report positive findings promptly.
- Administer parenteral antibiotics in a timely fashion. Reschedule antibiotics if a dosage is delayed for more than 1 h. Recognize that failure to administer antibiotics on schedule may result in inadequate drug blood levels and treatment failure. Aminoglycosides are used frequently; therefore monitor patient for hearing loss. Older adults are especially susceptible to the ototoxic effects of aminoglycosides. Check BUN and creatinine levels, and monitor

urinary output to ensure that patient has adequate renal function, inasmuch as aminoglycosides are potentially nephrotoxic. Measure peak and trough levels of aminoglycosides, and consult physician for levels that are above or below therapeutic range.

- To minimize microbial growth, facilitate drainage of pus, GI secretions, old blood, necrotic tissue, foreign material such as feces, and other body fluids from wounds (Table 2-14, p. 191).
- Evaluate wounds for evidence of infection (e.g., erythema, warmth, swelling, unusual drainage). Culture any unusual drainage (see Table 2-14 for a description of normal drainage).
- Evaluate patient's orientation to time, place, and person and LOC q2-4h. Document and report significant deviations from baseline.

NIC Medication Management; Hemodynamic Regulation; Vital Signs Monitoring; Temperature Regulation; Intravenous (IV) Therapy; Wound Care

- See discussion of sepsis in "Septic Shock," p. 593, for additional information.

Hyperthermia related to infectious process, increased metabolic rate, and dehydration secondary to peritonitis

Desired outcomes: Patient's temperature remains within acceptable limits (36°-38.9° C [97°-102° F]) or returns to acceptable limits within 4-6 h of this diagnosis. An open airway is secured in the event of hyperthermic seizures.

- Monitor rectal or core temperature q2-4h.
- If a hypothermia blanket is required, perform the following interventions:
  - ☐ Protect the skin that is in contact with the blanket by placing a sheet between the blanket and patient.
  - ☐ Inspect patient's skin q2h for evidence of tissue damage caused by local vasoconstriction. Massage patient's skin q2h to promote circulation and minimize tissue damage.
  - ☐ Check patient's temperature at frequent intervals to ensure that sudden decreases (along with shivering) do not occur, which could increase metabolic demand.
- If patient has a high fever (i.e., >38.9° C [102° F]), administer tepid baths, which may be helpful in reducing the fever.
- Administer antipyretics as prescribed.
- Keep an appropriate-size oral airway and suction equipment in the patient's room for use in the event of seizure activity.

NIC Fever Treatment; Temperature Regulation; Vital Signs Monitoring

ADDITIONAL NURSING DIAGNOSES

For other nursing diagnoses and interventions, see the following as appropriate: "Hemodynamic Monitoring," p. 28; "Prolonged Immobility," p. 74; "Psychosocial Support," p. 83; "Psychosocial Support for the Patient's Family and Significant Others," p. 95; and "Septic Shock," p. 593.

Acute gastrointestinal bleeding

PATHOPHYSIOLOGY

Bleeding can occur at any point along the alimentary tract. The following brief overview presents common GI bleeding sites or occurrences.

Esophagus: Esophageal varices (see p. 492) are the most common cause of massive esophageal hemorrhage. Esophagitis and esophageal ulcers and tumors also can cause acute bleeding, but they occur less frequently. Maneuvers that increase intraabdominal pressure (e.g., retching, vomiting, straining, coughing) can lead to Mallory-Weiss tear, a laceration at the esophagogastric junction, resulting in massive bleeding.

Stomach and duodenum: The most common causes of hematemesis and melena are duodenal and gastric ulcers, accounting for half of massive upper

GI bleeding disorders. Stress ulceration is a common and potentially life-threatening phenomenon that occurs in >85% of critically ill patients. Stress ulcers, also known as *erosive gastritis*, tend to be multiple, shallow lesions located in the proximal stomach. Cushing ulceration is a related condition occurring in patients who have sustained serious injury, major surgery, or critical CNS disorders. Curling ulcers occur in the esophagus, stomach, and duodenum and are associated with deeper mucosal invasion than stress ulcers. Curling ulcers are seen in patients with major burn injury. They are located in the duodenum and tend to be single, deep ulcers. Gastritis, another common cause of GI bleeding, usually occurs as slow, diffuse oozing that is difficult to control. Benign or malignant gastric tumors may initiate severe bleeding episodes, especially tumors located in the vascular system that supplies the GI tract.

Small intestine: This area of the alimentary tract accounts for only a small portion of GI bleeding episodes. Diverticular disease, arteriovenous malformation, intussusception of the small bowel, acute superior mesenteric artery occlusion, and Crohn disease are some of the possible causes for bleeding.

Large intestine: Arteriovenous malformation of the ascending colon and the cecum is the usual cause of massive colonic bleeding. Inflammatory bowel diseases such as ulcerative colitis and Crohn disease result in friable intestinal mucosa, which can lead to massive hemorrhage and other serious complications, including bowel obstruction and perforation. In addition, diverticular disease can cause serious, intermittent bleeding episodes. Other causes include benign or malignant neoplasms and congenital malformation such as hemangioma or telangiectasia.

Neighboring organs: Acute pancreatitis (see p. 526) and pancreatic pseudocyst are disorders associated with hemorrhage. Persons with intraabdominal vascular grafts are at risk for the development of aortoenteric fistulas with massive GI hemorrhage.

Systemic organ diseases: Hypoperfusion associated with decreased cardiac output or volume depletion can lead to GI ischemia, resulting in necrosis and hemorrhage. A high incidence of GI bleeding is associated with uremia because of platelet dysfunction. Collagen diseases can result in thrombosis of small vessels in the small intestine, eventually leading to ulceration. Many blood dyscrasias (e.g., DIC, thrombocytopenia) are associated with hematemesis and melena caused by decreased clotting.

Medications: Long-standing use of ASA, NSAIDs (even at low doses), steroids, or anticoagulants sometimes is associated with serious GI bleeding.

Other trauma: In addition to major abdominal trauma (see p. 183), foreign bodies (e.g., razors, screws, nails) may lacerate gastric or intestinal mucosa, causing bleeding.

ASSESSMENT

History and risk factors: Critical illness, especially that caused by major injury, surgery, CNS disorder, or burns; prolonged shock or hypoperfusion; organ failure; excessive alcohol, NSAID, or steroid ingestion; inflammatory bowel disease; foreign body ingestion; hiatal hernia; hepatic, pancreatic, or biliary tract disease; blood dyscrasias; penetrating or blunt trauma; familial cancer; recent abdominal surgery; and the presence of *Heliobacter pylori*, which is found in >90% of patients with duodenal ulcers and 70% of those with gastric ulcers. Identification of patients who are at risk for recurrent bleeding is essential to guide therapy and prevent poor outcomes. Risk factors associated with rebleeding are listed in Table 8-15.

Clinical presentation: Varies, depending on the amount of blood lost, rate of bleeding, and its effects on cardiovascular and other body systems. Adults can lose up to 500 ml of blood in 15 min and remain free of associated symptoms. A loss of 1000 ml in 15 min usually produces tachycardia, hypotension, nausea, weakness, and diaphoresis. Massive hemorrhage generally is defined as loss of

TABLE 8-15 Risk Factors to Predict Recurrent Bleeding

Large volume blood loss on admission with transfusion of >6 units
Shock
Age >60 yr
Hemetemesis as the initial sign of hemorrhage
Presence of stigmata of recent hemorrhage as identified endoscopically
Bleeding that occurs while hospitalized for another problem

>30% of total blood volume, or a bleeding episode that requires transfusion of 6 U of blood in 24 h. Syncope associated with hypotension also may occur. Hematemesis, melena (passage of black, shiny, fetid stools containing blood), and hematochezia (passage of bloody stools) usually are present. Blood can irritate the bowels, thereby increasing transit time and causing diarrhea. Mild to severe pain often is associated with ulcerative or erosive disease. As blood covers and protects the eroded tissue, pain may disappear. Severe hypovolemic shock and decreased cardiac output can lead to ischemia of various organs, especially the brain and kidneys. Alterations in LOC and diminished urinary output will result.

Physical assessment: With profuse, active bleeding, a fast assessment can determine if a shock state is present: the presence of tachycardia, hypotension, cool and diaphoretic extremities, decreased peripheral pulses, delayed capillary refill (>2 sec), pallor or cyanosis, restlessness, confusion, decreased urine output, and obvious bleeding. Auscultation of the abdomen may reveal hyperactive bowel sounds caused by mucosal irritation by blood, or it may reveal a silent abdomen, which suggests serious complications such as ileus, perforation, or vascular occlusion. Palpation may reveal epigastric tenderness, which is expected in peptic ulceration, or an epigastric mass or enlarged lymph nodes, which indicate gastric malignant disease. Jaundice, vascular spiders, ascites, and hepatosplenomegaly suggest liver disease. A careful digital rectal examination should be performed, along with testing vomitus and stool for occult blood. With upper GI bleeding, emesis or gastric aspirate contains obvious whole blood or coffee ground–appearing old blood. Stools usually are black and tarry (melena), with a distinctive fetid odor. With lower GI bleeding, stools may be dark or contain fresh blood. Massive lower GI bleeding is associated with dark red "currant jelly" stools or passing fresh blood with clots (hematochezia). Bleeding below the level of the duodenum is not associated with hematemesis.

Vital signs and hemodynamic measurements: HR and BP are quick indicators of a hypovolemic state. Systolic BP <100 mm Hg with an HR >100 bpm in a previously normotensive individual signals a 20% or greater reduction in blood volume. In addition, postural VS should be measured. A decrease in systolic BP >10 mm Hg or an increase in HR of 10 bpm indicates a recent blood loss of at least 1000 ml in the adult. Hemodynamic measurements usually reveal a decreased PAP and CO and an increased SVR. After major abdominal surgery a hyperdynamic state may exist similar to that seen in early septic shock, with an increased CO and decreased SVR (see "Septic Shock," p. 593). RR will be mildly elevated as a response to the diminished oxygen-carrying capacity of the blood. If abdominal pain is present, ventilatory excursion may be limited.

DIAGNOSTIC TESTS

Hematologic tests: Serial Hgb and Hct values will reflect the amount of blood lost. Because the ratio of blood cells to plasma remains unchanged initially, the first Hct value may be near normal. However, the Hct is expected to fall dramatically as volume is restored and extravascular fluid mobilizes into the vascular space. Platelet count rises within 1 h of hemorrhage, and leukocytosis follows.

Chemistry studies: Excessive vomiting or gastric suction may cause a hypochloremic, hypokalemic state accompanied by a rise in the serum bicarbonate level. Increases in BUN without corresponding creatinine increases occur because of excess intestinal protein from the digestion of RBCs. BUN increases are not seen with bleeding from the colon or the lower portion of the small intestine inasmuch as protein digestion occurs higher in the upper portion. Dehydration and renal insufficiency contribute to an elevated BUN level in affected patients. Plasma protein levels may rise in response to increased hepatic production. Mild hyperglycemia is the result of the body's compensatory response to a stressful stimulus. Hyperbilirubinemia is caused by the breakdown of reabsorbed blood and its pigments. Ammonia levels usually are elevated in patients with hepatic disease.

ABG values: If the shock state is severe, lactic acidosis occurs, reflected by low arterial pH and serum bicarbonate levels and the presence of an anion gap. With a low perfusion state, hypoxemia may be present.

Coagulation studies: Depending on preexisting disease, hypocoagulability may be present. Elevation of fibrinogen levels, FSP, PT, and PTT may be seen.

12/18-lead ECG: May reflect severe cardiac ischemia as a result of hypoperfusion. Ischemic changes include T-wave depression or inversion.

Esophagogastroduodenoscopy (EGD, panendoscopy): The most accurate means of determining source of upper GI bleeding. The esophagus, stomach, and duodenum are visualized directly with a fiberoptic endoscope, which is passed through the mouth. Attempts are made to identify the exact source and characteristics of the ulcer. Findings indicative of bleeding ulcers or ulcers at risk for rebleeding are referred to as stigmata of recent hemorrhage (SRH) (Table 8-16). EGD is usually performed within the first 12 h after the patient's admission. The procedure provides both critical diagnostic and prognostic information necessary to direct therapy and to identify patients at risk for recurrent bleeding (see Table 8-15). It may be necessary to clear the stomach of blood and clots by lavage before the procedure. Antacids and sucralfate should be withheld until after the procedure, because they alter the appearance of the lesions. Electrocautery, laser, and other therapeutic techniques may be employed during this procedure.

Proctosigmoidoscopy: The rectum and sigmoid colon are visualized directly through an endoscope, which is passed through the anus into the lower GI tract. Mucosal bleeding, polyps, hemorrhoids, and other lesions may be seen. Biopsy specimens may be obtained during this procedure.

T A B L E   8 - 1 6   Stigmata of Recent Hemorrhage (SRH)

Characteristic endoscopic findings of recent upper gastrointestinal, nonvariceal hemorrhage
- Active bleeding
- Nonbleeding visible vessel or pigmented protuberance (red, blue, purple, or white elevated mound protruding from the base of the ulcer)
- Adherent or overlying clot without oozing
- Flat, dark slough or spot on the ulcer base

These findings are indicative of high risk for rebleed, requiring more aggressive therapy. For patients who do not exhibit these findings, the risk of rebleeding is significantly lower.

Radiologic procedures: Flat-plate abdominal x-ray may reveal free air under the diaphragm, which suggests perforation. A chest x-ray is taken to establish baseline pulmonary status. Barium studies usually are reserved for nonemergent situations to verify the presence of tumors or other large GI lesions.

Angiography: If the bleeding is rapid and suspected of being arterial or from a large vein, selective angiography of various GI arterial systems may aid in the visualization of bleeding site(s). If the bleeding site is clearly identified, therapeutic embolization may be attempted during angiography.

COLLABORATIVE MANAGEMENT

Fluid and electrolyte management: Volume replacement in acute GI bleeding must be performed as quickly as possible. Two large-bore IV lines (14- or 16-gauge) are inserted, and rapid fluid resuscitation is initiated. Crystalloid replacement therapy is initiated until dramatic blood loss or differential diagnosis warrants the use of colloids or blood products. In addition to GI blood loss, sequestration of fluid into the peritoneum and interstitium depletes intravascular volume. Packed cells and fresh-frozen plasma should be balanced to provide replacement of cells and clotting components. Generally, fresh-frozen plasma is required after 6 U of packed RBCs are infused. All blood components should be warmed to prevent hypothermia. Large transfusions will cause Ca^{++} to bind with the citrate from the stored blood and deplete free Ca^{++} levels. In addition, large-volume blood transfusions can lead to coagulopathy disorders. If bleeding is massive, lactated Ringer's solution is the preferred crystalloid volume expander because electrolyte disturbances are minimized. Vasopressors and inotropic agents should be used *only* if tissue perfusion remains compromised despite adequate intravascular volume replacement. Hemodynamic monitoring is essential for continuous evaluation of the patient's volume status, especially in patients >50 yr of age or those with chronic illnesses such as cardiovascular, pulmonary, renal, or hepatic disease. Overaggressive volume resuscitation results in fluid volume excess with complications of cardiac failure and pulmonary edema. Electrolyte levels are closely monitored, especially in patients with renal or hepatic disease.

Respiratory support: Because of a decrease in the oxygen-carrying capacity of the RBCs in massive blood loss, oxygen therapy by nasal cannula or face mask is initiated. Continuous or frequent pulse oximetry monitoring is recommended in actively bleeding patients to ensure adequate oxygenation. More aggressive ventilatory support may be required for patients with persistent hypoxemia and other evidence of early respiratory failure or impending ARDS (see p. 243).

Nutritional support: As soon as the patient's hemodynamic status stabilizes, nutritional support must be considered. Total parenteral nutrition (TPN) is started for patients whose status is likely to remain NPO for days to weeks. Enteral or oral feedings are started when there is no further evidence of GI hemorrhage and bowel function has returned.

Gastric intubation: Gastric intubation often is necessary, especially with upper GI bleeding. Gastric lavage is performed using room-temperature saline to clear blood and clots from the stomach and to allow for estimation of ongoing blood loss. A lavage free of blood suggests a lower GI source of bleeding. Gastric intubation is avoided if esophageal varices are the suspected bleeding source, because variceal tearing may occur.

Endoscopic electrocoagulation or laser photocoagulation: May be successfully employed in the treatment of bleeding ulcers.

Pharmacotherapy: Gastric alkalization with antacids, histamine H_2-receptor antagonists, and other agents is effective in preventing and controlling ulceration, but this therapy in critically ill patients is associated with a higher incidence of nosocomial pneumonia because of increase in bacterial counts and the possibility of aspiration. Some clinicians recommend sucralfate therapy over gastric alkalization because sucralfate does not affect gastric pH. Gastric pH monitoring (see below) can be used to guide therapy.

Antacids: Raise the gastric pH level and decrease the corrosiveness of gastric acid. Appropriately dosed antacids will help control pain.

Histamine H_2-receptor antagonists (e.g., famotidine and ranitidine):   Block gastric acid and pepsin secretion and are employed in the treatment of erosive and ulcerative disease. Cimetidine usually is avoided in critically ill patients because it inhibits certain liver enzymes, resulting in potential drug interactions.

Sucralfate (Carafate):   Oral sucralfate may be prescribed for patients with gastric erosions. The sucralfate combines with gastric acid and forms an adhesive protective coating over damaged mucosa. This drug is not absorbed from the GI tract and frequently leads to constipation.

Misoprostol (Cytotec):   Synthetic prostaglandin E_1 that enhances the body's normal mucosal protective mechanisms and decreases acid secretion. Aspirin and other NSAIDs inhibit natural prostaglandin synthesis, and therefore misoprostol is especially effective for ulceration associated with long-term administration of these drugs.

Omeprazole (Prilosec):   Deactivates the enzyme system that pumps hydrogen ions from the parietal cells, thus inhibiting gastric acid secretion. Omeprazole is highly effective in reducing gastric acid and may completely inhibit gastric acid secretion.

Gastric pH monitoring: Performed to assess the pH of gastric contents (intraluminal pH) or of gastric mucosal tissue (intramural pH). The goal of therapy is to maintain gastric pH within a given range, usually 4-5. Intraluminal pH is measured by aspirating gastric secretions and testing the aspirate with a pH indicator paper. Some gastric tubes have an electronic pH meter attached to the distal end that permits continuous monitoring of intraluminal pH. A more sophisticated device is the gastrointestinal tonometer and sump tube, which measures gastric mucosal pH. Because the gut is especially vulnerable to ischemia associated with hypoperfusion and septic shock states, the intramural pH is a valuable early predictor of intestinal ischemia, sepsis, and multisystem organ dysfunction.

Surgical management: Many surgical techniques are used, depending on the location and severity of the lesion. Ulcerative disease requires surgery if the lesions continue to bleed despite aggressive medical therapy or if complications such as perforation or obstruction develop. Oversewing of the bleeding vessel usually is followed by an acid-reducing procedure. In the unstable patient, vagotomy and pyloroplasty are performed. Antrectomy or parietal cell vagotomy may be performed in patients who are more stable. A common procedure for duodenal ulcers is gastrojejunostomy (Billroth II procedure). Massive lower GI bleeding is difficult to control and may require aggressive surgical procedures such as a colectomy with the creation of a permanent ileostomy or internal ileal pouch. If GI bleeding is caused by gastroesophageal varices, see "Bleeding Esophageal Varices," p. 492.

NURSING DIAGNOSES AND INTERVENTIONS

Fluid volume deficit related to active loss secondary to hemorrhage from the GI tract

Desired outcome: Within 8 h of this diagnosis, patient becomes normovolemic as evidenced by MAP ≥70 mm Hg; HR 60-100 bpm; CVP 2-6 mm Hg; PAWP 6-12 mm Hg; CI ≥2.5 L/min/m^2; Hgb approximately 10 g/dl or greater, and urinary output ≥0.5 ml/kg/h.

- Monitor BP q15min during episodes of rapid active blood loss or unstable VS. Be alert to MAP decreases of >10 mm Hg from previous reading.
- Monitor postural VS on patient's admission, q4-8h, and more frequently if recurrence of active bleeding is suspected: measure BP and HR with patient in a supine position, followed immediately by measurement of BP and HR

with patient in a sitting position (as tolerated). A decrease in systolic BP >10 mm Hg or an increase in HR of 10 bpm with patient in a sitting position suggests a significant intravascular volume deficit, with approximately 15%-20% loss of volume.

- Monitor HR, ECG, and cardiovascular status hourly, or more frequently in the presence of active bleeding or unstable VS. Be alert to a sudden increase in HR, which suggests hypovolemia.

> **Note:** Increases in HR may be caused by other factors, such as pain and anxiety.

- Measure central pressures and thermodilution CO q1-4h. Be alert to low or decreasing CVP, PAWP, and CO. Calculate SVR q4-8h, or more frequently in unstable patients. An elevated HR, decreased PAWP, decreased CO (CI <2.5 L/min/m^2), and increased SVR suggest hypovolemia and the need for volume restoration.
- Replace volume with prescribed fluids (usually a combination of crystalloid and blood products) via large-bore IV (18-gauge or larger) catheter.
- Measure urinary output hourly. Be alert to output <0.5 ml/kg/h for 2 consecutive hours. Increase fluid intake if decreased output is caused by hypovolemia and hypoperfusion.
- Monitor Hct; consult physician for values <28%-30%.
- Measure and record all GI blood losses from hematemesis, hematochezia, melena.
- Check all stools and gastric contents for occult blood.
- Ensure proper function and patency of gastric tubes. Do not occlude the air vent of double-lumen tubes, because this may result in vacuum occlusion. Confirm placement of gastric tube at least q8h, and reposition as necessary.
- Teach patient signs and symptoms of actual or impending GI hemorrhage: pain, nausea, vomiting of blood, dark stools, lightheadedness, and passage of frank blood in stools. Reinforce the importance of seeking medical attention promptly if signs of bleeding occur.
- Teach patient the importance of avoiding medications/agents with the potential for gastric irritation: aspirin, NSAIDs, ethanol.

NIC Bleeding Reduction: Gastrointestinal; Blood Products Administration; Fluid/Electrolyte Management; Shock Management: Volume; Hemodynamic Regulation; Gastrointestinal Intubation; Bleeding Precautions; Teaching: Individual; Surgical Preparation

Decreased cardiac output related to decreased preload secondary to acute blood loss

Desired outcome: Within 8 h of this diagnosis, cardiac output returns to or approaches normal limits as evidenced by CI ≥2.5 L/min/m^2; MAP ≥70 mm Hg; urinary output ≥0.5 ml/kg/h; normal sinus rhythm on ECG; distal pulses >2+ on a 0-4+ scale; and brisk capillary refill (<2 sec).

- Administer oxygen as prescribed to facilitate maximal oxygen delivery to the tissues.
- Monitor continuous or frequent pulse oximetry and ABG values for hypoxemia. Consult physician if arterial Pao$_2$ is <80 mm Hg or if oxygen saturation falls below 92%.
- Monitor ECG for evidence of myocardial ischemia (i.e., T-wave depression, QT prolongation, ventricular dysrhythmias).
- Monitor for physical indicators of diminished cardiac output, including pallor, cool extremities, capillary refill delayed for >2-3 sec, and decreased or absent amplitude of distal pulses.
- Monitor VS and thermodilution CO, and replace volume as indicated (see the first five entries under **Fluid volume deficit** in preceding nursing diagnosis).

- Monitor urine output hourly; document and report urine output <0.5 ml/kg/h for 2 consecutive hours.

NIC Cardiac Care: Acute; Oxygen Therapy; Respiratory Monitoring; Invasive Hemodynamic Monitoring; Dysrhythmia Management

Pain related to chemical or physical injury of GI mucosal surfaces caused by digestive juices and enzymes or tissue trauma

Desired outcomes: Within 2 h of this diagnosis, patient's subjective evaluation of discomfort improves, as documented by a pain scale. Nonverbal indicators of discomfort, such as grimacing, are absent.

- Monitor and document presence of abdominal pain or discomfort. Devise a pain scale with patient, rating discomfort from 0 (no pain) to 10 (severe). Be aware that pain may disappear concomitant with a bleeding episode inasmuch as blood covers and protects eroded tissue.
- Administer gastric alkalizing agents and sucralfate as prescribed to relieve pain caused by upper GI disorders.
- Measure gastric pH q2-4h or continuously. If measuring by gastric aspirate, be sure to use a clean syringe and discard the first aspirate to ensure accurate results. Adjust gastric alkalizing therapy to maintain pH of 4-5 or other prescribed range. Avoid excessive alkalization, which has been associated with increased risk of nosocomial pneumonia. As available, use NG tonometer to measure gastric mucosal pH.
- If opiate analgesics are prescribed for postoperative or severe pain, administer with caution. Many opiate analgesics cause vasodilation, thereby decreasing preload and afterload. For patients with GI bleeding and markedly reduced preload, opiate administration can result in dramatic hypotension.
- Monitor respiratory rate and depth to avoid opiate-induced respiratory depression.
- Because anxiety reduction contributes to pain relief, ensure consistency and promptness in delivering analgesic.
- Supplement analgesics with nonpharmacologic maneuvers to aid in pain reduction. Modify patient's body position to optimize comfort. Patients who have pain associated with gastric reflux may be more comfortable with HOB elevated, if this position does not compromise hemodynamic status.

NIC Analgesic Administration; Pain Management; Distraction; Environmental Management; Vital Signs Monitoring

- See "Pain," p. 61, for additional interventions.

Altered nutrition: less than body requirements, related to inability to ingest or digest food secondary to vomiting, medically prescribed restrictions, or disease process

Desired outcome: Within 7 days of this diagnosis (or by the time of hospital discharge) patient has adequate nutrition as evidenced by stable weight, thyroxine-binding prealbumin 20-30 mg/dl, and a state of nitrogen balance on nitrogen studies.

- Collaborate with physician, dietitian, and pharmacist to estimate patient's individual metabolic needs on the basis of activity level, underlying disease process, and nutritional status before hospitalization.
- Provide parenteral nutrition during acute phase of the bleeding, as prescribed.
- Begin enteral therapy when acute hemorrhagic episode has subsided and bowel function has returned. This may take several weeks in some patients.
- Monitor thyroxine-binding prealbumin, and report decreasing levels.
- Weigh patient daily at the same time of day, using the same scale. Weight can be a practical indicator of nutritional status if patient's weight changes are interpreted on the basis of the following factors: fluid shifts (edema, diuresis, third spacing), surgical resection, and weight of dressings and equipment.

NIC Nutrition Management; Nutritional Monitoring; Total Parenteral Nutrition (TPN) Administration; Enteral Tube Feeding; Aspiration Precautions

- For additional information, see "Nutritional Support," p. 1.

Diarrhea related to irritation and increased motility secondary to the presence of blood in the GI tract

Desired outcome: By the time of hospital discharge, patient's stools are normal in consistency and frequency and negative for occult blood.

- Monitor and record the amount, frequency, and character of patient's stools.
- Provide or have bedpan or bedside commode (only for hemodynamically stable patients) readily available.
- Minimize embarrassing odor by removing stool promptly and using room deodorizers.
- Use matter-of-fact approach when assisting patient with frequent bowel elimination. Reassure patient that frequent elimination is a common problem for most patients with GI bleeding.
- Evaluate bowel sounds q4-8h. Anticipate normal to hyperdynamic bowel sounds. Absence of bowel sounds (especially in association with severe pain or abdominal distention) may signal serious complications such as ileus or perforation.
- Monitor serum sodium, potassium, and calcium levels, and consult physician for abnormalities. Normal values are serum sodium 137-147 mEq/L, serum potassium 3.5-5.0 mEq/L, and serum calcium 8.5-10.5 mg/dl.
- Keep patient on NPO status until diarrhea episodes have subsided.

NIC Diarrhea Management; Electrolyte Monitoring; Fluid/Electrolyte Management

ADDITIONAL NURSING DIAGNOSES

See other nursing diagnoses and interventions as appropriate: "Hemodynamic Monitoring," p. 28; "Prolonged Immobility," p. 74; "Psychosocial Support," p. 83; and "Psychosocial Support for the Patient's Family and Significant Others," p. 95.

Enterocutaneous fistulas

PATHOPHYSIOLOGY

Enterocutaneous fistulas are formed when trauma, surgery, infection, neoplastic disease, or other pathologic condition results in a gastrointestinal-cutaneous communication. High-output proximal small bowel fistulas, which generally are defined as having an output >500 ml/24 h, are the most difficult to manage. Drainage from proximal fistulas is hypertonic; rich in enzymes, electrolytes, and proteins; thin in consistency; and tends to be copious. Losses as high as 2 L/24 h are not uncommon. Extensive skin and tissue breakdown often occur because of the presence of activated pancreatic enzymes in fistula drainage. Electrolyte and protein loss is great with high-output proximal fistulas. Drainage from distal sites, such as the ileum and colon, is thick and of less volume than is proximal fistula drainage.

Three factors are associated with mortality in patients with enterocutaneous fistulas: (1) fluid and electrolyte imbalance, (2) malnutrition, and (3) sepsis. Fluid, potassium, sodium, and bicarbonate may be lost in great quantities. Replacement by enteral or parenteral nutrition is complex, and proper balance often is difficult to achieve. Sepsis frequently is associated with bowel fistulization, as either a cause or a result of anastomotic breakdown or as a result of local wound contamination or inadequate drainage. Hypercatabolism and malnutrition are associated with both sepsis and fistulization, creating a great demand for calories and protein. Aggressive nutritional support and meticulous local wound management are critical to patient survival.

ASSESSMENT

History and risk factors: Direct trauma to the GI system, especially to the bowel; infection of surgical wound, drainage tract, or peritoneum; prolonged catabolic state in association with bowel injury, GI neoplasm, GI abscess, or severely inflammatory bowel disease; and complex GI surgical procedures, such as lysis of adhesions for intestinal obstruction or complicated intestinal anastomosis.

Clinical presentation: Varies, according to cause and location of fistula. Discharge of obvious bile, enteric contents, or gas through a surgical incision is an obvious sign of fistulization, as is a sudden increase in the amount of drainage from a surgical incision or drainage catheter. A change in the nature of drainage from serous or serosanguineous to yellow, green, brown, or foul smelling may indicate a fistula. With pancreatic drainage, a change to milky white suggests a pancreatic fistula. Mental confusion often is present as a result of electrolyte imbalance, dehydration, or early sepsis. Dry mouth, loss of tissue turgor, sunken eyes, and a decreasing urinary output with increasing specific gravity are expected if excessive fluid loss results in dehydration. Erythema, maceration, and edema may be present because of irritating fistula drainage. With persistent fistulization, loss of weight and muscle mass is anticipated because of protein loss and hypercatabolism.

Physical assessment: Sunken eyes, poor skin turgor, and dry oral mucosa, which are associated with dehydration; peripheral edema and muscle wasting related to protein loss; diminished or absent bowel sounds if peritonitis or ileus is present; discomfort and guarding on abdominal palpation over an abdominal mass (abscess) or near a drain site or surgical incision; tenderness, erythema, and possibly pain at the incision/fistula site caused by irritation from fistula output or infection; and muscle weakness and irregular HR if hypokalemia is present. Other assessment findings related to the underlying disease state (e.g., trauma, neoplasm, infection, pancreatitis) may be present.

Vital signs and hemodynamic monitoring parameters: Increased temperature and tachycardia due to infection or dehydration; and decreased BP, PAP, and CO if dehydration is present. If early sepsis is present, expect elevated CO and decreased SVR. Oxygen demand is increased and may exceed supply. Svo_2 will fall without aggressive pulmonary and cardiovascular support. The patient will exhibit general hemodynamic instability until fluid balance and infection are controlled.

DIAGNOSTIC TESTS

Radiography: Water-soluble contrast medium may be injected into the suspected fistula (fistulography) to identify the tract. An upper GI series may be indicated if the suspected fistula is proximal. CT may be used to identify and direct the drainage of abscesses associated with fistulization.

Biopsy: In patients with neoplastic disease a biopsy specimen of the fistula tract may be obtained to identify the presence of malignancy within the tract.

Culture: Fistula effluent from the stomach, duodenum, biliary tree, and pancreas may be cultured for evidence of infection. Small and large bowel fistulas generally are not cultured because of the expected presence of bacteria.

COLLABORATIVE MANAGEMENT

Nutritional support: With distal small bowel and colonic fistulas, enteral elemental diets may be infused into the proximal small bowel if the patient is capable of proximal absorption. Enteral diets sometimes are used if the fistula is extremely proximal. In these patients the feeding is infused distal to the fistula into the jejunum via a fine, weighted intestinal feeding tube. Enteral feedings are slowed or discontinued if fistula output increases after initiation of feedings. Patients with proximal small bowel fistulas, prolonged adynamic ileus, or extensive intraabdominal sepsis usually require TPN. Providing sufficient calories, protein, electrolytes, and fluids for patients with high-output fistulas can be challenging (see "Nutritional Support," p. 1).

Fluid and electrolyte replacement: Balanced salt solutions, usually containing potassium, are administered to maintain fluid and electrolyte balance. Often the amount to be delivered is prescribed in direct relation to fistula output,

TABLE 8-17   Nursing Assessment of the Enterocutaneous Fistula

- Evaluate size, shape, and location of the fistula. Reposition or lift skinfolds as necessary.
- Identify any potential leakage tracks created by skinfolds or body hollows.
- Examine the condition of adjacent skin and tissue. Note the presence and spread of both erythema and excoriation, which suggest leakage tracks.
- Note the consistency and character of fistula output.
- Assess each fistula separately.
- Document all findings, and compare them with baseline assessment made at the time of initial evaluation.

especially when the output is widely variable. Effluent from each fistula is measured separately for accurate estimation of specific electrolyte and fluid losses. In general, fistulas that are more proximal result in greater fluid, electrolyte, and protein losses than those that are distal.

Local fistula management: Ideally, drainage from each fistula is collected separately to assess individual fistula activity and healing. Individualized systems of gravity or gentle suction drainage and barrier skin protection are devised for each patient. Good local management reduces the incidence of wound-related bacteremias and increases the rate of wound healing.

Antibiotics: Indicated for infection, which frequently is present. Administration of aminoglycosides requires careful monitoring of peak and trough plasma levels to achieve adequate therapeutic results.

Surgery: A large percentage of patients with gastrocutaneous fistulas require surgery. Surgery is indicated in the following instances: (1) to close fistulas that continue to drain significant amounts despite absence of infection and appropriate nutritional support, (2) to explore and drain fistula tracts that could not be identified or drained by less invasive techniques, and (3) if overwhelming sepsis fails to respond to antibiotics and supportive therapy. In these cases immediate surgery is planned as a life-saving measure. The usual operation to close persistently draining fistulas is resection with end-to-end anastomosis. Postoperatively, parenteral nutrition and antibiotic coverage are continued. A gastrostomy usually is created to allow for prolonged intestinal decompression and drainage. The patient is expected to remain on NPO status for 1-2 wk after surgery, depending on the rate of healing and the return of bowel function.

NURSING DIAGNOSES AND INTERVENTIONS

Impaired tissue integrity related to chemical trauma, infection, or malnutrition
Desired outcome: Within 72 h of this diagnosis, patient's tissue adjacent to the fistula is free of erythema, excoriation, and edema.

- Assess the extent of the local problem (Table 8-17). Consult physician for signs of extensive damage to the tissue adjacent to the fistula (i.e., severe local erythema, excoriation, edema, maceration).
- Establish drainage and collection system for each fistula (Table 8-18). Consult physician regarding use of continuous wound suction device(s).
- Note character, color, odor, and volume of output from each fistula. Consult physician for significant changes in any of these indicators.
- If increased fistula output results from oral or enteral feedings, eliminate or modify the feedings as prescribed.
- Consult ostomy nurse or enterostomal therapist for recommendations in pouching complex or multiple fistulas.

TABLE 8-18 Recommendations for Containing Fistula Drainage

- Clean the intact skin surrounding the fistula with a nonirritating antibacterial cleanser.
- Clip body hair (if present) around the fistula.
- Remove pooled drainage from the wound and surrounding area by using sterile absorbent pads or gentle suction. The help of an assistant may be necessary to maintain a dry field during application of the collection device.
- Apply a barrier powder (e.g., karaya or Orahesive) to any excoriated skin. A flexible transparent dressing (e.g., Op-Site) can be used to protect intact skin.
- Use a skin paste (e.g., Stomahesive or karaya) to fill in any grooves surrounding recessed fistulas.
- Apply a sized barrier sheet (e.g., Stomahesive, HolliHesive) to the surrounding skin, being careful not to overlap the fistula.
- Attach a collecting bag to the barrier sheet base. For high-output fistulas, a urostomy bag and collecting system may be necessary. Transparent appliances enable observation of drainage. Devices that have a drainage opening permit emptying and measurement of output.
- Reposition the patient frequently to optimize gravity drainage of fistula output. For example, it sometimes is necessary to use a rotating bed frame or a bed modified with foam blocks to facilitate prone positioning.

NIC Wound Care; Dressing; Ostomy Care; Tube Care; Fluid/Electrolyte Management
- See **Altered nutrition,** which follows, and **Risk for infection,** see below, for interventions that optimize nutrition and prevent infection.

Altered nutrition: less than body requirements, related to protein loss via fistula output, disruption of GI tract continuity, or absorptive disorder

Desired outcome: By the time of hospital discharge, patient has adequate nutrition as evidenced by food intake that increases to his or her recommended daily allowance and body weight that returns to baseline or within 10% of patient's ideal weight.

- Collaborate with physician, dietitian, and pharmacist to estimate patient's metabolic needs on the basis of activity level, estimated metabolic rate, and baseline nutritional status.
- Monitor for the presence of bowel sounds q8h. If bowel sounds are absent, withhold oral or enteral feedings.
- If fistula output increases in response to enteral feedings, slow the rate of infusion or reduce the strength of the feeding. If the patient tolerates oral feedings but they increase fistula output, increase the frequency of the feedings and decrease the amount consumed at each feeding.
- Be aware that when the entire intestine is not available for normal absorption, elemental feeding formulas (see p. 6) may be more readily absorbed.
- Prepare patient for parenteral feedings if oral/enteral feedings are inadequate for patient's requirements.

NIC Nutrition Management; Nutritional Monitoring; Fluid/Electrolyte Management; Total Parenteral Nutrition (TPN) Administration; Enteral Tube Feeding
- For additional information, see "Nutritional Support," p. 1.

Risk for infection related to inadequate primary defenses (altered integumentary system, disruption in continuity of GI system), hypercatabolic state, presence of invasive lines, and protein loss/malnutrition

---

TABLE 8-19 **Aminoglycoside Antibiotics: Nursing Applications**

- Administer prepared solution over 30-60 min, according to recommendations for specific agent. Too-rapid administration increases the risk of toxicity.
- Reschedule if dosage is delayed >1 h.
- Obtain serum specimen in a timely fashion so that peak and trough levels can be evaluated adequately.
- Monitor patient for evidence of hearing loss.
- Monitor BUN and creatinine levels and urinary output, which are indicators of renal function.
- Be aware that older adults are especially susceptible to ototoxic and nephrotoxic effects of these medications.
- To avoid potential incompatibilities/interactions, administer at separate sites and stagger schedules when penicillin and cephalosporins also are prescribed.

Desired outcome: Patient remains free of infection as evidenced by core or rectal temperature <37.8° C (100° F); negative culture results; HR 60-100 bpm; RR 12-20 breaths/min; BP within patient's normal range; and orientation to time, place, and person.

- Check rectal or core temperature q4h for increases.
- If temperature suddenly rises, assess patient for potential sources, noting presence of purulent secretions; erythema around wound, drain, or fistula site; and pain, tenderness, or masses with abdominal palpation. Consult physician for temperature elevation and assessment findings. Obtain specimens for culture of likely sites for infection as prescribed by physician or unit protocol.
- Evaluate orientation and LOC q4h. Document and report significant deviations from baseline values.
- Monitor BP, HR, RR, CO, and SVR q4h. Be alert to increases in HR and RR associated with temperature elevations. As available, monitor Svo_2 continuously or at scheduled intervals. An elevated CO and a decreased SVR suggest early septic shock (see Table 4-22, p. 345, for a complete hemodynamic profile; also see "Septic Shock," p. 593).
- Administer parenteral antibiotics in a timely fashion. Reschedule antibiotics if a dosage is delayed for more than 1 h. Recognize that failure to administer antibiotics on schedule can result in inadequate blood levels and treatment failure. Aminoglycosides are used frequently; administer agents promptly, and monitor patient for potential complications (Table 8-19).
- Optimize gravity drainage of fistula by prone or upright positioning as tolerated by patient.
- Wear gloves when contact with drainage is possible. Prevent transmission of potentially infectious agents by washing hands thoroughly before and after caring for patient and carefully disposing of dressings and drainage.

NIC Medication Management; Hemodynamic Regulation; Vital Signs Monitoring; Temperature Regulation; Intravenous (IV) Therapy; Wound Care

Fluid volume deficit related to active loss secondary to fistula drainage

Desired outcome: Within 8 h of this diagnosis, patient becomes normovolemic as evidenced by balanced daily I&O; urinary output ≥0.5 ml/kg/h; moist mucous membranes; good skin turgor; HR ≤100 bpm; CVP 2-6 mm Hg; and PAWP 6-12 mm Hg.

- Evaluate patient's fluid balance by calculating and comparing daily I&O. In patients with high-output fistulas, evaluate total I&O q8h. Record all sources of output, including drainage from each fistula. Replace fistula output with prescribed fluid (usually a balanced salt solution containing potassium) q2-8h.

- Measure urine output q1-4h. Consult physician if urine output is <0.5 ml/kg/h or if specific gravity increases and urine volume decreases.
- Assess and document condition of mucous membranes and skin turgor. Dry membranes and inelastic skin indicate inadequate fluid volume and the need for increase in fluid intake (PO or IV route).
- Measure and evaluate VS, CVP, and PAP (when available) q1-4h, depending on hemodynamic stability. Be alert to increasing HR, decreasing CVP, and decreasing PAP, which indicate inadequate intravascular volume. Encourage increased oral intake (if possible), or consult with physician regarding increase in IV fluid intake.
- Control sources of insensible fluid loss by humidifying oxygen, maintaining comfortable environment, and controlling fever (if present) with antipyretics such as acetaminophen.

NIC Fluid/Electrolyte Management; Fluid Monitoring; Hemodynamic Regulation; Hypovolemia Management; Invasive Hemodynamic Monitoring; Shock prevention

Body image disturbance related to biophysical change secondary to presence of external fistula

Desired outcome: By the time of hospital discharge, patient acknowledges body changes as evidenced by viewing fistula and not exhibiting preoccupation with or depersonalization of fistula.

- Evaluate the patient's reaction to the fistula by observing and noting evidence of body image disturbance (see Table 1-40, p. 92).
- Anticipate feelings of shock and repulsion initially. Be aware that the development of an external fistula usually is an unanticipated complication and patients are not emotionally prepared for the disfigurement.
- Anticipate and acknowledge normalcy of feelings of rejection, isolation, and uncleanliness (because of odor and possible presence of feces).
- Offer patient opportunity to view fistula/wound as desired. Use mirrors if necessary.
- Encourage patient and significant others to verbalize feelings regarding fistula/wound.
- If possible, offer the patient an opportunity to participate in wound care. Patient may be able to perform simple tasks, such as holding the bag into which you will deposit the soiled dressing or applying the pouch that collects drainage.
- Convey an accepting attitude toward the patient. Many fistulas that require critical care involve open and infected wounds. If the attending nurse is inexperienced in dressing these complex wounds, another more experienced nurse should be present during the initial dressing change.
- Reassure patient that the fistula is not permanent. Acknowledge that a scar will be visible but the fistula will close with appropriate care.

NIC Body Image Enhancement; Coping Enhancement; Self-Care Assistance; Support System Enhancement

Altered oral mucous membrane related to prolonged NPO status

Desired outcome: Within 24 h of this diagnosis, patient's oral mucosa is intact, moist, and free of pain and oral lesions.

- Inspect the patient's oral cavity, noting the degree of moisture, inflammation, bleeding, or lesions. Consult physician for open lesions and bleeding.
- Assist patient with brushing teeth with a soft-bristle toothbrush. Irrigate the oral cavity with a solution of 500 ml normal saline and 15 ml sodium bicarbonate. Provide mouth care q4h.
- For patients with altered LOC, massage gums and teeth with saline-moistened, sponge-tipped applicator and brush teeth gently if there is no evidence of bleeding. Place patient in a side-lying position, and irrigate the

mouth with small amounts of a saline and bicarbonate solution (per second entry). Carefully suction the solution from the oral cavity throughout the procedure with a Yankauer tonsil suction device.

• Keep the lips moist with emollients, such as lanolin or Eucerin cream. Take care to apply emollient to external tissue only. Oil-containing emollients are harmful if aspirated or otherwise introduced into the respiratory tract.

NIC Oral Health Promotion; Oral Health Maintenance

ADDITIONAL NURSING DIAGNOSES

See "Nutritional Support," p. 1, for additional information about the patient with extra nutritional needs. See "Psychosocial Support," p. 83, for psychosocial nursing diagnoses and interventions. Also see nursing diagnoses and interventions related to sepsis under "Septic Shock," p. 593.

Bibliography

Al-Saden PC: Cirrhosis. In Daly-Gawenda D, editor: *Manual of medical-surgical nursing: med-surg fact finder,* Boston, 1997, Little, Brown.

Al-Saden PC et al: Hepatitis C: an emerging dilemma, *Am Assoc Occupat Health Nurses* 47:217-222, 1999.

Alter H et al: Viral hepatitis. In *Advances in therapeutic hepatology: a world view*, Chicago, 1998, Course booklet at the International Association for the Study of Liver Diseases.

Amann ST, DiMangno E, Rubin W: Pancreatitis diagnostic and therapeutic interventions, *Patient Care*, June 15, 1997, pp. 200-216.

Barron TH, Morgan DE: The diagnosis and management of fluid collections associated with pancreatitis, *Am J Med* 102:555-563, 1997.

Bezzarro ER: Changing perspectives of H_2-antagonists for stress ulcer prophylaxis, *Crit Care Nurs Clin North Am* 5(2):325-331, 1993.

Brown A: Acute pancreatitis: pathophysiology, nursing diagnoses, and collaborative problems, *Focus Crit Care* 18(2):121-130, 1991.

Brozenec SA: Gastrointestinal hemorrhage. In Daly-Gawenda D, editor, *Manual of medical-surgical nursing: med-surg fact finder*, Boston, 1997, Little, Brown.

Butler R: Managing the complications of cirrhosis, *Am J Nurs* 94(3):46-49, 1994.

Chase SL: Even low doses of NSAIDs pose a GI threat, *RN* 61(3):78, 1998.

Covington J: Nursing care of patients with alcoholic liver disease, *Crit Care Nurse* 13(3):47-57, 1993.

Generali J: *Heliobacter pylori* update, *Drug Newsletter* 13(5):39-40, 1994.

George-Gay B: Disorders of the biliary tract and exocrine pancreas. In Burrell LO, Gerlach MJ, Pless BS, editors: *Adult nursing: acute and community care*, ed 2, Stamford, Conn, 1997, Appleton Lange.

Halm M: Acute gastrointestinal complications after cardiac surgery, *Am J Crit Care* 5(2):109-117, 1996.

Hashizume M et al: Laparoscopic gastric devascularization and splenectomy for sclerotherapy-resistant esophagogastric varices with hypersplenism, *J Am Coll Surg* 187(3):263-270, 1998.

Hoofnagle JH: Chronic viral hepatitis. In *Clinical and pathological correlations in liver disease: approaching the next millennium*, Chicago, 1998, Postgraduate course booklet at the American Association for the Study of Liver Diseases.

Horne M, Heitz UE, Swearingen PL: *Pocket guide to fluid, electrolyte, and acid-base balance,* ed 3, St Louis, 1996, Mosby.

International Society for Peritoneal Dialysis, 1996, The Advisory Committee on Peritonitis Management of the International Society of Peritoneal Dialysis [On-line], Available: www.horus-medical.fr/ispd/perit.htm

Interqual: *The ISD-A review system with adult ISD criteria,* North Hampton, NH, and Marlboro, Mass, Aug, 1992, Interqual.

Jackson MM, Rymer T: Viral hepatitis: anatomy of a diagnosis, *Am J Nurs* 94(1):43-48, 1994.

Kajmowicz L: Viral hepatitis. In Daly-Gawenda D, editor, *Manual of medical-surgical nursing: med-surg fact finder*, Boston, 1997, Little, Brown.

Keen JH: Hepatic failure. In Swearingen PL, Keen JH, editors: *Manual of critical care: applying nursing diagnoses to adult critical illness,* ed 3, St Louis, 1995, Mosby.

Kerber K: The adult with bleeding esophageal varices, *Crit Care Nurs Clin North Am* 5(1):153-162, 1993.

Kim MJ, McFarland GK, McLane AM, editors: *Pocket guide to nursing diagnoses,* ed 7, St Louis, 1997, Mosby.

Kovacs OG, Jensen DM: Therapeutic endoscopy for nonvariceal upper gastrointestinal bleeding. In Taylor MB, editor: *Gastrointestinal emergencies,* ed 2, Baltimore, 1997, Williams & Wilkins.

Krumberger JM: Acute pancreatitis, *Crit Care Nurs Clin North Am* 5(1):169-185, 1993.

Kucharski S: Fulminant hepatic failure, *Crit Care Nurs Clin North Am* 5(1):141-151, 1993.

Laine L, Stein C, Sharma V: Randomized comparison of ligation versus ligation plus sclerotherapy in patients with bleeding esophageal varices, *Gastroenterology* 110(2):529-533, 1996.

Lancaster S, Stockbridge J: PV shunts relieve ascites, *RN* 55(8):58-60, 1992.

Lee WM: Medical management of acute liver failure. In Lee WM, Williams R, editors: *Acute liver failure,* Cambridge, 1997, Cambridge University Press.

Lichenstein DR, Berman MD, Wolfe MM: Approach to the patient with acute upper gastrointestinal hemorrhage. In Taylor MB, editor: *Gastrointestinal emergencies,* ed 2, Baltimore, 1997, Williams & Wilkins.

Lindor KO, Dickson ER, editors: Pbc, psc, and adult cholangiopathies, *Clin Liver Dis* 2(2):217-449, 1998.

McCloskey JC, Bulechek GM, editors: *Nursing interventions classification (NIC),* ed 2, St Louis, 1996, Mosby.

Meguid MM, Campos ACL: Nutritional management of gastrointestinal fistulas, *Surg Clin North Am* 76(5):1035-1080, 1996.

Mergenger K, Baillic J: Fortnightly review: acute pancreatitis, *Br Med J* 316(7124):44-48, 1998.

Ockner RK et al: Diseases of the liver, gallbladder and bile ducts. In Bennett JC, Plum F, editors: *Cecil textbook of medicine,* Philadelphia, 1996, Saunders.

Pessoa MG et al: Quantitation of hepatitis G and C virus in the liver: evidence that hepatitis G virus is not hepatotropic, *Hepatology* 27:877-880, 1998.

Petrini J: Acute upper gastrointestinal tract bleeding. In Snape WJ: *Consultations in gastroenterology,* Philadelphia, 1996, Saunders.

Pien ECT, Hume KE, Pien FD: Gastrostomy tube infections in a community hospital, *Am J Infect Control* 24(5):353-358, 1996.

Portmann B, Saxena R: Pathology of acute liver failure. In Lee WM, Williams R, editors: *Acute liver failure,* Cambridge, 1997, Cambridge University Press.

Prevost SS, Overle A: Stress ulceration in the critically ill patient, *Crit Care Nurs Clin North Am* 5(1):163-169, 1993.

Qadir MT et al: Penicillium peritonitis in a patient receiving continuous ambulatory peritoneal dialysis, *Heart Lung* 27(1):67-68, 1998.

Roberts LR, Kamath PS: Pathophysiology and treatment of variceal hemorrhage, *Mayo Clin Proc* 71:973-982, 1996.

Schwartz SI et al, editors: *Principles of surgery,* ed 7, New York, 1999, McGraw-Hill.

Selvey LA et al: Is there evidence for vector transmission of GBV-C? *Lancet* 351:1104-1105, 1998.

Shakil AO, Mazariegos GV, Kramer DJ: Fulminant hepatic failure. In Fung JJ, Rakela J, editors: *Surg Clin North Am* 79:77-108, 1999.

Sherlock S: *Diseases of the liver and biliary system,* ed 9, Boston, 1992, Blackwell.

Smith SL, Ciferni M: Liver transplantation for acute hepatic failure: a review of clinical experience and management, *Am J Crit Care* 2(2):137-144, 1993.

Trupp R: Case presentation: a gastroventricular fistula resulting from peptic ulcer disease, *Heart Lung* 27(1):71-73, 1998.

Williams R: Classification and clinical syndromes of acute liver failure. In Lee WM, Williams R, editors: *Acute liver failure,* Cambridge, 1997, Cambridge University Press.

Wright JA: Seven abdominal assessment signs every emergency nurse should know, *J Emerg Nurs* 23(5):446-450, 1997.

Hematologic Dysfunctions

The hematologic or hematopoietic system involves the blood, lymph, and components that form and circulate blood and lymph. Blood-forming organs include the bone marrow, thymus gland, liver, spleen, and lymph nodes. Lymph is derived from the interstitial fluid passing into the lymphatic capillaries. The primary functions of the hematologic system are:

   Respiratory gas exchange (oxygen [O_2] and carbon dioxide [CO_2])
   Delivery of nutrients to the body cells
   Elimination of wastes from the body cells

In addition, blood also has a role in:

   Temperature regulation
   Delivery of hormones
   Fluid and electrolyte balance
   Acid-base balance
   Protection from foreign antigens and infectious organisms

   Blood is composed of plasma, erythrocytes (red blood cells [RBCs]), leukocytes (white blood cells [WBCs]), and thrombocytes (platelets). Dysfunctions of the hematologic system lead to problems performing the eight functions listed above. Hematologic dysfunctions can be classified as anemias and bleeding and thrombotic disorders.

Profound anemias/hemolytic crisis

PATHOPHYSIOLOGY

For anemias

Anemia reflects a reduction in total body hemoglobin concentration, potentially caused by hemoglobinopathies (abnormal hemoglobin, including hemoglobin S, which occurs with sickle cell disease); various other hemolytic anemias (e.g., hereditary spherocytosis, glucose-6-phosphate dehydrogenase [G6PD] deficiency, pyruvate kinase [PK] deficiency, thalassemias [Cooley or Mediterranean anemia], erythroblastosis fetalis); anemia of renal failure (erythropoietin deficiency); aplastic anemia (lack of bone marrow production of RBCs related to malignancy, increased immunoglobulin G [IgG] antibodies, drugs, or thymoma); megaloblastic anemia (decreased vitamin B_{12} or other B vitamins, folic acid, or intrinsic factors; includes pernicious anemia); and anemia related to blood loss/hemorrhage.

As the hemoglobin decreases, the oxygen-carrying capacity of the blood is reduced, resulting in tissue hypoxia unless compensatory mechanisms are adequate to assist the body with oxygen delivery. The anemias just discussed originate from one of three main problems:

- *Acute or chronic blood loss:* Chronic GI bleeding, excessive menstruation, trauma, ruptured blood vessel(s), and other various disorders.
- *Decreased production of erythrocytes:* Iron deficiency, lead poisoning, thalassemias, megaloblastic/pernicious anemia, renal failure, aplastic/hypoplastic anemia.
- *Increased destruction of erythrocytes:* Hemolytic anemias caused by abnormal hemoglobin (hemoglobin S, C, D, E), RBC membrane anomalies (spherocytosis, hemolytic uremic syndrome), physical trauma to blood (extracorporeal "bypass" circulation, balloon counterpulsation, prosthetic heart valves), abnormal RBC-related antibodies (e.g., drug-induced hemolysis), and presence of bacterial endotoxins (malaria, clostridia).

For hemolytic crisis

Hemolytic crisis is an acute disorder that frequently accompanies hemolytic anemias. It is characterized by premature pathologic destruction (hemolysis) of RBCs. As RBC destruction accelerates, the oxygen-carrying capacity of the blood decreases, which results in a reduction in the amount of oxygen delivered to the tissues. This hypoxic state produces tissue ischemia and can progress to tissue infarction. Hemolytic episodes can be triggered by both emotional and physiologic states, including stress, trauma, surgery, acute infectious processes, and abnormal immune responses.

ASSESSMENT

For anemias

Clinical presentation (chronic indicators):   Pallor, melena, hematochezia, fatigue, weight loss, dyspnea on exertion, uremia, sensitivity to cold, intermittent dizziness, excessive menstruation, paresthesias, and history of iron deficiency, folic acid deficiency, and vitamin B_{12} deficiency.

- *Chronic hemolytic anemia:* Jaundice, renal failure, hematuria, arthritis, increased incidence of gallstones, skin ulcers.

Clinical presentation (acute indicators):   Fever, chest pain, acute heart failure, confusion, irritability, tachycardia, orthostatic hypotension, dyspnea, tachypnea, frank bleeding.

Physical assessment: Inspection may reveal tachypnea, orthopnea, tachycardia, weight loss, altered mental status, spider angiomas, electrocardiogram (ECG) changes, unusual fatigue or weakness, smooth tongue, unusual bleeding (stool, urine, emesis), monoarticular or polyarticular arthritis, and skin ulcers. Palpation may detect bone tenderness (especially sternal), enlargement of the liver and/or spleen, and joint tenderness. Auscultation may reveal crackles associated with heart failure.

For hemolytic crisis

Risk factors: Individuals with mild or chronic hemolytic anemia may be asymptomatic until they are exposed to a severe stressor, such as an acute infectious process, profound emotional upset, critical illness, surgery, or trauma. With added stress, hemolysis can accelerate to a crisis state wherein patients experience organ congestion from massive amounts of hemolyzed blood cells, precipitating multiple organ dysfunction syndrome (MODS) and shock.

Clinical presentation (acute):   Fever; abdominal, chest, joint, and back pain; jaundice; headache; dizziness; palpitations; shortness of breath (SOB); hemoglobinuria; lymphadenopathy; splenomegaly; and signs of peripheral nerve damage, including paresthesias, paralysis, chills, and vomiting.

Clinical presentation (chronic):   Anemia; pallor; fatigue; dyspnea on exertion; icterus; bone infarctions; monoarticular and polyarticular arthritis; hematuria; renal failure; increased gallstone formation; and skin ulcers.

Physical assessment: Depending on severity and duration of the anemia, the patient may exhibit impaired growth and development. Inspection may reveal the presence of jaundice, SOB, monoarticular or polyarticular arthritis, retinal detachment and associated vitreous hemorrhage, and hemiplegia. Palpation may demonstrate splenomegaly, lymphadenopathy, hepatomegaly, or abdominal guarding. Chronic skin ulcers may be seen, particularly in the ankle area.

DIAGNOSTIC TESTS

RBCs: Reduced. In hemolytic crisis an increased number of premature RBCs will be present.

Reticulocyte count: RBC precursors; elevated because of increased bone marrow production of RBCs.

Hemoglobin (Hgb) and hematocrit (Hct):   Decreased.

Morphologic classification of RBCs: Mean corpuscular volume (MCV).
- *Macrocytic:* MCV >100 μ^3
- *Microcytic:* MCV <80 μ^3
- *Normocytic:* MCV 80-100 μ^3

Sickle cell test: Screens for the presence of hemoglobin S, which is indicative of sickle cell anemia.

Hemoglobin electrophoresis: Screens for abnormal hemoglobins often present in hemolytic anemias:
- *Hemoglobins A_1, A_2, and F:* Normally found in the body.
- *Hemoglobin C:* Causes RBCs to sickle.
- *Hemoglobins D and E:* Rarely occur "singly"; sometimes present with sickle cell disease or thalassemias.
- *Hemoglobin H:* Causes premature destruction of RBCs and abnormal binding of O_2 to the RBC.
- *Hemoglobin S:* Most common abnormal hemoglobin, occurring in 10% of the black population; causes sickle cell disease or seen with sickle cell trait.

Erythrocyte sedimentation rate (ESR):   Elevated in hemolytic anemia more often than in other anemias.

C_3 proactivator: Increased in hemolytic anemia.

Total iron-binding capacity (TIBC):   Normal or reduced, depending on the type of anemia.

Unconjugated bilirubin: Elevated in hemolytic anemia as a result of the liver's inability to process increasing bilirubin released during hemolysis.

Serum lactic dehydrogenase isoenzymes (LDH$_1$ and LDH$_2$):   Elevated in hemolytic anemia because of the release of these enzymes when the RBC is destroyed.

Haptoglobin level: Decreased in hemolytic anemia as a result of increased binding of haptoglobin (a plasma protein) to facilitate removal of increased amounts of hemoglobin from the bloodstream.

Peripheral blood smear: May reveal abnormally shaped RBCs, such as spherocytes. Red cell hyperplasia is present in nearly all cases of chronic hemolysis with intact bone marrow.

Bone marrow aspiration: May reveal abnormal size, shape, or amounts of erythrocytes or reticulocytes in various anemias.

Coombs test: Positive in antibody-mediated/immunologic hemolysis.

Immunoglobulin levels: Frequently elevated with sickle cell disease.

G6PD levels: Decreased in G6PD deficiency but cannot be tested while hemolysis is active.

Radiologic examinations/tests
- *X-rays and bone scans:* May reveal increased density or aseptic necrosis of the bones.

- *Liver/spleen scans:* May reveal disease or dysfunction of either organ, which may contribute to anemia.

COLLABORATIVE MANAGEMENT

All anemias

Volume replacement: If patient is hypovolemic, aggressive fluid and/or blood replacement is mandatory to prevent profound hypotension and shock. Fluid challenges/boluses also assist in prevention of deposition of hemolyzed RBCs in the microvasculature.

Transfusions/blood component replacement: Packed RBCs are necessary in the management of profound anemia to assist with increasing the oxygen-carrying capacity of the blood.

Oxygen therapy: To relieve SOB or dyspnea. Methods of oxygen delivery range from nasal cannulas, to various face masks, to mechanical ventilation in severe cases.

Selected anemias

Vitamin B$_{12}$: Injections or IV infusion is necessary for management of pernicious anemia, a type of megaloblastic anemia caused by failure of the gastric mucosa to absorb vitamin B$_{12}$.

Iron supplements: For iron-deficiency states to help increase production of normal-size RBCs.

Folic acid supplement: Necessary for RBC production. Supplements of 1 mg/day are used to treat megaloblastic anemia and, theoretically, to prevent hemolytic crisis in patients with hemolytic anemia. It is not effective in all patients with hemolytic anemia.

Epoetin alfa: erythropoietin, recombinant (Epogen/Procrit): Stimulates production of RBCs in patients with bone marrow hypofunction/lack of production of RBCs, particularly when related to renal failure.

Bone marrow transplantation: Recommended for some patients with sickle cell disease or aplastic anemia to provide a mechanism for regenerating normal RBC production.

Elimination of causative factor: Certain drugs and chemicals, cold temperatures, and stress can worsen many anemias, but most profoundly hemolytic and aplastic anemias. Identifying and removing the causative agent can prevent life-threatening crisis.

Hemolytic anemias only

Red cell exchange therapy for sickle cell crisis: Cytapheresis procedure for patients who are unresponsive to other treatments for sickle cell disease.

Thrombocytapheresis: Cytapheresis procedure for patients experiencing symptoms of excessive thrombosis, to reduce platelets rapidly in an attempt to decrease clotting before onset of MODS.

Corticosteroids: Therapy used with limited success in management of hemolytic anemia.

Pain management: Aspirin, acetaminophen, nonsteroidal antiinflammatory drugs (NSAIDs), narcotics, and sedatives may be necessary for relief of pain and anxiety associated with hemolytic anemia, particularly during hemolytic crisis.

Splenectomy: Sometimes recommended for patients suspected of having splenic sequestration crisis related to hemolytic anemia.

Antisickling agents: Some clinical trials are underway to evaluate the efficacy of these agents in ablating the sickling phenomenon.

NURSING DIAGNOSES AND INTERVENTIONS

Impaired gas exchange related to lack of RBCs; hemoglobin abnormalities
Desired outcome: Within 48-96 h of onset of treatment, patient has adequate gas exchange as evidenced by heart rate (HR) and respiratory rate (RR) within

10% of patient's baseline (or HR 60-100 beats per minute [bpm] and RR 12-20 breaths/min); Hgb and Hct returned to patient's baseline (or Hgb >12 mg/dl and Hct >37%); oxygen saturation >90%; and blood pressure (BP) returned to patient's baseline (or >90 mm Hg systolic within 24 h of initiation of treatment).

- Administer supplemental oxygen as needed, using appropriate device (i.e., nasal cannula, face mask/shield, or mechanical ventilation as necessary).
- Monitor rate, rhythm, depth of respirations.
- Monitor for increased restlessness, anxiety, air hunger.
- Monitor oxygen saturation using pulse oximeter continuously. Consult with physician for persistent values <90% or, if oxygen saturation is chronically decreased, a sustained drop of >10% of baseline.
- Note changes in Sao_2, Svo_2, end-tidal CO_2 and changes in arterial blood gas (ABG) values, as appropriate.
- Monitor oxygen liter flow.
- Provide for oxygen when patient is transported.
- Maintain large-bore (18-gauge) intravenous (IV) catheter(s) in case transfusion or rapid volume expansion is necessary.
- Transfuse with packed cells (RBCs) (Table 9-1) as prescribed to facilitate oxygen delivery and assist in volume expansion.
- Describe the purpose of blood product transfusion therapy to the patient and significant others.
- Carefully evaluate dyspnea and chest pain in patients with sickle cell disease because of the possibility of pulmonary infarction.

You may also wish to refer to the following interventions from the Nursing Interventions Classification (NIC):

NIC Airway Management; Oxygen Therapy; Respiratory Monitoring
Activity intolerance related to anemia/lack of oxygen-carrying capacity of the blood
Desired outcomes: Within 48 h of onset of treatment, patient's activity tolerance improves as evidenced by HR and RR returning to within 10% of baseline (or HR 60-100 bpm and RR 12-20 breaths/min) and BP returning to within 10% of patient's baseline (or systolic BP >90% mm Hg). Within 24 h of initiation of treatment patient is able to assist minimally with self-care activities.

- Alternate periods of rest and activity to avoid physically stressing the patient and increasing oxygen demand.
- Collaborate with occupational therapy (OT), physical therapy (PT), and/or recreational therapy personnel in planning and monitoring an activity program as appropriate.
- Assist to focus on what patient can do, rather than on deficits.
- Determine patient's physical limitations.
- Reposition patient slowly to evaluate the effects of position change on myocardial and cerebral perfusion.
- Reduce fear, pain, and anxiety to decrease oxygen demand.
- Determine causes of fatigue (e,g., treatments, pain, medications).
- Monitor nutritional intake to ensure adequate energy resources.
- Teach patient to avoid physically and psychologically stressful situations, which can exacerbate symptoms of anemia and precipitate hemolytic crisis in patients with hemolytic anemia.
- Teach patient and significant others to recognize impending hypoxemia: altered mental status, activity intolerance, SOB, chest pain, and weakness.
- Teach patient and significant others about the etiology of the specific anemia that is affecting the patient.
- See this diagnosis in "Prolonged Immobility," p. 74.

NIC Activity Therapy; Energy Management; Positioning
Risk for impaired skin integrity related to impaired oxygen transport secondary to chronic anemia

T A B L E 9 - 1   Blood and Blood Products*

Product	Volume	Infusion time	Contents	Possible complications
Whole blood (rarely used)	500 ml/U	2-4 h or <1 h in emergency	All blood components. If fresh, processed with citrate-phosphate-dextrose (CPD)	Hepatitis, transmission of HIV (human immunodeficiency virus), CMV (cytomegalovirus), EBV (Epstein-Barr virus), and other organisms; transfusion reactions: all types
Packed red blood cells	200-250 ml/U	1-4 h or <1 h in emergency	Red blood cells	See whole blood
Fresh-frozen plasma	200-250 ml/U	20 min to thaw ½ to 1 h or <½ h in emergency	All clotting factors except platelets	See whole blood
Platelets	35-50 ml/U	Direct IV push at 30-50 ml/min. May combine or "pool" several bags into one; given in multiple units	Platelets	Transfusion reaction: febrile or mild allergic; may need to premedicate with acetaminophen (Tylenol) or diphenhydramine HCl (Benadryl); rare instance of septic reaction
Cryoprecipitate	10-20 ml/U	May need 10-30 U infused at 1 U/min or 10-20 ml/min	Factor VIII; factor XIII and fibrinogen	Small possibility of febrile or mild allergic reaction; rare instance of septic reaction

*Use correct filter with each blood product; most filters can be used to administer 2-4 U; either piggyback or flush products with normal saline solution *only.*

Continued

TABLE 9-1   Blood and Blood Products—cont'd

Product	Volume	Infusion time	Contents	Possible complications
Granulocytes	300 ml/U	1-2 h; administer slowly for 5 min as test dose	White blood cells (WBC) extracted from 1 U of whole blood	Transfusion reactions: all types; often ineffective in elevating WBC count
Leukocyte-poor and washed, frozen red blood cells	250-300 ml/U	2 h or 1-2 h in emergency	Red cells washed with saline (and possibly irradiated) to remove WBCs and protein from RBCs	Markedly reduced possibility of transfusion reactions: all types
Factor VIII concentrate	10-20 ml/U	May need >10 U infused at 1 U/min	Factor VIII (pooled from possibly thousands of donors)	Small possibility of febrile or mild allergic reaction; rare instance of septic reaction
Factor IX concentrate	20-30 ml/U	May need >10 U infused at 1 U/min	Factor IX (pooled from possibly thousands of donors)	Small possibility of febrile or mild allergic reaction; rare instance of septic reaction
Volume expanders Albumin (5% or 25%) Plasma protein fraction (PPF) Salt-poor albumin	Varies with each product	1 ml/min or as rapidly as tolerated in shock states	Reconstituted from human blood, plasma, or serum	Possible hypervolemia with rapid infusions, particularly with 25% albumin

Desired outcome: Patient's skin remains intact during hospitalization.
- Keep extremities warm to promote circulation and help prevent tissue hypoxia.
- Perform a comprehensive appraisal of peripheral circulation (e.g., check peripheral pulses, edema, capillary refill, color and temperature of extremity).
- Monitor for sources of pressure and friction.
- Monitor for infection, especially of edematous areas.
- Use a bed cradle to reduce pressure of covers on extremities.
- Monitor skin and mucous membranes for areas of discoloration and bruising.
- Monitor skin for rashes, abrasions, excessive dryness, moisture.
- Provide adequate nutrition and nutritional supplements as appropriate. Negative nitrogen state or low serum protein or albumin increases the risk for skin breakdown.
- Teach patient the signs of skin breakdown, since it can occur at any time with chronic anemia.
- Instruct the patient on the importance of preventing venous stasis.
- Teach patient about appropriate nutrition as discussed in "Nutritional Support," p. 1.
- Apply appropriate skin-saving dressing (e.g., Duoderm) or initiate aggressive skin care regimen to areas of breakdown.
- For additional interventions, see "Wound and Skin Care," p. 55.

NIC Pressure Management; Pressure Ulcer Prevention; Skin Surveillance; Nutrition Management

For hemolytic crisis

Altered tissue perfusion: peripheral, cardiopulmonary, gastrointestinal, renal, and cerebral, related to interruption of arterial or venous blood flow secondary to microthrombi formation

Desired outcome: Within 24 h of onset of treatment, patient has adequate perfusion as evidenced by warm extremities; pink nail beds; peripheral pulses at least 2+ on a scale of 0-4+ or patient's baseline; capillary refill <2 sec; BP within 10% of patient's normal range (or systolic BP >90 mm Hg); HR and RR within 10% of patient's baseline (or HR 60-100 bpm, RR 12-20 breaths/min with a normal depth and pattern [eupnea]); oxygen saturation >90%; urinary output ≥0.5 ml/kg/h; and patient oriented to time, place, and person.
- Initiate aggressive IV fluid volume replacement as prescribed to prevent deposition of hemolyzed RBCs in the microvasculature.
- Assess extremities for coolness, pallor, and prolonged capillary refill, which are signals of inadequate peripheral perfusion.
- Assess amplitude of peripheral pulses as an indicator of peripheral perfusion. Use Doppler device if unable to palpate pulses.
- Evaluate chest pain.
- Document cardiac dysrhythmias.
- Monitor vital signs frequently.
- Note signs and symptoms of decreased cardiac output.
- Monitor respiratory status for symptoms of heart failure.
- Monitor for signs of impending shock, including increased HR and RR, increased restlessness and anxiety, and cool and clammy skin, followed by a decrease in BP.
- Monitor abdomen for signs of decreased perfusion.
- Keep lower extremities elevated slightly to promote venous blood flow.
- Monitor for decreased oxygen saturation using continuous pulse oximetry. Consult physician for sustained decreases.
- Monitor ABG values for signs of acidosis (i.e., pH <7.35 and hypercarbia/CO_2 retention [$Paco_2$ >45 mm Hg]), indicating hypoperfusion, hypoxemia, and respiratory insufficiency.

- Monitor urinary output for decrease, which can signal decreased renal perfusion. Consult physician for urine output <0.5 ml/kg/h for 2 consecutive hours.
- Monitor neurologic status q2-4h, using the Glasgow coma scale (see Appendix 3).
- Teach patient and significant others about hemolytic anemia, including the signs of impending hemolytic crisis, rendering information on the following:
  - ☐ *Indicators of impending hemolytic crisis:* Fever, abnormal pain, headache, dizziness, palpitations, paresthesias, and paralysis.
  - ☐ *Sensorimotor impairment:* Unsteady gait, paresthesias, blurring of vision, weakness, and paralysis.
  - ☐ *Support groups:* Names, phone numbers, and addresses of other persons/ groups that can assist with support of people with hemolytic anemias.
  - ☐ *Smoking cessation:* Support groups and programs that assist in stopping cigarette smoking to decrease vasoconstriction associated with nicotine intake.
  - ☐ *Medications:* Drug name, dosage, frequency, and possible side effects, especially related to steroids: increased appetite, weight gain, "moon face," "buffalo hump," increased possibility of infection, headaches, and increased BP. In addition, discuss the possibility of steroid-induced diabetes mellitus with long-term therapy.
  - ☐ *Prevention of infection:* Especially important if patient is on long-term steroid therapy or has had a splenectomy. The patient should obtain an annual flu vaccine; practice good personal hygiene; obtain regular dental check-ups; and get adequate rest, sleep, and relaxation. If a splenectomy has been performed, patients should have a pneumococcal vaccine and wear a medical-alert identification bracelet.

NIC Cardiac Care: Acute; Circulatory Care: Arterial Insufficiency; Circulatory Care: Venous Insufficiency; Respiratory Monitoring; Shock Management: Cardiac; Cerebral Perfusion Promotion; Neurologic Monitoring; Peripheral Sensation Management; Fluid/Electrolyte Management; Fluid Management; Vital Signs Monitoring

Pain related to tissue ischemia secondary to vessel occlusion; inflammation/ injury secondary to blood within the joints

Desired outcomes: Within 1-2 h of initiating treatment, patient's subjective evaluation of discomfort improves as documented by a pain scale; nonverbal indicators of discomfort are reduced or absent.

- Monitor patient for signs of discomfort, including guarded positioning, muscle spasm, and increases in HR, BP, and RR. Devise a pain scale with patient, rating discomfort from 0 (no pain) to 10.
- Perform a comprehensive assessment of pain to include location, characteristics, onset/duration, frequency, quality, intensity or severity of pain, and precipitating factors.
- Medicate for pain as prescribed, and assess effectiveness of medication on the basis of the pain scale. Confer with physician if pain relief is ineffective; devise an alternate plan for analgesia.
- If pain medication injections are frequent, choose the IV route rather than the intramuscular (IM), when possible.
- Administer adjuvant analgesics and/or medications when needed to potentiate analgesia.
- Consider use of continuous infusion, either alone or in conjunction with bolus opioids, to maintain serum levels.
- Collaborate with the physician if drug, dose, route of administration, or interval changes are indicated, making specific recommendations based on equianalgesic principles.
- Consider alternate method of pain control such as relaxation techniques: guided imagery, controlled breathing, meditation, and listening to soft, soothing music.

- Control environmental factors that may influence the patient's response to discomfort (e.g., room temperature, light, noise).
- Use therapeutic/healing touch to relieve pain if practitioner is trained and patient agrees to participate. Or consult trained practitioner.
- Apply warm compresses to joints to increase circulation and thereby improve tissue oxygenation.
- Apply elastic stockings to promote venous return and enhance circulation.
- Encourage patient to perform isometric or range-of-motion (ROM) exercises of the extremities to promote circulation.
- Help allay fears by reassuring patient that pain will decrease as the crisis subsides.
- Provide emotional support to patient during the crisis episode. Reassure patient that the crisis is time limited, and enable significant others to be with patient, if possible, during the crisis.
- Teach patient to assess extremities daily for evidence of tissue breakdown or blood sequestration (i.e., swelling, erythema, tenderness) so that early interventions can be implemented in an attempt to prevent severe pain.

NIC Analgesic Administration; Pain Management; Medication Administration; Medication Administration: Intravenous (IV); Heat/Cold Application; Anxiety Reduction

Risk for fluid volume deficit or excess related to failure of renal regulatory mechanisms of fluid and electrolyte balance secondary to microthrombi occluding the nephrons

Desired outcome: Patient's volume status returns to normal/baseline as evidenced by urinary output $\geq$0.5 ml/kg/h; stable weight; BP within patient's normal range; HR 60-100 bpm; RR 12-20 breaths/min; good skin turgor; moist mucous membranes; urine specific gravity 1.005-1.025; pulmonary artery wedge pressure (PAWP) 6-12 mm Hg (or patient's baseline); pulmonary artery diastolic (PAD) 8-15 mm Hg (or patient's baseline); and central venous pressure (CVP) 2-6 mm Hg (5-12 cm H_2O).

- Monitor intake and output (I&O) hourly. Consult physician for a urinary output <0.5 ml/kg/h for 2 consecutive hours.
- Recognize presence of blood pressure alterations.
- Monitor and document heart rate, rhythm, pulses.
- Evaluate efficacy of volume expansion by closely comparing CVP, PAWP, and PAD. Overzealous volume expansion can lead to heart failure and pulmonary edema with CVP >20%-25% normal values and PAD and/or PAWP >16 mm Hg.
- Administer diuretics as prescribed in the well-hydrated or overhydrated patient with urine output <0.5 ml/kg/h.
- Insert urinary catheter if appropriate.
- Assess patient for indicators of volume depletion, including poor skin turgor; dry mucous membranes; hypotension; tachycardia; and decreasing urine output, PAWP, PAD, and CVP.
- Monitor electrolytes and serum osmolality. A universal increase in electrolytes and osmolality is indicative of dehydration. A universal decrease signals fluid overload.
- Assess pH (normal range is 7.35-7.45) before replacing electrolytes, because acidosis and alkalosis alter electrolyte values. Replace potassium cautiously if the patient's pH is outside the normal range.

NIC Electrolyte Monitoring; Fluid Management; Fluid Monitoring; Intravenous (IV) Therapy; Hypervolemia Management; Shock Management: Volume

ADDITIONAL NURSING DIAGNOSES

Uncontrolled bleeding and complications of hemolysis can be terrifying to the patient and significant others, who may fear that the patient may die. See "Psychosocial Support," p. 83, and "Psychosocial Support for the Patient's Family and Significant Others," p. 95, accordingly.

Bleeding and thrombotic disorders

Bleeding can result from qualitative (dysfunctional) or quantitative (lack of) abnormalities of platelets and/or coagulation factors in the plasma. Thrombocytopenia is common in the critically ill and, like anemia, requires differential diagnosis. The *cause* of thrombocytopenia, rather than simply the decreased platelets, poses the greatest threat to the critically ill patient. The four main causes of thrombocytopenia are as follows:

1. *Hemodilution:* related to administration of large amounts of crystalloids, colloids, or red cell concentrates.

2. *Increased platelet destruction:* includes heparin-induced thrombocytopenia (HIT), antiphospholipid antibody syndrome (APAS) or lupus anticoagulant syndrome, idiopathic thrombocytopenic purpura (ITP), thrombotic thrombocytopenic purpura (TTP), hemolytic-uremic syndrome (HUS), and HELLP syndrome (hemolysis, elevated liver enzymes, and low platelet count). Disseminated intravascular coagulation (DIC) presents with a combined coagulopathy and platelet consumption.

3. *Platelet sequestration:* related to hypersplenism, and hypothermia.

4. *Decreased production of platelets:* caused by alcohol (ETOH) abuse, bone marrow irradiation, bone marrow/stem cell disease, graft vs. host disease, aplastic anemia, vitamin B_{12} or folate deficiencies, metastatic carcinoma, some renal diseases, leukemia, and myeloproliferative disorders.

Platelet destruction may be mediated by either congenital autoimmune or alloimmune disorders or acquired immunologic or nonimmunologic mechanisms. Causative or related factors include septicemia, systemic inflammatory response syndrome, pulmonary hypertension, extracorporeal circulation, thrombotic disorders, acute transplant rejection, severe allergic reactions, rheumatic disorders, intravascular catheters and prosthetics, fat emboli, acute respiratory distress syndrome (ARDS), and human immunodeficiency virus (HIV) infection. The most diagnostic finding associated with severe thrombocytopenia is presence of petechiae in dependent areas (back, posterior thighs of bedridden patients). Larger purpura such as ecchymoses and hematomas may also be present but are nonspecific for diagnosis of platelet disorders. Patients must be assessed for risk of bleeding with thrombocytopenia, considering the severity and cause along with co-morbid factors.

Coagulopathies may be caused by liver disease, vitamin K deficiency, pregnancy-induced hypertension associated with HELLP syndrome, or other defects related to blood coagulation factors, such as hemophilia, von Willebrand disease, and DIC. Other disorders that may lead to thromboembolic conditions include roughened surface of vascular endothelium (as seen with arteriosclerosis, trauma, and infection) and slow/stagnant blood flow through the vessels.

Normal blood coagulation is activated most often as a result of injury to blood vessels, causing the following series of events:

- *Reflex vasoconstriction:* Vascular spasm that decreases blood flow to the site of injury.
- *Platelet aggregation:* Leads to formation of a platelet plug to help repair the injury. If the damage to the vessel is small, the plug is sufficient to seal the injury. If the hole is large, a blood clot is necessary to stop the bleeding.
- *Activation of plasma clotting factors:* Leads to the formation of a fibrin clot. The pathways that initiate clotting factors (Figure 9-1) include:
  - ☐ *Intrinsic system:* Initiated by "contact activation" subsequent to an endothelial injury. The problem is "intrinsic" to the circulation, or begins with an injury to the blood or circulatory system itself.
  - ☐ *Extrinsic system:* Initiated by tissue thromboplastin released from injured tissue. The problem is "extrinsic" to the circulation, or begins with an injury to tissue rather than within the blood system itself.

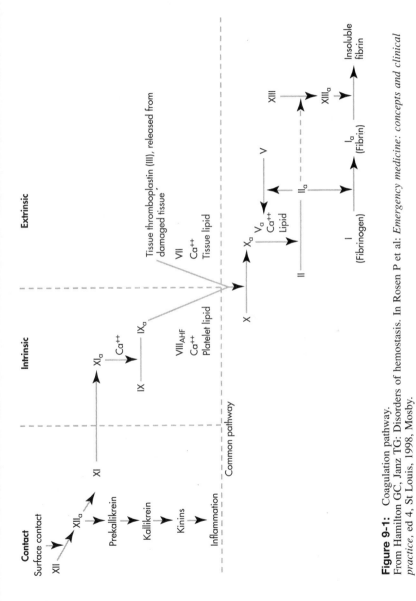

Figure 9-1:   Coagulation pathway.
From Hamilton GC, Janz TG: Disorders of hemostasis. In Rosen P et al: *Emergency medicine: concepts and clinical practice*, ed 4, St Louis, 1998, Mosby.

☐ *Common pathway:* The final part of the coagulation system, which completes the clot formation process begun by either the intrinsic or extrinsic pathway.

☐ *Clot retraction:* Several minutes after its formation, the clot contracts for 30-60 min to express most of the fluid from within the clot. The expressed fluid is called *serum,* because most of the clotting factors have been used/removed by the clot formation process. Serum is unable to clot. The absence of clotting factors differentiates *serum* from *plasma.*

• *Growth of fibrous tissue:* Tissue that completes the organization of the clot within approximately 7-10 days after injury. This process results in permanent closure of the vessel injury.

Both the intrinsic and extrinsic pathways are activated after rupture of a blood vessel. Tissue thromboplastin from the vessel initiates the extrinsic pathway, while contact of factor XII and platelets with the injured vessel wall traumatizes the blood, which initiates the intrinsic pathway. The extrinsic pathway is able to form clots in as little as 15 sec with severe trauma, whereas the intrinsic pathway requires 2-6 min for clot formation.

HEPARIN-INDUCED THROMBOCYTOPENIA

PATHOPHYSIOLOGY

Heparin is a widely used anticoagulant that prevents the conversion of fibrinogen to fibrin. Heparin-induced thrombocytopenia (HIT), also called *heparin-induced thrombocytopenic thrombosis (HITT),* "white clot syndrome," or *heparin-associated thrombocytopenia (HAT types I and II),* results when heparin therapy causes either a mild to moderate (HAT type I) or severe (HAT type II) decrease in the number of freely circulating platelets. Platelets in these patients manifest unusual aggregation, which can result in heparin resistance, arterial and venous thrombosis, and subsequent emboli in extreme cases (Figure 9-2). Incidence of HAT type I is about 10% of all patients receiving heparin. Incidence of HAT type II ranges from 0.5%-5% in patients receiving subcutaneous (SC) or IV heparin, with a higher incidence reported with IV use. Bovine (beef-based) heparin has been associated with HIT more frequently than other heparins. Incidence of HAT is not related to the heparin dosage and has been seen in patients receiving low-dose SC heparin, as well as in patients receiving simple heparin "flushes" to maintain patency of IV lines.

There are two types of HIT:

Mild to moderate, low morbidity (HAT type I):   Generally occurs 1-2 days after initiation of heparin. It may resolve in 5 days after symptoms begin. Platelets may decrease to as low as $100,000/mm^3$ or may remain in the low-normal range. No treatment is required, and heparin therapy may be continued.

Severe, high morbidity (HAT type II):   Generally occurs 5-22 days after initiation of heparin. Symptoms persist until heparin is discontinued. Platelets decrease to $<100,000/mm^3$. Thrombosis with subsequent embolization and bleeding is apparent. Complications include pulmonary emboli, myocardial infarction, cerebral infarction, and circulatory impairment resulting in limb amputations. Mortality rate is 29%. Overall, 0.6% of all patients receiving heparin therapy develop thromboembolization. *Heparin must be discontinued immediately* and subsequent complications managed as they occur.

ASSESSMENT

Risk factors: Prior drug-induced immunologic thrombocytopenia.

Clinical presentation

Mild to moderate, low morbidity (HAT type I):   Slight decrease in platelet count without clinical symptoms.

Severe, high morbidity (HAT type II):   Hemorrhage, ecchymosis, gingival bleeding, hemoptysis, epistaxis, and possible chest pain, SOB, and strokelike

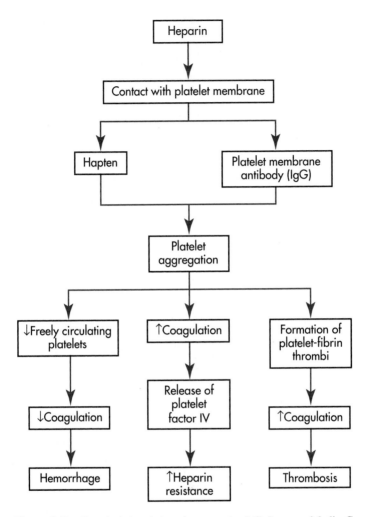

Figure 9-2: Heparin-induced thrombocytopenia. *IgG,* Immunoglobulin G.

symptoms. Extreme cases: arterial thrombosis of the distal aorta and proximal lower limb arteries.

Physical assessment (severe, or HAT type II): Presence of petechiae, purpura, bruising from mucosal surfaces or wounds. The patient also may manifest signs of arterial occlusion: cold, pulseless extremities; severe chest pain and SOB, indicative of myocardial ischemia; paresthesias; paralysis; and diminished level of consciousness (LOC), indicative of cerebral ischemia.

DIAGNOSTIC TESTS

Platelet count: Mild to moderate: 100,000-150,000/mm^3; severe: <100,000/mm^3 caused by severe clumping or aggregation of platelets.

Bleeding time: Prolonged if platelets are <100,000/mm^3.

Platelet antibody screen: Positive findings because of the presence of IgG platelet antibodies.

Coagulation screening (prothrombin time [PT]; partial thromboplastin time [PTT], thromboplastin time):   Normal, inasmuch as the clotting factors that govern these test results are normal.

Fibrinogen: May be low normal or low because of increased consumption. Normal is 200-400 mg/dl.

Fibrin degradation products: Elevated to ≥40 μg/ml because of fibrinolysis of platelet-fibrin thrombi. Normal is <10 μg/ml.

Platelet aggregation: Results will be >100% (or high value of specific laboratory) because of release of platelet membrane antibody.

Heparin-induced platelet aggregation: Reflects abnormal aggregation curve with decrease in the optical density in the aggregometer.

Clinical trials of serotonin release testing and ELISA heparin PF4:   Both tests are being studied to assist in the differential diagnosis of HAT.

Bone marrow aspiration: Normal or increased number of megakaryocytes (platelet precursors), indicative of normal bone marrow production of platelets.

COLLABORATIVE MANAGEMENT

Heparin therapy: If the platelet count is >100,000/mm^3 and the patient is symptom free, heparin may be continued. Oral anticoagulation should begin immediately, if possible. If the platelet count is <100,000/mm^3 and the patient develops bleeding or thrombosis, *all heparin should be discontinued immediately, including heparin "flushes."*

Monitoring heparin therapy: A preheparin platelet count is done to establish baseline values. Daily platelet counts should be done for at least the first 4 days of heparin therapy. Subsequent counts are done q2days. If increasing amounts of heparin are needed to maintain therapeutic levels (i.e., PTT 40-60 sec), heparin resistance should be suspected, which sometimes precedes HIT (see Figure 9-2).

Administration of defibrinogenating agents: Ancrod (Arvin) may be given to reduce the possibility of thrombosis.

Administration of direct thrombin inhibitors: Recombinant hirudin may be given for anticoagulation.

Vena caval filter: If patient experiences thrombosis with decrease or loss of perfusion to an extremity, the physician may consider surgical insertion of a vena caval filter to reduce the risk of pulmonary emboli caused by clot migration from an extremity. See "Pulmonary Emboli," p. 232.

Platelet transfusions: May be initiated after heparin therapy is discontinued if bleeding fails to subside.

Plasma exchange: In severe cases, 2-3 L of plasma is removed and replaced with albumin, crystalloids, or fresh-frozen plasma to assist in decreased bleeding by removing bound heparin from the body.

Alternate anticoagulant: If the patient is in need of further anticoagulation, an alternate medication, such as warfarin sodium (Coumadin), acetylsalicylic

Research Brief 9-1   Hirudin can be used to correct the complications of arterial and venous thrombosis associated with HAT type II. Dosage should be titrated by carefully monitoring activated partial thromboplastin time (aPTT) with a target range of aPTT prolongation of 50-70 sec. aPTT prolongation of >100 sec has been associated with increased incidence of hemorrhage and should be avoided.

Challapalli R, Lefkovits J, Topol EJ: Clinical trials of recombinant hirudin in acute coronary syndrome, *Coron Artery Dis* 7(6):429-437, 1996.

acid (aspirin), dipyridamole (Persantine), or dextran, should be considered. Streptokinase, urokinase, and alteplase (rt-PA) have been used successfully to manage pulmonary emboli in HIT. Low-molecular-weight heparin also has been used successfully in many patients.

NURSING DIAGNOSES AND INTERVENTIONS

Altered protection related to decreased platelet count with risk of bleeding and thromboembolization

Desired outcome: Within 24 h of discontinuing heparin therapy, patient exhibits no signs of new bleeding, bruising, or thrombosis as evidenced by HR 60-100 bpm or within 10% of patient's baseline; RR 12-20 breaths/min with normal depth and pattern; systolic BP ≥90 mm Hg; and all peripheral pulses at patient's baseline or >2+ on a 0-4+ scale.

- Assess patient at least q2h for signs of bleeding, including hemoptysis, gastrointestinal (GI) bleeding, hematuria, and bleeding from invasive sites or mucous membranes.
- Monitor the patient closely for hemorrhage.
- Note Hgb and Hct levels before and after blood loss, as indicated.
- Monitor for signs of persistent bleeding (e.g., check all secretions for frank or occult blood).
- Assess patient at least q2h for signs of thrombosis, including decreased peripheral pulses, altered sensation in extremities (i.e., paresthesias, numbness), pallor, coolness, cyanosis, or capillary refill time >2 sec.
- Perform a comprehensive assessment of peripheral circulation (e.g., check peripheral pulses, edema, capillary refill, color and temperature of extremities).
- Monitor extremities for areas of heat, pain, redness, or swelling.
- Maintain adequate hydration to prevent increased blood viscosity.
- Avoid IM injections and venous and arterial punctures as much as possible until bleeding time returns to normal.
- Protect the patient from trauma that may cause bleeding.
- Avoid taking rectal temperatures.
- Monitor platelet count daily for significant changes. Consult physician for values that remain <150,000/mm^3 or below patient's baseline.
- Assess ECG for heart rate and rhythm, respiratory rate and pattern, and BP for evidence of active bleeding. Be alert to sustained increase in HR and RR or ECG changes, such as ST depression or elevation, since these indicators may precede hypotension.
- Monitor heparin dosage carefully. If increasing doses are required to maintain a therapeutic level (PTT 40-60 sec or 2-2½ times patient's baseline), consult physician for possible heparin resistance, an early indicator of HIT.
- Monitor Hgb and Hct values daily in patients with recent or active bleeding.
- At least q8h assess patient's mental status (orientation to time, place, person, and self) and sensation and strength of movement of extremities.
- Monitor for signs of MODS secondary to thrombosis or prolonged hypotension if patient has hemorrhaged. Be alert for respiratory distress, chest pain, elevated temperature, decreasing urine output, vomiting or intolerance of diet, abdominal distention, decreasing bowel sounds, and elevated liver enzymes.
- Teach patient and significant others basic pathophysiology of HIT, and instruct them to report this problem to all subsequent health care providers. Teach patient to wear a medical-alert bracelet to alert health care providers if patient becomes unable to speak.

NIC Surveillance: Safety; Bleeding Precautions

Fluid volume deficit (or risk for same) related to active blood loss

Desired outcomes: Patient becomes normovolemic within 24 h of onset of treatment as evidenced by HR within patient's normal range or 60-100 bpm; RR 12-20 breaths/min with normal depth and pattern; and urinary output

≥ 0.5 ml/kg/h; absence of abdominal pain/tenderness, back pain, or pain from invasive sites.

- Monitor patient for signs of hypovolemia, including increased HR and RR, decreased BP, increased restlessness or fatigue, and decreased urine output.
- Weigh daily, and monitor trends.
- Maintain accurate I&O record.
- Insert urinary catheter if appropriate.
- Monitor vital signs as appropriate.
- Administer IV therapy as prescribed.
- Administer supplemental oxygen if patient is actively bleeding.
- Assess for abdominal pain, tenderness, guarding, or back pain, which may signal intraabdominal bleeding.
- Check excretions for occult blood, and observe for blood in emesis, sputum, feces, urine, nasogastric (NG) drainage, and wound drainage as appropriate.
- Instruct the patient and/or family on the need for blood replacement as appropriate.
- Replace lost volume with plasma expanders (albumin, hetastarch [Hespan]) or blood products as indicated. See Table 9-1 for more information.

NIC Electrolyte Management; Fluid Management; Fluid Monitoring; Hypovolemia Management; Intravenous (IV) Therapy; Shock Management: Volume; Blood Products Administration

ADDITIONAL NURSING DIAGNOSES

Uncontrolled bleeding or thrombotic complications can be terrifying for the patient and significant others, who may fear the patient will die. See nursing diagnoses and interventions in "Psychosocial Support," p. 83, and "Psychosocial Support for the Patient's Family and Significant Others," p. 95, accordingly.

IDIOPATHIC THROMBOCYTOPENIC PURPURA

PATHOPHYSIOLOGY

ITP is a disorder characterized by premature platelet destruction, resulting in a decrease in the platelet count to below $100,000/mm^3$. Normal platelet life span averages 1-3 wk, whereas in ITP the platelet life span averages 1-3 days because of the presence of antiplatelet IgG and IgM antibodies, which destroy platelets in the reticuloendothelial system of the spleen. The coagulopathy is believed to be an autoimmune response and manifests as both an acute and a chronic problem.

Primarily acute ITP is a childhood disease, characterized by an abrupt onset of severe thrombocytopenia with evident purpura. Usually it occurs <21 days after a viral infection. At the onset, platelets decrease to $<20,000/mm^3$. The chronic form is typically a disease of adults ages 20-50 yr, but it has occurred in a small percentage of children and elders. The disease rarely resolves spontaneously, sometimes responds to treatment of the underlying disorder, and usually is not associated with infection but can be related to autoimmune (systemic lupus erythematosus, rheumatoid arthritis) and neoplastic (chronic lymphocytic leukemia, Hodgkin's/non-Hodgkin's lymphoma) disorders. Women are affected 3 times more often than are men. Petechiae and purpura are commonly seen on the distal upper and lower extremities. Patients may feel symptom free until actual bleeding begins. Intracranial hemorrhage is a potential complication. Platelet counts decrease to as low as $5,000/mm^3$ in some patients but may be as high as $75,000/mm^3$ in others.

ASSESSMENT

Risk factors: In acute ITP there usually is a history of antecedent viral infection occurring about 3 wk before the hemorrhagic episode. The chronic form usually is insidious and sometimes is seen in association with autoimmune hemolytic anemia, HIV disease, hemophilia, Hodgkin's lymphoma, chronic lymphocytic leukemia, systemic lupus erythematosus, sarcoidosis, high-titer anticardiolipin antibodies, and thyrotoxicosis.

Clinical presentation: Petechiae, purpura, and prolonged bleeding are commonly seen. Occasionally, epistaxis, GI and gingival bleeding, and increased menstrual flow are present. The rarest complication is intracranial hemorrhage, occurring in <1% of patients. Signs of an autoimmune process, such as fever, splenomegaly, or lymphadenopathy, may occur, but because they are not specific to ITP, they require further evaluation.

Physical assessment: Presence of petechiae and purpura anywhere on the skin or mucous membrane, most commonly on the distal upper and lower extremities. Ecchymosis is apparent in traumatized areas, along with generalized bruising. Neurologic signs should be monitored closely in patients with acute ITP. Joint tenderness and visual (retinal) disturbances may be noted because of bleeding into these areas.

DIAGNOSTIC TESTS

Platelet count: Decreased to 5,000-75,000/mm^3 because of premature destruction. Normal range is 150,000-400,000/mm^3.

Bleeding time: Prolonged when platelet count is <100,000/mm^3.

Screening coagulation tests (PT, PTT, thrombin time): Normal because these tests measure nonplatelet components of the coagulation pathway.

Platelet antibody screen: Positive findings because of the presence of IgG and IgM antiplatelet antibodies.

Complete blood cell count (CBC) with differential: Hgb and Hct may be decreased because of insidious blood loss or simultaneous hemolytic anemia (Evans syndrome); WBC count will be normal unless the ITP is associated with another disease that alters the differential leukocyte count.

Bone marrow aspiration: Biopsy will reveal megakaryocytes (platelet precursors) in normal or increased numbers with a "nonbudding" appearance, possibly indicating defective maturation or failure of platelet production.

Capillary fragility test: Will show >1+, which signals that more than 11 petechiae were present in a 2.5-cm radial area on the skin after prolonged application of a BP cuff. Normal is 1+ or <10 petechiae.

COLLABORATIVE MANAGEMENT

Platelet transfusions: Platelets are given only in cases of life-threatening hemorrhage. The shortened platelet life span renders prophylactic transfusions ineffective.

Glucocorticoid therapy: Adrenocorticosteroids (e.g., prednisone 0.25-1.0 mg/kg/day) are effective in increasing the platelet count in 1-3 wk after initiation of treatment. Effectiveness is attributed to suppression of phagocytic activity of the macrophage system (particularly the spleen), which increases the life span of the antibody-coated platelets. If improvement does not occur within 2-3 wk or excessive doses of steroids are required or patient cannot tolerate tapering of steroids, splenectomy should be considered. "Normal" responders are able to have steroid dosage tapered over several weeks until platelets reach a sustained value of 50,000/mm^3. Relapse during or after tapering prednisone is a common occurrence.

Splenectomy: Treatment of choice in cases that are refractory to glucocorticoid therapy. The condition stabilizes in 70%-90% of patients who undergo splenectomy. The positive results are attributed to the removal of the site of destruction of the antibody-sensitized platelets. Prospective splenectomy candidates should have pneumococcal, meningococcal, and possibly *Haemophilus influenzae* type b vaccinations before planned splenectomy, to reduce the risk of septicemia after surgery.

IV infusions of gamma globulin: Given 400 mg/kg/day for 5 days, resulting in increased platelet count in 60%-70% of patients. It is less effective in patients with long-standing chronic ITP. The platelet level at initiation of treatment is unrelated to the patient's response. Duration of response may be longest in individuals who achieve the highest initial platelet increases.

Anti-Rh immunoglobulin: Low dose (200-1000 μg) given IV for 1-5 days has been effective in limited studies. Success of treatment is attributed to sensitization of recipient RBCs, which results in low-grade hemolysis and blockade of the platelet destruction by the reticuloendothelial system.

Immunosuppression: Various immunosuppressive drugs, including azathioprine, cyclophosphamide, vincristine, and cyclosporine, given alone or in combination with prednisone, have been used successfully in limited situations. A trial of immunosuppression therapy may be indicated in patients who fail to respond to splenectomy or in those who are too unstable to be surgical candidates.

Vinca "alkaloid-loaded" platelets: Transfusions of platelets "loaded" with vinblastine may reduce the phagocytic destruction of platelets in patients who fail to respond to other treatments.

Colchicine: A small percentage of patients refractory to other treatments may improve with 1.2 mg colchicine daily for ≥2 wk. The drug has been used successfully in limited studies.

Danazol: 400-800 mg/day has resulted in complete remission or partial improvement in 60%-70% of patients in several studies. Use is controversial because other researchers have reported poor results and many untoward side effects.

Plasmapheresis: Several days of machine-assisted plasma exchange to remove approximately 1-1½ times the patient's total plasma volume per procedure and replace it with a suitable solution (e.g., colloids, crystalloids, plasma). Therapy is reserved for patients with life-threatening hemorrhage unresponsive to other measures. It is costly and of marginal benefit.

NURSING DIAGNOSES AND INTERVENTIONS

Altered protection related to decreased platelet count resulting in increased risk of bleeding

Desired outcomes: Within 72 h of onset of treatment, patient exhibits no clinical signs of new bleeding or bruising episodes. Secretions and excretions are negative for blood, and VS are within 10% of patient's normal range. Within the 24-h period before discharge from intensive care, patient and significant others verbalize understanding of the indicators of impending bleeding.

- Monitor patient for signs of bleeding, including elevated HR and RR, oozing from invasive sites, bleeding mucous membranes, hematuria, and GI bleeding (i.e., emesis, gastric aspirate, stool with frank or occult blood).
- Monitor the patient closely for hemorrhage.
- Note Hgb and Hct levels before and after blood loss, as indicated.
- Avoid IM and SC injections and all unnecessary venous or arterial punctures to minimize oozing from invasive sites.
- Protect the patient from trauma that may cause bleeding.
- Avoid taking rectal temperatures.
- Monitor skin for areas of breakdown and redness.
- Monitor skin and mucous membranes for areas of discoloration and bruising.
- Monitor coagulation studies, including PT, PTT, fibrinogen, fibrin degradation products (FDP), fibrin split products (FSP), and platelet counts as appropriate.
- Consult physician for sustained low platelet values ($<100,000/mm^3$).
- Avoid administering NSAIDs (e.g., aspirin, ibuprofen). Teach patient to avoid all medications that potentially decrease platelet aggregation, especially aspirin.
- If severe menorrhagia is present, confer with physician regarding need for progestational hormones (e.g., norethindrone acetate, 5-10 mg PO, qd) for

suppression of menses. Assess volume of blood loss by weighing perineal pads or tampons.
- During the acute (bleeding) phase of ITP, teach patient to perform oral hygiene using sponge-tipped applicators soaked in water or dilute mouthwash to help prevent gum bleeding.
- Teach patient that it is safer to use an electric razor for shaving, both during and after the bleeding phase of ITP.
- Instruct family member/caregiver about signs for skin breakdown, as appropriate.
- Teach patient and significant others to recognize the signs of impending hemorrhage, including increased pulse rate, rapid breathing, increased bruising, painful joints, "spitting up" blood, blood in the urine, and tarry stools.

NIC Bleeding Precautions; Skin Surveillance

Decreased adaptive capacity: intracranial (or risk for same), related to potential for intracranial hemorrhage (<1% of patients) secondary to decreased platelet level

Desired outcomes: Throughout the hospitalization, patient remains free of symptoms of intracranial hemorrhage as evidenced by orientation to time, place, and person; normoreactive pupils and reflexes; patient's normal visual acuity, motor strength, and coordination; and absence of headache and other clinical indicators of increased intracranial pressure (IICP).

- Assess patient for initial signs of IICP, including diminished LOC, pupillary responses (unequal; sluggish/absent response to light), visual disturbances, weakness and paralysis, slow HR, and change in respiratory rate and pattern.
- Monitor trend of Glasgow coma scale.
- Monitor ICP and cerebral perfusion pressure (CPP).
- Increase frequency of neurologic monitoring as appropriate.
- Avoid activities that increase intracranial pressure.
- Space required nursing activities that increase intracranial pressure.
- Monitor patient for the presence of headaches, visual disturbances, or motor dysfunction, which are symptoms of IICP.
- If initial signs of IICP are noted, consult physician immediately. Severe intracranial bleeding can lead to herniation. ICP can increase rapidly with severe bleeding, sometimes causing death within 1 h of onset. Signs of impending herniation include unconsciousness, failure to respond to deeply painful stimuli, decorticate or decerebrate posturing, Cushing triad (bradycardia, increased systolic BP, widening pulse pressure), nonreactive/fixed pupils, unequal pupils, or fixed and dilated pupils. See p. 119 for more information about herniation.
- Consult with physician regarding use of diuretics for occurrence of IICP (see p. 125 for collaborative interventions for IICP).
- Position patient with HOB slightly elevated (30-40 degrees) and neck in neutral position to decrease ICP. For additional interventions for IICP, see Table 2-5.
- Teach patient to avoid Valsalva maneuver (e.g., straining at stool or when lifting; forceful and sustained coughing or nose blowing), which could cause intracranial bleeding.
- Teach the importance of avoiding tobacco products (particularly cigarettes) and excessive caffeine, which may cause vasoconstriction. Constricted vessels may prevent platelets from circulating through portions of the capillary network.
- Confer with physician regarding use of stool softeners or cough suppressants as necessary.

NIC Cerebral Edema Management; Cerebral Perfusion Promotion; Intracranial Pressure (ICP) Monitoring; Neurologic Monitoring

Risk for fluid volume deficit related to active loss secondary to intraabdominal bleeding or postsplenectomy intraabdominal bleeding

Desired outcome: Patient remains normovolemic as evidenced by HR, RR, and BP within 10% of patient's normal range (or HR 60-100 bpm, RR 12-20 breaths/min with normal depth and pattern [eupnea], systolic BP ≥90 mm Hg); urinary output ≥0.5 ml/kg/h; and absence of abdominal pain or tenderness, back pain, and frank bleeding from the splenectomy incision.

- Monitor patient for signs of hypovolemia, including increases in HR and RR, decreases in BP and urinary output, and restlessness and fatigue.
- Monitor fluid status, including I&O, as appropriate.
- Inspect for bleeding from mucous membranes, bruising after minimal trauma, oozing from puncture sites, and presence of petechiae.
- Note tachycardia, decreased BP, or abnormally low systemic arterial pressure, as well as decreased refill and diaphoresis.
- Monitor orthostatic vital signs, including BP.
- Maintain patent IV access.
- Monitor for symptoms of inadequate tissue oxygenation (e.g., pallor, cyanosis, sluggish capillary refill).
- Administer supplemental oxygen as necessary for postoperative status or active bleeding.
- Assess for abdominal pain, tenderness, guarding, or back pain, any of which may signal intraabdominal bleeding.
- Replace lost volume with plasma expanders (albumin, hetastarch [Hespan]) and/or blood products as indicated. See Table 9-1 for information about blood products.
- Inform patient of the importance of wearing a medical-alert bracelet and obtaining a pneumococcal vaccination if a splenectomy has been performed.

NIC Bleeding Precautions; Electrolyte Management; Fluid Management; Fluid Monitoring; Hypovolemia Management; Intravenous (IV) Therapy; Shock Management: Volume; Blood Products Administration

Pain   related to joint inflammation and injury secondary to bleeding into the synovial cavity of the joint(s); postsplenectomy pain

Desired outcomes: Within 4 h of initiating treatment, patient's subjective evaluation of discomfort improves as documented by a pain scale; nonverbal indicators of discomfort are absent or decreased. HR, RR, and BP are within 10% of patient's baseline.

- Devise a pain scale with patient, rating discomfort from 0 (no pain) to 10. Monitor patient for signs of fatigue and malaise. As appropriate, instruct patient to decrease or eliminate those activities that cause fatigue and malaise.
- Perform a comprehensive assessment of pain to include location, characteristics, onset/duration, frequency, quality, intensity or severity, and precipitating factors.
- Elevate patient's legs to decrease joint pain in the lower extremities. Avoid knee flexion.
- Decrease stress on joints by supporting extremities with pillows, making sure bed is not "gatched" at the knee.
- Ensure that patient receives appropriate analgesic care.
- Provide information about the pain, such as causes of the pain, how long it will last, and anticipated discomforts from procedures.
- Reduce or eliminate factors that precipitate or increase the pain experience.
- Teach patient to splint abdomen when coughing postsplenectomy.
- Consult with physician regularly until patient's pain is controlled. Avoid use of meperidine for pain relief in elders because adverse effects are common.
- Evaluate patient's anxiety level, and provide emotional support to control fear and anxiety. If patient becomes agitated, evaluate potential causes, including hypoxemia, poor pain or anxiety control, fluid and electrolyte imbalance, and alcohol or drug withdrawal, and intervene appropriately.

- Teach the use of nonpharmacologic techniques (e.g., biofeedback, transcutaneous electrical nerve stimulation [TENS], hypnosis, relaxation, guided imagery, acupressure, hot/cold application, massage) before, after, and during painful activities before pain occurs or increases and along with other pain relief measures.
- See p. 61 for additional pain interventions. Also see "Prolonged Immobility," p. 74, for patients who are unable to move or who have limited movement.

NIC Analgesic Administration; Pain Management; Coping Enhancement; Anxiety Reduction

Impaired tissue integrity related to intradermal bleeding

Desired outcome: Within 48 h of initiating treatment, patient has no symptoms of further tissue injury (e.g., bruising, petechiae, purpura).

- Apply ice pack or manual pressure over sites of intradermal bleeding to promote hemostasis.
- Monitor skin for areas of breakdown and redness.
- Monitor skin and mucous membranes for areas of discoloration and bruising.
- Move/transfer patient carefully and gently to avoid tissue trauma.
- Avoid IM injections and all venous and arterial punctures, which may cause intradermal bleeding. Hold pressure on invasive sites for ≥5 min, and subsequently apply a small pressure dressing or collagen-coated adhesive dressing (e.g., Tipstop) over sites from which needles or IV catheters have been removed.
- Inspect and document appearance of patient's skin q8-12h. Consult physician for new or increased petechiae, purpura, or bruising.
- Monitor for sources of pressure and friction.
- Explain chronic skin/tissue problems associated with steroids, such as increased vascular fragility, ulceration, "moon face," "buffalo hump," and increased possibility of infections.
- Teach patient the importance of regular check-ups and medical follow-through in managing chronic illness.
- See "Wound and Skin Care," p. 55, for additional interventions.

NIC Wound Care; Skin Surveillance; Pressure Management

ADDITIONAL NURSING DIAGNOSES

Uncontrolled bleeding can be terrifying for the patient and significant others, who may fear the patient will die. Refer to nursing diagnoses in "Psychosocial Support," p. 83, and "Psychosocial Support for the Patient's Family and Significant Others," p. 95, for appropriate interventions.

DISSEMINATED INTRAVASCULAR COAGULATION

PATHOPHYSIOLOGY

DIC is a syndrome characterized by overstimulation of the normal coagulation cascade. DIC is a commonly acquired coagulopathy with the potential to cause both profuse bleeding and widespread thrombosis leading to MODS. Inherent bodily control of bleeding requires a balance between procoagulants and thrombus formation, along with anticoagulants, inhibitors, and thrombolysis (Figure 9-1, Table 9-2). The delicate balance may be upset by disease processes (Table 9-3), resulting in a cascade of uncontrolled coagulation and fibrinolysis. The abnormal clotting cascade that develops during DIC is as follows:

- Platelets and coagulation factors are activated by a disease stimulus and are rapidly consumed, particularly factors V and XIII and fibrinogen.
- Thrombin is formed very rapidly, and inherent inhibitors cannot stop the formation of the vast amounts of thrombin generated. Thrombin directly activates fibrinogen.

TABLE 9-2 Clotting Factors: Primary Actions

Coagulation factor	Thrombin sensitive/promotes vasoconstriction	Vitamin-K sensitive	Sites of heparin activity
I Fibrinogen	✔		
II Prothrombin		✔	✔ IIa
III Tissue thromboplastin (tissue factor)			
IV Calcium			
V Proaccelerin (AC globulin [AC-g])	✔		
VI Not assigned			
VII Proconvertin stable factor (prothrombin accelerator)		✔	
VIII Antihemophilic factor A (antihemophilic factor [AHF], antihemophilic globulin [AHG])	✔		
IX Antihemophilic factor B (plasma thromboplastin component [PTC], Christmas factor)		✔	✔ IXa
X Stuart-Prower factor (Stuart factor)		✔	✔ Xa
XI Plasma thromboplastin antecedent (antihemophilic factor C)			✔ XIa
XII Hageman factor (contact factor)			
XIII Fibrin stabilizing factor	✔		
Other factors:			
Prekallikrein (Fletcher factor)			
High-molecular-weight kininogen (HMWK-Fitzgerald factor)			
Platelets			

- Fibrin is deposited throughout the capillary beds of organs and tissues.
- The fibrinolytic system lyses fibrin and impairs thrombin formation.
- FDPs (or FSPs) result from fibrinolysis, which changes platelet aggregation and inhibits fibrin polymerization. See Figure 9-1 for the normal coagulation pathway.

A predisposing event, such as damage to the vascular endothelium, initiates the clotting cascade. Studies reflect that both the intrinsic and extrinsic pathways are activated initially, resulting in an abnormal acceleration of the clotting process. Thrombocytopenia occurs because of thrombin production and microvascular thrombus formation.

TABLE 9 - 3   Clinical Conditions That Can Activate Disseminated Intravascular Coagulation (DIC)

Obstetric	GI disorders	Tissue damage	Infections	Hemolytic processes	Vascular disorders	Miscellaneous
Abruptio placentae	Cirrhosis	Surgery	Viral	Transfusion reaction	Shock	Fat or pulmonary embolism
Toxemia	Hepatic necrosis	Trauma	Bacterial	Acute hemolysis secondary to infection or immunologic disorder	Aneurysm	Snake bite
Amniotic fluid embolism	Acute fulminant hepatitis	Burns	Rickettsial		Giant hemangioma	Neoplastic disorder
Septic abortion	Pancreatitis	Prolonged extra-corporeal circulation	Protozoal			Acute anoxia
Retained dead fetus	Peritoneovenous shunts	Transplant rejection	Fungal			
Hydatid mole	Necrotizing enterocolitis	Heat stroke				

ASSESSMENT

Risk factors: Any clinical state or pharmacologic therapy (e.g., chemotherapy) that inhibits the removal of activated clotting factors, FDPs, and thromboplastin by the reticuloendothelial system. DIC may manifest as a profound bleeding/clotting disorder in the *acute* phase or as a less symptomatic *chronic* disorder.

In chronic (compensated) DIC, activation of coagulation and fibrinolysis does not occur rapidly enough to exceed the rate of production of clotting factors or inhibitors. The course of DIC depends on the intensity of the stimulus, coupled with the status of the liver, bone marrow, and vascular endothelium. Bleeding vs. thrombosis in DIC is profoundly affected by the underlying disease process.

Clinical presentation: *Abrupt onset of bleeding* or oozing of blood from all invasive sites and mucosal surfaces (e.g., oral, nasal, tracheal, gastric, urethral, vaginal, rectal). In addition, the patient may have hematuria, petechiae, stools or gastric aspirate positive for occult blood, pallor, tachycardia, tachypnea, vertigo, hypotension, ecchymoses (e.g., on palate, gums, skin, conjunctivae), lethargy, irritability, or feeling of impending doom, and possible back pain and abdominal tenderness.

Abnormal thrombosis may manifest with extremity pain, diminished pulses, oliguria or anuria, diminished or absent bowel sounds, severe chest pain with SOB (indicative of either myocardial infarction or pulmonary embolism), or paresis or paralysis (indicative of cerebral thrombus).

Physical assessment: Bleeding from invasive sites and mucosal surfaces, petechiae, ecchymoses, acrocyanosis, bruising, mottling, SOB, tachypnea, possible Grey Turner sign (flank ecchymosis), purpura, diminished or absent bowel sounds, weakened/absent peripheral pulses, confusion, decreased responsiveness, abdominal tenderness, weakness, ST-segment elevation or depression, and T-wave inversion.

DIAGNOSTIC TESTS

Also see Table 9-4.

FDP or FSP: Increased (>10 µg/ml) because of widespread fibrinolysis, which produces FDPs as the end product of clot lysis. Critical value: >40 ng/ml.

D-dimer assay: Increased to >500 because of increased thrombin and plasmin generation. This is a rapid measurement technique, less sensitive than FDPs, and not recommended as a substitute for FDPs and fibrinogen determinations.

Fibrinogen levels: May remain normal or decrease in the early acute phase. As the process continues, fibrinogen levels will decrease. Normal range is 150-400 mg/dl.

PTT or aPTT: Prolonged (>40 sec) because of activation of the intrinsic pathway, causing consumption of coagulation factors. Critical value: >70 sec. In chronic DIC the value may be normal (25-35 sec) or less than normal.

PT: Prolonged (>15 sec) because of activation of the extrinsic pathway, causing consumption of the extrinsic clotting factors. Critical value: >40 sec.

Thrombin time: Prolonged (>1.5 times the control value or >2 sec in excess of a 9- to 13-sec control value) because of rapid conversion of fibrinogen into fibrin.

Antithrombin III (AT-III):   Decreased (<50% of control value using a plasma sample, or <80% using functional values) because of rapid consumption of this thrombin inhibitor. The action of AT-III is catalyzed by heparin.

Euglobulin clot lysis time: This test measures fibrinogen activity via measurement of plasminogen and plasminogen activator, which assist in prevention of fibrin clot formations. Decreased time is seen with DIC. Normal: lysis in 2-4 h. Critical value: 100% lysis in 1 h.

T A B L E 9 - 4   Blood Coagulation Screen in Disseminated Intravascular Coagulation (DIC)

Parameter	Normal	Acute DIC	Chronic DIC
Fibrinogen	150-400 mg/dl (adult)	Decreased	Normal or increased
Fibrin degradation	<10 μg/ml	Positive (increased)	Positive (increased)
Platelet count	150,000-400,000/mm^3 (adult)	Decreased	Normal or increased
Partial thromboplastin time (PTT); also known as activated partial thromoplastin time (aPTT)	25-35 sec	Increased	Normal
Prothrombin time (PT)	11-15 sec	Increased	Normal
Thrombin time	$1.5 \times$ control value	Increased	Increased

Platelet count: Decreased ($<140,000$/mm^3) because of rapid rate of platelet aggregation to form clots during DIC. Aggregation decreases the freely circulating platelets.

Alpha$_2$- (α_2-) antiplasmin: Decreased because of rapid consumption of same in response to large amounts of plasmin generated. When all α_2-antiplasmin is depleted, excessive hyperfibrinolysis (massive, rapid clot lysis) occurs.

Protamine sulfate test, FSP: Results are positive (normal: negative), indicative of presence of fibrin strands. It is associated with the formation of excessive amounts of thrombin and secondary fibrinolysis.

Peripheral blood smear: For visualization during microscopic examination of schistocytes and burr cells, which indicate the deposition of fibrin in the small blood vessels.

COLLABORATIVE MANAGEMENT

Treatment of the underlying disease process often corrects the secondary DIC. Other treatments may vary in effectiveness, depending on the underlying disease. Use of heparin and antifibrinolytic agents in DIC is controversial, inasmuch as these agents have not improved survival in DIC and may exacerbate bleeding (heparin) or thrombosis (antifibrinolytic agent). The following treatments have been effective in individual patients.

Treatment of the primary pathology: A primary disease generally promotes the development of DIC. When DIC occurs without apparent cause, the possibility of undiagnosed malignancy (e.g., prostate cancer), a large abdominal aortic aneurysm, a progressive gram-negative bacterial infection, or hepatic cirrhosis should be explored. Idiopathic DIC is extremely rare but has been reported in infants and several adults.

Continuous IV heparin therapy: There are three conditions associated with DIC in which heparin generally is effective:

Underlying malignancy/carcinoma

Acute promyelocytic leukemia (APML)

Purpura fulminans/extreme purpura, often seen with severe sepsis

Low-dose therapy (5-10 U/kg/h) is considered. Heparin binds to antithrombin, which then inhibits proteases involved in both the intrinsic and common coagulation pathways, resulting in a strong anticoagulant effect. Use of higher-dose heparin in DIC is associated with a high risk of bleeding, and greater efficacy has not been documented. Heparin may be considered for other instances of serious bleeding or clotting when the condition underlying the DIC is not rapidly reversible and the patient's vascular system is surgically intact.

> **Note:**   APML patients with DIC often accelerate symptoms of fibrinolysis (declotting) when receiving chemotherapy. If these individuals receive heparin, an antifibrinolytic agent such as epsilon- (ϵ-) aminocaproic acid (Amicar) may be added to decrease bleeding.

Antifibrinolytic agents: ϵ-Aminocaproic acid (Amicar) and tranexamic acid (Cyklokapron) are used to inhibit fibrinolysis in patients who are bleeding as a result of a variety of causes. In patients with DIC, these agents should be used with extreme caution because they may convert a bleeding disorder into a thrombotic problem. When used in DIC, these agents are used in combination with heparin to minimize the potential for thrombosis.

Thrombolytic agents: Use of streptokinase, urokinase, and tissue plasminogen activator (TPA) is not indicated for patients with thrombosis because these agents may facilitate excessive bleeding.

Blood component replacement: Clotting factors and inhibitors are replaced in the form of fresh-frozen plasma. The PT is suggested as the most accurate parameter for guiding plasma replacement. Patients with markedly decreased fibrinogen levels may be given cryoprecipitate, which contains 5-10 times more fibrinogen than plasma contains. Thrombocytopenia in DIC generally is not severe, and the platelet count usually is $>50,000/mm^3$. General replacement therapy guidelines indicate that approximately 10 U of cryoprecipitate should be given for every 2-3 U of plasma. Platelet transfusions rarely are needed unless the patient has impaired platelet production and profuse bleeding. AT-III concentrate has been used on a limited basis in clinical trials (see Table 9-1). Clinical trials are underway wherein DIC is being managed with activated protein C (APC), tissue factor pathway inhibitor (TFPI), and synthetic serine protease inhibitors (e.g., aprotinin).

Red blood cell replacement: Packed RBCs may be administered to increase oxygen-carrying capacity with a hemoglobin value <9 mg/dl or >20% below the patient's baseline if the patient is chronically anemic.

Vitamin K_1 (phytonadione) and folate: Patients with DIC are at high risk for deficiency of these substances, and administration of both vitamins is recommended for most patients.

Protease inhibitors: Investigational medications, including gabexate, nafamostat, and transylol, have been used in limited clinical trials.

Vasoactive drugs: If patient becomes severely hypotensive, the following drugs may be considered: amrinone, dobutamine, dopamine, epinephrine, and nitroprusside (see Appendix 7).

> **Research Brief 9-2**   Protein C deficiency is associated with increased mortality and morbidity. By minimizing microvascular coagulopathy and inflammation, protein C replacement may improve organ perfusion, prevent multiple organ dysfunction, and decrease mortality. It does not act as a blockade to the pathology but, rather, provides a supplement to a naturally occurring substance that is deficient in some people.

Hartman DL: *N Engl J Med* 336:912-918, 1997.

NURSING DIAGNOSES AND INTERVENTIONS

Altered protection related to bleeding resulting from overstimulation of the clotting cascade and rapid consumption of clotting factors

Desired outcome: Within 48-72 h of initiation of treatment, patient is free of symptoms of bleeding as evidenced by absence of frank bleeding from invasive sites and mucosal surfaces; secretions and excretions that are negative for blood; absence of large or increasing ecchymoses; decreasing purpura; and HR, RR, and BP within 10% of patient's baseline (or HR 60-100 bpm, RR 12-20 breaths/min, systolic BP >90 mm Hg).

- Discuss bleeding history with patient or significant others as possible, assessing prior incidence of a bleeding problem, gingival bleeding, skin bleeding, hematuria, tarry/bloody stools, muscle bleeding, bleeding into joints, hemoptysis, vomiting of blood, epistaxis, prolonged bleeding from small wounds or after tooth extraction, and unusual bruising or tendency to bruise easily.
- Question patients who have no previous history of bleeding regarding current medications, including over-the-counter (OTC) preparations, since many medications promote bleeding (Table 9-5).
- Monitor coagulation/clotting tests daily. Consult physician for values that exceed normal ranges by 15% (see Table 9-4).
- Protect the patient from trauma, which may cause bleeding.
- Use soft-bristle toothbrush for oral care.
- Monitor closely for increased bleeding, bruising, petechiae, and purpura. Assess for internal bleeding by testing suspicious secretions (i.e., sputum, urine, stool, emesis, gastric drainage) for the presence of blood.
- Monitor the patient closely for hemorrhage.
- Maintain bed rest during active bleeding.
- Monitor neurologic status (see Glasgow coma scale, Appendix 3) q2h by assessing LOC, orientation, pupillary reaction, and movement and strength of extremities. Changes in status can indicate intracranial bleeding.
- Use alcohol-free mouthwash and swabs for oral care to minimize the risk of bleeding from gum injury. Use normal saline solution (NSS) or solution of NSS and sodium bicarbonate (500 ml NSS with 15 ml bicarbonate) to irrigate the oral cavity. Massage gums gently with a sponge-tipped applicator to help remove debris. Do not attempt to remove large clots from the mouth, inasmuch as profuse bleeding may ensue.
- Use electric rather than safety razor for shaving patient.
- Avoid unnecessary venipunctures and IM injections.
- Avoid taking rectal temperatures.
- Refrain from inserting objects into a bleeding orifice.
- If patient undergoes an invasive procedure, manually hold pressure over the insertion site for 3-5 min for IV catheters and 10-15 min for arterial catheters or until bleeding subsides.
- Instruct the patient and/or family on signs of bleeding and appropriate actions (e.g., notify the nurse) should bleeding occur.
- Teach patient the importance of avoiding vitamin K–inhibiting and platelet aggregation–inhibiting medications (see Table 9-5), which promote bleeding.

NIC Infection Control; Infection Protection; Bleeding Precautions; Surveillance: Safety

Risk for fluid volume deficit related to bleeding/hemorrhage

Desired outcomes: Patient remains normovolemic as evidenced by HR and RR within patient's baseline (or HR 60-100 bpm and RR 12-20 breaths/min with normal depth and pattern); BP within patient's baseline (or systolic BP >90 mm Hg); warm extremities; distal pulses >2+ on a 0-4+ scale; urinary output ≥0.5 ml/kg/h; and capillary refill <2 sec. Within 24 h of initiating treatment, patient verbalizes orientation to time, place, person, and self.

- Monitor VS at least q2h, noting increases in HR and RR, decreased BP, and decreasing pulse pressure.

TABLE 9-5   Medications That May Promote Bleeding

Medications that inhibit platelets or cause thrombocytopenia		Medications that inhibit vitamin K

Analgesics

Nonsteroidal antiinflammatory agents (NSAIDs)
Aspirin
Acetaminophen
Antipyrine
Ibuprofen
Indomethacin
Fenoprofen
Sodium salicylate

Antirheumatic agents

Oxyphenbutazone
Phenylbutazone
Hydroxychloroquine
Gold salts

Antimicrobials

Ampicillin
Cephalothin
Methicillin
Penicillin
Pentamidine
Streptomycin

Diuretic agents

Sulfonamide derivatives
Acetazolamide
Chlorpropamide
Chlorothiazide
Chlorthalidone
Clopamide
Diazoxide
Furosemide
Bumetanide
Hydrochlorothiazide
Tolbutamide
Spironolactone
Mercurial diuretics

Glycoprotein IIB IIIA inhibitors

Abciximab
Eptifibatide
Tirofiban

Phenothiazines

Chlorpromazine
Promethazine
Trifluoperazine

Other

Antihistamines
Ethanol
Heparin
Beta-adrenergic
  blocking agents
General anesthetics
Local anesthetics
Chemotherapeutic
  agents
Vitamin E
Estrogens
Digitoxin
Cimetidine
Levodopa
Propylthiouracil

Salicylates

Aspirin and aspirin combination drugs
Other salicylates

Coumarins

Anisindione
Dicumarol
Warfarin

Broad-spectrum antibiotics

Sulfonamides
  Triple sulfa
  Sulfamethoxazole
  Sulfasalazine
  Sulfisoxazole
  Sulfamethoxazole-trimethoprim
Clindamycin
Gentamicin
Neomycin
Tobramycin
Vancomycin
Imipenem
Cefamandole
Cefoxitin

Sulfonamides (antibiotics)
Chloramphenicol
Isoniazid
Nitrofurantoin
Rifampin
Trimethoprim
Anticoagulants
Heparin
Enoxaparin
Dalteparin
Thrombolytics
Alteplase
Reteplase
Streptokinase
Urokinase (currently
  unavailable)
Anisoylated plasminogen
  streptokinase

Phosphodiesterase inhibitors
Caffeine
Dipyridamole
Theophyllines
Antiplatelet drugs
Aspirin
Ticlopidine
Clopidogrel
Prostaglandins
I_2
D_2
E
Sedative-hypnotics
Benzodiazepines
Clonazepam
Diazepam
Vasodilators
Nitroglycerin
Nitroprusside

Vitamins
A
E

- Measure urinary output q2-4h. Consult physician for output <0.5 ml/kg/h.
- Maintain accurate I&O record.
- Weigh daily, and monitor trends.
- Increase frequency of measurement of VS and urine output to at least q30min if patient is bleeding actively. For profuse bleeding, check VS at least q15min. Consider insertion of an arterial line for continuous monitoring of BP.
- Monitor CBC daily for significant alterations in Hct, Hgb, and platelets (Table 9-6).
- Arrange for availability of blood products (e.g., check blood with patient identification; prepare infusion setup as appropriate).
- Ensure that patient has typed and crossmatched blood available for transfusion in the hospital's blood bank.
- Monitor coagulation studies, including PT, PTT, fibrinogen, FDP/FSP, and platelet counts, as appropriate.
- Assess patient for signs of impending shock if HR and RR increase or if BP decreases: pallor, diaphoresis, cool extremities, delayed capillary refill, diminished intensity of peripheral pulses, restlessness, agitation, and disorientation.

TABLE 9-6   Complete Blood Count Values

Parameters	Common measurement value	Population
Red blood cells (RBCs)	4-5.5 million/mm^3	Adult females
	4.5-6.2 million/mm^3	Adult males
Hemoglobin (Hgb)	12-16 g/dl	Adult females
	14-18 g/dl	Adult males
Hematocrit (Hct)	37%-47%	Adult females
Mean corpuscular volume (MCV)	83-93 μ^3	Adults
Mean cell hemoglobin (MCH)	26-34 pg	Adults
Mean cell hemoglobin concentration (MCHC)	31%-38%	Adults
White blood cells (WBCs)	4,500-11,000/mm^3	Adults
Differential white blood cells		
Granulocytes		
Segmented neutrophils (Segs)	54%-62%	Adults
Band neutrophils (Bands)	3%-5%	Adults
Eosinophils (Eos)	1%-3%	Adults
Basophils (Basos)	0-0.75%	Adults
Monocytes (Monos)	3%-7%	Adults
Lymphocytes (Lymphs)	25%-33%	Adults
Platelets	150,000-400,000/mm^3	Adults

- Inspect all invasive sites for frank bleeding, including a thorough assessment of all dressings that are covering wounds.
- Inspect for bleeding from mucous membranes, bruising after minimal trauma, oozing from puncture sites, and presence of petechiae.
- Maintain at least one 18-gauge or larger IV catheter for use during shock management, at which time rapid infusion of blood products or IV fluids may be necessary. For more information, see Advanced Cardiac Life Support (ACLS) algorithms, Appendix 1.
- Evaluate the effects of fluid therapy.

NIC Electrolyte Management; Fluid Management; Fluid Monitoring; Hypovolemia Management; Intravenous (IV) Therapy; Shock Management: Volume

Altered tissue perfusion (or risk for same): peripheral, cardiopulmonary, cerebral, gastrointestinal, and renal, related to blood loss or presence of microthrombi

Desired outcomes: Patient has adequate perfusion as evidenced by peripheral pulses >2+ on a scale of 0-4+; brisk capillary refill (<2 sec); BP within patient's normal range; CVP ≥5 cm H_2O or ≥2 mm Hg; PAWP 6-12 mm Hg; and HR regular and ≤100 bpm. Patient is oriented to time, place, person, and self and has urinary output ≥30 ml/h (0.5 ml/kg/h) and oxygen saturation >90%.

- Assess and document peripheral perfusion q2h, including temperature, sensation, pulses, and movement in extremities. Consult physician for coolness and pallor of extremities, decreased sensation/numbness, localized weakness, and delayed capillary refill.
- Monitor vital signs frequently.
- Evaluate chest pain.
- Document cardiac dysrhythmias.
- Recognize presence of blood pressure alterations.
- Monitor BP and assess for early signs of perfusion deficit at least q2h, including dizziness, confusion, and decreased urinary output.
- Perform a comprehensive assessment of peripheral circulation (e.g., check peripheral pulses, edema, capillary refill, color and temperature of extremities).
- Monitor for decreased myocardial or pulmonary perfusion as evidenced by chest pain, ST-segment depression or elevation, T-wave inversion, SOB, dyspnea, and decreased oxygen saturation using continuous pulse oximetry.
- Monitor PAWP frequently, observing for both high and low readings. Decreased pressures are indicative of hypovolemia/ hemorrhage. Elevated PAD pressures may signal pulmonary embolus.
- Monitor cardiac output (CO), and calculate systemic vascular resistance (SVR), pulmonary vascular resistance (PVR), and cardiac index (CI). Anticipate vasoconstriction with hypovolemia. SVR will be elevated >1400 dynes/sec/cm^{-5}. CO may increase or decrease from normal range of 4-7 L/min, depending on cardiac contractility. PVR will be elevated >240 dynes/sec/cm^{-5} in the presence of pulmonary emboli.
- Monitor effects of medications.
- Monitor GI status by observing tolerance to diet or tube feedings, bowel habits (constipation, diarrhea), character of stool (tarry, bloody), and presence or absence of bowel sounds. Palpate for abdominal tenderness and monitor abdominal girth q8h.

NIC Cardiac Care: Acute; Circulatory Care: Arterial Insufficiency; Circulatory Care: Venous Insufficiency; Respiratory Monitoring; Shock Management: Cardiac; Cerebral Perfusion Promotion; Neurologic Monitoring; Peripheral Sensation Management; Fluid/Electrolyte Management; Fluid Management; Vital Signs Monitoring

Impaired gas exchange (or risk for same) related to loss of oxygen-carrying capacity through hemorrhage or pulmonary microembolus formation

Desired outcome: Patient's gas exchange is adequate as evidenced by Pao_2 ≥80 mm Hg; $Paco_2$ 35-45 mm Hg; pH 7.35-7.45; RR 12-20 breaths/min with normal depth and pattern (eupnea); oxygen saturation >90%; HR 60-100 bpm; Svo_2 >60%; and orientation to time, place, and person.

- Assess respiratory status q2h, noting rate, rhythm, depth, and regularity of respirations.
- Monitor for increased restlessness, anxiety, and air hunger.
- Monitor for dyspnea and events that improve and worsen it.
- Monitor chest x-ray reports.
- Monitor oxygen saturation via pulse oximetry. Consult physician for persistent values ≤90%, which may signal inadequate oxygenation.
- Monitor ABG values, being alert to an increase in $Paco_2$ and decrease in pH, which can signal hypoventilation. Consult physician accordingly.
- If BP is stable, place patient in high Fowler's position or in a comfortable, upright position to promote lung expansion.
- Assess lungs for the presence of bibasilar crackles (rales), which can occur with fluid accumulation.
- Institute respiratory therapy treatments (e.g., nebulizer) as needed.
- Monitor patient's respiratory secretions.
- Monitor for signs of pulmonary embolus, including sharp, stabbing chest pain; dyspnea; pallor; cyanosis; pupillary dilation; rapid, irregular pulse; profuse diaphoresis; and anxiety. Assess need for supplemental oxygen, and consult physician immediately. Patients with severe pulmonary emboli may require mechanical ventilation. See "Pulmonary Emboli," p. 232.
- Assess patient for changes in sensorium (confusion, lethargy, somnolence), which can indicate either inadequate cerebral oxygenation or carbon dioxide retention (respiratory insufficiency). Notify physician accordingly.
- Monitor for diaphragmatic muscle fatigue (paradoxic motion).

NIC Airway Management; Oxygen Therapy; Respiratory Monitoring

Risk for injury related to blood product administration

Desired outcome: Throughout transfusion and up to 8 h after transfusion, patient does not exhibit signs of a blood transfusion reaction as evidenced by absence of fever and chills; normal appearance of skin (no flushing, rash, lesions); and baseline RR, BP, and HR.

- Check blood to be given with another professional to ensure that the crossmatch report and requisition form match the blood unit information. Verify the following: patient's name and hospital number, blood unit number, blood expiration date, blood group, and blood type.
- When blood products are infusing, check VS q15min for the first hour. Check patient frequently throughout the first 15 min of the transfusion to observe for signs of an acute intravascular hemolytic transfusion reaction, including fever, chills, dyspnea, hypotension, flushing, tachycardia, back pain, hematuria, and shock.
- Observe for transfusion reactions throughout the transfusion and during the 8-h period afterward. If a transfusion reaction (Table 9-7) occurs, implement the following:
  1. If the transfusion is in progress, stop the infusion immediately.
  2. Maintain IV access with NSS.
  3. Maintain BP with a combination of volume infusion and vasoactive drugs, if indicated. See ACLS algorithms, Appendix 1, accordingly.
  4. Monitor HR and ECG for changes. Consult physician, and treat symptomatic dysrhythmias as prescribed.
  5. Administer diuretics and fluids as prescribed to promote diuresis (urine output approximately 100 ml/h).
  6. Obtain blood and urine for a transfusion workup per institution blood bank protocol.
  7. Perform blood cultures if patient exhibits signs of sepsis.
- If an intravascular hemolytic reaction is confirmed, implement the following:
  ☐ Monitor coagulation studies, including PT, PTT, and fibrinogen levels (see Table 9-4).

TABLE 9-7   Acute Transfusion Reactions

Type	Symptoms	Time frame
Acute intravascular hemolytic	Fever, chills, dyspnea, tachycardia hypotension, back pain, flushing, hematuria, shock	After start of transfusion Within 5-30 min
Acute extravascular hemolytic	Fever, elevated bilirubin, unusually low post-transfusion hematocrit and hemoglobin	Usually within 8 h Delayed: 7-10 days
Allergic (mild)	Rash, hives pruritus	Within 1 h
Anaphylactic	Dyspnea, shortness of breath, bronchospasms, tachycardia, flushing, hypotension, shock	Within 30 min-1 h
Febrile	Fever, chills	Within 4 h
Hypervolemic	Dyspnea, tachycardia, bibasilar crackles, jugular venous distention, possible hypertension, headache	Within 1-2 h
Septic	Fever, chills, tachycardia, hypotension, vomiting, shock, muscle pain, cardiac arrest	Within 5 min-4 h

☐ Monitor renal status, noting blood urea nitrogen (BUN), creatinine, potassium, and phosphate levels.
☐ Monitor laboratory values indicative of hemolysis, including lactate dehydrogenase (LDH), bilirubin, and haptoglobin.
• With massive transfusion for severe bleeding, patients also can develop hypocalcemia caused by citrated blood; hyperkalemia of uncertain etiology; hypothermia from refrigerated blood; ARDS; coagulopathy; and hemochromatosis (iron overload).

NIC Bleeding Precautions; Bleeding Reduction; Blood Products Administration

ADDITIONAL NURSING DIAGNOSES

The uncontrolled bleeding related to DIC can be terrifying to the patient and significant others, who may fear the patient will die. Refer to nursing diagnoses in "Psychosocial Support," p. 83, and "Psychosocial Support for the Patient's Family and Significant Others," p. 95. For patients who manifest activity intolerance, see that nursing diagnosis in "Prolonged Immobility," p. 74.

Bibliography

Ansell JE: Acquired bleeding disorders. In Rippe JM et al: *Intensive care medicine,* ed 3, Boston, 1996, Little, Brown.

Aster RH: Heparin-induced thrombocytopenia and thrombosis, *N Engl J Med* 332(20):1374-1376, 1995 (editorial).

Balk R et al: Therapeutic use of antithrombin concentrate in sepsis, *Semin Thromb Hemost* 24(2):183-194, 1998.

Colvin BT: Management of disseminated intravascular coagulation, *Br J Haematol* 101(suppl 1):15-17, 1998.

Eisenstaedt RS: Transfusion therapy: blood components and transfusion complications. In Rippe JM et al: *Intensive care medicine*, ed 3, Boston, 1996, Little, Brown.

Esmon CT et al: The protein C pathway: new insights, *Thromb Haemost* 78(1):70-74, 1997.

Fahey VA: Heparin-induced thrombocytopenia, *J Vasc Nurs* 13(4):112-116, 1995.

Griffiths E, Dzik WH: Assays for heparin induced thrombocytopenia, *Transfus Med* 7(1):1-11, 1997.

Harenberg J et al: Dosage, anticoagulant and antithrombotic effects of heparin and low-molecular-weight heparin in the treatment of deep vein thrombosis, *Semin Thromb Hemost* 23(1):83-90, 1997.

Kelton, JG, Warkentin TE: Heparin-induced thrombocytopenia: diagnosis, natural history and treatment options, *Postgrad Med* 103(2):169-171, 175-178, 1998.

Keriakes DJ et al: Abciximab-associated profound thrombocytopenia: therapy with immunoglobulin and platelet transfusion, *Am J Cardiol* 78:1161-1163, 1996.

Lechner DL: A standardized weight-based heparin protocol: improving clinical outcomes, *Nurs Manage* 28(4):29-32, 1997.

Mayer DM, Docktor WJ: Abciximab: a novel platelet blocking drug: pharmacology and nursing implications, *Crit Care Nurse* 18(2):29-37, 1998.

Murkin JM: Cardiopulmonary bypass and the inflammatory response: a role for serine protease inhibitors? *J Cardiothorac Vasc Anesth* 11(2 Suppl 1):19-23, 1997 (review).

Pechet L: The hemolytic anemias. In Rippe JM et al: *Intensive care medicine*, ed 3, Boston, 1996, Little, Brown.

Penner JA: Disseminated intravascular coagulation in patients with multiple organ failure of non-septic origin, *Semin Thromb Hemost* 24(1):45-52, 1998.

Ray MJ, Marsh NA: Aprotinin reduces blood loss after cardiopulmonary bypass by direct inhibition of plasmin, *Thromb Haemost* 78(3):1021-1026, 1997.

Riewald M, Reiss H: Treatment options for clinically recognized disseminated intravascular coagulation, *Semin Thromb Hemost* 24(1):53-59, 1998.

Schmidt OH, Lang W: Heparin-induced thrombocytopenia with thromboembolic arterial occlusion treated with recombinant hirudin (case study), *N Engl J Med* 337(19):1389, 1997.

Simko LC, Lockhart JS: Action STAT: heparin-induced thrombocytopenia and thrombosis, *Nursing* 26(3):33, 1996.

Warkentin TE, Kelton JG: Thrombocytopenia. In Rippe JM et al: *Intensive care medicine*, ed 3, Boston, 1996, Little, Brown.

CHAPTER 10

Multisystem Stressors

Septic shock

PATHOPHYSIOLOGY

Sepsis is an acute systemic clinical syndrome caused by bacteria, viruses, or fungi in the blood. It can be described as a continuum from bacteremia to profound septic shock. Septic shock is present when sepsis results in hypotension and perfusion abnormalities. Impaired perfusion may cause lactic acidosis, oliguria, or acute alterations in mental status. Microorganisms commonly involved in infections in patients in the intensive care unit (ICU) include gram-negative enteric pathogens (e.g., *Escherichia coli, Klebsiella* spp., *Enterobacter* spp., *Pseudomonas aeruginosa),* *Staphylococcus aureus,* coagulase-negative staphylococci, *Enterococcus* spp., and *Candida* spp. Antibiotic-resistant bacteria such as MRSA are common causes of infection in critically ill patients.

In early sepsis, infection causes a generalized inflammatory response, or systemic inflammatory response syndrome (SIRS) (see p. 604). Uncontrolled systemic inflammation leads to vasodilation, hypotension, increased microvascular obstruction, and greatly accelerated coagulation. Severe sepsis occurs when sepsis is accompanied by dysfunction of one or more vital organs. Severe sepsis accompanied by hypotension that does not respond to volume infusion is called *septic shock.* Multiple organ dysfunction syndrome (MODS) ensues if the uncontrolled systemic inflammatory response continues and two or more vital organ systems fail.

See Figure 10-1 for a depiction of the pathophysiologic process of sepsis.

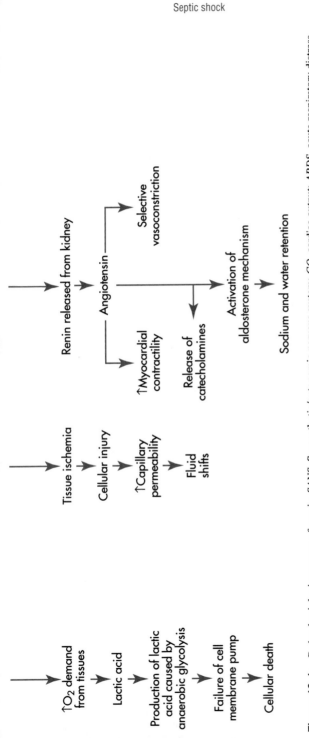

Figure 10-1: Pathophysiologic process of sepsis. *SANS,* Sympathetic/autonomic nervous system; *CO,* cardiac output; *ARDS,* acute respiratory distress syndrome; *SVR,* systemic vascular resistance.

Research Brief 10-1　The records of 41 patients who developed septic shock were analyzed to determine if the patient's location (general ward vs. intensive care unit [ICU]) at time of onset of shock influenced the mortality rate. All patients were treated in the ICUs, but there was a 67-min delay before the patients on the ward were transferred to an ICU. The ICU patients received a fluid bolus after a 15-min delay, whereas 27 min lapsed before the patients on the ward received a fluid bolus. In addition, the patients on the ward had a delay of 310 min before inotropic support was started, compared with 22.5 min for patients in the ICU. Even though the ICU patients were older and more ill than the general ward patients, they had a lower crude mortality than the non-ICU patients. The authors conclude that delays in initiation of fluid bolus and inotropic support have clinical significance for general ward patients who experience septic shock.

From Lundberg JS et al: Septic shock: an analysis of outcomes for patients with onset on hospital wards versus intensive care units, *Crit Care Med* 26(6):1020-1024, 1998.

ASSESSMENT

History and risk factors:　Malnutrition, immunosuppression, chronic health problems (e.g., liver or renal disease), bone marrow suppression, advanced age, recent traumatic injuries, or surgical or invasive procedures; sequential infections. Underlying diseases or conditions such as splenectomy, injecting drug use, and rheumatic heart disease are other risk factors.

Clinical presentation:　Early stages: fever, restlessness, confusion, flushed and warm skin, tachypnea, hypotension, hyperglycemia. Later stages: pallor, cool skin, peripheral cyanosis, hypoventilation, hypoglycemia. Elders may present with altered level of consciousness (LOC), weakness, anorexia, hypothermia.

Physical assessment:　See Tables 10-1 and 10-2.

Hemodynamic measurements:　*Early stages:* Increased respiratory rate (RR) and heart rate (HR); decreased blood pressure (BP). Temperature >38.3° C (101° F) but sometimes normal or even decreased, especially in elders. Pulmonary artery wedge pressure (PAWP) <6 mm Hg; systemic vascular resistance (SVR) <900 dynes/sec/cm^{-5}; cardiac output (CO) >7 L/min; cardiac index (CI) >4 L/min/m^2; Svo$_2$ reflects the decreased oxygen use by cells and is >80%.

Late stages: Decreased RR; increased HR; decreased BP and temperature. PAWP >12 mm Hg; SVR >1200 dynes/sec/cm^{-5}; CO <4 L/min; CI <2.5 L/min/m^2; and Svo$_2$, reflecting decreased oxygen binding to hemoglobin (Hgb) caused by profound acidosis, is ≤60%.

DIAGNOSTIC TESTS

Complete blood cell count (CBC):　White blood cells (WBCs) usually increase early, with increased immature neutrophils (bands) or "shift to the left." Later, WBCs may decrease as a result of sequestration within organs and bone marrow exhaustion.

Chemistries:　Early increase in serum glucose levels results from glucogenesis; later decrease results from hepatic failure. Venous lactate levels increase if tissue perfusion is inadequate. Hepatic, renal, or other organ failure is reflected in electrolyte and enzyme abnormalities.

Blood cultures and antibiotic sensitivity testing of isolates:　Identify causative organism(s).

Culture and antibiotic sensitivity testing of suspect infection sites (e.g., urine, sputum, blood, intravenous (IV) lines, incisions):　Correlate with blood cultures to identify source(s) of the sepsis.

TABLE 10-1   Assessment Guidelines for the Patient With Sepsis in the Early, Hyperdynamic Stage

Clinical indicator	Cause
Cardiovascular	
Increased HR (≥100 bpm)	Sympathetic/autonomic nervous system (SANS) stimulation
Decreased BP (<90 mm Hg systolic)	Vasodilation
CO >7 L/min; CI >4 L/min/m^2	Hyperdynamic state secondary to SANS stimulation
Svo$_2$ >80%	Decreased utilization of oxygen by cells
PAWP usually <6 mm Hg	Venous dilation; decreased preload
SVR <900 dynes/sec/cm^{-5}	Vasodilation
Strong, bounding peripheral pulses	Hyperdynamic cardiovascular system
Respiratory	
Tachypnea (>20 breaths/min) and hyperventilation	Decreases in cerebrospinal fluid pH that stimulate the central respiratory center
Crackles	Interstitial edema occurring with increased vascular permeability
Paco$_2$ <35 mm Hg	Tachypnea and hyperventilation
Dyspnea	Increased respiratory muscle work
Renal	
Decreased urine output (<0.5 ml/kg/h)	Decreased renal perfusion
Increased specific gravity (1.025-1.035)	Decreased glomerular filtration rate
Cutaneous	
Flushed and warm skin	Vasodilation
Metabolic	
Increasing body temperature (usually >38.3° C [100.9° F])	Increased metabolic activity; release of pyrogens secondary to invading microorganisms; release of interleukin-I by macrophages
pH <7.35	Metabolic acidosis occurring with accumulation of lactic acid
↑ Blood sugar	Release of glucagon; insulin depletion
Neurologic	
Changes in LOC	Decreased cerebral perfusion and brain hypoxia
Fluid	
↑ Fluid retention	↑ ADH, ↑ aldosterone

HR, Heart rate; *bpm*, beats per minute; *BP*, blood pressure; *CO*, cardiac output; *CI*, cardiac index; *PAWP*, pulmonary artery wedge pressure; *SVR*, systemic vascular resistance; *LOC*, level of consciousness; *ADH*, antidiuretic hormone.

TABLE 10-2   **Assessment Guidelines for the Patient With Sepsis in the Late Stage**

Clinical indicator	Cause
Cardiovascular	
Extreme tachycardia with S_3 sound	Compensatory attempt by sympathetic nervous system to maintain CO
Profound hypotension	Decreased stroke volume. Diastolic BP may remain high because of vasoconstriction
CO <4 L/min; CI <2.5 L/min/m²	Failure of compensatory mechanisms
PAWP usually >12 mm Hg	Increased left ventricular end-diastolic pressure (LVEDP) because of increased residual volume from decreased stroke volume
SVR >1200 dynes/sec/cm⁻⁵	Vasoconstriction
Weak or absent peripheral pulses	Decreased peripheral perfusion because of decreased CO
$S\overline{v}o_2$ ≤60%	Decreased oxygen binding to hemoglobin because of acidosis
Respiratory	
Decreased respiratory rate (<12 breaths/min) and depth	Central respiratory center depression
Crackles, rhonchi, wheezes	Accumulation of lung secretions
Increased Fio_2 required to maintain Pao_2 (possible ARDS)	Ventilation/perfusion mismatch and decreased lung compliance
Increased $Paco_2$ (>45 mm Hg)	Decreased tidal volume
Renal	
Decreased urine output progressing to anuria	Decreased renal perfusion and tubular ischemia
Decreased fractional excretion of sodium	Activation of the aldosterone mechanism and release of ADH, which stimulate sodium and water retention
Cutaneous	
Cool, pale skin or cyanosis	Sustained vasoconstriction
Neurologic	
Decreased LOC, coma	Severe hypoxia
Hematologic	
Oozing from previous venipuncture sites	Development of DIC caused by stimulation of coagulation process, and fibrinolysis
Acid-base status	
pH <7.35; $Paco_2$ ≥45 mm Hg; HCO_3^- ≤22 mEq/L (or less than expected)	Mixed acid-base disorder: respiratory acidosis and metabolic acidosis

CO, Cardiac output; *CI,* cardiac index; *PAWP,* pulmonary artery wedge pressure; *SVR,* systemic vascular resistance; *ARDS,* acute respiratory distress syndrome; *LOC,* level of consciousness; *ADH,* antidiuretic hormone; *DIC,* disseminated intravascular coagulation.

ABG values: Will reflect metabolic acidosis (low HCO_3^-). Early in septicemia a low $Paco_2$ may reflect hyperventilation. As shock progresses, however, respiratory acidosis (retention of CO_2) will occur and hypoxemia will be present because of respiratory failure.

Clotting studies: Will demonstrate an increased prothrombin time (PT), increased partial thromboplastin time (PTT), increased bleeding time, thrombocytopenia, and increased fibrin split products. These results all reflect activation of the clotting cascade and may signal development of disseminated intravascular coagulation (DIC).

Liver studies: Aspartate aminotransferase (AST) (serum glutamic-oxaloacetic acid transaminase [SGOT]); alanine aminotransferase (ALT) (serum glutamic pyruvic transaminase [SGPT]); and lactate dehydrogenase (LDH) will be elevated secondary to liver ischemia.

Imaging

X-rays: Chest x-ray to check for pneumonia or acute respiratory distress syndrome (ARDS). Other x-rays as indicated according to underlying condition.

Computed tomography (CT): To check for abnormalities such as intraabdominal abscess or perforated viscus.

COLLABORATIVE MANAGEMENT

Antibiotic therapy (specific to causative organism): Therapy usually is begun immediately after culture specimens are obtained and before sensitivity studies are completed (usually 24-48 h). Empiric treatment depends on the suspected source of infection.

Supplemental oxygen: Administered to support oxygen delivery to the tissues. The amount and method of oxygen administered are guided by ABG results. Intubation and mechanical ventilation may be necessary.

Fluid administration: Intravenous volume expansion is implemented to maintain adequate ventricular filling pressures and volume, which become compromised with increased capillary permeability and vasodilation. Lactated Ringer's solution, normal saline, albumin, and fresh-frozen plasma are used.

Positive inotropic drugs (e.g., dopamine, dobutamine): May be given to augment cardiac contractility and cardiac output. In the late stages of sepsis, positive inotropic drugs may be given along with *vasodilators,* such as nitroprusside and nitroglycerin, which decrease preload and afterload by dilating veins and arteries.

> **Note:** Dopamine hydrochloride dosages of 2-5 µg/kg/min will increase renal and mesenteric blood flow. For additional information about inotropic agents and vasodilators, see Appendix 7.

Vasopressors (e.g., dopamine, epinephrine, norepinephrine, phenylephrine): May be administered in cases when optimal left ventricular preload fails to restore adequate tissue perfusion (e.g., the initial mean arterial pressure (MAP) is very low or MAP is persistently <60 mm Hg). Goal of therapy is to optimize CI.

Sodium bicarbonate: Administered judiciously to patients with severe metabolic acidosis (pH <7.25). Measures to increase oxygen delivery should be attempted before sodium bicarbonate is administered.

Steroid therapy: Benefit of steroids for septic shock is not clearly established. Steroid use is indicated if adrenal insufficiency is present or suspected.

Nutritional support: Short- and medium-chain fatty acids and branched-chain amino acids are administered to stop protein catabolism. The short- and medium-chain fatty acids are absorbed more readily and metabolized more easily than long-chain fatty acids. They may be given orally, such as MCT Oil (proprietary name meaning triglycerides of medium-chain fatty acids), or given

IV (e.g., intralipid solutions). Branched-chain amino acid solutions are used in sepsis because they are metabolized by muscle rather than by the liver and therefore can be used in the presence of organ failure.

Antipyretic agents, cooled IV fluid, or cooling blanket: To normalize temperature.

Naloxone hydrochloride (Narcan):   May be used to reverse some of the vasodilation effects of sepsis.

Glucose-potassium-insulin (GKI):   This combination may be given to increase cardiac performance during sepsis.

NURSING DIAGNOSES AND INTERVENTIONS

Fluid volume deficit related to active loss from vascular compartment secondary to increased capillary permeability and shift of intravascular volume into interstitial spaces

Desired outcomes: Within 4 h of initiation of therapy, patient is normo-volemic as evidenced by peripheral pulses >2+ on a 0-4+ scale; stable body weight; urine output ≥0.5 ml/kg/h; systolic BP ≥90 mm Hg or within patient's normal range; and absence of edema and adventitious lung sounds. PAWP is 6-12 mm Hg, CO is 4-7 L/min, and SVR is 900-1200 dynes/sec/cm^{-5}.

- Monitor hemodynamic pressures, particularly PAWP, CO, and SVR. During the early (warm) stage of sepsis, PAWP usually is decreased to <6 mm Hg but will be increased to >12 mm Hg in the late (cold) stage. CO usually is >7 L/min in the early stage and decreased to <4 L/min in the late stage. SVR can be <900 dynes/sec/cm^{-5} in the early stage but usually increases to >1200 dynes/sec/cm^{-5} in the late stage.
- Administer crystalloid and colloid fluid replacement as prescribed. Often fluid replacement therapy will be given to maintain a PAWP of 6-12 mm Hg. Assess PAWP and lung sounds at frequent intervals during fluid replacement to detect evidence of fluid overload: crackles and increasing PAWP.
- Administer positive inotropic agents as prescribed to maintain adequate cardiac output in the presence of massive vasodilation.
- Assess fluid volume by monitoring BP and peripheral pulses hourly. Report systolic BP <90 mm Hg (or 20-30 mm Hg less than presepsis level) and decreasing amplitude of peripheral pulses.
- Weigh patient daily; monitor intake and output (I&O) every shift, noting 24-h trends. Report urine output <0.5 ml/kg/h. The patient's weight actually may increase with fluid volume deficit because of shift of intravascular volume into interstitial spaces.
- Monitor specific gravity, being alert to increases >1.030, which indicate a dehydration state, or a fixed specific gravity of 1.010, which may signal inadequate glomerular filtration.
- Assess for interstitial edema as evidenced by pretibial, sacral, ankle, and hand edema, as well as crackles on auscultation of lung fields.
- As prescribed, administer vasopressor agents to help maintain perfusion.
- Position patient supine with legs elevated to increase venous return and preload.

You may also wish to refer to the following interventions from the Nursing Interventions Classification (NIC):

NIC Invasive Hemodynamic Regulation; Fluid/Electrolyte Management; Hypovolemia Management; Fluid Management; Shock Management: Volume

Decreased cardiac output related to negative inotropic changes in the heart (late stage) secondary to effects of tissue hypoxia

Desired outcome: Within 8 h of initiation of therapy, patient has adequate cardiac output as evidenced by systolic BP ≥90 mm Hg (or within patient's normal range); HR ≤100 beats per minute (bpm); peripheral pulses >2+ on a scale of 0-4+; urine output ≥0.5 ml/kg/h; PAWP ≤12 mm Hg; CO ≥4 L/min; CI ≥2.5 L/min/m^2; and Svo$_2$ 60%-80%.

- Assess patient for signs of decreased cardiac output: decreasing BP, increasing HR, decreasing amplitude of peripheral pulses, restlessness, decreasing urinary output, and increasing PAWP.
- Administer positive inotropic agents as prescribed to augment cardiac contractility.
- Position patient supine with legs elevated to optimize preload and enhance stroke volume.
- Assess CO at least q4h. Optimally, CO will be $\geq$4 L/min and CI will be $\geq$2.5 L/min/m^2.
- Monitor cardiac rhythm per monitor at frequent intervals. Observe for development of dysrhythmias, such as premature ventricular complexes (PVCs), which may occur with hypoxia, and extreme tachycardia, both of which will potentiate a decreased cardiac output.
- Minimize myocardial oxygen demand by assisting patient with activities of daily living (ADL) and ensuring uninterrupted periods of rest.
- Monitor Svo_2 continuously; report values outside of normal range.

NIC Cardiac Care: Acute; Hemodynamic Regulation; Invasive Hemodynamic Monitoring; Fluid/Electrolyte Management

Altered tissue perfusion: cerebral, renal, and gastrointestinal, related to hypovolemia secondary to vasodilation (early stage); interruption of arterial and venous blood flow secondary to vasoconstriction and thrombus obstruction (late stage)

Desired outcomes: Within 24 h of initiating therapy, patient has adequate perfusion as evidenced by orientation to time, place, and person; peripheral pulses >2+ (on a scale of 0-4+); brisk capillary refill (<2 sec); urine output $\geq$0.5 ml/kg/h; and $\geq$5 bowel sounds/min. BP is 110-120/70-80 mm Hg (or within patient's normal range); Svo_2 is 60%-80%; SVR is 900-1200 dynes/sec/cm^{-5}; CO is 4-7 L/min; and CI is 2.5-4 L/min/m^2.

- Assess for changes in LOC as an indicator of decreasing cerebral perfusion.
- Assess for the following signs of decreasing renal perfusion: urine output <0.5 ml/kg/h and increased blood urea nitrogen (BUN), serum creatinine, and serum potassium levels. Normal laboratory values are as follows: BUN $\leq$20 mg/dl; serum creatinine $\leq$1.5 mg/dl; and serum potassium $\leq$5 mEq/L.
- Monitor arterial BP continuously. Be alert to decreased systolic BP, normal or increased diastolic BP, and decreased pulse pressures, which occur in the presence of decreasing perfusion.

> **Note:** Systolic BP will be decreased because of decreased cardiac output, and the diastolic BP may be high secondary to compensatory vasoconstriction.

- Assess peripheral pulses, temperature, color of skin, and capillary refill. With hypoperfusion, pulse amplitude decreases, extremities are cool because of vasoconstriction, skin color is pale or mottled because of decreased perfusion, and capillary refill is delayed.
- Monitor cellular oxygen consumption (Svo_2) as an indicator of tissue perfusion. With sepsis, cellular oxygen delivery is decreased (precapillary vasoconstriction) and thus cellular oxygen use is decreased. Therefore the mixed venous blood oxygen saturation (Svo_2) will be abnormally high.
- Administer vasoactive drugs as prescribed, and assess SVR and CO during administration to determine the effect of these drugs. Optimally, SVR will increase to $\geq$900 dynes/sec/cm^{-5}, CO will be 4-7 L/min, and CI will be 2.5-4 L/min/m^2.

> **Note:** Vasoactive drugs probably will include vasopressors (e.g., norepinephrine) early in sepsis and vasodilators (e.g., nitroprusside) late in sepsis. Vasopressors always are accompanied by fluid resuscitation as needed.

- Assess for evidence of decreasing splanchnic (visceral) circulation, including decreased or absent bowel sounds, elevated serum amylase level, and decreased platelet count. Normal values are as follows: serum amylase ≤180 Somogyi units/dl; platelet count ≥150,000/mm^3.

NIC Cerebral Perfusion Promotion; Circulatory Care; Fluid/Electrolyte Management; Oxygen Therapy; Hemodynamic Regulation; Shock Management; Nutrition Management; Hemodialysis Therapy

Impaired gas exchange related to alveolar-capillary membrane changes secondary to interstitial edema, alveolar destruction, and endotoxin release with activation of histamine and kinins

Desired outcomes: Within 4 h of initiation of therapy, patient's Pao$_2$ is ≥80 mm Hg; Paco$_2$ is ≤45 mm Hg; pH is 7.35-7.45, and the lungs are clear.

- Assess for and maintain a patent airway by assisting patient with coughing or suctioning trachea as necessary.
- Assess all ABG values. Be alert to decreasing Pao$_2$, increasing Paco$_2$, and acidosis (decreasing pH). Monitor patient for the presence of dyspnea, shortness of breath (SOB), and restlessness.
- Listen to breath sounds hourly. The presence of crackles may indicate fluid accumulation.
- If patient exhibits evidence of inadequate gas exchange (e.g., Pao$_2$ <60 mm Hg on 100% oxygen via nonrebreathing mask), prepare for the probability of endotracheal intubation.
- If patient has been placed on mechanical ventilation, monitor inspiratory peak pressures for increasing trends, which may signal decreasing compliance and development of ARDS. Also, assess for and document mode of ventilation, tidal volume, Fio$_2$, rate of respirations, and level of positive end-expiratory pressure (PEEP). Typically, as ARDS develops, an increasing Fio$_2$ (>0.50) and increasing levels of PEEP are required to maintain adequate Pao$_2$ (>60 mm Hg). Consult physician if inspiratory peak pressures increase with each breath or if the following signs of hypoxia occur at the prescribed Fio$_2$ and level of PEEP: increased HR (≥100 bpm), anxiety, cool extremities, change in mentation, or skin color changes (pallor or cyanosis). (See "Mechanical Ventilation," p. 17.)
- Turn patient q2h to maintain optimal ventilation-perfusion ratios and to prevent atelectasis.

NIC Acid-Base Management: Metabolic Acidosis; Oxygen Therapy; Respiratory Monitoring; Artificial Airway Management; Invasive Hemodynamic Regulation

Ineffective breathing pattern related to decreased lung expansion secondary to central respiratory depression occurring in late shock

Desired outcome: Within 2 h of treatment/intervention, patient has an effective breathing pattern as evidenced by normal limits of inspiratory-expiratory ratio (1:1-1:2); tidal volume (≥4ml/kg); and maximal inspiratory pressures (≥20 cm H$_2$O).

- Monitor patient's rate and depth of respirations. Be alert to decreasing rate, depth, and air movement. Ensure that patient demonstrates adequate air movement by noting presence of breath sounds over all lung fields.
- Assist patient into a position for comfort to facilitate respirations. Depending on patient's hemodynamic stability, the optimal position may be having the head of bed (HOB) elevated 15-30 degrees.
- Assess/measure tidal volume and inspiratory force. Be alert to tidal volume <4-5 ml/kg and inspiratory force <20 cm H$_2$O as indicators of ineffective breathing pattern.
- If patient exhibits respiratory depression/ineffective breathing pattern, prepare for the probability of endotracheal intubation.

NIC Respiratory Monitoring; Oxygen Therapy; Mechanical Ventilation

Ineffective thermoregulation related to illness with concomitant endotoxin effect on hypothalamic temperature-regulating center
Desired outcome: Within 24 h of initiation of treatment, patient becomes normothermic.
- Monitor patient's temperature continuously or at frequent intervals. Use temperature probe (rectal or tympanic) for continuous monitoring of core temperature. Body temperature can range from 38.3°-40.6° C (101°-105° F) in the early stage of sepsis and can be <35.6° C (96° F) in the late stage. Be alert to shaking chills early in sepsis as temperature increases and to profuse diaphoresis as temperature decreases late in sepsis. The following are weighed for each patient to determine the extent of treatment that should be employed to decrease fever (e.g., acetaminophen):
  - ☐ Useful effects of a fever: Decreased viral and bacterial replication.
  - ☐ Harmful effects of a fever: Increased cardiac workload and increased oxygen consumption.
- Administer antimicrobials as prescribed. Observe for untoward effects, including renal toxicity, ototoxicity, allergic reactions, anaphylaxis, pseudo-membranous colitis, overgrowth of normal flora, and superimposed infectious processes of the skin, urinary tract, or respiratory tract. Large doses of antibiotics may cause the release of endotoxins from dying bacteria, which may potentiate the progression of septic shock.
- Administer antipyretic agents as prescribed.
- For patients with hyperthermia, use tepid baths, which decrease body temperature by releasing internal heat. Cooled IV fluids also may decrease core temperature. In addition, a cooling blanket may be prescribed to reduce the metabolic rate, thereby decreasing myocardial oxygen demand. Avoid "chilling," which will cause shivering and thus increase myocardial oxygen demand and cardiac workload.
- In the presence of hypothermia, use warm blankets to increase body temperature. Heating devices can damage ischemic cells in peripheral tissues and usually are avoided.

NIC Fever Treatment; Temperature Regulation; Environmental Management
Altered nutrition: less than body requirements, related to increased need secondary to increased metabolic rate
Desired outcome: Within 48 h of initiation of treatment, patient has adequate nutrition as evidenced by stable weight; serum albumin 3.5 g/dl; thyroxine-binding prealbumin 20-30 mg/dl; retinol-binding protein 4-5 mg/dl; urine urea nitrogen 10-20 mg/dl; and a state of nitrogen balance as determined by nitrogen studies.
- Administer nutritional supplements as prescribed.

> **Note:**   Standard total parenteral nutrition (TPN) solutions are not metabolized well in the septic state. Branched-chain amino acid solutions and short- to medium-chain fatty acid solutions may be used (e.g., MCT Oil or FreAmine HBC).

- Observe for and document areas of tissue breakdown, which can indicate a negative nitrogen state.
- Monitor laboratory findings for serum albumin, thyroxine-binding prealbumin, retinol-binding protein, and nitrogen studies.
- Assess and record weight and nutritional intake daily. Consult with nutritional services for calorie count.
- If patient is receiving oral feedings, assess for the presence of bowel sounds at least q2h. Paralytic ileus can occur secondary to an ischemic bowel.
- If the patient is receiving continuous gastric tube feedings, assess for residual feeding q2h. Assess for residual before intermittent tube feedings. If residual

is ≥100 ml (or 1½ times the hourly rate of infusion), hold the feeding and consult with physician.

NIC TPN Administration; Enteral Tube Feeding

ADDITIONAL NURSING DIAGNOSES

Also see nursing diagnoses and interventions in "Hemodynamic Monitoring," p. 28 ; "Psychosocial Support," p. 83; "Psychosocial Support for the Patient's Family and Significant Others," p. 95; and "Acute Respiratory Distress Syndrome," p. 229. See "Disseminated Intravascular Coagulation" for **Altered protection,** p. 585, and **Altered tissue perfusion,** p. 589. Also see "SIRS/MODS," p. 604.

Systemic inflammatory response syndrome (SIRS) and multiple organ dysfunction syndrome (MODS)

PATHOPHYSIOLOGY

Inflammation is a complex response that is started when mechanical, ischemic, chemical, or microbial sources trigger immediate inflammatory and immune processes. The purpose of the inflammatory response is to protect the body from further injury and promote rapid healing. Vasodilation, increased microvascular permeability, neutrophil activation and adhesion, and enhanced coagulation occur. The vascular response is initiated at the cellular level by histamine, prostaglandins, bradykinin, and numerous other mediators. In some instances, regulatory mechanisms fail and uncontrolled systemic inflammation over-whelms the body's normal protective response. This leads to systemic vasodilation, hypotension, a generalized increase in vascular permeability, extravascular fluid sequestration, increased cellular aggregation with microvascular obstruction, and greatly accelerated coagulation. If allowed to progress, SIRS leads to widespread organ inflammation and impairment, ultimately resulting in MODS.

SIRS is characterized by signs of systemic inflammation such as fever and leukocytosis. When an infectious process is the underlying cause of SIRS, the condition is known as *sepsis.* Impaired functioning of two or more vital organ systems in a patient with SIRS is called *MODS.* Mortality increases as additional organ systems fail. When four or more organ systems fail, the mortality exceeds 80%. MODS is characterized by ARDS, DIC, acute tubular necrosis (ATN), liver failure, hyperdynamic circulatory failure, and metabolic encephalopathy.

History and risk factors: SIRS and MODS are not primary illnesses—they are systemic manifestations of other diseases. SIRS may be initiated by infection, ischemia, reperfusion injury, intestinal endotoxin, thermal injury, pancreatitis, shock state, and multisystem injury. Patients with immunosuppression are more susceptible to SIRS/MODS. Factors such as chronic illness, sequential infections, steroid therapy, HIV infection, bone marrow depression, and advanced age contribute to immunosuppression.

Clinical presentation: According to the American College of Chest Physicians/Society of Critical Care Medicine (ACCP/SCCM) (1992), diagnosis of SIRS is based on the following laboratory and clinical findings: tachypnea (RR >20 breaths/min); hypocarbia (<32 torr); tachycardia (HR >90 bpm); temp >38° C (100.4° F) or < 36° C (96.8° F); WBCs >12,000/mm³ or <4000/mm³; or >10% immature (band) forms.

Early: Findings reflect compensatory hypermetabolic state. Restlessness, confusion, fever, SOB, tachypnea, tachycardia, hyperglycemia.

Late: Findings are consistent with impaired perfusion. Diminished LOC, coma, respiratory failure requiring mechanical ventilation, heart failure refractory to inotropes, jaundice, hypoglycemia, oliguria/anuria, bruising, uncontrolled bleeding.

ASSESSMENT

Physical assessment

Neurologic: Decreased cerebral blood flow with central nervous system (CNS) depression, stupor, progressing to coma.

Respiratory: Tachypnea, hyperventilation, to compensate for metabolic acidosis (early); later, crackles and respiratory depression/acidosis caused by CNS depression, increased lung water.

Gastrointestinal (GI): Decreased or absent bowel sounds; jaundice.

Genitourinary (GU): Oliguria, anuria.

Vital signs/hemodynamics: Early stages characterized by a hyperdynamic hypotension with venous pooling. In advanced stages there is transudation of fluid ("third spacing"), vasoconstriction, reduced blood flow, and a generalized hypodynamic state.

RR: Increased (>20 breaths/min).

HR: Increased (>90 bpm).

BP: Decreased.

Temperature: Increased to >38° C (100.4° F) or decreased to <36° C (96.8° F); fever (early); thermoregulatory failure and hypothermia (late).

Central venous pressure (CVP): Decreased, caused by relative fluid deficit.

Pulmonary artery pressure (PAP): Decreased initially; later increased, caused by pulmonary vasoconstriction occurring with hypoxemia, pulmonary edema.

PAWP: Decreased initially, caused by relative fluid deficit; later increased if heart failure present.

SVR: Decreased because of mediator-induced vasodilation.

CO/CI: Early increase as a result of tachycardia; later decreased if heart failure present.

Cerebral perfusion pressure (CPP): Decreased as direct effect of chemical mediators and decreased cerebral blood flow.

DIAGNOSTIC TESTS

CBC: WBCs usually increase early, with increased bands (left shift). ACCP/SCCM definition of SIRS includes WBCs >12,000/mm^3 or <4000/mm^3; >10% immature neutrophils (bands). With MODS, WBCs may decrease as a result of sequestration within organs and bone marrow exhaustion. Anemia, if present, contributes to tachycardia, hyperdynamic state, and impaired tissue oxygenation.

Chemistries: Early increase in serum glucose results from gluconeogenesis; later, decrease results from hepatic failure. Venous lactate levels increase if tissue perfusion is inadequate. Renal, cardiac, pulmonary, hepatic, or other organ failure is reflected in electrolyte, enzyme abnormalities.

Culture and sensitivities (C&S): Blood, sputum, urine, surgical, or other site; obtained if infection suspected.

ABGs: Usually show pH <7.35 and hypocarbia (<32 torr), because of metabolic acidosis.

Imaging: Chest x-ray to check for pulmonary edema, ARDS; other x-rays as indicated according to underlying condition.

COLLABORATIVE MANAGEMENT

Oxygenation: Humidified oxygen for all patients; mechanical ventilation may be necessary if pulmonary edema, ARDS, or other ventilatory impairment is present.

Fluids: Crystalloids, colloids administered to sustain adequate intravascular volume; hyperdynamic state supported until patient stabilized. Goal is CVP

8-10 mm Hg; or pulmonary capillary wedge pressure (PCWP) 16-18 mm Hg. Ranges may be higher or lower for specific patients.

Hemodynamic monitoring and oxygen transport: To maximize Do_2, Vo_2, and CI. Goal is to maintain Vo_2 above 100 ml/min/m². Some literature supports the maintenance of supranormal levels of Do_2, Vo_2. Fluid adjustment, inotropes, vasopressors, and ensuring adequacy of oxygen-carrying capacity via optimal hematocrit (Hct) and oxygen administration are mainstays of management.

Urinary drainage: To monitor hourly urinary output.

Pharmacotherapy

Inotropes and vasopressors: Inotropes such as digitalis, dopamine, dobutamine, or norepinephrine help increase CO. Dopamine, epinephrine, norepinephrine stimulate alpha receptors and may be used for refractory hypotension. Intramucosal gastric monitoring is recommended, if available, to evaluate tissue oxygenation during vasopressor therapy.

Antibiotics: Broad-spectrum antibiotics if infection suspected.

Analgesia, sedation: To relieve pain and agitation, which increase oxygen consumption.

Antioxidant therapy: Used to limit inflammatory organ injury. Limited clinical experience and not in widespread use.

Antiinflammatory antibodies: Antibodies against inflammatory mediators such as endotoxin, tumor necrosis factor, interleukin-1 used to block the inflammatory response. Their use is controversial and not widespread.

Hemofiltration and hemodialysis: To remove mediators of the inflammatory response and waste products of the hypermetabolic state. Also removes excess fluid if necessary.

Nutritional support: Enteral nutrition optimal but often not possible. Short- and medium-chain fatty acids (absorbed more readily and metabolized more easily than long-chain fatty acids) are given parenterally. Branched-chain amino acids, metabolized by muscle rather than by the liver, may be used if there is evidence of hepatic failure.

NURSING DIAGNOSES AND INTERVENTIONS

Altered tissue perfusion: cerebral, renal, GI, related to hypovolemia secondary to vasodilation (early) or interrupted arterial/venous blood flow secondary to microvascular obstruction (late)

Desired outcomes: Within 24 h of initiating therapy, patient has adequate perfusion as evidenced by orientation × 3; peripheral pulses >2+ on 0-4+ scale; brisk capillary refill (<2 sec); urinary output ≥ 0.5 ml/kg/h; and ≥5 bowel sounds/min. BP 110-120/70-80 mm Hg (or within normal level for patient); Svo_2 60% to 80%; SVR 900-1200 dynes/sec/cm⁻⁵; CO 4-7 L/min; and CI 2.5-4 L/min/m².

- Assess for decreased cerebral perfusion: decreased level of consciousness, restlessness.
- Assess for decreased renal perfusion: urinary output <0.5 ml/kg/h; increased BUN, creatinine, and serum potassium levels.

- Monitor BP continuously for decreased systolic BP, normal or increased diastolic BP, decreased pulse pressures occurring with decreased perfusion.
- Assess for hypoperfusion: decreased pulse amplitude, cool extremities, pallor or mottling, delayed capillary refill.
- Monitor Svo_2 as an indicator of tissue perfusion. Be aware that cellular oxygen delivery may be decreased because of precapillary vasoconstriction and thus cellular oxygen use is decreased (shunting). This condition results in abnormally high Svo_2 that does not reflect true tissue oxygenation.
- Administer fluids, inotropes, and/or vasodilators or vasopressors to optimize SVR and CO/CI. Be aware that increased filling pressures may be necessary for optimal CO.
- Assess for decreased splanchnic (visceral) circulation, including decreased or absent bowel sounds, increased amylase, increased liver enzymes, and decreased platelet count.
- Consult physician for failure to respond to therapy as evidenced by signs and symptoms of inadequate tissue perfusion: altered mental status, restlessness; decreased BP, peripheral pulses; urinary output <0.5 ml/kg/h × 2 h; Svo_2 80%; decreased or absent bowel sounds.
- Treat underlying infection with appropriate antimicrobial therapy, being certain to administer precisely as scheduled to optimize blood levels.

NIC Cerebral Perfusion Promotion; Circulatory Care; Fluid/Electrolyte Management; Oxygen Therapy; Hemodynamic Regulation; Shock Management; Nutrition Management; Hemodialysis Therapy

Fluid volume deficit related to loss from vascular compartment secondary to increased capillary permeability and shift of intravascular volume into interstitial spaces

Desired outcomes: Within 8 h of therapy initiation, patient is normovolemic as evidenced by peripheral pulses >2+ on 0-4+ scale; stable body weight; urinary output ≥0.5 ml/kg/h; systolic BP ≥90 mm Hg or within normal limits for patient; and absence of edema and adventitious lung sounds. PAWP 6-12 mm Hg, CO 4-7 L/min, and SVR 900-1200 dynes/sec/m^{-5}.

- Assess fluid volume by monitoring BP, HR, and peripheral perfusion qh or more often if unstable. Continuous direct arterial pressure monitoring is optimal.
- During acute hypotension, position patient supine with legs elevated to optimize preload.
- Give crystalloids and colloids to maintain PAWP or 6-12 mm Hg or ≤18 mm Hg with left ventricular (LV) failure. Assess PAWP and lung sounds frequently during fluid replacement to detect overload: crackles and increased PAWP. As indicated, administer packed RBCs to increase oxygen-carrying capacity of the blood.
- Monitor hemodynamic pressures and Svo_2 as available.
- In early stage, anticipate decreased BP, PAWP, and SVR; increased CO/CI. Give fluids, inotropes as necessary.
- In late stage, decreased BP, increased PAWP and SVR, and decreased CO/CI may occur. In general, use vasodilators if MAP >100 mm Hg or use vasopressors if MAP <70 mm Hg. Fluids, inotropes, vasopressors, and vasodilators all may be necessary because of MODS and desensitization to endogenous catecholamines. Titrate carefully to optimize CI and maintain Svo_2 of at least 60% to 80%.
- Weigh q day; monitor I&O every shift and urinary output qh, noting 24-h trends. Weight may increase despite actual fluid volume deficit as a result of shift of intravascular volume into interstitial spaces.
- Assess for interstitial edema as evidenced by pretibial, sacral, ankle, and hand edema, as well as lung crackles. Take measures to protect skin integrity.

NIC Invasive Hemodynamic Regulation; Fluid/Electrolyte Management; Hypovolemia Management; Fluid Management; Shock Mangement: Volume

Impaired gas exchange related to alveolar-capillary membrane changes secondary to interstitial edema, alveolar destruction, and endotoxin release with activation of histamine and kinins

Desired outcomes: Within 4 h of therapy initiation, patient's Pao_2 ≥80 mm Hg; $Paco_2$ ≤45 mm Hg; pH 7.35-7.45; and lungs clear.

- Administer supplemental oxygen to maximize oxygen available to tissues.
- If patient exhibits inadequate gas exchange (e.g., Pao_2 <60 mm Hg on 100% oxygen via nonrebreathing mask), prepare for probability of endotracheal (ET) intubation.
- Assess for/maintain patent airway by assisting with coughing or suctioning as necessary.
- Assess ABGs. Be alert to decreased Pao_2, increased $Paco_2$, acidosis. Monitor for dyspnea, SOB, crackles, restlessness. Adjust supplemental oxygen, ventilator settings as indicated.
- Closely monitor PAWP; keep as low as possible to avoid contributing to excess lung water. Be aware that a narrow range of optimal PAWP exists because of complex pathophysiology, including intravascular fluid volume deficit, increased capillary permeability, and possible LV failure.
- If patient is on mechanical ventilation, monitor for evidence of ARDS: increased peak inspiratory pressures (e.g., decreased lung compliance); Fio_2 >0.50; increased PEEP necessary to maintain adequate Pao_2; and diffuse, bilateral pulmonary infiltrates ("white out") on chest x-ray.
- Turn q2h to maintain optimal ventilation-perfusion (V/Q) ratios and prevent atelectasis.

NIC Acid-Base Management: Metabolic Acidosis; Oxygen Therapy; Respiratory Monitoring; Artificial Airway Management; Invasive Hemodynamic Regulation

ADDITIONAL NURSING DIAGNOSES

See also nursing diagnoses and interventions in "Hemodynamic Monitoring," p. 1; "Psychosocial Support," p. 83; "Psychosocial Support for the Patient's Family and Significant Others," p. 95; and "Acute Respiratory Distress Syndrome," p. 229. See "Disseminated Intravascular Coagulation" for **Altered protection**, p. 585, and **Altered tissue perfusion**, p. 589.

Anaphylactic shock

PATHOPHYSIOLOGY

Systemic anaphylactic shock (anaphylaxis) is a potentially life-threatening situation. It is the result of an exaggerated or a hypersensitivity response to an antigen (or allergen). The classic form of anaphylaxis occurs in a sensitized person (i.e., someone who has been exposed previously to the same antigen), usually 1-20 min after introduction of the antigenic substance. The most common substances that cause anaphylaxis are drugs, foods, insect stings or bites, antisera, and blood products.

The hypersensitivity response occurs on the surface of the mast cells, which are located primarily in the lungs, in small blood vessels, and in connective tissue. There the antigen combines with sensitized antibodies from previous exposure (usually immunoglobulin E [IgE] type). The antigen also attaches to basophils circulating in the blood. This triggers release of substances from the granules within the cells, including histamine, serotonin, kinins, and eosinophil and neutrophil chemotactic factors. In addition, the antigen-antibody complex activates a cellular process that produces prostaglandins and leukotrienes, which are termed *slow-reacting substances of anaphylaxis (SRSA)*. These chemical mediators produce systemic effects that can have deleterious results, including profound shock.

Histamine is the primary mediator in an anaphylactic response. Activation of histamine receptors has many effects, including increased capillary permeability, increased pulmonary secretions, bronchoconstriction, and systemic vasodilation. The *leukotrienes* produce bronchoconstriction that is more severe than that caused by histamine. They also cause venule dilation and increased vascular permeability. The *prostaglandins* exaggerate the bronchoconstriction and potentiate the effects of histamine on vascular permeability and pulmonary secretions. *Kinins* contribute to the bronchoconstriction, vasodilation, and increased vascular permeability. The combined effects of these substances cause (1) airway obstruction and respiratory distress, which can lead to respiratory arrest and (2) relative hypovolemia caused by massive vasodilation and the fluid shift from the vascular to interstitial spaces, which can lead to vasogenic shock and end-organ dysfunction because of tissue hypoxia.

Finally, eosinophilic chemotactic factor of anaphylaxis (ECFA) is released. ECFA attracts eosinophils, which work to neutralize mediators such as histamine. However, this response cannot by itself reverse the anaphylaxis. (See Figure 10-2 for a depiction of the pathophysiologic process of anaphylaxis.)

ASSESSMENT

History and risk factors: Recent exposure to pharmacologic agents (e.g., penicillin, anesthetics, vaccines), contrast medium, blood transfusions, food (e.g., seafood, shellfish, nuts, grains, dairy products), insect bites or stings (e.g., wasps, hornets, bees, fire ants), or latex.

Clinical presentation: Depends on several factors and varies with the means of antigen entry, the amount absorbed, the rate of absorption, and the degree of hypersensitivity. Dramatic symptoms develop rapidly, usually within minutes, and progress swiftly. Usually, the quicker the onset the more severe the symptoms. *General early indicators* (which can occur within seconds to minutes) include uneasiness, lightheadedness, tingling feeling, flushing, and pruritus. *General late indicators* (which usually occur within minutes) include rapid progression of signs and symptoms (S&S): urticaria that involves large surface areas of the skin; angioedema (tissue swelling), especially of the eyes, lips, tongue, hands, feet, and genitalia; cough, hoarseness, dyspnea, and respiratory distress; lightheadedness or syncope; and abdominal cramps, diarrhea, and vomiting.

Ingestion: Cramping, diarrhea, nausea, vomiting may precede systemic shock symptoms.

Inhalation: Cough, hoarseness, wheezing, dyspnea.

Allergic: Edema, urticaria, itching at the site of a bee sting or drug injection.

Physical assessment: See Table 10-3.

Hemodynamic measurements: Decreased arterial BP and MAP caused by vasodilation; decreased CO (<4 L/min) if shock ensues; decreased CI (<2.5 L/min); decreased SVR (<900 dynes/sec/cm^{-5}) because of vasodilation; and low PAWP (<6 mm Hg) because of vasodilation, shift of intravascular fluid to interstitial spaces, and decreased venous return.

DIAGNOSTIC TESTS

The diagnosis of anaphylaxis is based on presenting signs and symptoms. There are no specific diagnostic tests for anaphylaxis, and treatment must be initiated before laboratory results are available. IgE levels may confirm allergic origin. ABG values may be assessed to evaluate respiratory status.

COLLABORATIVE MANAGEMENT

Airway maintenance: May require ET intubation. Early intubation is important because of the rapid progression of laryngeal edema. If laryngeal edema is severe and causes obstruction, a tracheostomy or emergency cricothyroidotomy may be necessary.

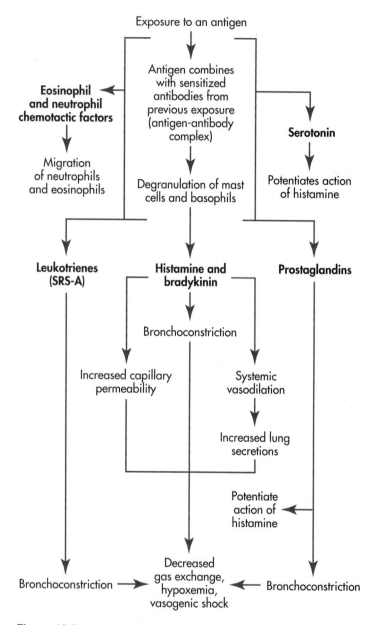

Figure 10-2: Pathophysiologic process of anaphylaxis. *(Major chemical mediators are in boldface print.)* SRS-A, Slow-reacting substance of anaphylaxis.

TABLE 10-3 Systemic Effects of Anaphylaxis

System	Effects	Cause
Neurologic	Apprehension; headache; confusion; decreased LOC progressing to coma	Vasodilation; hypoperfusion; cerebral hypoxia or cerebral edema occurring with interstitial fluid shifts
Respiratory	Dyspnea progressing to air hunger and complete respiratory obstruction; hoarseness; noisy breathing; high-pitched, "barking" cough; wheezes; crackles; rhonchi; decreasing breath sounds; pulmonary edema (some patients)	Laryngeal edema; bronchoconstriction; increased pulmonary secretions
Cardiovascular	Decreased BP leading to profound hypotension; increased HR; decreased amplitude of peripheral pulses; palpitations and dysrhythmias (atrial tachycardias, premature atrial beats, atrial fibrillation, premature ventricular beats progressing to ventricular tachycardia or ventricular fibrillation); lymphadenopathy	Increased vascular permeability; systemic vasodilation; decreased cardiac output with decreased circulating volume; reflex increase in HR; vasogenic shock
Renal	Decreased urine output; incontinence	Decreased renal perfusion; smooth muscle contraction of urinary tract
Gastrointestinal	Nausea, vomiting, diarrhea, abdominal cramping	Smooth muscle contraction of GI tract; increased mucus secretion
Cutaneous	Urticaria; angioedema (hands, lips, face, feet, genitalia); itching; erythema; flushing; cyanosis	Histamine-induced disruption of cutaneous vasculature; vasodilation, increased capillary permeability; decreased oxygen saturation

LOC, Level of consciousness; *BP,* blood pressure; *HR,* heart rate; *GI,* gastrointestinal.

Epinephrine: Counteracts the effects of anaphylaxis by increasing myocardial contractility, dilating bronchioles, constricting blood vessels, inhibiting histamine release, and counteracting histamine that already is circulating. Dosage and route vary. Generally, the following guidelines are used: Standard adult dosage administered by *IM or SC route* is 0.3-0.5 mg (0.3-0.5 ml of a 1:1000 solution), although an initial dose of 0.1 mg (0.1 ml of a 1:1000 solution) may be administered. May be repeated q10-15min PRN. The *IV route* is preferred if patient is in shock and/or has severe airway obstruction: Initially, a dose of 0.1 mg (0.1 ml of 1 : 1000 solution) diluted in 10 ml normal saline is infused over 5-10 min. The dose may be increased to 0.3-0.5 mg. After initial dosage, an IV drip of 1 μg of 1 : 1000 epinephrine in 250 ml D_5W is established. Initial infusion usually is 1 μg/min, which may be increased to 4 μg /min as necessary until desired response is achieved. May be given via *endotracheal* route, if needed, at a rate of 10 ml of 1:10,000 dilution.

Supplemental oxygen: May be administered to support oxygen delivery to the tissues. The amount and method of oxygen administration are guided by ABG results, although it usually is initiated at 6 L/min via nasal cannula or oxygen mask.

Fluid resuscitation: Crystalloids (e.g., lactated Ringer's solution, 0.9% normal saline [NS]) or colloids (e.g., albumin and plasma protein fraction [Plasmanate]) to increase intravascular colloid osmotic pressure and retain fluids within the vascular spaces, thus attaining adequate vascular volume. This may require a rapid infusion of 2-3 L.

Vasopressors: Necessary if fluid replacement does not reverse or prevent shock. Drugs such as dopamine hydrochloride, norepinephrine, or epinephrine are titrated for the desired response. (See Appendix 7.) Usual dosages:

☐ *Dopamine hydrochloride:* To increase cardiac contractility and systemic vascular resistance via its alpha (α) and beta (β) properties. Usual dosage is 5-20 μg/kg/min.

☐ *Norepinephrine:* α-Adrenergic stimulator. Initial dosage is 2-8 μg/min and can be increased to achieve the necessary BP.

☐ *Epinephrine:* α-Adrenergic agonist. Usual dosage is 2-4 μg/min.

Antihistamines: Usually given after the patient has been stabilized. Diphenhydramine, for example, may be given IV to relieve urticaria and abdominal cramping. Usual dosage is 20-50 mg. H_2-antagonists (e.g., cimetidine, ranitidine) also may be given.

Aminophylline (theophylline ethylenediamine):   May be given by IV drip to stimulate bronchodilation and relieve bronchospasm. Usual dosage is 2-4 mg/min (0.5 mg/kg).

Corticosteroids: May be given to decrease both capillary permeability and release of chemical mediators. The effect is not immediate. Usual loading dosages are hydrocortisone sodium succinate 250-1000 mg IV; or methylprednisolone sodium succinate 125-250 mg IV. The loading doses may be followed by IV or PO doses of corticosteroids for several days.

Inhaled bronchodilators such as albuterol or Terbutaline: May be given for continued bronchospasm.

Glucagon, 1 mg IV bolus: To counteract the effects of β-blocking drugs or in patients resistant to traditional therapy. Relaxes smooth muscle and has positive inotropic and chronotropic effects. Use is controversial.

Electrocardiogram (ECG) monitoring: To detect dysrhythmias.

NURSING DIAGNOSES AND INTERVENTIONS

Ineffective airway clearance related to tracheobronchial obstruction secondary to bronchoconstriction and increased secretions associated with histamine response and the presence of leukotrienes and prostaglandins

Desired outcome: Within 2 h of treatment/intervention, patient has adequate movement of air in and out of lungs as evidenced by ease of breathing; auscultated breath sounds in expected range (IER); and adventitious breath sounds not present.

• Assess patency of airway and respiratory effort continuously. Be alert to increased pulmonary secretions, cough, expiratory wheezing, SOB, and dyspnea. Keep suction equipment readily available. Suction PRN.

• Administer epinephrine by IV, intramuscular (IM), subcutaneous (SC), or ET route as prescribed.

> **Note:** Patients taking β-blocking drugs, such as propranolol, may not respond to epinephrine. Glucagon may be effective to counteract this effect.

- Auscultate breath sounds, noting areas of decreased or absent ventilation and presence of adventitious sounds. (As bronchoconstriction and obstruction progress, wheezing may decrease; therefore it is important to note decreasing air movement—not just adventitious sounds.)
- Identify patient requiring actual/potential airway insertion. Consult physician and prepare for ET intubation if lingual edema is present and/or respiratory distress continues.

> *Caution:* An oral airway provides airway support only as far as the posterior pharynx. If laryngeal edema is present, the oral airway will be ineffective because the obstruction is lower.

- If laryngeal edema prevents intubation, prepare for the possibility of a tracheostomy or cricothyroidotomy.
- Administer IV and inhaled bronchodilators as appropriate. Monitor for side effects such as dysrhythmias.
- Monitor ABG values for evidence of an improving or a worsening condition. Be alert to increasing $Paco_2$ (>50 mm Hg) and decreasing Pao_2 (<60 mm Hg).

Impaired gas exchange related to alveolar-capillary membrane changes secondary to increased capillary permeability associated with histamine response

Desired outcome: Within 2 h of initiation of treatment/intervention, patient has adequate alveolar exchange of CO_2 or O_2 as evidenced by ease of breathing; Pao_2 ≥80 mm Hg; and Spo_2 ≥90.

- Monitor patient for the presence of SOB or dyspnea. Assess ABG values for evidence of an improving or a worsening condition. Be alert to increasing $Paco_2$ (>50 mm Hg) and decreasing Pao_2 (<60 mm Hg).
- Administer supplemental oxygen as ordered.
- Monitor patient with continuous pulse oximetry. Be alert to levels <90%.
- Administer antihistamines as prescribed.
- Administer glucocorticoids as prescribed.
- Position to alleviate dyspnea. (If BP is stable, assist patient to sitting position to enhance gas exchange.)
- Stay with patient to promote safety and reduce fear. Use calm, reassuring approach.

Decreased cardiac output related to decreased preload and afterload secondary to release of vasoactive chemical mediators and associated vasodilation and increased capillary permeability

Desired outcome: Within 4 h of initiation of treatment, patient has adequate cardiac output as evidenced by BP ≥90/60 mm Hg; strong peripheral pulses; CO ≥4 L/min; CI ≥2.5 $L/min/m^2$; SVR ≥900 $dynes/sec/cm^{-5}$; urinary output ≥0.5 ml/kg/h; and normal sinus rhythm on ECG.

- Assess for physical and hemodynamic indicators of decreased cardiac output:
  - ☐ Palpate peripheral pulses for decreasing amplitude.
  - ☐ Assess arterial BP for decrease, an indicator of failed compensatory mechanisms.
  - ☐ Monitor SVR. A decrease (<900 $dynes/sec/cm^{-5}$) is associated with decreased afterload (vasodilation) and may precipitate decreased CO.
  - ☐ Monitor CO and CI if available. A CI of <2.5 $L/min/m^2$ usually is associated with hypoperfusion.
- Monitor for dysrhythmias, such as atrial tachycardias, PVCs, ventricular tachycardia, and ventricular fibrillation, which may signal hypoxemia or occur as side effects of drugs such as aminophylline or epinephrine.
- Monitor for increase and decrease in edema.

Note: Continued swelling, despite treatment, may indicate ineffective treatment, overaggressive fluid therapy, heart or kidney failure.

- Administer epinephrine as prescribed. Observe for therapeutic effects as evidenced by increased SVR, increased CO/CI, increased arterial BP and MAP, stronger peripheral pulses, warming of extremities, and increased urine output.
- Administer fluid replacement therapy as prescribed, using a large-bore IV catheter. Colloids and crystalloids may be given together.

Note: During fluid resuscitation, assess patient for indicators of fluid volume excess, including crackles with chest auscultation, presence of S_3 heart sounds, and jugular venous distention. If hemodynamic monitoring lines are present, be alert to increasing PAP, PAWP, and right atrial pressure (RAP).

- Prepare for possible vasopressor infusion if hypotension persists after fluid resuscitation and epinephrine administration.

Altered tissue perfusion: peripheral, renal, and cerebral, related to hypovolemia secondary to fluid shift from the vascular space to the interstitial space
Desired outcome: Within 4 h of initiation of treatment, patient has adequate perfusion as evidenced by strong proximal peripheral pulses; brisk capillary refill; warm extremity temperature; urinary output ≥0.5 ml/kg/h; uncompromised neurologic status; and no restlessness, listlessness, and unexplained anxiety.

- Assess peripheral pulses. Report decreased amplitude of pulses.
- Assess capillary refill. Delayed capillary refill (>2 sec) is likely with edema and decreased vascular volume.
- Assess degree of peripheral edema.
- Assess color and warmth of extremities. Report presence of coolness and pallor.
- Monitor BP at frequent intervals. Be alert for indicators of hypotension such as BP readings >20 mm Hg below patient's normal pressure, dizziness, restlessness, altered mentation, and decreased urinary output.
- Monitor urine output hourly.
- Observe for indicators of decreased cerebral perfusion such as anxiety, restlessness, confusion, and decreased LOC.

Note: Changes in LOC may signal either decreased cerebral perfusion (tissue hypoxia) or increasing intracranial pressure (ICP) caused by interstitial swelling from capillary permeability.

- Administer fluid and pharmacologic agents as prescribed (see previous nursing diagnosis).

Impaired skin integrity related to urticaria and angioedema secondary to allergic response
Desired outcomes: Within 4 h of initiation of treatment, patient states that urticaria is controlled. Skin remains intact.

- Assess patient for the presence of urticaria (hives) and itching of hands, feet, neck, and genitalia.
- Administer antihistamines as prescribed to relieve itching.
- Discourage patient from scratching the skin. If unavoidable, teach patient to use pads of fingertips rather than nails.
- Apply cool washcloths or covered ice as a soothing measure to irritated and edematous areas.

Knowledge deficit: severe hypersensitivity reaction, its causes, and its symptoms, related to no prior exposure or incomplete understanding

Desired outcome: By the time of discharge from the critical care unit, patient demonstrates increased knowledge of severe hypersensitivity reactions as evidenced by verbalization of potential causative factors, symptoms of allergic reaction, need to inform health care providers of allergies, importance of wearing medical-alert identification, prescribed treatment modalities when in contact with allergen, and the necessity of informing primary health care provider immediately of any allergic symptoms.

- Provide information about the antigenic agent that caused the anaphylaxis, including ways to avoid it in the future.
- Explain the purpose and necessity of wearing a medical-alert identification tag or bracelet to identify the allergy.
- Give information about anaphylaxis emergency treatment kits. Teach patient self-administration technique and the importance of prompt treatment.
- Stress the importance of seeking treatment immediately if symptoms of allergy occur, including flushing, warmth, itching, anxiety, and hives.
- Explain the importance of identifying and checking all over-the-counter (OTC) medications for the presence of potential allergens.

ADDITIONAL NURSING DIAGNOSES

Also see nursing diagnoses and interventions in "Hemodynamic Monitoring," p. 28; "Psychosocial Support," p. 83; "Psychosocial Support for the Patient's Family and Significant Others," p. 95; "Mechanical Ventilation," p. 17. See also "Hypovolemia" for **Altered cerebral, renal, and peripheral tissue perfusion,** p. 638.

Organ rejection

PATHOPHYSIOLOGY

The major problem with all types of organ transplantation is graft rejection. When the body detects the presence of a foreign substance, it mounts the defense of nonspecific inflammation and phagocytosis. The next level of immune response involves antibody-mediated (humoral) immunity and cell-mediated immunity. Both responses occur in a parallel fashion after exposure to an antigen. *Antibody-mediated immune response* is related to B-lymphocyte activity. When an antigen is encountered, the B lymphocyte enlarges, divides, and differentiates into a plasma cell that produces and secretes antigen-specific immunoglobulins, or antibodies. The formation of this antigen-antibody complex triggers events that augment the nonspecific responses of inflammation and phagocytosis. *Cell-mediated immune response* involves T lymphocytes. A T lymphocyte recognizes a foreign antigen on the surface of the macrophage, binds to the antigen, and enlarges and produces a sensitized clone, which migrates through the body to the site of the antigen. When the sensitized T cell combines with the antigen, chemicals are released that kill foreign cells directly and act to facilitate phagocytosis and the inflammatory response. (See Figure 10-3 for a delineation of this process.)

Because a transplanted organ originates from a donor who is genetically different from the recipient (the exception is a kidney from an identical twin), the organ contains foreign antigens that trigger an immune response in the recipient, which leads to organ rejection. Historically, rejection has been classified as hyperacute, accelerated acute, acute, and chronic (Table 10-4). An untreated rejection response results in complete destruction of the organ. Table 10-5 describes the clinical presentation for various types of acute organ rejection.

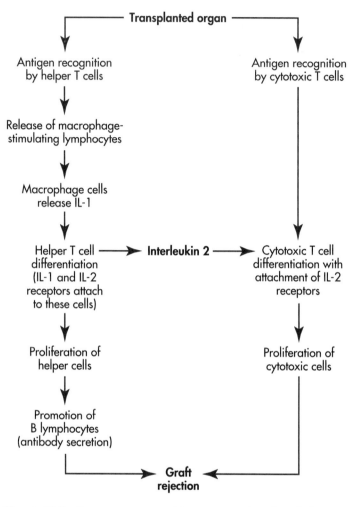

Figure 10-3: Immune response with organ transplantation. *IL-1,* Interleukin-1; *IL-2,* interleukin 2.

DIAGNOSIS AND ASSESSMENT OF REJECTION

Biopsy of the transplanted organ provides the means of diagnosing rejection, its severity, and the possibility of response to antirejection therapy. In addition, the following diagnostic tests are performed:

Cardiac
Chest x-ray: Will reveal increased dimension of the heart late in rejection.
ECG: Will show presence of atrial and ventricular dysrhythmias and decreased QRS voltage.
CBC: Will show increased total lymphocyte count.

TABLE 10-4   Characteristics of Organ Rejection by Category

Type of rejection	Characteristics	Outcome
Hyperacute	Described in "Renal Transplantation," p. 385 Occurs immediately Antibody mediated Result of preformed circulatory antibodies	Irreversible and untreatable
Accelerated acute	Occurs 3-5 days after transplant Antibody mediated Rapid loss of function Fever and oliguria	Irreversible and untreatable
Acute	Primarily T-cell mediated Possible presence of humoral component Occurs weeks, months, or years after transplant	Treatable and reversible multiple episodes affect long-term graft survival
Chronic	Develops slowly over months to years Probably a combination of cellular- and humoral-mediated processes	Untreatable; eventually leads to graft loss

VS and heart sounds: May reveal decreased stroke volume, cardiac output, cardiac tones, and BP; and presence of S_3 and S_4 sounds, pericardial friction rub, extrasystole, and crackles.

Liver
Serum bilirubin level: Total bilirubin will rise in relation to baseline postoperative level.
Transaminase level: Will increase from baseline; may be markedly elevated early in rejection.
Alkaline phosphatase level: Will increase from baseline.
Prothrombin time: Will be prolonged.
CBC: May reveal decreased platelet count and increased total lymphocyte count.

Pancreas
Open biopsy is the only means by which a definitive diagnosis can be made.
Fasting and 2-h postprandial plasma glucose: Levels will be increased above normal ranges.
Serum amylase: Levels may be elevated, indicating presence of pancreatitis, an inconsistent marker of rejection.
C peptide (serum and urine): Levels may be decreased.
Pancreas radioisotope flow scan: Determines organ viability. Decreased flow may indicate rejection.

Lung
Transbronchial biopsy is not helpful in detecting rejection; the morbidity risk increases with open biopsy.

TABLE 10-5   Clinical Presentation With Acute Organ Rejection

Organ	Clinical presentation	Treatment options
Heart	10-14 days after transplantation. Indicators include fever, anxiety, lethargy, low back pain, atrial or ventricular dysrhythmias, gallop, pericardial friction rub, jugular venous distention, hypotension, and decreased CO late in rejection.	Methylprednisolone sodium succinate (500 mg-1 g) daily for 2-4 days. Antilymphocyte sera (rabbit, horse, goat) IV for 6-14 days. Monoclonal antibody for 10-14 days. Retransplantation necessary for intractable acute rejection.
Liver	4-10 days after transplantation. Indicators include malaise; fever; abdominal discomfort; swollen, hard, tender graft; tachycardia; RUQ or flank pain; cessation of bile flow; change in bile fluid from golden to colorless; jaundice; elevated PT, bilirubin, transaminase, and alkaline phosphatase.	Methylprednisolone sodium succinate (500 mg-1 g) daily for 2-4 days. Antilymphocyte sera (rabbit, horse, goat) IV for 6-14 days. Retransplantation necessary for recurrent unresponsive rejection.
Pancreas	Time of rejection occurrence varies. Patient may have hyperglycemia, pancreatitis, pain over graft. Open biopsy may be necessary to diagnose rejection.	Methylprednisolone sodium succinate (250 mg-1 g) daily for 2-4 days. Antilymphocyte sera (rabbit, horse, goat) IV for 6-14 days. Monoclonal antibody for 10-14 days. Retransplantation for unresponsive rejection.
Lung	Expected during the first 21 postoperative days, with increased frequency and severity 6-8 wk after transplantation. *Classic rejection:* Decreased lung ventilation and perfusion alveolar exudate containing desquamated pneumocytes and inflammatory cells *Atypical rejection:* Decreased ventilation without blood flow reduction; ventilation-perfusion imbalances and respiratory insufficiency with shunting *Vascular rejection:* Increased vascular resistance; decreased blood flow to graft	Methylprednisolone sodium succinate (250 mg-1 g) daily for 2-4 days. Antilymphocyte sera (rabbit, horse, goat) IV for 6-14 days. Retransplantation for unresponsive rejection.

CO, Cardiac output; *IV,* intravenous; *RUQ,* right upper quadrant; *PT,* prothrombin time.

Leukocyte and absolute lymphocyte counts: Rise during rejection.
VS and hemodynamics: Can change suddenly with increases in the following: PVR, HR, BP, SVR, and CO.
ABG values: Decrease in Pao_2 and increase in $Paco_2$ occur with rejection.

Renal
See "Renal Transplantation," p. 385.

MECHANISMS OF IMMUNOSUPPRESSIVE AGENTS

The following drugs may be used in various combinations for additive effect in preventing or modifying the rejection response. The goal of therapy is to achieve enough immunosuppression to prevent graft rejection but not so much as to leave the patient in a defenseless state.

Azathioprine (Imuran): Interferes with deoxyribonucleic acid (DNA) synthesis and inhibits mitosis of immunologically competent cells. Cell division and proliferation occur in response to antigenic stimulation. Azathioprine affects rapidly replicating cells at an early stage of lymphocyte activation and is believed to block proliferation of helper T cells and cytotoxic T cells. Azathioprine is converted to mercaptopurine (6-MP) and further metabolized in the liver by xanthine oxidase.

> **Note:** Allopurinol inhibits xanthine oxidase-mediated metabolism and may result in increased activity and toxicity of azathioprine. If allopurinol must be used with azathioprine, the usual dose of azathioprine usually is reduced by one fourth to one third.

Mycophenolate mofetil: Inhibits denovo purine biosynthesis during cell division. It inhibits the proliferation of T and B lymphocytes, the production of antibodies, and the generation of cytotoxic T cells.

Corticosteroids: Suppress the production of cytotoxic T lymphocytes from noncytotoxic precursor cells. There is some evidence that steroids prevent the release of interleukin-1 (IL-1) and IL-2. IL-1, released by the macrophages, promotes the differentiation of helper T cells. The release of IL-2 promotes differentiation of cytotoxic cells.

Antilymphocyte sera (antilymphocytic globulin [ALG] or antithymocyte gamma-globulin [ATGAM]): The antilymphocyte antibodies in the sera are useful in the treatment of steroid-resistant rejection and potent suppressors of cell-mediated immunity. They are directed against many different antigens on the surface of human lymphocytes and affect immunity via reduction of T lymphocytes.

Monoclonal antibody (Orthoclone OKT3): This homologous antibody reacts with and blocks the function of the chemical (T3) complex on the surface of the T lymphocytes. The T3 complex is responsible for the T lymphocyte's identification of a transplanted organ as foreign and attempts to reject it. OKT3 binds to the T3 antigen on the surface of the T cells, enhancing phagocytosis and entrapment of the cells in the spleen and liver. The lymphocytes are removed from the circulation by this process in approximately 10-15 min.

Cyclosporine (Sandimmune or Neoral): Inhibits production and release of lymphokines and generation of cytotoxic and plasma cells by blocking the response of cytotoxic T lymphocytes to IL-2. Cyclosporine is metabolized by the cytochrome P-450 enzyme system in the liver. Careful monitoring of cyclosporine drug levels, with concomitant dose adjustments, is necessary when cyclosporine is used with other drugs (Table 10-6).

Tacrolimus (Prograf): Blocks T-cell activation genes by a similar mechanism to cyclosporine. It is also metabolized by the cytochrome P-450 enzyme system in the liver. Careful drug level monitoring and awareness of the

TABLE 10-6 Cyclosporine (CyA) Drug Interactions

Drugs causing decreased blood levels of CyA*	Drugs causing increased blood levels of CyA†
Carbamazepine	Cimetidine
Isoniazid	Danazol
Phenobarbital	Diltiazem
Phenytoin	Erythromycin
Rifampin	High-dose corticosteroids
Sulfamethoxazole	Ketoconazole
Trimethoprim	Methyltestosterone
	Nicardipine
	Oral contraceptives
	Ranitidine

NOTE: Careful monitoring of CyA blood levels and adjusting dosage as indicated are necessary when these drugs are used in patients taking cyclosporine.
*Decreased blood levels may precipitate organ rejection.
†Increased blood levels may cause nephrotoxicity.

interactions of concomitant medications and the potential for dose adjustment are imperative.

NURSING DIAGNOSES AND INTERVENTIONS

Anxiety/fear related to threat of change in health status secondary to potential loss of transplanted organ because of rejection

Desired outcomes: Patient expresses anxieties and fears regarding possibility of organ loss and verbalizes accurate information about the signs and symptoms of organ rejection. Within 12 h of this diagnosis, patient's fear and anxiety are controlled as evidenced by BP within patient's normal range; HR ≤100 bpm; and RR ≤20 breaths/min with normal depth and pattern (eupnea).

- Encourage patient to discuss concerns and fears.
- Assess patient's knowledge about the rejection process and the signs and symptoms that occur.
- Use short, simple sentences to explain patient's current organ function and the signs and symptoms of organ rejection (see Table 10-5).
- Reassure patient that appropriate medications are being given to prevent ongoing rejection. Review medication names, dosage, and action (see p. 619).
- Explain to patient that rejection does not necessarily mean organ loss. Under most circumstances, rejection can be reversed.
- Reassure patient that retransplantation is a viable option if organ loss occurs.

Fluid volume excess (or risk for same) related to compromised regulatory mechanism secondary to diminished organ function associated with rejection episode

Desired outcome: Patient is normovolemic as evidenced by stable weight; urine output ≥0.5 ml/kg/h; BP within patient's normal range; HR 60-100 bpm; RR 12-20 breaths/min with normal depth and pattern (eupnea); and absence of edema, crackles, and other clinical indicators of fluid overload.

- Measure weight daily. Remember that a 1-kg weight gain can signal approximately 1 L of fluid retention.

- Measure I&O q1-2h; note 24-h trends.
- Assess BP, pulse, and respirations q1-2h. Be alert to increased BP, tachycardia, and tachypnea, which are indicators of fluid overload.
- Auscultate for the presence of crackles (rales) and pericardial friction rub at least q8h.
- Assess and document the presence of peripheral, sacral, and periorbital edema on a scale of 0-4+.
- Consult physician promptly for any significant findings from the aforementioned assessments.

Powerlessness related to actual and perceived helplessness with controlling organ rejection episodes
Desired outcome: Within 72 h of this diagnosis, patient relates that he or she can control aspects of daily care, as well as assume responsibility for taking medications appropriately and obtaining follow-up care.

- Encourage patient to express feelings of frustration and powerlessness regarding organ rejection.
- Enable and encourage patient to participate in decisions about care routines. Help patient identify areas of the care plan he or she can control, such as timing of morning care or initiating rest periods.
- Reinforce that taking medications appropriately and keeping appointments for follow-up care *are* within patient's control and are significant in the prevention of rejection and organ destruction.
- Solicit comments and opinions from patient. Honor patient's opinions and preferences.

Body image disturbance related to biophysical changes secondary to side effects from immunosuppressive medications
Desired outcome: Within 48-72 h of this diagnosis, patient verbalizes understanding of body changes that may occur with immunosuppression medications, along with interventions to minimize their effect on body image.

- Identify body changes associated with steroid therapy: profuse diaphoresis, changes in fat distribution, moon face, acne, bruising.
  - ☐ Suggest that patient try different brands of deodorants or talcs to help counteract the odor from profuse diaphoresis and wear cotton clothing, which absorbs perspiration.
  - ☐ If patient usually wears makeup, suggest that to minimize the effects of facial swelling, patient apply makeup that highlights the eyes.
  - ☐ Suggest that patient refrain from wearing prints and stripes, which may increase attention to fat distribution in the trunk area.
  - ☐ Advise patient to use facial astringents to keep skin clean and to minimize acne.
  - ☐ Suggest that patient wear long sleeves and slacks to cover bruised arms and legs.
- Teach patient about body changes that are associated with cyclosporine: hirsutism, gum hyperplasia.
  - ☐ Suggest that female patient use facial depilatories.
  - ☐ Teach patient to use a soft-bristle toothbrush and mouthwash for frequent, gentle mouth care.

ADDITIONAL NURSING DIAGNOSES

See "Renal Transplantation" for **Knowledge deficit: immunosuppressive medications and their side effects,** p. 392; **Risk for infection,** p. 393; **Altered oral mucous membrane,** p. 394; and **Impaired skin integrity,** p. 394. For other nursing diagnoses and interventions, see the following, as appropriate:"Prolonged Immobility," p. 74; "Psychosocial Support," p. 83; and "Psychosocial Support for the Patient's Family and Significant Others," p. 95.

Drug overdose

Drug overdose is a widespread problem that affects all ages, races, and socioeconomic levels. There is no one single clinical profile of individuals who overdose with either street, medically prescribed, or over-the-counter (OTC) drugs. Drug overdose can be categorized in several ways, including deleterious reactions to street drugs during a first-time use, chronic abuse of street drugs, chronic abuse of medically prescribed drugs, and overdose experienced by the elderly related to untoward effects of prescribed medications. Overdose may be intentional or nonintentional in all categories.

No organ or body system is immune to the detrimental effects of drug overdose. The type, amount, and route of the drug affect the outcome, prognosis, and physical presentation. The following discussion considers the illicit and medically prescribed drugs commonly involved in drug overdose, the effects of these substances on the body systems, the laboratory tests and collaborative management, and general nursing diagnoses and interventions.

OVERVIEW OF TREATMENT OPTIONS

Treatment of drug overdose depends on five factors: the type of drug ingested, the amount, the rate of absorption, the route of administration, and the time span between ingestion and delivery of care. These factors determine the specific time frames for resolution of the drug's effects. Removal of the orally ingested substance may be accomplished through the following emerging trends in treatment.

Ipecac: Use of this gastric decontamination agent depends on the length of time from ingestion to treatment and on the patient's mental status.

- May be inappropriate in patients who ingested the drug >1 h before seeking treatment. This is especially true with ingestion of drugs in liquid form, because these are rapidly absorbed.
- Contraindicated if patient has altered mental status, because aspiration of gastric contents is a possibility. Commonly ingested agents likely to result in serious alteration of mental status are antihistamines, barbiturates, benzodiazepines, β-blockers, cyclic antidepressants, ethanol, and opioids.
- May cause bradycardia. In combination with vomiting, this side effect may cause deleterious hemodynamic compromise, particularly if cardiotoxic drugs such as digoxin or cyclic antidepressants are involved.
- Other considerations when assessing the use of ipecac:
  - ☐ Has the patient already vomited?
  - ☐ Has the patient ingested a hydrocarbon or caustic substance?
  - ☐ Is there another oral antidote?
- When ipecac is administered, vomiting should be expected within 20 min. If this does not occur, repeat dose. If ineffective, proceed to gastric lavage.

Research Brief 10-3   Gender-specific research is providing insight into how the characteristics and course of alcohol and illicit drug use differ in women and men. Health care professionals have more opportunity to screen adolescent, adult, and geriatric women for substance abuse since women use the health care system more frequently than men do. The incidence of a "worsening depression" is a significant indicator for alcohol abuse. It is also suggested that women who experiment with heroin are at higher risk than men to evolve into users of this substance daily and at higher amounts. Their life-style changes involve inclusion of high-risk behaviors, making them more susceptible for human immunodeficiency virus (HIV) infection and suicide.

From Stein M et al: *Med Clin North Am* 81(4):979-998, 1997.

Activated charcoal: Effectiveness is enhanced when this chemical is mixed with sorbitol cathartic but diminished when food is present in the GI tract. If multidose administration is necessary, provide subsequent doses within 2-6 h. Activated charcoal does not bind with lithium, potassium, potassium chloride, ethanol, or iron.

Gastric lavage: Important adjunct in the treatment of ingested overdose because it results in prompt emptying of gastric contents. It is essential to protect the airway when using this therapy. Lavage should continue until the fluid is clear of fragments, which may take 10-30 min.

ACETAMINOPHEN

Acetaminophen (Tylenol) is one of the drugs most commonly ingested in overdose. Most patients will admit to having taken this medication.

Routes of administration
Oral (most common); rectal per suppository.

Effects on body systems
Cardiovascular: May cause myocardial damage secondary to hepatic damage, which may lead to ischemia and injury (as manifested by chest pain/pressure, nausea, SOB, T-wave inversion and ST-segment elevation on ECG). Cardiac dysrhythmias have been reported.

Respiratory: Bronchospasm (as manifested by increased RR, wheezes, and difficulty breathing) has been reported as a hypersensitivity reaction or as a side effect of N-acetylcysteine. See "Collaborative Management."

Neurologic: Coma and seizures.

Hepatic: Acute ingestion will cause hepatic necrosis, which can lead to hepatic failure. Hypoglycemia, right-sided abdominal pain, and nausea with vomiting may be noted, usually 1-2 days after ingestion.

Renal: Renal tubular necrosis (manifested by oliguria and increased BUN and creatinine values) is seen in some cases but tends to be transient.

Associated findings: Hypophosphatemia, metabolic acidosis, hypothermia, thrombocytopenia, and hemorrhagic pancreatitis.

Diagnostic tests
Serum blood levels for acetaminophen: The first serum blood levels usually are drawn 4 h after ingestion, if possible. Subsequent levels are drawn periodically (e.g., q4h) until levels are below the predicted hepatotoxic range.

Additional tests: Serum Na^+, K^+, CO_2, BUN, blood glucose, creatinine, liver enzyme, and bilirubin; PT, coagulation studies; CBC; protein; amylase; ABGs; and renal function tests.

Collaborative management
Support of cardiovascular and respiratory systems: Oxygen supplementation. If ABG values indicate a trend toward respiratory failure or if the patient has an ineffective or absent breathing effort, mechanical ventilation is provided. Serial ECGs monitor for evidence of dysrhythmias. Ventricular dysrhythmias are treated with antidysrhythmic agents, and bradyarrhythmias are treated with atropine, dopamine, epinephrine, or a pacemaker.

Removal of acetaminophen from the system: A combination of activated charcoal and N-acetylcysteine (Mucomyst) administered orally or via a gastric tube is the preferred treatment. Treatment with these agents is most effective when it is initiated as soon after ingestion as possible but may be effective up to 8-10 h after ingestion. These agents bind with acetaminophen until the toxin is passed via the GI tract. Lavage also may be initiated to remove the drug or assess the stomach contents for evidence of drug ingestion. Activated charcoal, especially if administered within 1 h of ingestion, is highly effective in absorbing acetaminophen. Ipecac may not be prescribed because the vomiting it induces will delay use of activated charcoal and N-acetylcysteine. Ipecac may be a treatment option if ingestion is recent (e.g., within 1-2 h).

Treatment of nausea and vomiting: Fluid replacement therapy with lactated Ringer's solution or D_5NS; antiemetics, usually promethazine hydrochloride (Phenergan).

Rewarming: A heating blanket is applied if patient has hypothermia.

Treatment of hypoglycemia: Usually with a bolus of D_{50} and continuous infusion of D_5W, based on serum glucose results. Hypoglycemia occurs because of the potent hepatotoxic effects of acetaminophen.

ALCOHOL

Route of administration
Oral.

Effects on body systems

Cardiovascular: Tachycardia, atrial fibrillation, cardiac arrest.

Respiratory: Hypoventilation with acute intoxication; respiratory failure.

Neurologic: Confusion, aggressive behavior, irritability, tremors, hallucinations (especially auditory), memory loss, stupor, coma, seizures related to hypoglycemia, loss of deep tendon reflexes (DTRs).

Renal: May have significant output initially; will demonstrate dehydration with acute intoxication.

Associated findings: Dry oral mucosa, odor of alcohol on breath, hypoglycemia, hypothermia, lactic acidosis, hypokalemia.

Diagnostic tests

Blood alcohol level and urine drug screen are performed, along with serum K^+, Na^+, CO_2, BUN, glucose, and creatinine. In addition, the following may be evaluated: CBC, liver and renal function studies, and blood gas values.

Collaborative management

Support of cardiovascular and respiratory systems to prevent collapse: Oxygen supplementation; treatment of ventricular dysrhythmias with antidysrhythmic agents; treatment of bradyarrhythmias with atropine.

Fluid/potassium replacement: See discussions, pp. 639 and 650.

Removal of substance from system: The body can remove alcohol from its system via its own metabolic process. Blood alcohol concentration will decrease 20-30 mg/dl/h (legal limit is <100 mg/dl). Coma usually occurs if the level is >300 mg/dl, but this is influenced by each individual's metabolic process and tolerance. In life-threatening intoxication, in which large amounts of alcohol have been absorbed into the system, the liver and kidneys may not be able to break down and excrete the alcohol. Thus hemodialysis (see p. 399) may be of substantial benefit.

Prevention of emesis: Antiemetics are given for nausea and vomiting, and a gastric tube is inserted and maintained at low continuous suction.

Anticipation and treatment of withdrawal: Usually with short-acting benzodiazepines such as oxazepam (Serax) or lorazepam (Ativan). These patients must be medicated with an amount of medication equivalent to their usual 24-h alcohol intake; for example, 60 ml (2 oz) of 80% liquor equals 10 mg diazepam (Valium), 10 mg oxazepam, 30 mg phenobarbital, 25 mg chlordiazepoxide (Librium), or 2 mg lorazepam. Individuals who have been drinking 0.95 L (1 qt) of vodka per day will need 400 mg chlordiazepoxide or 160 mg diazepam. Cautious use of benzodiazepines with long half-lives (see Table 10-8) in patients with chronic alcohol consumption is important because of the likelihood of cirrhosis in these individuals. Oxazepam is the drug of choice because of its shorter half-life.

Treatment of hypoglycemia: Usually with a bolus of D_{50} and continuous infusion of D_5W, based on serum glucose results. If thiamine deficiency is suspected, thiamine should be administered before glucose to avoid sudden precipitation of heart failure and worsening neurologic impairment.

Treatment of delirium tremens (DTs): The most severe progression of withdrawal, which can result in death. Signs and symptoms develop 72-96 h after cessation of drinking and can include disorientation with loss of touch with reality, delirium, agitation, severe diaphoresis, tachycardia, cardiovascular collapse, and fever. Generally, DTs resolve within 3-5 days. Patients are sedated with benzodiazepines (usually IV diazepam), allowed to rest and sleep, and oriented frequently to reality.

Treatment/prevention of seizures: Because alcohol withdrawal seizures occur during the first 6-48 h after abstinence, benzodiazepines are given to raise the seizure threshold during the withdrawal period. Alcohol withdrawal seizures mandate the use of a heparin lock and IV diazepam (drug of choice) to achieve control over the seizure(s). Additional seizure management should reflect institution protocol. If the patient has a history of a primary seizure disorder, an anticonvulsant agent, such as phenytoin (Dilantin), is indicated.

IM thiamine on admission; supplemental oral thiamine; and multivitamins and multiminerals high in C, B-complex, zinc, and magnesium: Thiamine is given to prevent Wernicke-Korsakoff syndrome (discussed next); multivitamins and multiminerals are given because of the potential for malnutrition related to inadequate food intake and malabsorption caused by alcohol's irritating effect on the GI tract.

Wernicke-Korsakoff syndrome: Caused by thiamine deficiency and manifested by diplopia (the first real diagnostic clue), confusion, excitation, peripheral neuropathy, severe recent memory loss, impaired thought processes, and confabulation. Prophylactic administration of thiamine is recommended.

Caution: Ingestion of carbohydrates, either orally or parenterally, increases the body's demand for thiamine. For patients with a history of chronic alcohol ingestion, administration of thiamine should precede administration of glucose to prevent sudden profound thiamine deficiency and irreversible neurologic impairment.

AMPHETAMINES

Street names
Methamphetamine, speed, crystal, meth, white crosses, ice.

Routes of administration
Oral, IV, IM, smoked.

Effects on body systems
Cardiovascular: Tachycardia, atrial and ventricular dysrhythmias, hypertension, myocardial ischemia and infarction, cardiovascular collapse.
Respiratory: Hyperventilation and respiratory failure related to cardiovascular collapse.
Neurologic: Confusion, aggressive behavior, hyperactivity, convulsions, delusions, irritability, tremors, hallucinations, memory loss, stupor, stroke, coma.
Renal: Renal failure related to dehydration and rhabdomyolysis.
Associated findings: Mydriasis, fasciculations, hyperthermia, thrombocytopenic purpura.

Diagnostic tests
Blood and urine specimens are tested for substances of abuse. In addition to serum K^+, Na^+, CO_2, BUN, glucose, and creatinine, the CBC and liver and renal studies also are evaluated. Cardiac enzyme levels with isoenzyme fractionations are monitored to evaluate presence and degree of myocardial injury.

Collaborative management
Support of cardiovascular and respiratory systems to prevent collapse:
Antidysrhythmic agents, verapamil, and digitalis are given for atrial dysrhythmias. If origin of dysrhythmia is unknown, adenosine triphosphate is administered to convert or diagnose the site of origin. Ischemia is treated with nitrates; myocardial infarction is treated with thrombolytic therapy (see p. 254), PTCA (see p. 253), or CABG (see p. 255).
Removal of substance from the system: For oral ingestion, activated charcoal is administered orally or via gastric tube to bind with the ingested substance in the stomach, often followed by gastric lavage. Ipecac is not recommended.
Treatment of hypertension: Usually with antihypertensives, such as nitroprusside (Nipride), which is titrated to decrease BP.
Prevention/treatment of seizures: IV diazepam 0.1-0.2 mg/kg is administered slowly and repeated q5min until sedation is achieved. Haldol can be used via the IM route at a dosage of 0.1-0.2 mg/kg.
Treatment of hyperthermia: Cooling blanket, antipyretics.
Treatment of dehydration: Fluid replacement, such as lactated Ringer's solution and D_5NS.
Anticipation and treatment of rhabdomyolysis: Usually treated with sodium bicarbonate, mannitol, or furosemide (Lasix).

BARBITURATES
See Table 10-7.

Street names
Yellow jackets, reds, barbs.

Routes of administration
Oral, IV, IM.

Effects on body systems
Cardiovascular: Hypotension, bradycardia, cardiac arrest.
Respiratory: Respiratory depression leading to hypoventilation, apnea, respiratory failure, and respiratory arrest.
Neurologic: Symptoms may include headache, vertigo, dizziness, lethargy, ataxia, stupor, flaccidity, seizures, absent doll's-eye reflex, coma, loss of DTRs, and nystagmus (see coma scale, which follows).

TABLE 10-7   Common Barbiturates

Generic name	Common brand name	Half-life (h)
Amobarbital	Amytal	8-42
Secobarbital	Seconal	19-34
Pentobarbital	Nembutal	15-48
Phenobarbital	Luminal and others	24-140
Butabarbital	Butisol	34-42
Secobarbital/amobarbital	Tuinal	8-42

Drug half-life: Withdrawal symptoms can be correlated with the half-life of the drug that was used. Withdrawal from drugs with shorter half-lives produces intense symptoms that last for shorter periods, whereas withdrawal from drugs with longer half-lives produces less intense symptoms that can be prolonged. Moreover, the severity of the withdrawal is directly related to the drug's dosage.

Renal: Acute renal failure is possible.
Associated findings: Hypothermia, nausea, vomiting. Patient may experience opposite reactions of euphoria and excitability before the normal sedative effects occur. Withdrawal symptoms of tremors and convulsions may occur.

Classification of barbiturate intoxication
Alert: No signs of CNS depression.
Drowsy: CNS depression from alert to stuporous.
Stuporous: Markedly sedated; responsive to verbal and tactile stimuli.
COMA 1: Responsive to painful but not to verbal and tactile stimuli; no change in respirations or BP.
COMA 2: Unconscious; unresponsive to pain; no change in respirations or BP.
COMA 3: Unresponsive to pain; slow, shallow, or rapid spontaneous respirations; low but adequate BP.
COMA 4: Unresponsive to pain; apnea or inadequate BP or both.

Diagnostic tests
Serum drug screen is analyzed. In addition to serum K^+, Na^+, CO_2, BUN, glucose, and creatinine, the CBC, ABGs, and liver and renal function studies are evaluated.

Collaborative management
Support of cardiovascular and respiratory systems to prevent collapse: Electrical rhythm is monitored; bradyarrhythmias are treated with atropine, L-dopamine, epinephrine, and possibly isoproterenol, as well as pacing. After fluids are replaced, vasopressor therapy (see Appendix 7), including dopamine and norepinephrine bitartrate (Levophed), may be initiated for hypotension. Mechanical ventilation may be required, depending on the degree of hypoxia and CO_2 retention.
Removal of substance from system: Ipecac to promote vomiting; activated charcoal administered orally or via gastric tube to bind with the substance in the stomach; gastric lavage; and hemodialysis, which may be used if patient is in COMA 4 stage.
Prevention/treatment of seizures: Phenytoin or diazepam may be given.
Sedation for withdrawal symptoms: Typically the barbiturate that was ingested is tapered gradually to zero.
Prevention of aspiration: Insertion of gastric tube, which is then connected to low suction.
Treatment of nausea and vomiting: Antiemetics, usually IV promethazine hydrochloride.
Treatment of hypothermia: Warming blanket.

BENZODIAZEPINES
See Table 10-8.

Routes of administration
Oral, IM, IV.

Effects on body systems
Cardiovascular: Hypotension, tachycardia.
Respiratory: Respiratory arrest.
Neurologic: Drowsiness, ataxia, slurred speech, coma. Withdrawal may be manifested by seizures.
Renal: Renal failure because of rhabdomyolysis.
Associated findings: Hypothermia.

TABLE 10-8 Common Benzodiazepines

Generic name	Common brand name	Half-life (h)
Chlordiazepoxide	Librium and others	7-28
Diazepam	Valium and others	20-90
Lorazepam	Ativan	10-20
Oxazepam	Serax	3-21
Prazepam	Centrax	24-200*
Flurazepam	Dalmane	24-100*
Chlorazepate	Tranxene	30-100
Temazepam	Restoril	9.5-12.4
Clonazepam	Klonopin	18.5-50
Alprazolam	Xanax	12-15
Halazepam	Paxipam	14

*Includes half-life of major metabolites.
Drug half-life: Withdrawal symptoms can be correlated with the half-life of the drug that was used. Withdrawal from drugs with shorter half-lives produces intense symptoms that last for shorter periods, whereas withdrawal from drugs with longer half-lives produces less intense symptoms that can be prolonged. Moreover, the severity of the withdrawal is directly related to the drug's dosage.

Diagnostic tests
Serum and urine drug screens are analyzed. In addition to serum K^+, Na^+, CO_2, BUN, glucose, and creatinine, the CBC and liver and renal studies are evaluated.

Collaborative management
Support of cardiovascular system to prevent collapse: Electrical rhythm is monitored; tachyarrhythmias are treated with verapamil. Hypotension is treated with fluid replacement, followed by dopamine or norepinephrine bitartrate (Levophed).
Support of respiratory system: Apnea monitoring and mechanical ventilation (see p. 17) may be indicated.
Removal of substance from system: Ipecac to induce vomiting; activated charcoal to bind with the substance in the stomach; gastric lavage.
Prevention of seizures: Administration of phenytoin and diazepam.
Prevention of aspiration: Insertion of gastric tube, which is then connected to low intermittent suction.
Identification of rhabdomyolysis: The accumulation of protein in the kidneys, detected by increased BUN, creatinine, and protein values in the urine. Seizure activity and breakdown of muscle cause protein to precipitate in the kidneys, leading to renal failure. Prevention of seizures (see above) is the best treatment for prevention of rhabdomyolysis.
Treatment of hypothermia: Warming blanket if indicated.
Treatment of diazepam overdose: Sedative and respiratory depressant effects may be reversed by flumazenil (Romazicon). Repeat doses may be necessary.

COCAINE

Street names
Crack, rock, freebase, snow.

Routes of administration
Nasal or IV (cocaine, snow); smoked (crack, rock, freebase).

Effects on body systems
Cardiovascular: Hypertension; sinus tachycardia and sinus bradycardia; ventricular dysrhythmias, such as PVCs, ventricular tachycardia, and ventricular fibrillation; myocardial infarction; heart failure; cardiomyopathy; acute endocarditis; and aortic dissection. Acute intoxication also may result in profound hypotension and shock.

Respiratory: Sharp pleuritic pain, hemoptysis, pneumothorax, bronchospasm, pulmonary edema, and respiratory failure. Both lactic acidosis and metabolic acidosis have been associated with cocaine overdose.

Neurologic: The degree of CNS stimulation depends on the route and amount of drug taken, but it can include hyperexcitable state, paranoia, delirium, hallucinations, tremors, and aggression. Mentation may vary from stimulated, euphoric, and excited states to delirium, stupor, and coma. Seizures are common, usually of a tonic-clonic nature, and may last for hours. Initially the individual may seem well coordinated but may deteriorate to tremors and fasciculations. Headache is common.

Renal: Renal failure can occur and has been related to profound hypotension and rhabdomyolysis.

Associated findings: Hyperthermia is common, and rectal temperatures may be elevated to as high as 43° C (109.4° F). In addition, perforated nasal septum, track marks related to IV use, and mydriasis (dilated pupils) occur.

Indicators of withdrawal: Poor concentration, anergia, anhedonia, bradykinesis, sleep disturbance, decreased libido, intense cocaine craving, depression, and suicidal tendencies.

Indicators of cocaine psychosis: Tactile and visual hallucination and paranoia.

Peak action
Intranasal: 20-60 min.
Oral: 60-90 min.
IV: 5 min.
Smoked: <5 min.

Cutting agents
Cutting agents are substances that are used to increase bulk in pure cocaine. These include procaine, phencyclidine (angel dust), amphetamine, quinine, talc, and strychnine. Agents used in the preparation of crack include powdered cocaine, water, baking soda, and lidocaine. Cutting agents can become emboli that shower into cerebral and pulmonary circulation, with subsequent effects.

Diagnostic tests
Assessing blood levels of cocaine usually is of little diagnostic value. Urinalysis provides a quantitative method for identifying the presence of a cocaine metabolite. In addition to serum K^+, Na^+, CO_2, BUN, glucose, and creatinine, the CBC and renal function studies also are analyzed.

Collaborative management
Support of cardiovascular system to prevent collapse: Electrical rhythm is monitored. Supraventricular tachycardia may be treated with propranolol (Inderal) or verapamil; ventricular dysrhythmias are treated with antidysrhythmics such as lidocaine, procainamide (Pronestyl), and bretylium. Monitor patient's ECG for changes that signal ischemic or infarction pattern. Be alert to T-wave inversion or ST-segment elevation or depression.

Support of respiratory system: Comatose patients are placed on mechanical ventilation (see p. 17).

Identification of route of administration and removal of substance from system if ingested orally: An x-ray of the GI tract may reveal the presence of a cocaine-filled condom. If present, surgery may be performed to remove it. Activated charcoal may be administered to bind with cocaine in the stomach, or a laxative or suppository may be given to facilitate rectal excretion. An approach under investigation to flush cocaine from the system is the administration of IV ammonium chloride.

Treatment of hypotension or hypertension: Antihypertensives or vasopressors as indicated.

Treatment of volume deficiency: IV fluid replacement, such as lactated Ringer's solution or D_5NS.

Prevention/treatment of seizures: Administration of diazepam, phenytoin, or phenobarbital.

Treatment of hyperthermia: Cooling blanket, ice, acetaminophen. Core temperature is monitored for the most accurate measurements.

Prevention of aspiration: Insertion of gastric tube, which is then connected to low continuous suction.

HALLUCINOGENS

Common agents
Lysergic acid diethylamide (LSD), mescaline, morning glory seeds, nutmeg, ecstasy.

Routes of administration
Oral, IV, nasal, smoked.

Effects on body systems
Effects will depend on the amount and type of drug ingested.
Respiratory: Apnea, respiratory arrest.
Neurologic: Hallucinations and paranoid behavior patterns, tremors, seizures, coma.
LSD: Description of tasting or hearing colors, mental dissociation.
Mescaline: Sense of being followed by moving geometric shapes.
Ecstasy: Heightened sexual libido.
Associated findings: Hyperthermia and diaphoresis. In addition, visual hallucinations may occur.

Diagnostic tests
Serum plasma is analyzed for the presence of the drug. In addition to serum K^+, Na^+, CO_2, BUN, glucose, and creatinine, the CBC and liver and renal studies also are evaluated.

Collaborative management
Support of cardiovascular system to prevent collapse.
Removal of substance from system: If orally ingested, ipecac to induce vomiting; activated charcoal administered orally or via gastric tube to bind with the substance in the stomach; gastric lavage.
Prevention of seizures: Administration of anticonvulsants such as phenytoin or diazepam.

OPIOIDS

Examples of opioids include codeine, fentanyl, heroin, hydrocodone, hydromorphone hydrochloride (Dilaudid), levorphanol tartrate (Levo-Dromoran), meperidine hydrochloride (Demerol), methadone (Dolophine), morphine, opium, oxycodone hydrochloride (Percocet-5, Tylox), and oxymorphone (Numorphan).

Routes of administration
Oral, IV, IM, smoked.

Effects on body systems
Cardiovascular: Profound hypotension, bradycardia, cardiovascular collapse, sudden death.
Respiratory: Atelectasis, acute pulmonary edema, infiltrates related to aspiration complications, respiratory depression, apnea, hypoventilation, and bronchospasm.
Neurologic: Range from decreased mental alertness to stupor and coma, pinpoint pupils, seizures.
Renal: Renal failure has been associated with profound hypotension and rhabdomyolysis.
Associated findings: Track marks and scarring on arms and in hidden locations of the body, including between the toes and in the vessels underneath the tongue.

Diagnostic tests
Urine sampling for drug detection is the best way to identify the drug. In addition to serum K^+, Na^+, CO_2, BUN, glucose, and creatinine, the CBC and liver and renal studies also are evaluated.

Collaborative management
Support of cardiovascular system to prevent collapse: Electrical rhythm is monitored; bradyarrhythmias are treated with atropine and pacemaker. Vasopressor therapy is initiated for hypotension after fluids have been replaced.
Removal of drug from system: If oral ingestion is suspected, ipecac is used to induce vomiting; activated charcoal is administered orally or via gastric tube to bind with the substance in the stomach.
Reversal of opioid effects: Administration of naloxone hydrochloride (Narcan). After the initial dose of naloxone, the patient must be monitored closely, since additional doses may be required. Respiratory depression and coma may occur when the effects of naloxone wear off and the opiate effects predominate. The half-life of naloxone is 60-90 min, and effects last 2-3 h. If the narcotic effects last longer than the effects of the naloxone, the patient may slip into coma once the naloxone wears off. In this case a continuous naloxone infusion may be considered.
Treatment of drug withdrawal symptoms: Hallucinations are treated with haloperidol (Haldol).
Support of respiratory system: Pulmonary edema is treated with diuretics and restriction of IV fluid intake. An individual whose respiratory system is deteriorating is placed on apnea monitoring or mechanical ventilation (see p. 17).
Prevention of aspiration: Insertion of gastric tube, which is then connected to low continuous suction.
Prevention/treatment of seizure activity: Anticonvulsant therapy, such as phenytoin.
Prevention of rhabdomyolysis: See discussion, p. 628.

PHENCYCLIDINE
Street names
PCP, angel dust, mist.

Routes of administration
Oral, nasal, smoked.

Effects on body systems
Cardiovascular: Hypertension, hypertensive crisis, tachycardia.

Respiratory: Respiratory depression, respiratory arrest, laryngeal stridor (manifested by crowing sounds), bronchospasm.

Neurologic: Can range from hyperexcitability, hyperreflexia, muscle rigidity, and paranoid and psychotic behavior to stupor, seizures, and coma. Coma state may be accompanied by eyes open in a blank stare, nystagmus, and pinpoint pupils.

Renal: Renal failure precipitated by rhabdomyolysis and myoglobinuria.

Associated findings: Hypothermia or hyperthermia, hypoglycemia.

Diagnostic tests

Blood and urine samples are tested for the presence of the drug. In addition to serum K^+, Na^+, CO_2, BUN, glucose, and creatinine, the CBC and liver and renal studies also may be evaluated.

Collaborative management

Support of cardiovascular system to prevent collapse: Electrical rhythm is monitored and tachyarrhythmias are treated with verapamil. Nitroprusside is used for antihypertensive therapy. Nitroglycerin may be given to dilate myocardial vasculature.

Removal of drug from the system: No specific antidote is available, although multiple administrations of charcoal to bind with the ingested substance in the stomach is standard practice. The first dose of charcoal should be accompanied with sorbitol.

Prevention/treatment of seizure activity: Phenytoin and diazepam are given. Diazepam is administered IV at an initial dose of 2-5 mg. This may be repeated q30min until sedation is achieved. Haldol may be given 5-10 mg IV to control psychosis. The effects of Haldol usually occur within 5-10 min of administration.

Respiratory support: Pulmonary edema is treated with diuretics and restriction of IV fluid intake. Persons with hypoxia and deteriorating respiratory integrity are placed on apnea monitoring and potentially on mechanical ventilation.

Prevention of aspiration: Insertion of gastric tube, which is then connected to intermittent low suction.

Prevention of rhabdomyolysis: See discussion, p. 628.

Treatment of hypothermia or hyperthermia: Warming or cooling blanket as appropriate.

SALICYLATES

Examples include aspirin, bismuth subsalicylate, fendosal.

Routes of administration

Oral, rectal (suppository).

Effects on body systems

Respiratory: Hyperventilation, hyperpnea, pulmonary edema.

Neurologic: Coma, cerebral edema (manifested by indicators of IICP [see Table 6-3]).

Renal: Renal failure secondary to rhabdomyolysis.

Hepatic: Liver dysfunction, hepatitis.

Associated findings: Hyperthermia, bleeding, anemia, thrombocytopenia, hypokalemia, and tinnitus.

Diagnostic tests

Blood plasma is analyzed for the presence and amount of the salicylate and repeated q4-6h. This repetition is helpful, especially if the patient ingested salicylates in a sustained-release form. In addition to serum K^+, Na^+, CO_2,

BUN, glucose, and creatinine, the CBC and liver and renal studies also are evaluated.

Collaborative management
Support of cardiovascular system to prevent collapse: Electrical rhythm is monitored. Ventricular dysrhythmias are treated with lidocaine, procainamide hydrochloride (Pronestyl), and bretylium. Bradyarrhythmias are treated with atropine.
Removal of substance from the system: Ipecac to induce vomiting; activated charcoal administered orally or via gastric tube to bind with the substance in the stomach; gastric lavage; and hemodialysis, which may be necessary if the substance has been absorbed into the system. Several doses of activated charcoal may be necessary to achieve a 10:1 ratio of charcoal to salicylate.
Fluid replacement: Replace with lactated Ringer's solution or D_5NS 20 ml/kg over 1-2 h. Sodium bicarbonate may be added at a rate of 1 mEq/kg/h to promote forced alkaline diuresis.
Potassium replacement: See discussion, p. 649.
Treatment of hyperthermia: Cooling blanket or applications of ice.
Treatment of cerebral edema: Hyperventilation (via mechanical ventilation), mannitol.
Respiratory support: Mechanical ventilation (p. 17) as indicated.
Treatment of pulmonary edema: Nitrates, morphine, diuretics, potassium replacement, intermittent positive pressure breathing (IPPB). See discussion, p. 265.
Prevention of aspiration: Insertion of gastric tube, which is then connected to low suction.
Replacement of blood loss: Delivery of blood and blood products.

CYCLIC ANTIDEPRESSANTS
Examples include amitriptyline hydrochloride (Elavil), doxepin hydrochloride (Sinequan), imipramine hydrochloride (Presamine, Tofranil), and trimipramine maleate (Surmontil).

Route of administration
Oral.

Effects on body systems
Cardiovascular: Hypotension, sinus tachycardia, supraventricular tachycardia, ventricular dysrhythmias, conduction defects, myocardial infarction, cardiopulmonary arrest. Hypertension also has been noted. Monitor for widening of the QRS complex. Progressive widening of this complex signals worsening toxicity.
Respiratory: Respiratory arrest, pulmonary edema, ARDS. Hyperventilation also has been noted.
Neurologic: Coma, seizures, delirium, hallucinations.
Renal: Acute tubular necrosis; renal failure secondary to rhabdomyolysis.
Pancreatic: Pancreatitis.
Associated findings: Hyperthermia or hypothermia.

Diagnostic tests
Blood plasma, urine, and gastric contents are analyzed to determine the presence and amount of the drug. In addition to serum K^+, Na^+, CO_2, BUN, glucose, and creatinine, the CBC and liver and renal studies are evaluated. Cardiac enzymes and isoenzyme fractionations are assessed to determine presence and degree of myocardial damage.

Collaborative management
If the patient is symptom free, monitor for a minimum of 6-8 h, noting VS and width of QRS complex.

Support of cardiovascular system to prevent collapse: Electrical rhythm is monitored for at least 6 h to enable assessment for a widening QRS complex, which is a signal of worsening toxicity. Supraventricular tachycardias are treated with verapamil; ventricular dysrhythmias are treated with antidysrhythmics such as lidocaine. Atropine and pacing may be indicated in the presence of symptomatic conduction defects.

Removal of the substance from the system: Activated charcoal is administered via gastric tube to bind with the ingested substance in the stomach, facilitating its removal via gastric lavage. Ipecac to promote vomiting is not recommended.

Reversal of the effects of the drugs: IV sodium bicarbonate. An alternative approach is to promote a state of respiratory alkalosis by increasing respiratory rate via mechanical ventilation.

Prevention/treatment of seizures: Phenytoin and diazepam.

Respiratory support: Mechanical ventilation (see p. 17). Pulmonary edema is treated with nitrates, morphine, diuretics, potassium replacement, and IPPB treatments.

Treatment of hypotension: Fluid replacement, followed by dopamine and norepinephrine bitartrate (Levophed) as indicated.

Treatment of hyperthermia or hypothermia: Cooling or warming blanket as indicated.

Prevention of aspiration: Insertion of gastric tube, which is then connected to low intermittent suction.

FOR ALL DRUG OVERDOSES

Nursing diagnoses, interventions, and outcomes

Ineffective airway clearance related to presence of tracheobronchial secretions or obstruction; decreased sensorium

Desired outcome: Chest x-ray clear. Within 2-24 h of intervention/treatment, patient has a clear airway as evidenced by clear breath sounds over the upper airways and lung fields; RR 12-20 breaths/min with normal depth and pattern (eupnea); $Pao_2 \geq 80$ mm Hg; $Paco_2$ 35-45 mm Hg; pH 7.35-7.45; and $Spo_2 \geq 92\%$.

- Assess respiratory function hourly and prn. Be alert to secretions; stridor; gurgling; shallow, irregular, or labored respirations; use of accessory muscles of respiration; restlessness and confusion; and cyanosis (a late sign of respiratory distress).
- Suction oropharynx or via ET tube PRN.
- Administer bronchodilators as appropriate.
- Monitor ABG values for evidence of hypoxia (Pao_2 <80 mm Hg) and respiratory acidosis ($Paco_2$ >45 mm Hg; pH <7.35).
- Monitor respiratory patterns; provide continuous apnea monitoring if available.
- If patient has been placed on mechanical ventilation, monitor for indicators of airway obstruction (see "Mechanical Ventilation," p. 17).
- Monitor oxygen saturation continuously. Be alert to values <92%, depending on patient's baseline and clinical presentation.
- Administer and evaluate effects of antiemetics.

Hyperthermia related to overdose of cocaine, hallucinogens, phencyclidine, salicylates, or cyclic antidepressants

Desired outcome: Optimally, within 24-72 h of intervention, patient becomes normothermic.

Note: With massive overdose, temperature regulation may never be achieved.

- Monitor for signs of hyperthermia: temperature >38.3° C (>101° F), pallor, absence of perspiration, and torso that is warm to the touch. If available, provide continuous monitoring of temperature. Otherwise, measure rectal, core, or tympanic temperature hourly and PRN.
- Provide and monitor effects of cooling blanket, cooling baths, and ice packs to the axillae and groin.
- Maintain fluid replacement as prescribed. Monitor hydration status and trend of I&O.
- Monitor neurologic status hourly and PRN until stabilized.
- Monitor VS continuously or hourly and PRN until stabilized. Be alert to increased BP, HR, and RR.
- Administer and evaluate effects of antipyretic medications.

Risk for fluid volume deficit related to altered intake or excessive losses secondary to vomiting or diaphoresis and shock conditions
Desired outcome: Patient remains normovolemic as evidenced by urine output >0.5 ml/kg/h; moist mucous membranes; balanced I&O; BP within patient's normal range; HR <100 bpm; stable weight; CVP 2-6 mm Hg; and PAWP 6-12 mm Hg.

- Monitor hydration status on an ongoing basis. Be alert to continuing dehydration as evidenced by poor skin turgor, dry mucous membranes, complaints of thirst, weight loss >0.5 kg/day, urine specific gravity >1.020, weak pulse with tachycardia, and postural hypotension.
- If the patient has a PA line:
  - ☐ Monitor systemic and pulmonary vascular resistance as appropriate.
  - ☐ Monitor cardiac output as appropriate.
  - ☐ Monitor pulmonary capillary/artery wedge pressure and central venous/ right atrial pressure if appropriate.
  - ☐ Administer positive inotropic/contractility medications.
- Evaluate the effects of fluid therapy.
- Assess for indicators of electrolyte imbalance, especially the presence of hypokalemia. Be alert to irregular pulse, cardiac dysrhythmias, and serum potassium level <3.5 mEq/L.
- Monitor I&O hourly; assess for output elevated disproportionate to intake, bearing in mind the insensible losses.
- Monitor laboratory values, including serum electrolyte levels and serum and urine osmolality. Be alert to BUN values elevated disproportionate to the serum creatinine (indicator of dehydration rather than renal disease), high urine specific gravity, low urine sodium, and rising Hct and serum protein concentration. Optimal values are: serum osmolality 275-300 mOsm/kg; urine osmolality 300-1090 mOsm/kg; BUN 10-20 mg/dl; serum creatinine 0.7-1.5 mg/dl; urine sodium 40-180 mEq/24 h (diet dependent); Hct 37%-47% (female), or 40%-54% (male); and serum protein 6-8.3 g/dl.
- Maintain fluid intake as prescribed; administer prescribed electrolyte supplements.

Sensory/perceptual alterations related to chemical alterations secondary to ingestion of mind-altering drugs
Desired outcome: Within 48 h of intervention, patient verbalizes orientation to time, place, and person.

- Establish and maintain a calm, quiet environment to minimize patient's sensory overload. Dim the lights when possible.
- At frequent intervals, assess patient's orientation to time, place, and person. Reorient as necessary.
- Orient patient to the unit, and explain all procedures before performing them. Include significant others in orientation process.
- Do not leave patient alone if he or she is agitated or confused.
- Administer antianxiety agents as prescribed.
- If patient is hallucinating, intervene in the following ways:
  - ☐ Be reassuring. Explain that hallucinations may be very real to patient but

that they are not real, that they are caused by the substance patient consumed, and that they will go away eventually.

☐ As appropriate, try to involve family and significant others, because patient may have more trust in them.

☐ Explain that restraints are necessary to prevent harm to patient and others. Reassure patient that restraints will be used only as long as they are needed. As indicated, suggest to patient that you may release one restraint at a time as patient's condition improves.

☐ Tell patient that you will check on him or her at frequent intervals (e.g., q5-10min) or that you will stay at patient's side.

Risk for violence: self-directed, related to mind-altering drugs or depressed state

Desired outcome: Patient, staff, and patient's significant others remain free of either self-inflicted injury or injury by the patient.

• If patient's condition is stable, provide auxiliary staff member, such as orderly or nursing assistant, to watch patient when awake.

• Speak with patient in a quiet and calm voice, using short sentences.

• Establish a therapeutic relationship with patient.

• Encourage patient to take control over own behavior.

• Facilitate support by significant others.

• Limit interventions.

• Administer and evaluate effectiveness of sedation to calm patient.

• Keep all sharp instruments out of patient's room. Follow agency protocol accordingly.

• If necessary, restrain patient. Start with soft restraints but progress to leather restraints if the patient is threatening to self or staff. Communicate risk to other health care professionals, family, and significant others.

• Develop appropriate behavior expectations and consequences, given the patient's level of cognitive functioning and capacity for self-control.

NIC Substance Use Treatment: Alcohol Withdrawal; Substance Use Treatment: Overdose

ADDITIONAL NURSING DIAGNOSES

See nursing diagnoses and interventions in the following as appropriate: "Nutritional Support," p. 1; "Mechanical Ventilation," p. 17; "Hemodynamic Monitoring," p. 28; "Prolonged Immobility," p. 74; "Psychosocial Support," p. 83; "Psychosocial Support for the Patient's Family and Significant Others," p. 95; "Acute Respiratory Distress Syndrome," p. 229; "Acute Respiratory Failure," p. 243; "Acute Coronary Syndromes," p. 247; "Heart Failure/Pulmonary Edema," p. 265; "Cardiomyopathy," p. 272; "Dysrhythmias and Conduction Disturbances," p. 277; "Aortic Aneurysm/Dissection," p. 340; "Acute Renal Failure," p. 371; "Renal Replacement Therapies," p. 395; "Status Epilepticus," p. 441; "Hepatic Failure," p. 503; "Acute Pancreatitis," p. 536; "Fluid and Electrolyte Disturbances," p. 636; and "Acid-Base Imbalances," p. 670. In addition, see "Traumatic Brain Injury" for **Impaired corneal tissue integrity,** p. 132.

Fluid and electrolyte disturbances

The major constituent of the human body is water. The average male adult is approximately 60% water by weight, and the average female adult is 55% water by weight. Typically, body water decreases with both age and increasing body fat. Body water is distributed between two fluid compartments: approximately two-thirds is located within the cells (intracellular fluid [ICF]) and the remaining one-third is located outside the cells (extracellular fluid [ECF]). The ECF is further divided into *interstitial fluid,* which surrounds the cells; *intravascular fluid,* which is contained within blood

TABLE 10-9 Primary Constituents of Body Water Compartments*

Element	Intravascular	Interstitial	Intracellular (skeletal muscle cell)
Na^+	142 mEq/L	145 mEq/L	12 mEq/L
Cl^-	104 mEq/L	117 mEq/L	4 mEq/L
HCO_3^-	24 mEq/L	27 mEq/L	12 mEq/L
K^+	4.5 mEq/L	4.5 mEq/L	150 mEq/L
HPO_4^-	2 mEq/L	2 mEq/L	40 mEq/L

*This is a partial list. Other constituents include calcium (Ca^{++}), magnesium (Mg^{++}), and proteins.
Na^+, Sodium; Cl^-, chloride; HCO_3^-, bicarbonate; K^+, potassium; HPO_4^-, phosphate.

vessels; and *transcellular fluid*, the fluid produced by specialized cells (e.g., gastric secretions, cerebrospinal fluid [CSF], and pericardial fluid). The body gains water through oral intake, fluid therapy, and oxidative metabolism. Water is lost from the body via the kidneys, GI tract, skin, and lungs.

In addition to water, body fluids contain two types of dissolved substances: electrolytes and nonelectrolytes. *Electrolytes* are substances that dissociate in solution and will conduct an electrical current. They dissociate into positive and negative ions and are measured by their capacity to combine (milliequivalents/liter [mEq/L]) or by the molecular weight in milligrams (millimoles/liter [mmol/L]). *Nonelectrolytes* are substances, such as glucose and urea, that do not dissociate in solution and are measured by weight (milligrams per 100 milliliters, or mg/dl). The body fluid compartments are separated by a semipermeable membrane, which allows movement of these dissolved substances to occur. However, the unique composition of each compartment is maintained (Table 10-9).

The composition and concentration of ECF are regulated by a combination of renal, metabolic, and neurologic functions, providing an optimal bath for the body's cells. Although ECF is altered and then modified as the body reacts with its surrounding environment, ICF remains relatively stable, which is important for maintaining normal cellular function. Composition of ECF is determined by measuring the individual electrolytes and nonelectrolytes. Osmolality (i.e., the number of particles in solution) reflects the concentration. Two important mechanisms for maintaining volume and concentration of ECF are thirst and the release of antidiuretic hormone (ADH). ADH is released in response to a reduction in intravascular volume or an increase in extracellular osmolality. It acts on the kidney to increase urine concentration, thereby conserving water. Thirst is stimulated by similar changes in volume and osmolality.

Aldosterone is another important regulator of fluid volume. It is released by the adrenal cortex in response to an increased plasma renin level and acts on the kidney to conserve sodium and thus water and to increase potassium and hydrogen excretion. In contrast, atrial natriuretic peptide (ANP) is a hormone released by the cardiac atria in response to conditions that increase atrial pressure (e.g., acute volume expansion). ANP acts to reduce blood pressure and vascular volume by increasing excretion of sodium and water by the kidneys, by decreasing the release of aldosterone and ADH, and by direct vasodilation.

Fluid Disturbances

HYPOVOLEMIA
Pathophysiology
Depletion of ECF volume is termed *hypovolemia*. It occurs because of abnormal skin, GI, or renal losses; bleeding; decreased intake; or movement of fluid into a nonequilibrating third space. Depending on the type of fluid lost, hypovolemia may be accompanied by acid-base, osmolar, or electrolyte imbalances. Severe ECF volume depletion can lead to hypovolemic shock. Compensatory mechanisms in hypovolemia include increased sympathetic nervous system stimulation (increased HR, increased inotropy-cardiac contraction, increased vascular resistance), increased thirst, increased release of ADH, and increased release of aldosterone. Prolonged hypovolemia may lead to acute renal failure.

Hypovolemic shock develops when the intravascular volume decreases to the point that compensatory mechanisms cannot maintain adequate tissue perfusion and normal cellular function. Altered cellular metabolism results in acidosis, cardiac depression, intravascular coagulation, increased capillary permeability, and release of toxins. If shock is allowed to progress too long without treatment or with inadequate treatment, it may become irreversible and no amount of intervention will prevent death.

Assessment
History and risk factors
Abnormal GI losses: Vomiting, NG suctioning, diarrhea, intestinal drainage.
Abnormal skin losses: Excessive diaphoresis secondary to fever or exercise; burns.
Abnormal renal losses: Diuretic therapy, diabetes insipidus, renal disease (polyuric forms), adrenal insufficiency, osmotic diuresis (e.g., uncontrolled diabetes mellitus, post-dye study).
Third spacing or plasma-to-interstitial fluid shift: Peritonitis, intestinal obstruction, burns, ascites.
Hemorrhage: Major trauma, GI bleeding, obstetric complications.
Altered intake: Coma, fluid deprivation.
Clinical presentation: Dizziness, weakness, fatigue, syncope, anorexia, nausea, vomiting, thirst, confusion, constipation.
Physical assessment: Decreased BP, especially when standing (orthostatic hypotension); increased HR; decreased urine output; poor skin turgor; dry, furrowed tongue; dry mucous membranes; sunken eyeballs; flat neck veins; increased temperature; and acute weight loss (Table 10-10), except with third spacing.
Hemodynamic measurements: Decreased CVP, decreased PAP, decreased CO, decreased MAP, increased SVR.

TABLE 10-10   Weight Loss as an Indicator of ECF Deficit in the Adult

Acute weight loss	Severity of deficit
2%-5%	Mild
5%-10%	Moderate
10%-15%	Severe
15%-20%	Fatal

ECF, Extracellular fluid.

Diagnostic tests
BUN values: May be elevated because of dehydration, decreased renal perfusion, or decreased renal function. BUN/plasma creatinine ratio of >20:1 suggests hypovolemia.
Hct levels: Elevated with dehydration; decreased in the presence of bleeding, although not initially.
Serum electrolyte levels: Variable, depending on type of fluid lost. Hypokalemia often occurs with abnormal GI or renal losses. Hyperkalemia occurs with adrenal insufficiency. Hypernatremia may be seen with increased insensible or sweat losses and diabetes insipidus. Hyponatremia occurs in most types of hypovolemia because of increased thirst and ADH release, which lead to increased water intake and retention, thus diluting the serum sodium. (See individual electrolyte imbalances, p. 670.)
Serum total CO_2 (also known as CO_2 content): Decreased with metabolic acidosis and increased with metabolic alkalosis (see "ABG values," p. 671).
ABG values: Metabolic acidosis (pH <7.35 and HCO_3^- <22 mEq/L) may occur with lower GI losses, shock, or diabetic ketoacidosis. Metabolic alkalosis (pH >7.45 and HCO_3^- >26 mEq/L) may occur with upper GI losses and diuretic therapy.
Urine specific gravity: Increased because of kidneys' attempt to conserve water; may be fixed at approximately 1.010 in the presence of renal disease.
Urine sodium: Demonstrates kidneys' ability to conserve sodium in response to an increased aldosterone level. In the absence of renal disease, osmotic diuresis, or diuretic therapy, value should be <20 mEq/L.
Serum osmolality: Variable, depending on the type of fluid lost and the body's ability to compensate with thirst and ADH.
Urine osmolality: Indicates kidneys' ability to produce a concentrated urine. Level should be increased as the kidneys attempt to conserve water, usually >450 mOsm/kg.

Collaborative management
Restoration of normal fluid volume and correction of acid-base and electrolyte disturbances: The type of fluid replacement depends on the type of fluid lost and the severity of the deficit, serum electrolytes, serum osmolality, and acid-base status. Fluid should be administered at a rate that will induce positive fluid balance (e.g., 50-100 ml *in excess* of the sum of all hourly losses).
Isotonic saline: Expands ECF only; does not enter ICF. Appropriate for rapid volume replacement, especially in shock.
Hypotonic saline solutions: Expand the ECF and provide some free water to the cells. Useful in the management of the patient who is both volume depleted and hyperosmolar (e.g., hypernatremia or hyperglycemia).
Dextrose and water: Provides free water only and will be distributed evenly through both ICF and ECF; used to treat water deficit.
Mixed saline/electrolyte solutions: Provide additional electrolytes (e.g., potassium and calcium) and a buffer (lactate or acetate).
Blood and albumin: Expand only the intravascular portion of the ECF.
Dextran or hetastarch: Colloid solutions that expand the intravascular portion of the ECF.
Restoration of tissue perfusion (hypovolemic shock): Treatment includes rapid volume replacement with crystalloids. Generally, fluid may be given rapidly as long as cardiac filling pressures and BP remain low. Overaggressive fluid resuscitation in uncontrolled hemorrhage is avoided, because there is an increased risk of secondary hemorrhage as the intravascular hydrostatic pressure increases. The use of colloids (e.g., albumin) to prevent the development of pulmonary edema secondary to rapid volume replacement remains controversial. Blood is administered only as necessary to maintain

oxygen-carrying capacity. Hct should not be raised >35%. Vasopressors may be used to augment volume restoration if endotoxic, anaphylactic, or neurogenic shock is also present.
Treatment of underlying cause.

Nursing diagnoses and interventions

Fluid volume deficit related to abnormal loss of body fluids; reduced intake
Desired outcome: Within 24 h of initiation of fluid therapy, patient becomes normovolemic as evidenced by urine output ≥0.5 ml/kg/h; specific gravity 1.010-1.030; stable weight; no clinical evidence of hypovolemia (e.g., furrowed tongue); BP within patient's normal range; CVP 2-6 mm Hg; PAP 20-30/8-15 mm Hg; CO 4-7 L/min; MAP 70-105 mm Hg; HR 60-100 bpm; and SVR 900-1200 dynes/sec/cm^{-5}.

- Monitor I&O hourly. Initially, intake should exceed output during therapy. Consult physician for urine output <0.5 ml/kg/h for 2 consecutive hours. Measure urine specific gravity q4h as available. Normal range is 1.010-1.030. Expect it to decrease with therapy.
- Monitor VS and hemodynamic pressures for signs of continued hypovolemia. Be alert to decreased BP, CVP, PAP, CO, and MAP and to increased HR and SVR.
- Place patient who is in shock in a supine position with the legs elevated to 45 degrees to increase venous return. Avoid Trendelenburg position because it causes abdominal viscera to press on the diaphragm, thereby impairing ventilation.
- Weigh patient daily. Daily weight measurements are the single most important indicator of fluid status, because acute weight changes usually indicate fluid changes. For example, in the individual who is being fed, a decrease in daily weight of 1 kg is equal to the loss of 1 L of fluid. The adult who is not eating or receiving any enteral or parenteral nutrition will lose 0.25 kg of weight daily because of actual loss of body tissue. Weigh patient at the same time of day (preferably before breakfast) on a balanced scale, with patient wearing approximately the same clothing. Document type of scale used (i.e., standing, bed, chair).
- Administer PO and IV fluids as prescribed. Ensure adequate intake, especially in an older adult because of the increased risk of volume depletion in this population. Document response to fluid therapy. Monitor for signs and symptoms of fluid overload or too-rapid fluid administration: crackles (rales), SOB, tachypnea, tachycardia, increased CVP, increased PA pressures, neck vein distention, and edema. Ensure a patent IV access and availability of blood products if needed.
- Monitor patient for hidden fluid losses. For example, measure and document abdominal girth or limb size if indicated.
- Consult physician for decreases in Hct that may signal bleeding. Remember that Hct will decrease in the dehydrated patient as he or she becomes rehydrated. Decreases in Hct associated with rehydration may be accompanied by decreases in serum sodium and BUN values.
- Hypocalcemia may develop in rapidly transfused patients because of the citrate in stored blood. Monitor patient for sudden symptoms of hypocalcemia (see p. 654). As prescribed, administer 10 ml calcium chloride or gluconate for every 2 U of blood transfused.

You may also wish to refer to the following interventions from the Nursing Interventions Classification (NIC):
NIC Fluid Monitoring; Hypovolemia Management; Fluid Resuscitation; Intravenous (IV) Therapy; Invasive Hemodynamic Monitoring; Shock Management: Volume
Altered tissue perfusion: cerebral, renal, and peripheral, related to hypovolemia

Desired outcome: Within 12 h after initiation of therapy, patient has adequate perfusion as evidenced by alertness; warm and dry skin; BP within patient's normal range; HR ≤100 bpm; urinary output ≥0.5 ml/kg/h; and capillary refill <2 sec.

- Monitor for signs of decreased cerebral perfusion: vertigo, syncope, confusion, restlessness, anxiety, agitation, excitability, weakness, nausea, and cool, clammy skin. Consult physician for worsening symptoms. Document response to fluid therapy.
- Protect patients who are confused, dizzy, or weak. Keep side rails up and bed in lowest position with wheels locked. Assist with ambulation in step-down units. Raise patient to sitting or standing positions slowly. Monitor for indicators of orthostatic hypotension: decreased BP, increased HR, dizziness, and diaphoresis. If symptoms occur, return patient to supine position.
- To avoid unnecessary vasodilation, treat fevers promptly. Cover patient with a light blanket to maintain body temperature.
- Reassure patient and significant others that sensorium changes will improve with therapy.
- Evaluate capillary refill, noting whether it is brisk (<2 sec) or delayed (≥2 sec). Consult physician if refill is delayed.
- Palpate peripheral pulses bilaterally in arms and legs (radial, brachial, dorsalis pedis, posterior tibial). Use a Doppler ultrasonic device if unable to palpate pulses. Rate pulses on a 0-4+ scale. Consult physician if pulses are absent or barely palpable.

Note: Abnormal pulses also may be caused by a local vascular disorder.

- Consult physician for urinary output <0.5 ml/kg/h for 2 consecutive hours.

NIC Neurologic Monitoring; Circulatory Care

Additional nursing diagnoses
For additional nursing diagnoses, see specific medical disorder, electrolyte imbalance, or acid-base disturbance.

HYPERVOLEMIA
Pathophysiology
Expansion of ECF volume is termed *hypervolemia.* It occurs in four situations: (1) with excessive retention of sodium and water caused by a chronic renal stimulus to conserve sodium and water; (2) with abnormal renal functioning that involves reduced excretion of sodium and water; (3) with excessive administration of IV fluids; or (4) with interstitial-to-plasma fluid shift. Hypervolemia can lead to heart failure and pulmonary edema, especially in the patient with cardiovascular dysfunction.

Assessment
History and risk factors
Retention of sodium and water: Heart failure, hepatic failure, nephrotic syndrome, excessive administration of glucocorticosteroids.
Abnormal renal function: Acute or chronic renal failure with oliguria or anuria.
Excessive administration of IV fluids.
Interstitial-to-plasma fluid shift: Remobilization of fluid after treatment of burns, excessive administration of hypertonic solutions (e.g., mannitol, hypertonic saline) or colloid oncotic solutions (e.g., albumin).
Clinical presentation: SOB, orthopnea.
Physical assessment: Edema, weight gain, increased BP (decreased BP as the heart fails), bounding pulses, ascites, crackles, rhonchi, wheezes, distended neck veins, moist skin, tachycardia, gallop rhythm.

TABLE 10-11 Foods High in Sodium	
Bouillon	Olives
Celery	Pickles
Cheeses	Preserved meat
Dried fruits	Salad dressings and prepared sauces
Frozen, canned, or packaged foods	Sauerkraut
Monosodium glutamate (MSG)	Snack foods (e.g., crackers, chips, pretzels)
Mustard	Soy sauce

Hemodynamic measurements: Increased CVP, PAP, and PAWP. MAP is increased unless left heart failure is present.

Diagnostic tests
Laboratory findings are variable and usually nonspecific.
Hct levels: Decreased because of hemodilution.
BUN levels: Increased in renal failure.
ABG values: May reveal hypoxemia (decreased Pao_2) and alkalosis (increased pH and decreased $Paco_2$) in the presence of pulmonary edema. Respiratory acidosis (decreased $Paco_2$) may be present in severe pulmonary edema.
Serum sodium and serum osmolality: Will be decreased if hypervolemia occurs as a result of excessive retention of water (e.g., in chronic renal failure).
Urinary sodium: Elevated if the kidney is attempting to excrete excess sodium. Urinary sodium will not be elevated in conditions with secondary hyperaldosteronism (e.g., heart failure, cirrhosis, nephrotic syndrome) because hypervolemia occurs secondary to a chronic stimulus to the release of aldosterone.
Urine specific gravity: Decreased if the kidney is attempting to excrete excess volume. May be fixed at 1.010 in acute renal failure.
Chest x-ray: May reveal signs of pulmonary vascular congestion.

Collaborative management
The goal of therapy is to treat the precipitating problem and return ECF to normal. Treatment may include the following measures.
Restriction of sodium and water: Oral, enteral, or parenteral. Table 10-11 lists some common foods high in sodium.
Diuretics: May be given IV or PO. Loop diuretics (e.g., furosemide) are indicated in severe hypervolemia or renal failure.
Dialysis or continuous renal replacement therapy: In renal failure or life-threatening fluid overload (see "Renal Replacement Therapies," p. 395).

Note: Also see specific discussions under "Burns," p. 193; "Acute Respiratory Distress Syndrome," p. 229; and "Acute Renal Failure," p. 371.

Nursing diagnoses and interventions
Fluid volume excess related to excessive fluid intake; excessive sodium intake; compromised regulatory mechanism
Desired outcome: Within 24 h after initiation of treatment, patient becomes normovolemic as evidenced by absence of edema; BP within patient's normal range; HR 60-100 bpm; CVP 2-6 mm Hg; PAP 20-30/8-15 mm Hg; MAP 70-105 mm Hg; and CO 4-7 L/min.
- Monitor I&O hourly. With the exception of oliguric renal failure, urine output should be ≥0.5 ml/kg/h. Measure urine specific gravity q4h. If patient is receiving diuretic therapy, specific gravity should be <1.010-1.020.

- Observe for and document presence of edema (pretibial, sacral, periorbital); rate pitting on a 0-4+ scale.
- Weigh patient daily. Daily weight measurements are the single most important indicator of fluid status. For example, a 2-kg acute weight gain is usually indicative of a 2-L fluid gain. Weigh patient at the same time each day (preferably before breakfast) on a balanced scale, with patient wearing approximately the same clothing. Document type of scale used (i.e., standing, bed, chair).
- Limit oral, enteral, and parenteral sodium intake as prescribed. Be aware that medications may contain sodium (e.g., penicillins, bicarbonate). See Table 10-11 for some foods high in sodium.
- Limit fluids as prescribed. Offer a portion of allotted fluids as ice chips to minimize patient's thirst. Teach patient and significant others the importance of fluid restriction and how to measure fluid volume.
- Provide oral hygiene at frequent intervals to keep oral mucous membrane moist and intact.
- Document response to diuretic therapy (e.g., increased urine output, decreased CVP/PAP, decreased adventitious breath sounds, decreased edema). Many diuretics (e.g., furosemide, thiazides) cause hypokalemia. Observe for indicators of hypokalemia: muscle weakness, dysrhythmias (especially PVCs and ECG changes such as flattened T wave, presence of U waves). See "Hypokalemia," p. 649. Potassium-sparing diuretics (e.g., spironolactone, triamterene) may cause hyperkalemia: weakness, ECG changes (e.g., peaked T wave, prolonged PR interval, widened QRS complex). See "Hyperkalemia," p. 651. Consult physician for significant findings.
- Observe for physical indicators of overcorrection and dangerous volume depletion secondary to therapy: vertigo, weakness, syncope, thirst, confusion, poor skin turgor, flat neck veins, acute weight loss. Monitor VS and hemodynamic parameters for signs of volume depletion occurring with therapy: decreased BP, CVP, PAP, MAP, and CO; increased HR. Consult physician for significant changes or findings.
- Monitor appropriate laboratory tests (e.g., BUN and creatinine in renal failure). Consult physician for abnormal trends.

NIC Fluid Monitoring; Hypervolemia Management; Fluid/Electrolyte Management; Invasive Hemodynamic Monitoring; Hemodialysis Therapy

Impaired gas exchange (or risk for same) related to alveolar-capillary membrane changes secondary to pulmonary vascular congestion occurring with ECF expansion

Desired outcomes: Within 12 h of initiation of treatment, patient has adequate gas exchange as evidenced by RR ≤20 breaths/min with normal depth and pattern (eupnea); HR ≤100 bpm; Pao_2 ≥80 mm Hg; pH 7.35-7.45; $Paco_2$ 35-45 mm Hg; and Spo_2 ≥92%. Patient does not exhibit crackles, gallops, or other clinical indicators of pulmonary edema. PAP is ≤30/15 mm Hg and PAWP is ≤12 mm Hg.

- Acute pulmonary edema is a potentially life-threatening complication of hypervolemia. Monitor patient for indicators of pulmonary edema, including air hunger, anxiety, cough with production of frothy sputum, crackles, rhonchi, tachypnea, tachycardia, gallop rhythm, and elevation of PAP and PAWP. As prescribed, administer diuretics such as furosemide or other medications that reduce venous return to the heart.
- Monitor ABG values for evidence of hypoxemia (decreased Pao_2) and respiratory alkalosis (increased pH and decreased $Paco_2$). As available, monitor Spo_2 for oxygen saturation levels. Administer oxygen as prescribed to maintain Spo_2 at ≥92%. Increased oxygen requirements may indicate increasing pulmonary vascular congestion.
- Keep patient in semi-Fowler's position or position of comfort to minimize dyspnea. Avoid restrictive clothing.

NIC Respiratory Monitoring

Impaired skin and tissue integrity (or risk for same) related to edema secondary to fluid volume excess

Desired outcome: Patient's skin and tissue remain intact.

- Assess and document circulation to extremities at least each shift. Note color, temperature, capillary refill, and peripheral pulses. Determine whether capillary refill is brisk (<2 sec) or delayed (≥2 sec). Palpate peripheral pulses bilaterally in arms and legs (radial, brachial, dorsalis pedis, posterior tibial). Use Doppler device if unable to palpate pulses. Consult physician if capillary refill is delayed or if pulses are diminished or absent.
- Turn and reposition patient at least q2h to minimize tissue pressure.
- Check tissue areas at risk with each position change (e.g., heels, sacrum, other areas over bony prominences).
- Use pressure-relief mattress as indicated.
- Support arms and hands on pillows and elevate legs to decrease dependent edema. Do not elevate legs in the presence of pulmonary congestion.
- Treat pressure ulcers with occlusive dressings (e.g., Duoderm, Op-Site, Tegaderm) per unit protocol. Consult physician if sores, ulcers, or other areas of tissue breakdown are present in patients who are at increased risk for infection (e.g., individuals with diabetes mellitus or renal failure; those who are immunosuppressed).
- Consult a skin/wound care nurse specialist, as available, for advanced tissue breakdown or any alteration in tissue integrity in high-risk patients (e.g., advanced age, debilitation).

NIC Circulatory Care; Skin Surveillance

ELECTROLYTE DISTURBANCES

SODIUM IMBALANCE

Sodium plays a vital role in maintaining concentration and volume of ECF. It is the main cation of ECF and the major determinant of ECF osmolality. Under normal conditions ECF osmolality can be estimated by doubling the serum sodium value. Sodium imbalances usually are associated with parallel changes in osmolality. Sodium also is important in maintaining irritability and conduction of nerve and muscle tissue and assisting in the maintenance of acid-base balance.

Sodium concentration is maintained via regulation of water intake and excretion. If serum sodium concentration is decreased (hyponatremia), the kidneys respond by excreting water. Conversely, if serum sodium concentration is increased (hypernatremia), serum osmolality increases, stimulating the thirst center and causing an increased release of ADH by the posterior pituitary gland. ADH acts on the kidneys to conserve water. The adrenal cortical hormone, aldosterone, is an important regulator of sodium and ECF volume. The release of aldosterone causes the kidneys to conserve sodium and thus water, thereby increasing ECF volume. Because changes in serum sodium levels typically reflect changes in water balance, gains or losses of total body sodium are not necessarily reflected by the serum sodium level. Normal serum sodium is 137-147 mEq/L.

HYPONATREMIA

Pathophysiology

Hyponatremia (serum sodium <137 mEq/L) can occur because of a net gain of water or a loss of sodium-rich fluids that are replaced by water. Clinical indicators and treatment depend on the cause of the hyponatremia and whether it is associated with a normal, decreased, or increased ECF volume. For more information, see "Burns," p. 193; "Heart Failure," p. 265; "Acute Renal Failure," p. 371; and "Syndrome of Inappropriate Antidiuretic Hormone (SIADH)," p. 484.

Assessment
History and risk factors
Decreased ECF volume
- GI losses: Diarrhea, vomiting, fistulas, NG suction.
- Renal losses: Diuretics, salt-wasting kidney disease, adrenal insufficiency.
- Skin losses: Burns, wound drainage.

Normal/increased ECF volume
- Hypothyroidism or syndrome of inappropriate antidiuretic hormone (SIADH).
- Edematous states: Heart failure, cirrhosis, nephrotic syndrome.
- Excessive administration of hypotonic IV fluids or excessively dilute enteral feedings.
- Oliguric renal failure.
- Primary polydipsia.
- Any patient with impaired ability to excrete free water (e.g., thiazide diuretics) is at risk for hyponatremia if given hypotonic fluids.

> **Note:** Hyperlipidemia, hyperproteinemia, and hyperglycemia may cause a pseudohyponatremia. Hyperlipidemia and hyperproteinemia reduce the total percentage of plasma that is water. The sodium-to-water ratio of the plasma does not change, but the amount of sodium in plasma is reduced. With hyperglycemia the osmotic action of the elevated glucose causes a shift of water out of the cells and into the ECF, thus diluting the existing sodium. For every 100 mg/dl that glucose is elevated, sodium is diluted by 1.6 mEq/L.

Clinical presentation: Neurologic symptoms usually do not occur until the serum sodium level has dropped to approximately 120-125 mEq/L, and they are more likely to develop with a sudden decrease than with a gradual decrease. Seizures, coma, and permanent neurologic damage may occur when the plasma sodium level is <115 mEq/L.
Hyponatremia with decreased ECF volume: Irritability, apprehension, dizziness, personality changes, poor skin turgor, postural hypotension, dry mucous membranes, cold and clammy skin, tremors, seizures, coma.
Hyponatremia with normal or increased ECF volume: Headache, lassitude, apathy, confusion, weakness, edema, weight gain, elevated BP, hyperreflexia, muscle spasms, convulsions, coma.
Hemodynamic measurements
Decreased ECF volume: Evidence of hypovolemia, including decreased CVP, PAP, CO, MAP; increased SVR.
Increased ECF volume: Evidence of hypervolemia, including increased CVP, PAP, MAP.

Diagnostic tests
Serum sodium: Will be <137 mEq/L.
Serum osmolality: Decreased, except in cases of pseudohyponatremia.
Urine specific osmolality: Usually >100 mOsm/kg H_2O but less than the plasma level. In SIADH the urine will be inappropriately concentrated.
Urine sodium: Decreased (usually <20 mEq/L) except in SIADH, salt-wasting kidney disease, and adrenal insufficiency.

Collaborative management
The goals of therapy are to raise the serum sodium at a safe rate, correct any volume abnormality, and treat the underlying cause. The presence of acute symptomatic hyponatremia requires more aggressive treatment than chronic, asymptomatic hyponatremia. Overly rapid correction of chronic hyponatremia may result in permanent neurologic damage.

Hyponatremia with reduced ECF volume

Replacement of sodium and fluid losses: Adequate replacement of fluid volume is essential to *turn off* the physiologic stimulus to ADH release and enable the kidneys to restore the balance between sodium and water.

Replacement of other electrolyte losses: For example, potassium, bicarbonate.

IV hypertonic saline: If serum sodium is dangerously low or the patient has extreme symptoms. The goal is to give enough 3% NaCl to correct symptoms—*not* to return the sodium level to normal.

Hyponatremia with expanded ECF volume

Removal or treatment of underlying cause.

Diuretics.

Water restriction: Restricting fluid intake to 1000 ml/day will establish negative water balance and increase serum sodium levels in most adults.

> **Note:**   See "Syndrome of Inappropriate Antidiuretic Hormone," p. 484, for specific treatment.

Nursing diagnoses and interventions

Fluid volume deficit related to active fluid loss; excessive intake of hypotonic solutions; compromised regulatory mechanisms

Desired outcome: Within 24 h of initiating treatment, patient becomes normovolemic as evidenced by HR 60-100 bpm; RR 12-20 breaths/min; BP within patient's normal range; CVP 2-6 mm Hg; and PAP 20-30/ 8-15 mm Hg.

- If patient is receiving hypertonic saline, assess carefully for signs of intravascular fluid overload: tachypnea, tachycardia, SOB, crackles (rales), rhonchi, increased CVP, increased PAP, gallop rhythm, and increased BP.
- For other interventions, see "Hypovolemia," p. 638, for **Fluid volume deficit.**

NIC Fluid Monitoring; Electrolyte Management: Hyponatremia; Fluid/Electrolyte Management; Intravenous (IV) Therapy; Invasive Hemodynamic Monitoring

Altered protection related to neurosensory alterations secondary to sodium level <120-125 mEq/L

Desired outcomes: Within 48 h of treatment, patient verbalizes orientation to time, place, and person and does not exhibit signs of physical injury caused by altered sensorium. Serum sodium level increases to >125 mEq/L in the first 48 h after treatment.

- Assess and document LOC, orientation, and neurologic status with each VS check. Reorient patient as necessary. Consult physician for significant changes.
- Inform patient and significant others that altered sensorium is temporary and will improve with treatment.
- Keep side rails up and bed in lowest position with wheels locked.
- Use reality therapy, such as clocks, calendars, and familiar objects; keep these items at the bedside within patient's visual field.
- If seizures are expected, pad side rails and keep an appropriate-size airway at the bedside.
- Monitor serum sodium levels closely. Permanent neurologic damage may occur with untreated, severely symptomatic hyponatremia secondary to cerebral edema. However, overly aggressive or inappropriate treatment of hyponatremia can also cause permanent neurologic damage secondary to osmotic demyelination syndrome. Initially, sodium levels should not increase at a level >0.5-1.0 mEq/L/h in patients being treated for symptomatic hyponatremia with hypertonic NaCl. After an initial 6-8 mEq/L increase in the serum sodium level, the rate of increase should not be >0.5 mEq/L/h. As well, levels should not increase at an average rate of >0.5 mEq/L/h in patients without symptoms. The overall increase during the first 24 h of treatment should not exceed 12 mEq/L.

NIC Neurologic Monitoring; Electrolyte Management: Hyponatremia; Seizure Precautions

HYPERNATREMIA

Pathophysiology

Hypernatremia (serum sodium level >147 mEq/L) may occur with water loss or sodium gain. Because sodium is the major determinant of ECF osmolality, hypernatremia always causes hypertonicity. In turn, hypertonicity causes a shift of water out of the cells, which leads to cellular dehydration and increased extracellular fluid volume.

Assessment

History and risk factors

Sodium gain: IV administration of hypertonic saline or sodium bicarbonate, increased oral intake, primary aldosteronism, drugs such as sodium polystyrene sulfonate (Kayexalate).

Water loss: Increased diaphoresis, respiratory infection, mechanical ventilation, diabetes insipidus, osmotic diuresis (e.g., hyperglycemia), osmotic diarrhea.

Clinical presentation: Intense thirst, fatigue, restlessness, agitation, coma. Symptoms of hypernatremia occur only in individuals who do not have access to water or who have an altered thirst mechanism (e.g., infants, older adults, those who are comatose).

> **Note:** Symptoms are most likely to develop with a sudden increase in plasma sodium. After approximately 24 h, brain cells adjust to ECF hypertonicity by increasing intracellular osmolality. The exact mechanism by which this occurs is unclear, but it is known that this increased osmolality helps to rehydrate the cells. Thus individuals with chronic hypernatremia may exhibit few symptoms. This adaptive mechanism has great significance in the treatment of hypernatremia. If the plasma sodium is reduced too quickly via administration of water, there will be a rapid and dramatic movement of water into the cells because of increased osmolality, which will cause dangerous cerebral edema.

Physical assessment: Low-grade fever, flushed skin, peripheral and pulmonary edema (sodium gain); postural hypotension (water loss)—usually mild.

Hemodynamic measurement: Variable.

Sodium excess: Increased CVP and PAP.

Water loss: Decreased CVP and PAP, although these changes may be minimized by the extracellular shift of fluid that occurs with hypernatremia.

Diagnostic tests

Serum sodium: Will be >147 mEq/L.

Serum osmolality: Increased because of elevated serum sodium.

Urine specific gravity: Increased because of kidneys' attempt to retain water; will be decreased in diabetes insipidus and osmotic diuresis (e.g., hyperglycemia).

Collaborative management

IV or oral water replacement: For water loss. If sodium is >160 mEq/L, IV D_5W or hypotonic saline is given to replace pure water deficit. (See "Diabetes Insipidus," p. 479, for specific treatment.)

Diuretics and oral or IV water replacement: For sodium gain.

> **Note:** Hypernatremia is corrected slowly, over approximately 2 days, to avoid too great a shift of water into brain cells.

Nursing diagnoses and interventions

Altered protection related to neurosensory alterations secondary to primary hypernatremia or cerebral edema occurring with too-rapid correction of hypernatremia

Desired outcomes: Within 48 h after treatment, patient verbalizes orientation to time, place, and person and does not exhibit evidence of injury caused by altered sensorium or seizures. Serum sodium level is ≤147 mEq/L.

- Cerebral edema may occur if hypernatremia is corrected too rapidly. Monitor serial serum sodium levels (sodium should not decrease at a rate greater than 0.5-1.0 mEq/L/hr); consult physician for rapid decreases.
- Assess patient for indicators of cerebral edema: lethargy, headache, nausea, vomiting, increased BP, widening pulse pressure, decreased HR, altered sensorium, and seizures.
- Assess and document LOC, orientation, and neurologic status with each VS check. Reorient patient as necessary. Consult physician for significant changes.
- Inform patient and significant others that altered sensorium is temporary and will improve with treatment.
- Keep side rails up and bed in lowest position with wheels locked.
- Use reality therapy, such as clocks, calendars, and familiar objects; keep these items at the bedside within patient's visual field.
- If seizures are anticipated, pad side rails and keep an airway at the bedside.
- Provide comfort measure to decrease thirst.

NIC Neurologic Monitoring; Electrolyte Management: Hypernatremia; Seizure Precautions

Additional nursing diagnoses

See "Hypovolemia," p. 638, for **Fluid volume deficit;** and "Hypervolemia," p. 641, for **Fluid volume excess.**

POTASSIUM IMBALANCE

Potassium is the primary intracellular cation, and thus it plays a vital role in cell metabolism. Because it affects the resting membrane potential of nerve and cardiac cells, abnormal serum potassium levels adversely affect neuromuscular and cardiac function. A relatively small amount of potassium is located within the ECF and is maintained within a narrow range. The vast majority of the body's potassium is located within the cells. Distribution of potassium between ECF and ICF is maintained by the sodium-potassium pump located in the membrane of all body cells and is affected by ECF pH, glucose and protein metabolism, insulin levels, and stimulation of β_2-adrenergic receptors. Acute changes in serum pH are accompanied by reciprocal changes in serum potassium concentration.

The body gains potassium through foods (primarily meats, fruits, and vegetables) and medications. In addition, ECF gains potassium any time there is a breakdown of cells or movement of potassium out of the cell. Because the kidneys are the primary regulators of potassium balance, an elevated serum potassium level usually does not occur unless there is a reduction in renal function. Potassium is lost from the body through the kidneys, GI tract, and skin. Potassium also may be lost from ECF because of an intracellular shift. Normal serum potassium level is 3.5-5 mEq/L.

Note: Disorders of potassium balance are potentially life threatening because of the effects of altered potassium levels on neuromuscular and cardiac function. Suspected alterations in potassium balance require prompt consultation with physician.

HYPOKALEMIA

Pathophysiology

Hypokalemia (serum potassium level <3.5 mEq/L) occurs because of a loss of potassium from the body or a movement of potassium into the cells.

Note: Changes in serum potassium levels reflect changes in ECF potassium—not necessarily changes in total body levels.

Assessment

History and risk factors

Reduction in total body potassium

- Hyperaldosteronism.
- Diuretic therapy or abnormal urinary losses (e.g., hypomagnesemia).
- Increased GI losses.
- Increased loss through diaphoresis.
- Decreased intake.
- Dialysis.

Note: A poorly balanced or inadequate diet may contribute to, but rarely will cause, hypokalemia because significant amounts of potassium are contained in a variety of foods. Hypokalemia may develop, however, in individuals who are maintained on parenteral fluid therapy with inadequate replacement of potassium or when reduced intake is combined with increased losses.

Intracellular shift

- Increased insulin (e.g., from TPN or treatment of diabetic ketoacidosis [DKA]).
- Acute alkalosis.

Stress: Any condition causing physical or emotional stress may result in hypokalemia because of increased loss of potassium in the urine secondary to increased release of aldosterone; or an intracellular shift of potassium secondary to increased stimulation of β_2-adrenergic receptors.

Clinical presentation: Muscle weakness and cramps, soft and flabby muscles, nausea, vomiting, ileus, paresthesias, enhanced digitalis effect.

Physical assessment: Decreased bowel sounds, weak and irregular pulse, decreased reflexes, and decreased muscle tone.

ECG findings: Because of the effects of hypokalemia on the shape and slope of the action potential, the heart muscle is slow to return to its fully resting or repolarized state. During this slow return to resting, weak impulses from an irritable myocardium may initiate abnormal beats. Dangerous ventricular tachycardia may develop in severe hypokalemia.

Diagnostic tests

Serum potassium levels: Values will be <3.5 mEq/L.

ABG values: May show metabolic alkalosis (increased pH and HCO_3^-) because hypokalemia usually is associated with this condition. Hypokalemia also may be associated with metabolic acidosis (e.g., DKA, diarrhea, renal tubular acidosis).

ECG findings: ST-segment depression, flattened T wave, presence of U wave, ventricular dysrhythmias. With severe hypokalemia there will be increased amplitude of the P wave, prolonged PR interval, and widening of the QRS complex.

Note: Hypokalemia potentiates the effect of digitalis. ECG may reveal signs of digitalis toxicity in spite of a normal serum digitalis level.

Collaborative management
Treatment of underlying cause.
Replacement of potassium: Accomplished either PO (via increased dietary intake or medication) or IV, with the usual dosage 40-80 mEq/L/day in divided doses. IV potassium is necessary if hypokalemia is severe or if the patient is unable to take potassium orally. Potassium is *never* administered by IV push. It *must* be appropriately diluted and administered at rates ≤10-20 mEq/h or in concentrations ≤30-40 mEq/L (when added to IV solutions) unless hypokalemia is severe. Too-rapid administration can result in life-threatening hyperkalemia. If potassium is administered via a peripheral line, the rate of administration may require reduction to prevent irritation of vessels. Patients receiving 10-20 mEq/h should be on a continuous cardiac monitor. The development of peaked T waves suggests the presence of hyperkalemia and requires immediate consultation with a physician. IV potassium may be administered as potassium chloride or potassium phosphate. Table 10-12 lists some foods high in potassium.
Potassium-sparing diuretics: May be given in place of oral potassium supplements.

Nursing diagnoses and interventions
Decreased cardiac output (or risk for same) related to altered conduction secondary to hypokalemia or too-rapid correction of hypokalemia, with resulting hyperkalemia
Desired outcome: Within 2 h of treatment, patient has adequate cardiac conduction as evidenced by normal T-wave configuration and normal sinus rhythm without ectopy on ECG.

- Administer potassium supplement as prescribed. Avoid giving IV potassium chloride at a rate faster than recommended, inasmuch as this can lead to life-threatening hyperkalemia. Potassium supplementation for symptomatic hypokalemia usually is given in isotonic saline because D_5W will increase insulin-induced intracellular shift of potassium. Concentrated solutions of potassium may be administered in limited volumes (e.g., 20 mEq in 100 ml of isotonic NaCl), but it should be administered no more rapidly than 20 mEq/h. Concentrated solutions and infusion rates of >10 mEq/h are used only with severe hypokalemia. Do not add potassium chloride to IV solution containers in the hanging position, because this can cause layering of the medication. Instead, invert the solution container before adding the medication and mix well.
- Be aware that IV potassium chloride can cause local irritation of veins and chemical phlebitis. Assess IV insertion site for erythema, heat, or pain. Alert

TABLE 10-12 Foods High in Potassium	
Apricots	Nuts
Artichokes	Oranges, orange juice
Avocados	Peanuts
Bananas	Potatoes
Cantaloupes	Prune juice
Carrots	Pumpkins
Cauliflower	Spinach
Chocolate	Swiss chard
Dried beans, peas	Sweet potatoes
Dried fruit	Tomatoes, tomato juice, tomato sauce
Mushrooms	

physician to symptoms. Irritation may be relieved by applying an ice bag, giving mild sedation, or numbing insertion site with a small amount of local anesthetic. Phlebitis may necessitate changing of IV site. Oral supplements may cause GI irritation. Administer with a full glass of water or fruit juice; encourage patient to sip slowly. Consult physician for symptoms of abdominal pain, distention, nausea, or vomiting. Do not switch potassium supplements without physician prescription.

- Monitor I&O hourly. Consult physician for urine output <0.5 ml/kg/h. Unless severe symptoms of hypokalemia are present, potassium supplements should not be given if the patient has an inadequate urine output because hyperkalemia can develop rapidly in patients with oliguria (<15-20 ml/h). Increased urine output increases the risk of hypokalemia.
- Physical indicators of abnormal potassium levels are difficult to identify in the patient who is critically ill. Monitor ECG for signs of continuing hypokalemia (ST-segment depression, flattened T wave, presence of U wave, ventricular dysrhythmias) or hyperkalemia (tall, thin T waves; prolonged PR interval; ST depression; widened QRS complex; loss of P wave), which may develop during potassium replacement.
- Monitor serum potassium levels carefully, especially in individuals at risk for hypokalemia, such as patients taking diuretics or undergoing gastric suction.
- Administer potassium cautiously in patients receiving potassium-sparing diuretics (e.g., spironolactone or triamterene) or angiotensin-converting enzyme (ACE) inhibitors (e.g., captopril) because of the potential for the development of hyperkalemia.
- Because hypokalemia can potentiate the effects of digitalis, monitor patients receiving digitalis for signs of increased digitalis effect: multifocal or bigeminal PVCs, paroxysmal atrial tachycardia with varying AV block, and other heart blocks.

NIC Electrolyte Management: Hypokalemia; Medication Administration; Dysrhythmia Management

Ineffective breathing pattern (or risk for same) related to weakness or paralysis of respiratory muscles secondary to sudden, *severe* hypokalemia (potassium <2-2.5 mEq/L)

Desired outcome: Within 2 h of treatment, patient has effective breathing pattern as evidenced by normal respiratory depth and pattern (eupnea) and rate of 12-20 breaths/min.

- If patient is exhibiting signs of worsening hypokalemia, be aware that severe hypokalemia can lead to weakness of respiratory muscles, resulting in shallow respirations and eventually apnea and respiratory arrest. Assess character, rate, and depth of respirations. Consult physician promptly if respirations become rapid and shallow.
- Keep manual resuscitator at patient's bedside if severe hypokalemia is suspected.
- Reposition patient q2h to prevent stasis of secretions; suction airway as needed.
- Encourage deep breathing (and coughing if indicated) q2h in conscious patients.

NIC Respiratory Monitoring

HYPERKALEMIA

Pathophysiology

Hyperkalemia (serum potassium level >5 mEq/L) occurs because of an increased intake of potassium, a decreased urinary excretion of potassium, or sudden movement of potassium out of the cells.

Note: Changes in serum potassium levels reflect changes in ECF potassium—not necessarily changes in total body levels of potassium.

Assessment
History and risk factors
Inappropriately high intake of potassium: Usually, IV potassium delivery. Symptomatic hyperkalemia may develop when appropriate doses of IV potassium chloride (KCl) are administered too rapidly.
Decreased excretion of potassium
  • Renal disease, especially acute and chronic renal failure.
  • Potassium-sparing diuretics, ACE inhibitors.
  • Addison disease (hypoaldosteronism).
Movement of potassium out of the cells
  • Acidosis.
  • Insulin deficiency, particularly in dialysis patients.
  • Tissue catabolism (e.g., with fever, sepsis, trauma, surgery).
Clinical presentation: Irritability, abdominal cramping, diarrhea, ascending weakness, paresthesias.
Physical assessment: Irregular pulse and abdominal distention; cardiac standstill may occur at levels >8.5 mEq/L.

Diagnostic tests
Serum potassium: Will be >5 mEq/L.

> **Note:** Pseudohyperkalemia may occur with mechanical trauma during venipuncture or incorrect handling of the laboratory specimen. It is the result of potassium moving out of the cells during or after the blood specimen has been drawn.

ABG values: May show metabolic acidosis (decreased pH and HCO_3^-) because hyperkalemia often occurs with acidosis.
Diagnostic ECG: Progressive changes include tall, thin T waves; prolonged PR interval; ST depression; widened QRS complex; loss of P wave. Eventually, QRS complex becomes widened further and cardiac arrest occurs.

Collaborative management
The goal is to treat the underlying cause and return the serum potassium level to normal.
Subacute
Cation exchange resins (e.g., Kayexalate):   Given either orally or via retention enema to exchange sodium for potassium in the gut. Oral Kayexalate usually is combined with sorbitol to promote rapid transit through the gut and induce diarrhea and thus increase potassium loss in the bowels. The recommended rectal dose for adults is 30-50 g q6h.
Acute
IV calcium gluconate: To counteract the neuromuscular and cardiac effects of hyperkalemia. Serum potassium levels will remain elevated.
IV glucose and insulin: To shift potassium into the cells. This reduces serum potassium temporarily.
Sodium bicarbonate: To shift potassium into the cells. Reduces serum potassium temporarily.
β_2-*Adrenergic agonists (albuterol):*   To shift potassium into the cells. This reduces serum potassium temporarily.

> **Note:**   The effects of calcium, glucose and insulin, sodium bicarbonate, and β_2-adrenergic agonists are temporary, lasting only a few hours. Usually it is necessary to follow these medications with a therapy that removes potassium from the body (e.g., dialysis or administration of cation exchange resins).

Dialysis: For rapid removal of potassium from the body.

Nursing diagnoses and interventions

Decreased cardiac output (or risk for same) related to electrical factors (ventricular dysrhythmias) secondary to severe hyperkalemia or overcorrection of hyperkalemia, with resulting hypokalemia

Desired outcomes: Within 6 h after initiation of treatment, patient's cardiac output is adequate as evidenced by PAP 20-30/8-15 mm Hg; CVP ≤6 mm Hg; CO 4-7 L/min; HR ≤100 bpm; BP within patient's normal range; and absence of the clinical signs of heart failure or pulmonary edema (e.g., crackles, SOB). ECG shows normal sinus rhythm without ectopy or other electrical disturbances. Serum potassium levels are within normal range (3.5-5 mEq/L).

- Monitor I&O. Consult physician for urine output <0.5 ml/kg/h. Oliguria increases the risk for development of hyperkalemia.
- Monitor for indicators of hyperkalemia (e.g., irritability, anxiety, abdominal cramping, diarrhea, ascending weakness, paresthesias, irregular pulse). Also be alert to indicators of hypokalemia (e.g., muscle weakness and cramps, nausea, vomiting, decreased bowel sounds, paresthesias, weak and irregular pulse) after treatment. Assess for hidden sources of potassium: medications (e.g., potassium penicillin G), banked blood, salt substitute, GI bleeding, or conditions that cause increased catabolism such as infection or trauma.
- Monitor serum potassium levels, especially in patients at risk for hyperkalemia such as persons with renal failure. Consult physician for levels above or below normal range. Monitor other laboratory values that may affect potassium levels (e.g., BUN, creatinine, ABGs, glucose).
- Physical indicators of abnormal potassium levels are difficult to identify in a patient who is critically ill. Monitor ECG for signs of hypokalemia (ST-segment depression, flattened T waves, presence of U wave, ventricular dysrhythmias), which may result from therapy, or continuing hyperkalemia (tall, thin T waves, prolonged PR interval, ST depression, widened QRS complex, loss of P wave). Consult physician *stat* if ECG changes occur.
- Administer insulin and glucose in the order prescribed. When glucose is administered first, it stimulates endogenous insulin release and may potentiate the potassium, lowering the effect of the exogenous insulin.
- Administer calcium gluconate as prescribed, giving it cautiously in patients receiving digitalis because digitalis toxicity can occur. Do not add calcium gluconate to solutions containing sodium bicarbonate because precipitates may form. For more information about calcium administration, see "Hypocalcemia," p. 654.
- If administering cation exchange resins by enema, encourage patient to retain the solution for at least 30-60 min to ensure therapeutic effects. Administer Kayexalate (without sorbitol) via a Foley catheter inserted into the rectum. The balloon is filled with sterile water to keep the catheter in place, and the catheter is clamped. Cleansing enemas are recommended before administration to enhance absorption and afterward to reduce the risk of bowel complications.

NIC Electrolyte Management: Hyperkalemia; Dysrhythmia Management; Hemodialysis Therapy

CALCIUM IMBALANCE

Calcium, one of the body's most abundant ions, primarily is combined with phosphorus to form the mineral salts of the bones and teeth. In addition, calcium exerts a sedative effect on nerve cells and has important intracellular functions, including development of the cardiac action potential and contraction of muscles. Only 1% of the body's calcium is contained within ECF, yet this concentration is regulated carefully by the hormones *parathyroid hormone (PTH)* and *calcitonin*. PTH is released by the parathyroid gland in response to a low serum calcium level. It increases resorption of bone (movement of calcium and phosphorus out of the bone); activates vitamin D, which increases the absorption of calcium from the GI tract; and stimulates the kidneys to conserve calcium and excrete phosphorus. Calcitonin is produced by the thyroid gland when serum calcium levels are elevated. It inhibits bone resorption.

Slightly less than half of the plasma calcium is free, ionized calcium. Approximately 40% is bound to protein, primarily to albumin. The remaining percentage is complexed (i.e., it is combined with nonprotein anions such as phosphate, citrate, and carbonate). Only the ionized calcium is physiologically important. The percentage of calcium that is ionized is affected by plasma pH and albumin level. Patients with alkalosis may show signs of hypocalcemia because of increased calcium binding. Changes in plasma albumin level will affect total serum calcium level without changing the level of ionized calcium.

HYPOCALCEMIA

Pathophysiology
Symptoms of hypocalcemia may occur because of a reduction of total body calcium or a reduction of the percentage of calcium that is ionized. Total calcium levels may be decreased because of increased calcium loss, reduced intake secondary to altered intestinal absorption, or altered regulation (e.g., hypoparathyroidism). Elevated phosphorus levels and decreased magnesium levels may precipitate hypocalcemia.

Assessment
History and risk factors
Decreased ionized calcium
- Alkalosis.
- Rapid administration of citrated blood. Citrate added to the blood to prevent clotting may bind with calcium, causing hypocalcemia.
- Hemodilution (e.g., occurring with volume replacement with normal saline after massive hemorrhage).

Increased calcium loss in body fluids: As with loop diuretics.
Decreased intestinal absorption
- Decreased intake.
- Impaired vitamin D metabolism.
- Chronic diarrhea.
- After gastrectomy.

Acute and chronic renal failure: See p. 371.
Hypoparathyroidism
Hyperphosphatemia: As in renal failure.
Hypomagnesemia: Caused by decreased action of PTH.
Acute pancreatitis: See p. 529.
Clinical presentation: Numbness with tingling of fingers and circumoral region, hyperactive reflexes, muscle cramps, tetany, convulsions. Alterations in mental status may include anxiety, depression, and frank psychosis. In chronic hypocalcemia, fractures may be present because of increased bone porosity. Sudden precipitous drops in plasma calcium levels may cause hypotension secondary to vasodilation and heart failure secondary to decreased myocardial contractility.
Physical assessment
Positive Trousseau sign: Ischemia-induced carpopedal spasm. It is elicited by applying a BP cuff to the upper arm and inflating it past systolic BP for 2 min.
Positive Chvostek sign: Unilateral contraction of facial and eyelid muscles. It is elicited by stimulating the facial nerve during percussion of the face just in front of the ear.
ECG changes: Prolonged QT interval caused by elongation of ST segment.

Diagnostic tests
Total serum calcium level: Will be <8.5 mg/dl. Serum calcium levels should be evaluated with serum albumin. For every 1 g/dl drop in the serum albumin level, there is a 0.8-1 mg/dl drop in total calcium level. This drop, however, has little impact on the ionized calcium level. Symptomatic hypocalcemia can occur with normal total calcium levels when there is a sudden rise in serum pH.
Ionized serum calcium level: Will be <4.5 mg/dl.
PTH level: Decreased levels occur in hypoparathyroidism; increased levels may occur with other causes of hypocalcemia. Normal range is 150-350 pg/ml (varies among laboratories).
Magnesium and phosphorus levels: May be checked to identify potential causes of hypocalcemia.

Collaborative management
Treatment of underlying cause.
Calcium replacement: Hypocalcemia is treated with PO or IV calcium. Tetany is treated with 10-20 ml of 10% calcium gluconate administered IV or by continuous drip of 100 ml of 10% calcium gluconate in 1000 ml D_5W, infused over at least 4-6 h. Magnesium replacement should be initiated in the individual with magnesium depletion, inasmuch as hypomagnesemia-induced hypocalcemia is often refractory to calcium therapy alone.
Vitamin D therapy (e.g., dihydrotachysterol, calcitriol): To increase calcium absorption from the GI tract.
Phosphorus-binding antacids: To reduce elevated phosphorus before treating hypocalcemia.

Nursing diagnoses and interventions
Altered protection (risk of tetany and seizures) related to neurosensory alterations secondary to severe hypocalcemia
Desired outcome: Patient does not exhibit evidence of injury caused by complications of severe hypocalcemia.
- Monitor patient for evidence of worsening hypocalcemia: numbness and tingling of fingers and circumoral region, hyperactive reflexes, and muscle cramps. Consult physician promptly if these symptoms develop because they occur before overt tetany. In addition, consult physician if patient has positive Trousseau or Chvostek sign because they also signal latent tetany. Monitor total and ionized calcium levels as available.
- Administer IV calcium with caution. IV calcium should not be given faster than 0.5-1 ml/min, inasmuch as rapid administration can cause hypotension. Observe IV insertion site for evidence of infiltration because calcium will slough tissue. Concentrated calcium solutions should be administered through a central line. Do not add calcium to solutions that contain sodium bicarbonate or sodium phosphate because dangerous precipitates will form. Digitalis toxicity may develop in patients taking digitalis because calcium potentiates its effects. Monitor patient for signs and symptoms of hypercalcemia: lethargy, confusion, irritability, nausea, and vomiting.

Note: Always clarify type of IV calcium to be given. Both calcium chloride and calcium gluconate come in 10-ml ampules. One ampule of calcium chloride contains 13.6 mEq of calcium, whereas one ampule of calcium gluconate contains 4.5 mEq of calcium.

- For patients with chronic hypocalcemia, administer oral calcium supplements and vitamin D preparations as prescribed. Administer oral calcium 30 min before meals or at bedtime for maximal absorption. Administer phosphorus-binding antacids with meals. If calcium carbonate is being administered primarily to bind phosphorus, administer with food.

- Consult physician if response to calcium therapy is ineffective. Tetany that does not respond to IV calcium may be caused by hypomagnesemia.
- Maintain seizure precautions for patients with symptoms; decrease environmental stimuli.
- Avoid hyperventilation in patients in whom hypocalcemia is suspected. Respiratory alkalosis may precipitate tetany because of increased pH with a reduction in ionized calcium.
- Monitor for calcium loss (e.g., with loop diuretics, renal tubular dysfunction) or conditions that place the patient at risk (e.g., acute pancreatitis).
- Inform patient and significant others that neuropsychiatric symptoms of hypocalcemia will improve with treatment.

NIC Neurologic Monitoring; Electrolyte Management: Hypocalcemia; Seizure Precautions; Medication Administration

Decreased cardiac output related to altered conduction or negative inotropy secondary to hypocalcemia or digitalis toxicity occurring with calcium replacement therapy

Desired outcomes: Within 12 h of initiation of treatment, patient's cardiac output is adequate as evidenced by PAP 20-30/8-15 mm Hg; CVP ≤6 mm Hg; CO 4-7 L/min; HR ≤100; BP within patient's normal range; and absence of the clinical signs of heart failure or pulmonary edema (e.g., crackles, SOB). ECG shows normal sinus rhythm without ectopy or other electrical disturbances.

- Monitor ECG for signs of worsening hypocalcemia (prolonged QT interval) or digitalis toxicity with calcium replacement: multifocal or bigeminal PVCs, paroxysmal atrial tachycardia with varying AV block, and other heart blocks.
- Hypocalcemia may decrease cardiac contractility. Monitor patient for signs of heart failure or pulmonary edema: crackles, rhonchi, SOB, decreased BP, increased HR, increased PAP, or increased CVP.

NIC Dysrhythmia Management; Cardiac Care

Ineffective breathing pattern related to laryngeal spasm occurring with severe hypocalcemia

Desired outcome: Within 1 h of initiation of treatment, patient has an effective breathing pattern as evidenced by eupnea; RR 12-20 breaths/min; and absence of the indicators of laryngeal spasm: laryngeal stridor, dyspnea, or crowing.

- Assess patient's respiratory rate, character, and rhythm. Be alert to laryngeal stridor, dyspnea, and crowing, which occur with laryngeal spasm, a life-threatening complication of hypocalcemia.
- Keep an emergency tracheostomy tray at the bedside of all patients with symptoms of hypocalcemia.

NIC Respiratory Monitoring

HYPERCALCEMIA

Pathophysiology

Symptoms of hypercalcemia can occur because of an increase in total serum calcium or an increase in the percentage of free, ionized calcium. If hypercalcemia is accompanied by a normal or elevated serum phosphorus level, calcium phosphate crystals may precipitate in the serum and deposit throughout the body. Soft tissue calcifications usually occur when the product of the serum calcium and serum phosphorus (i.e., calcium times phosphorus) exceeds 70 mg/dl.

Assessment

History and risk factors: The two primary causes of hypercalcemia are hyperparathyroidism, which may be stress-related in the patient in ICU, and malignancy.

Increased intake of calcium: Excessive administration during cardiopulmonary arrest, milk-alkali syndrome.

Increased intestinal absorption: With vitamin D overdose or hyperparathyroidism.

Increased release of calcium from bone: Hyperparathyroidism, malignancies, prolonged immobilization, Paget disease.

Decreased urinary excretion: Renal failure, medications (e.g., thiazide diuretics), hyperparathyroidism.

Increased ionized calcium: Acidosis.

Clinical presentation: Symptoms are usually absent unless the serum calcium concentration is >11 mg/dl. Lethargy, weakness, anorexia, nausea, vomiting, polyuria, itching, bone pain, fractures, calculi, constipation, depression, confusion, paresthesias, personality changes, stupor, coma. Cardiovascular effects include hypertension, heart block, digitalis sensitivity, and cardiac arrest.

ECG findings: Shortening of ST segment and QT interval. PR interval is sometimes prolonged. Ventricular dysrhythmias can occur with severe hypercalcemia.

Diagnostic tests

Total serum calcium level: Will be >10.5 mg/dl. Serum calcium level should be evaluated with serum albumin level. For every 1 g/dl drop in serum albumin level, total calcium will drop 0.8-1 mg/dl.

Ionized calcium level: Will be >5.5 mg/dl.

Parathyroid hormone level: Increased levels occur in primary or secondary hyperparathyroidism.

X-ray findings: May reveal presence of osteoporosis, bone cavitation, or urinary calculi.

Collaborative management

Treatment of underlying cause or contributing factor: For example, antitumor chemotherapy for malignancy or partial parathyroidectomy for hyperparathyroidism; discontinuation of calcium supplements, vitamins A and D, and thiazide diuretics.

IV isotonic saline: Administered rapidly to increase urinary calcium excretion. Concomitant administration of furosemide prevents the development of fluid volume excess and further increases in urinary calcium excretion.

Low-calcium diet and cortisone: To reduce intestinal absorption of calcium. Steroids compete with vitamin D, thereby reducing intestinal absorption of calcium.

Decreased bone resorption: Accomplished via increased activity level, biphosphonates, or mithramycin. Etidronate and pamidronate are biphosphonates that act directly on bone to reduce decalcification and are used primarily to treat hypercalcemia associated with neoplastic disease. Biphosphonates take several days to work, but the effects may last for days to weeks. Mithramycin is a cytotoxic antibiotic that also decreases bones resorption. Compressional loads (e.g., weight bearing) stimulate bone deposition; thus increased activity decreases bone resorption.

Calcitonin: To reduce bone resorption, increase bone deposition of calcium and phosphorus, and increase urinary calcium and phosphate excretion.

Gallium nitrate: Inhibits osteoclasts and increases bone calcium. It is used in the treatment of malignancy-induced hypercalcemia.

Nursing diagnoses and interventions

Altered protection related to neurosensory alterations secondary to hypercalcemia

Desired outcomes: Within 24-48 h of initiating treatment, patient verbalizes orientation to time, place, and person. Patient does not exhibit evidence of injury caused by neurosensory changes.

- Monitor patient for worsening hypercalcemia. With each VS check, assess and document LOC; patient's orientation to time, place, and person; and neurologic status.
- Personality changes, hallucinations, paranoia, and memory loss may occur with hypercalcemia. Inform patient and significant others that altered sensorium is temporary and will improve with treatment. Use reality therapy: clocks, calendars, and familiar objects; keep them at the bedside within patient's visual field.
- Administer fluids and diuretics as prescribed. Evaluate response to therapy. Monitor serum calcium levels and albumin levels. Observe for signs of fluid volume excess with treatment.
- Hypercalcemia causes neuromuscular depression with poor coordination, weakness, and altered gait. Provide a safe environment. Keep side rails up and bed in lowest position with wheels locked. Assist patient with ambulation if it is allowed.
- Because hypercalcemia potentiates the effects of digitalis, monitor patient taking digitalis for signs and symptoms of digitalis toxicity: multifocal or bigeminal PVCs, paroxysmal atrial tachycardia with varying AV block, and other heart blocks.
- Monitor serum electrolyte values for changes in serum calcium as a result of therapy (normal range is 8.5-10.5 mg/dl); potassium (normal range is 3.5-5 mEq/L); and phosphorus (normal range is 2.5-4.5 mg/dl). Consult physician for abnormal values.
- Encourage increased mobility to reduce bone resorption. Ideally patient should be out of bed and up in a chair at least 6 h/day.

NIC Fluid Monitoring; Neurologic Monitoring; Electrolyte Management: Hypercalcemia; Dysrhythmia Management; Fluid Management

Altered urinary elimination related to dysuria, urgency, frequency, and polyuria secondary to administration of diuretics, calcium stone formation, or changes in renal function occurring with hypercalcemia

Desired outcome: Within 24 h of initiation of treatment, patient exhibits voiding pattern and urine characteristics that are normal for patient.

- Monitor I&O hourly. Consult physician for unusual changes in urine volume (e.g., oliguria alternating with polyuria, which may signal urinary tract obstruction, or continuous polyuria). Increased urinary calcium concentrations decrease the kidneys' ability to concentrate the urine, leading to polyuria and potentially to fluid volume deficit. This is a type of nephrogenic diabetes insipidus (see p. 479).
- Because hypercalcemia can impair renal function, monitor patient's renal function carefully: urine output, BUN, creatinine values (see "Acute Renal Failure," p. 371).
- Provide patient with a low-calcium diet, and avoid use of calcium-containing medications (e.g., antacids such as Tums). Encourage intake of fruits (e.g., cranberries, prunes, plums) that leave an acid ash in the urine. An acidic urine reduces the risk of calcium stone formation. Also increase fluid intake (at least 3 L in nonrestricted patients) to reduce the risk of renal stone formation.
- Assess patient for indicators of kidney stone formation: intermittent pain, nausea, vomiting, hematuria.
- Hypercalcemia leads to an increase in calcium in the urine, which inhibits the kidneys' ability to concentrate urine. This leads to polyuria and potential volume depletion. Be alert to polyuria. Also monitor for signs of volume depletion when giving diuretics: decreased BP, CVP, PAP; increased HR.

NIC Fluid Monitoring; Urinary Elimination Management; Electrolyte Management: Hypercalcemia

PHOSPHORUS IMBALANCE

Phosphorus, the primary anion of the ICF, has a wide variety of vital functions, including formation of energy-storing substances (e.g., adenosine triphosphatase); formation of red blood cell 2,3-diphosphoglycerate (DPG), which facilitates oxygen delivery to the tissues; metabolism of carbohydrates, protein, and fat; and maintenance of acid-base balance. In addition, phosphorus is critical to normal nerve and muscle function and provides structural support to bones and teeth.

Plasma phosphorus levels vary with diet and acid-base balance. Glucose, insulin, or sugar-containing foods cause a temporary drop in phosphorus because of a shift of serum phosphorus into the cells. Alkalosis, particularly respiratory alkalosis, may cause hypophosphatemia as a result of an intracellular shift of phosphorus. Although the exact mechanism for this shift is not fully understood, it may be related to an alkalosis-induced cellular glycolysis, with increased formation of phosphorus-containing metabolic intermediates. Respiratory acidosis may cause a shift of phosphorus out of the cells and contribute to hyperphosphatemia.

Although the level of ECF phosphate is affected by a combination of factors, including dietary intake, intestinal absorption, and hormonally regulated bone resorption and deposition, phosphorus balance depends largely on renal excretion. Normal range for serum phosphorus is 2.5-4.5 mg/dl (1.7-2.6 mEq/L).

HYPOPHOSPHATEMIA

Pathophysiology

Hypophosphatemia (serum phosphorus <2.5 mg/dl) may occur because of transient intracellular shifts, increased urinary losses, decreased intestinal absorption, or increased utilization (see "Assessment" in the next section for history and risk factors). Severe phosphorus deficiency also may develop because of a combination of factors in conditions such as chronic alcohol abuse and DKA.

Assessment

History and risk factors

Intracellular shifts: Carbohydrate load, respiratory alkalosis, treatment of DKA.

Increased utilization because of increased tissue repair: TPN with inadequate phosphorus content; recovery from protein-calorie malnutrition. Hypophosphatemia is common in the critical care patient largely because of nutritional deficiency.

Increased urinary losses: Hypomagnesemia, ECF volume expansion, hyperparathyroidism, use of thiazide diuretics, diuretic phase of ATN, glucosuria.

Reduced intestinal absorption or increased intestinal loss: Use of phosphorus-binding medications (e.g., aluminum-, magnesium-, or calcium-containing antacids; sucralfate); vomiting and diarrhea; malabsorption disorders such as vitamin D deficiency; prolonged gastric suction.

Mixed causes: Chronic alcohol abuse, DKA, severe burns, artificially ventilated patients, postsurgery status, post–renal transplant status, sepsis.

Clinical presentation: Patients may have acute symptoms caused by sudden decreases in serum phosphorus, or symptoms may develop gradually because of chronic phosphorus deficiency. The majority of symptoms are secondary to decreases in ATP and 2,3-DPG.

Acute: Confusion, seizures, coma, chest pain caused by poor oxygenation of the myocardium, muscle pain and weakness, increased susceptibility to infection, numbness and tingling of the fingers and circumoral region, incoordination, difficulty weaning from mechanical ventilation, respiratory failure.

Chronic: Memory loss, lethargy, weakness, bone pain.
Physical assessment
Acute: Decreased strength as evidenced by difficulty with speaking, weakness of respiratory muscles, and weakening hand grasp. Bruising and bleeding may occur because of platelet dysfunction. Rhabdomyolysis, hemolysis, and myocardial depression may occur in severe hypophosphatemia. Hypoxia may cause an increased RR and respiratory alkalosis because of hyperventilation.

> **Note:**   Respiratory alkalosis causes phosphorus to move intracellularly, aggravating the existing hypophosphatemia.

Chronic: Joint stiffness, arthralgia, osteomalacia, cyanosis, and pseudofractures may occur.
Hemodynamic measurements: Severely depleted patients may show signs of decreased myocardial function, including increased PAWP, decreased CO, and decreased BP with decreased response to pressor agents.

Diagnostic tests
Serum phosphorus level: Will be<2.5 mg/dl (1.7 mEq/L).
Mild hypophosphatemia: 1-2.5 mg/dl.
Severe hypophosphatemia: <1 mg/dl.
Parathyroid hormone level: Will be elevated in hyperparathyroidism.
Serum magnesium level: May be decreased because of increased urinary excretion of magnesium in hypophosphatemia.
X-ray findings: May reveal skeletal changes of osteomalacia.

Collaborative management
Identification and elimination of the cause: For example, avoiding use of phosphorus-binding antacids (aluminum, magnesium, or calcium gels or antacids); correction of respiratory alkalosis.
Phosphorus supplementation: Mild hypophosphatemia may be treated by increasing intake of foods high in phosphorus, especially milk (Table 10-13). Moderate hypophosphatemia usually can be treated with oral phosphate supplements such as Neutra-Phos (sodium and potassium phosphate) or Phospho-Soda (sodium phosphate). Administration of IV sodium phosphate or potassium phosphate is necessary in cases of severe hypophosphatemia or when the GI tract is nonfunctional.

Nursing diagnoses and interventions
Altered protection related to neurosensory alterations secondary to hypophosphatemia

---

TABLE 10-13   Foods High in Phosphorus

Dried beans and peas
Eggs and egg products (e.g., eggnog, soufflés)
Fish
Meats, especially organ meats (e.g., brain, liver, kidney)
Milk and milk products (e.g., cheese, ice cream, cottage cheese)
Nuts (e.g., Brazil, peanuts)
Poultry
Seeds (e.g., pumpkin, sesame, sunflower)
Whole grains (e.g., oatmeal, bran, barley)

Desired outcomes: Within 24 h of initiation of treatment, patient verbalizes orientation to time, place, and person. Patient does not exhibit evidence of injury caused by neurosensory changes.

- Monitor serum phosphorus levels in patients at increased risk. Consult physician for decreased levels. Monitor for associated electrolyte and acid-base imbalances: hypokalemia, hypomagnesemia, respiratory alkalosis, and metabolic acidosis.
- Apprehension, confusion, and paresthesias are signals of developing hypophosphatemia. Assess and document LOC, orientation, and neurologic status with each VS check. Reorient patient as necessary. Alert physician to significant changes.
- Inform patient and significant others that altered sensorium is temporary and will improve with treatment.
- Do not administer IV phosphate at a rate greater than that recommended by the manufacturer. Potential complications of IV phosphorus administration include *tetany* as a result of hypocalcemia (serum calcium levels may drop suddenly if serum phosphorus levels increase suddenly; see "Calcium Imbalance," p. 653, for additional information); *soft tissue calcification* (if hyperphosphatemia develops, the calcium and phosphorus in the ECF may combine and form deposits in tissue); and *hypotension,* caused by a too-rapid delivery. When IV phosphorus is administered as potassium phosphate, the infusion rate should not exceed 10 mEq/h. Monitor IV site for signs of infiltration, because potassium phosphate can cause necrosis and sloughing of tissue.
- Keep the side rails up and the bed in its lowest position with wheels locked.
- Use reality therapy, such as clocks, calendars, and familiar objects. Keep these articles at the bedside within patient's visual field.
- If patient is at risk for seizures, pad the side rails and keep an appropriate-size airway at the bedside.

NIC Neurologic Monitoring; Electrolyte Management: Hypophosphatemia; Medication Administration

Impaired gas exchange related to altered oxygen-carrying capacity of the blood secondary to decreased 2,3-DPG

> **Note:** With decreased 2,3-DPG levels, the oxyhemoglobin dissociation curve will shift to the left (i.e., at a given Pao_2 level, more oxygen will be bound to Hgb and less will be available to the tissues).

Desired outcome: Within 12 h of initiation of treatment, patient has adequate gas exchange as evidenced by RR 12-20 breaths/min with normal depth and pattern (eupnea); orientation to time, place, and person; Spo_2 ≥92%; and absence of the indicators of hypoxia (e.g., restlessness, somnolence).

- Assess patient for signs of hypoxia: restlessness, confusion, increased RR, complaints of chest pain, and cyanosis (a late sign).
- Monitor Spo_2 as available. Administer oxygen as prescribed to maintain Spo_2 at ≥92%.

NIC Respiratory Monitoring

Ineffective breathing pattern related to decreased strength of respiratory muscles secondary to hypophosphatemia

Desired outcome: Within 8 h of initiation of treatment, the nonventilated patient becomes eupneic. Optimally, for the ventilated patient, improved weaning is noted within 24 h of initiation of treatment.

- Monitor rate and depth of respirations in patients with severe hypophosphatemia. Assess for decreased tidal volume or decreased minute ventilation. Consult physician for changes.
- Monitor ABG values for evidence of hypoxemia or hypercapnia. Consult physician for significant changes.

- There is an increased incidence of hypophosphatemia in artificially ventilated patients. Monitor serum phosphate levels in these patients. Hypophosphatemia may contribute to difficulty in weaning patients from ventilators.
- Administer IV phosphorus as prescribed.

NIC Respiratory Monitoring

Impaired physical mobility related to musculoskeletal impairment (osteomalacia with bone pain and fractures) associated with movement of phosphorus out of the bone secondary to chronic hypophosphatemia; muscle weakness and acute rhabdomyolysis (breakdown of striated muscle) secondary to severe hypophosphatemia

Desired outcome: Within 24 h of initiation of therapy, patient exhibits ability to move purposefully and has full or baseline range of motion (ROM) and muscle strength.

- Monitor all patients with suspected hypophosphatemia for evidence of decreasing muscle strength. Perform serial assessments of hand grasp strength and clarity of speech. Consult physician for changes.
- Monitor serum phosphorus levels for evidence of worsening hypophosphatemia. Consult physician for changes.
- Assist the patient with ambulation and ADL. Keep personal items within easy reach.
- Encourage intake of foods high in phosphorus (see Table 10-13). Teach patient and significant others the importance of using phosphorus-binding antacids only as prescribed.
- Medicate for pain as prescribed.

NIC Neurologic Monitoring; Electrolyte Management: Hypophosphatemia

Decreased cardiac output related to negative inotropic changes associated with reduced myocardial functioning secondary to severe phosphorus depletion

Desired outcome: Within 12 h of initiation of treatment, patient's cardiac output is adequate as evidenced by CO ≥4 L/min; CI ≥2.5 L/min/m^2; CVP <6 mm Hg; PAP 20-30/8-15 mm Hg; HR ≤100 bpm; BP within patient's normal range; and absence of the clinical signs of heart failure or pulmonary edema.

- Monitor patient for signs of heart failure or pulmonary edema: crackles, rhonchi, SOB, decreased BP, increased HR, increased PAP, or increased CVP.
- Prevent patient from hyperventilating, if possible, inasmuch as metabolic alkalosis will cause an increased movement of phosphorus into the cells, which will negatively affect cardiac output.
- For additional interventions if decreased cardiac output develops, see "Cardiomyopathy," p. 272.

NIC Invasive Hemodynamic Monitoring; Cardiac Care

Risk for infection related to inadequate secondary defenses (impaired WBC functioning) secondary to reduced ATP

Desired outcome: Patient is free of infection as evidenced by normothermia and absence of erythema, swelling, warmth, and purulent drainage at invasive sites.

- Monitor temperature q4h for evidence of infection. Obtain cultures of wounds and drainage as prescribed if infection is suspected.
- Use meticulous aseptic technique when changing dressings or manipulating indwelling lines (e.g., TPN catheters, IV needles).
- Provide oral hygiene and skin care at regular intervals. Intact skin and membranes are the body's first line of defense against infection.

NIC Infection Protection

HYPERPHOSPHATEMIA

Pathophysiology

Hyperphosphatemia occurs most often in the presence of renal insufficiency caused by the kidneys' decreased ability to excrete excess phosphorus. In addition to renal failure, other causes of hyperphosphatemia include increased intake of phosphates, extracellular shifts (i.e., movement of phosphorus out of the cell and into the ECF), cellular destruction with concomitant release of intracellular phosphorus, and decreased urinary losses that are unrelated to decreased renal function. As serum phosphorus levels increase, serum calcium levels often drop, which may cause hypocalcemia to develop. Hypocalcemia is most likely to occur in sudden, severe hyperphosphatemia (e.g., after IV administration of phosphates) or when the patient already is prone to hypocalcemia (e.g., with chronic renal failure).

The primary complication of hyperphosphatemia is metastatic calcification (i.e., the precipitation of calcium phosphate in the soft tissue, joints, and arteries). Precipitation of calcium phosphate occurs when the product (calcium times phosphorus) exceeds 70 mg/dl. Chronic hyperphosphatemia in the patient with chronic renal failure may contribute to the development of renal osteodystrophy.

Assessment
History and risk factors
Renal failure: Acute and chronic. Hyperphosphatemia is an early feature of chronic renal failure secondary to declining glomerular filtration.
Increased intake: Excessive administration of phosphorus supplements; vitamin D excess with increased GI absorption; excessive use of phosphorus-containing laxatives or enemas; massive transfusion.
Extracellular shift: Respiratory acidosis; diabetic ketoacidosis (before treatment).
Cellular destruction: Neoplastic disease (e.g., leukemia, lymphoma) treated with cytotoxic agents; increased tissue catabolism (breakdown); rhabdomyolysis (breakdown of striated muscle).
Decreased urinary losses: Hypoparathyroidism; volume depletion.
Clinical presentation: Anorexia, nausea, vomiting, muscle weakness, hyperreflexia, tetany, tachycardia.

> **Note:** Usually patients experience few symptoms with hyperphosphatemia. The majority of symptoms that do occur relate to the development of hypocalcemia or soft tissue (metastatic) calcifications. Indicators of metastatic calcification include oliguria, corneal haziness, conjunctivitis, irregular heart rate, and papular eruptions.

Physical assessment: See "Hypocalcemia," p. 654. In addition, see preceding "Clinical Presentation" for indicators of metastatic calcifications.
ECG changes: See "Hypocalcemia," p. 654. Deposition of calcium phosphate in the heart may lead to dysrhythmias and conduction disturbances.

Diagnostic tests
Serum phosphate level: Will be >4.5 mg/dl (2.6 mEq/L).
X-ray: May show skeletal changes of osteodystrophy.
PTH level: Will be decreased in hypoparathyroidism.

Collaborative management
Identification and elimination of the cause.
Use of aluminum, magnesium, or calcium antacids: To bind phosphorus in the gut, thus increasing GI elimination of phosphorus. Calcium carbonate and calcium acetate are the preferred preparations for the patient with chronic renal failure. Magnesium antacids are avoided in renal failure because of the risk of hypermagnesemia, whereas aluminum-containing antacids are contraindicated because they may lead to aluminum accumulation and contribute to the development of bone disease. Serum phosphorus levels may be allowed to remain slightly elevated (4.5-6 mg/dl) in chronic renal failure to ensure adequate levels of 2,3-DPG. This helps to minimize the effects of chronic anemia on oxygen delivery to the tissues.

Dialytic therapy: May be necessary for acute, severe hyperphosphatemia accompanied by symptoms of hypocalcemia. See "Renal Replacement Therapies," p. 395.

Nursing diagnoses and interventions

Knowledge deficit: purpose of phosphate binders and the importance of reducing GI absorption of phosphorus to control hyperphosphatemia and prevent long-term complications

Desired outcome: Within the 24-h period before discharge from ICU, patient describes the potential complications of uncontrolled hyperphosphatemia and the ways in which they can be prevented.

> **Note:**   Because symptoms of hyperphosphatemia may be minimal, prevention of long-term complications relies primarily on adequate patient education.

- Teach patients the purpose of phosphate binders. Stress the need to take binders as prescribed with or after meals to maximize effectiveness.
- Prepare patients for the possibility of constipation as a result of binder use. Encourage use of bulk-building supplements or stool softener if constipation occurs. Phosphate-containing laxatives and enemas must be avoided.
- Phosphate binders are available in liquid, tablet, or capsule form. Confer with physician regarding an alternate form or brand for individuals who find binders unpalatable or difficult to take. Phosphate binders vary in their aluminum, magnesium, or calcium content, however, and one may not be exchanged for another without first ensuring that the patient is receiving the same amount of elemental aluminum, magnesium, or calcium.
- Encourage patient to avoid or limit foods high in phosphorus (see Table 10-13).
- Review the importance of avoiding phosphorus-containing OTC medications: certain laxatives, enemas, and mixed vitamin-mineral supplements. Instruct the patient and significant others to read the label for the words "phosphorus" and "phosphate."

NIC Teaching: Prescribed Medication; Electrolyte Management: Hyperphosphatemia

Risk for injury related to internal factors associated with precipitation of calcium phosphate in the soft tissue (e.g., corneas, lungs, kidneys, gastric mucosa, heart, blood vessels) and periarticular region of the large joints (e.g., hips, shoulders, elbows); development of hypocalcemic tetany

Desired outcome: Patient does not develop symptoms of physical injury caused by precipitation of calcium phosphate in the soft tissue or joints or hypocalcemic tetany.

- Monitor serum phosphorus and calcium levels. Calculate the calcium-phosphorus product (calcium times phosphorus). Values ≥70 mg/dl are associated with precipitation of calcium phosphate in the soft tissues. Consult physician for abnormal values. Remember that phosphorus values may be kept slightly higher (4-6 mg/dl) to ensure adequate levels of 2,3-DPG in patients with chronic renal failure, thereby minimizing effects of chronic anemia on oxygen delivery to the tissues.
- Vitamin D products and calcium supplements (taken between meals) may be limited until the serum phosphorus level approaches normal.
- Consult physician if patient develops indicators of metastatic calcification: oliguria, corneal haziness, conjunctivitis, irregular heart rate, and papular eruptions.
- Monitor patient for evidence of increasing hypocalcemia: numbness and tingling of the fingers and circumoral region, hyperactive reflexes, and muscle cramps. Consult physician promptly if these symptoms develop, because they occur before overt tetany. In addition, consult physician if

patient shows positive Trousseau or Chvostek sign, inasmuch as they signal latent tetany. (For a discussion of these signs and for additional information regarding treatment and prevention of hypocalcemia, see p. 654.)

- Because hyperphosphatemia can impair renal function, monitor patient's renal function carefully: urine output, BUN, and creatinine values.

NIC Neurologic Monitoring; Electrolyte Management: Hyperphosphatemia

MAGNESIUM IMBALANCE

Of the body's magnesium, approximately 60% is located in bone and approximately 1% is located in the ECF. The remaining magnesium is contained within the cells, thereby constituting the second most abundant intracellular cation after potassium. Magnesium is regulated by a combination of factors, including vitamin D–regulated GI absorption and renal excretion.

Because magnesium is a major intracellular ion, it plays a vital role in normal cellular function. Specifically, it activates enzymes involved in the metabolism of carbohydrates and protein, and it triggers the sodium-potassium pump, thus affecting intracellular potassium levels. Magnesium also is important in the transmission of neuromuscular activity, neural transmission within the CNS, and myocardial functioning. Normal serum magnesium level is 1.5-2.5 mEq/L.

HYPOMAGNESEMIA

Pathophysiology

Hypomagnesemia (serum magnesium level <1.5 mEq/L) usually occurs because of decreased GI absorption or increased urinary loss. It also may occur with excessive GI loss (e.g., vomiting, diarrhea) or with prolonged administration of magnesium-free parenteral fluids. Chronic abusers of alcohol (see "History and Risk Factors" in the next section) and patients undergoing critical care are the two most common patient populations. In the critical care setting, hypomagnesemia is associated with increased mortality. Dysrhythmias and sudden death increase when decreased magnesium levels occur in combination with myocardial infarction, heart failure, or digitalis toxicity. Hypomagnesemia usually is associated with hypocalcemia and hypokalemia (see "Diagnostic Tests," p. 666, for additional information). Symptoms of hypomagnesemia tend to develop once the serum magnesium level drops below 1 mEq/L. Decreased magnesium intake has been identified as a risk factor for hypertension, cardiac dysrhythmias, ischemic heart disease, and sudden cardiac death.

Assessment

History and risk factors

Chronic alcoholism: The most common cause of hypomagnesemia as a result of a combination of poor dietary intake, decreased GI absorption, and increased urinary excretion secondary to ethanol effect.

Decreased GI absorption: For example, as a result of cancer, colitis, pancreatic insufficiency, surgical resection of the GI tract, use of laxatives, diarrhea.

Increased GI loss: Prolonged vomiting or gastric suction.

Administration of low-magnesium or magnesium-free parenteral solutions: Especially with refeeding after starvation.

Poorly controlled diabetes including DKA: A result of movement of magnesium out of the cell and loss in the urine because of osmotic diuresis.

Increased urinary excretion: Resulting from medications such as diuretics, amphotericin, tobramycin, gentamicin, cisplatin, cyclosporine, or digoxin or from diuretic phase of ATN.

Protein-calorie malnutrition.

Cardiopulmonary bypass.

Clinical presentation: Lethargy, weakness, fatigue, mood changes, hallucinations, confusion, anorexia, nausea, vomiting, paresthesias.

Physical assessment: Increased reflexes, tremors, convulsions, tetany, and positive Chvostek and Trousseau signs (see p. 654), in part because of accompanying hypocalcemia. Skeletal and respiratory muscle weakness may be present. The patient also may have tachycardia, hypertension, and coronary spasm.

ECG findings: See "Hypokalemia," p. 649; and "Hypocalcemia," p. 654. PVCs and torsades de pointes.

Diagnostic tests

Serum magnesium level: <1.5 mEq/L. Hypomagnesemia is the most frequently undiagnosed electrolyte imbalance in hospitalized patients.

Magnesium tolerance test: Used to identify individuals with or at risk for magnesium deficiency. Results are based on the amount of magnesium retained after an infusion of magnesium.

Serum potassium level: May be decreased because of failure of the cellular sodium-potassium pump to move potassium into the cell and the accompanying loss of potassium in the urine. This hypokalemia may be resistant to potassium replacement until the magnesium deficit has been corrected.

Serum calcium level: Hypomagnesemia may lead to hypocalcemia because of a reduction in the release and action of parathyroid hormone. Parathyroid hormone is the primary regulator of serum calcium levels.

ECG evaluations: May reflect magnesium, as well as calcium and potassium, deficiencies: tachyarrhythmias, prolonged PR and QT intervals, widening of the QRS complex, ST-segment depression, and flattened T waves. Increased digitalis effect (as evidenced by multifocal or bigeminal PVCs, paroxysmal atrial tachycardia with varying AV block, and other heart blocks) also may occur. Dysrhythmias associated with hypomagnesemia include ventricular ectopy, torsades de pointes, and atrial fibrillation.

Collaborative management

Identification and elimination of the cause: For example, ensuring adequate replacement of magnesium in TPN solutions.

IV or IM magnesium sulfate (MgSO$_4$):   For severe hypomagnesemia or its symptoms.

Oral magnesium: Chronic magnesium loss is treated with oral magnesium salts (oxide or chloride). Magnesium-containing antacids (e.g., Mylanta, Maalox, Gelusil, Milk of Magnesia) also may be used. Some foods high in magnesium are listed in Table 10-14.

Nursing diagnoses and interventions

Altered protection related to neurosensory alterations secondary to hypomagnesemia

Desired outcomes: Within 8 h of initiation of treatment, patient verbalizes orientation to time, place, and person. Patient does not exhibit evidence of injury caused by complications of severe hypomagnesemia.

TABLE 10-14   Foods High in Magnesium

Bananas	Molasses
Chocolate	Nuts and seeds
Coconuts	Oranges
Green, leafy vegetables (e.g., beet greens, collard greens)	Refined sugar
Grapefruits	Seafood
Kelp	Soy flour
Legumes	Wheat bran

- Monitor serum magnesium levels in patient at risk for hypomagnesemia and its deleterious effects (e.g., those who are alcohol abusers or experiencing heart failure, recent myocardial infarction, or digitalis toxicity). Normal range for serum magnesium is 1.5-2.5 mEq/L. Consult physician for abnormal values.

> **Note:** Symptoms of hypomagnesemia may be mistakenly attributed to delirium tremens of chronic alcoholism. Be especially alert to indicators of magnesium deficit in these patients.

- Administer IV MgSO$_4$ with caution. Refer to manufacturer's guidelines. Too-rapid administration may lead to dangerous hypermagnesemia, with cardiac or respiratory arrest. Patients receiving IV magnesium should be monitored for decreasing BP, labored respirations, and diminished patellar reflex (knee jerk). An absent patellar reflex is a signal of hyporeflexia because of dangerous hypermagnesemia. Should any of these changes occur, stop the infusion and consult physician *stat* (see "Hypermagnesemia," p. 668). Keep calcium gluconate at the bedside in the event of hypocalcemic tetany or sudden hypermagnesemia.
- For patients with chronic hypomagnesemia, administer oral magnesium supplements as prescribed. All magnesium supplements should be given with caution in patients with reduced renal function because of an increased risk of the development of hypermagnesemia. Caution patient that oral magnesium supplements may cause diarrhea. Administer antidiarrheal medications as needed.
- When it is appropriate, encourage intake of foods high in magnesium (see Table 10-14). For most patients, a normal diet is usually adequate.
- Maintain seizure precautions for patients with symptoms (i.e., those who have hyperreflexia). Decrease environmental stimuli (e.g., keep the room quiet; use subdued lighting).
- For patients in whom hypocalcemia is suspected, caution against hyperventilation. Metabolic alkalosis may precipitate tetany as a result of increased calcium binding.
- Dysphagia may occur in hypomagnesemia. Test the patient's ability to swallow water before giving food or medications.
- Assess and document LOC, orientation, and neurologic status with each VS check. Reorient patient as necessary. Notify physician for significant changes. Inform patient and significant others that altered mood and sensorium are temporary and will improve with treatment.
- See "Hypokalemia," p. 649; "Hypocalcemia," p. 654; and "Hypophosphatemia," p. 659; for nursing care of patients with these disorders.

> **Note:** Because magnesium is necessary for the movement of potassium into the cell, intracellular potassium deficits cannot be corrected until hypomagnesemia has been treated.

NIC Neurologic Monitoring; Electrolyte Management: Hypomagnesemia; Electrolyte Management: Hypokalemia; Electrolyte Management: Hypocalcemia; Seizure Precautions; Medication Administration

Decreased cardiac output related to electrical alterations associated with tachyarrhythmias or digitalis toxicity secondary to hypomagnesemia

Desired outcomes: Within 24 h of initiating treatment, patient's cardiac output is adequate as evidenced by CO ≥4 L/min; CI ≥2.5 L/min/m^2; normal configurations on ECG; and HR within patient's normal range. Patient exhibits brisk capillary refill (<2 sec) and urinary output ≥0.5 ml/kg/h.

- Monitor heart rate and regularity with each VS check. Consult physician for changes. Be alert to decreased CO and CI.

- Assess ECG for evidence of hypomagnesemia. Consider hypomagnesemia as a cause in patients who develop sudden ventricular dysrhythmias.
- Because hypomagnesemia (and hypokalemia) potentiate the cardiac effects of digitalis, monitor patients taking digitalis for digitalis-induced dysrhythmias. ECG changes may include multifocal or bigeminal PVCs, paroxysmal atrial tachycardia with varying AV block, and other heart blocks.
- Monitor for and report decreased urinary output and delayed capillary refill.

NIC Cardiac Care; Dysrhythmia Management

Altered nutrition: less than body requirements of magnesium, related to history of poor intake or anorexia, nausea, and vomiting secondary to hypomagnesemia or starvation

Desired outcome: Within 24 h of resumption of oral feedings, patient receives diet adequate in magnesium.

- Encourage intake of small, frequent meals.
- Teach patient about foods high in magnesium content (Table 10-14), and encourage intake of these foods during meals.
- Administer antiemetics as prescribed.
- Include patient, significant others, and dietitian in meal planning as appropriate.
- Provide oral hygiene before meals to enhance appetite.
- As with the other major intracellular electrolyte levels, magnesium depletion may develop with refeeding after starvation. Anticipate hypomagnesemia with refeeding, and ensure increased dietary intake or supplementation.
- Consult physician for patients receiving magnesium-free solutions (e.g., TPN) for prolonged periods.

NIC Nutritional Monitoring; Nutrition Management; Nutrition Therapy; Nutritional Counseling

HYPERMAGNESEMIA

Pathophysiology

Hypermagnesemia (serum magnesium levels >2.5 mEq/L) occurs almost exclusively in individuals with renal failure who have an increased intake of magnesium (e.g., use of magnesium-containing medications). It also may occur in acute adrenocortical insufficiency (Addison disease) or in obstetric patients treated with parenteral magnesium for pregnancy-induced hypertension. In rare cases hypermagnesemia occurs because of excessive use of magnesium-containing medications (e.g., antacids, laxatives, enemas). The primary symptoms of hypermagnesemia are the result of depressed peripheral and central neuromuscular transmission. Symptoms usually do not occur until the magnesium level exceeds 4 mEq/L.

Assessment

History and risk factors

Decreased excretion of magnesium: As with renal failure or adrenocortical insufficiency.

Increased intake of magnesium: For example, excessive use of magnesium-containing antacids, enemas, and laxatives or excessive administration of magnesium sulfate (such as in the treatment of hypomagnesemia or pregnancy-induced hypertension).

Clinical presentation: Nausea, vomiting, flushing, diaphoresis, sensation of heat, altered mental functioning, drowsiness, coma, and muscular weakness or paralysis. Paralysis of the respiratory muscles may occur when the magnesium level exceeds 10 mEq/L.

Physical assessment: Hypotension, soft tissue (metastatic) calcification (see description, p. 656), bradycardia, and decreased deep tendon reflexes. The patellar (knee jerk) reflex is lost once the magnesium level exceeds 8 mEq/L.

TABLE 10-15 Magnesium-containing Medications

Antacids	*Laxatives*
Aludrox	Magnesium citrate
Camalox	Magnesium hydroxide (Milk of Magnesia,
Di-Gel	Haley's M-O)
Gaviscon	Magnesium sulfate (Epsom salts)
Gelusil and Gelusil II	Magnesium-containing mineral supplements
Maalox and Maalox Plus	
Mylanta and Mylanta-II	
Riopan	
Simeco	
Tempo	

Hemodynamic measurements: Decreased arterial pressure caused by peripheral vasodilation.

Diagnostic tests
Serum magnesium level: Will be >2.5 mEq/L.
ECG findings: Prolonged PR, QRS, and QT intervals occur with levels >5 mEq/L. Complete heart block and cardiac arrest may occur in severe hypermagnesemia (levels >15 mEq/L).

Collaborative management
Removal of cause: For example, discontinuing or avoiding use of magnesium-containing medications (Table 10-15) or supplements, especially in patients with decreased renal function.
Diuretics and 0.45% NaCl solution: To promote magnesium excretion in patients with adequate renal function.
IV calcium gluconate, 10 ml of a 10% solution: To antagonize the neuromuscular effects of magnesium for patients with potentially lethal hypermagnesemia.
Dialysis with magnesium-free dialysate: For patients with severely decreased renal function.

Nursing diagnoses and interventions
Altered protection related to neurosensory alterations secondary to hypermagnesemia
Desired outcomes: Within 12 h of initiation of treatment, patient verbalizes orientation to time, place, and person. Patient does not exhibit evidence of injury as a result of complications of hypermagnesemia. Patient has no symptoms of soft tissue (metastatic) calcifications: oliguria, corneal haziness, conjunctivitis, irregular heart rate, and papular eruptions.
• Monitor serum magnesium levels in the patient at risk for hypermagnesemia (e.g., those with chronic renal failure). Normal range for serum magnesium levels is 1.5-2.5 mEq/L. Obtain specimens for laboratory analysis as needed.
• Assess and document LOC, orientation, and neurologic status (e.g., hand grasp) with each VS check. Assess patellar (knee jerk) reflex in patients with a moderately elevated magnesium level (>5 mEq/L). With patient lying flat, support the knee in a moderately fixed position and tap the patellar tendon firmly just below the patella. Normally the knee will extend. An absent reflex suggests a magnesium level of ≥7 mEq/L. Consult physician for significant changes.

- Reassure patient and significant others that altered mental functioning and muscle strength will improve with treatment.
- Keep side rails up and the bed in its lowest position with the wheels locked.
- Assess patient for the development of soft tissue calcification. Consult physician for significant findings.
- Monitor for cardiopulmonary effects of hypermagnesemia: hypotension, flushing, bradycardia, respiratory depression.

NIC Neurologic Monitoring; Electrolyte Management: Hypermagnesemia

Knowledge deficit: importance of avoiding excessive or inappropriate use of magnesium-containing medications, especially for patients with chronic renal failure

Desired outcome: Within the 24-h period before discharge from ICU, patient verbalizes the importance of avoiding unusual magnesium intake and identifies potential sources of unwanted magnesium.

- Caution patients with chronic renal failure to review all OTC medications with physician before use.
- Provide a list of common magnesium-containing medications (see Table 10-15).
- Patients with renal failure usually are taking vitamin supplements. Caution these patients to avoid combination vitamin-mineral supplements because they usually contain magnesium.

NIC Teaching: Prescribed Diet; Teaching: Prescribed Medication

Acid-base imbalances

For optimal functioning of the cells, metabolic processes maintain a steady balance between acids and bases. Arterial pH is an indirect measurement of hydrogen ion (H^+) concentration and is a reflection of the balance between carbon dioxide (CO_2), a gaseous form of acid regulated by the lungs, and hydrogen ion (H^+), a nongaseous acid regulated by the kidney. H^+ is not measured but varies inversely to the bicarbonate (HCO_3^-), a base regulated by the kidneys. Carbon dioxide, when dissolved in water, becomes carbonic acid (H_2CO_3). Because H_2CO_3 cannot be measured directly, the amount of H_2CO_3 in the blood is reflected by the $Paco_2$ (see p. 672). The normal acid-base ratio is 1:20, representing one part acid (CO_2 [potential H_2CO_3]) to 20 parts base (HCO_3^-). If this balance is altered, derangements in pH occur. If extra acids are present or base is lost and the pH is <7.4, acidosis exists. If extra base is present or there is loss of acid and the pH is >7.4, alkalosis is present. Any alteration in gaseous (CO_2) or nongaseous acid (H^+) will affect the pH. Factors that increase H^+ are lipolysis resulting in ketosis, cellular hypoxia resulting in lactic acidosis, and failure to excrete H^+ and/or generate buffer.

Buffers

Buffers are present in all body fluids and act immediately (within 1 sec) after an abnormal acidotic pH level occurs. They combine with excess acid to form substances that do not greatly affect pH. Their effect, however, is limited. Some buffers have a strong affinity to acid; others are weak.

Bicarbonate: The most important buffer of acid, it is present in the largest quantity in body fluids. Its reabsorption, excretion, and generation are regulated by the kidneys.

Phosphate: Aids in the excretion of H^- in the renal tubules.

Ammonium: The kidneys produce an acidic urine by adding H^+ to ammonia (NH_3) to form ammonium (NH_4^+).

Protein: Present in cells, blood, and plasma. Hemoglobin is the most important protein buffer.

Evaluating Acid-Base Balance

ACID-BASE REGULATION

Several mechanisms regulate acid-base balance. These mechanisms are exceptionally sensitive to minute changes in pH. Usually the body is able to maintain pH levels without outside intervention—if not at a normal level, at least in a life-sustaining range.

Respiratory system

Hydrogen ions (H^+) exert direct action on the respiratory center in the brain as H^+ is released from the chemical reaction of CO_2 (which readily crosses the blood-brain barrier) and H_2O (H_2CO_3 yields $H_2O + CO_2$). Increased presence of acid increases alveolar ventilation (in the normal lung) to 4-5 times the normal level, whereas alkalemia decreases alveolar ventilation (in the normal lung) to 50%-75% of the normal level. The response occurs quickly—within 1-2 min, during which time the lungs eliminate or retain carbon dioxide in direct relation to arterial pH. Although the compensatory effect of the respiratory system cannot correct imbalances completely, it is 50%-75% effective. The compensatory effects of the respiratory system occur in response to an increase in tissue or metabolic acids and require an optimally functional respiratory system.

Renal system

This system regulates acid-base balance by increasing or decreasing H^+ and therefore bicarbonate (HCO_3^-) concentration in body fluids. This is accomplished through a series of complex reactions that involve H^+ secretion, sodium ion (Na^+) reabsorption, HCO_3^- conservation, and ammonia synthesis for excretion of H^+ in the urine. H^+ secretion is regulated by the amount of carbon dioxide in extracellular fluid: the greater the concentration of carbon dioxide, the greater the amount of H^+. If the kidneys are functional, there will be an increase in H^+ secretion, resulting in an acidic urine. When H^+ is secreted, HCO_3^- is generated by the kidneys, helping to maintain the $1:20$ balance of acids and bases, respectively. When extracellular fluid is alkalotic, the kidneys conserve H^+ and eliminate HCO_3^-, resulting in alkalotic urine. Although the kidneys' response to an abnormal pH level is slow—several hours to days—they are able to facilitate a nearly normal pH level because of their ability to excrete large quantities of excess HCO_3^- or H^+ from the body. Renal excretion of acid load and increase in circulating buffer is the major compensation for respiratory deficits and requires a normally functioning kidney.

ABG values: ABG analysis usually is based on arterial sampling. Venous values are given as a reference.

Arterial values	**Venous values**
pH: 7.35-7.45	pH: 7.32-7.38
$Paco_2$: 35-45 mm Hg	Pco_2: 42-50 mm Hg
Pao_2: 80-95 mm Hg	Po_2: 40 mm Hg
Saturation: 95%-99%	Saturation: 60%-80%
Base excess: 0 ± 2	
*Serum HCO_3^-: 22-26 mEq/L	Serum CO_2^-: 23-27 mEq/L

---

*Although serum bicarbonate is a buffer, it is usually reported in the venous blood sample as "CO_2 content" or "total CO_2" and not as serum bicarbonate. The serum HCO_3^- concentration usually is obtained separately from ABG analysis and is critical in the determination of acid-base status, although this value may be calculated from $Paco_2$ and pH results via the ABG analysis. HCO_3^- values should be obtained with the initial assessment and daily thereafter as indicated.

ABG analysis

pH: Measures H^+ concentration and reflects acid-base status of the blood. Values indicate whether arterial pH is perfect (7.4), acidic (<7. 4), or alkalotic (>7.4). When pH is <7.35 or >7.45, it will be considered acute, or uncompensated. Even though perfection is difficult to achieve, pH must be first evaluated as being perfect or within the range. Because of buffers and other compensatory mechanisms, a near-normal pH level does not exclude the possibility of an acid-base disturbance. However, it is rare to see a perfect pH with compensation for either a metabolic or respiratory deficit. One method for evaluation of causative effects on the pH is to determine the absence or presence of offending acids. An increase in respiratory acid will make the pH go down and vice versa. An increase in metabolic acid (assumed by the opposite change in HCO_3^-) will cause the pH to go down and vice versa. The change in pH is created by an opposite change in the circulating acid. Compensation will bring the pH into range but generally not back to perfect.

$Paco_2$:   Measures partial pressure of carbon dioxide in the arteries. $Paco_2$ is adjusted by changes in the rate and depth of alveolar ventilation. Hypercapnia ($Paco_2$ >45 mm Hg) signals alveolar hypoventilation and respiratory acidosis. Alveolar hyperventilation results in hypocapnia ($Paco_2$ <35 mm Hg) and respiratory alkalosis. Respiratory compensation occurs rapidly in metabolic acid-base disturbances. If any abnormality in $Paco_2$ exists, it is important to analyze pH and HCO_3^- (and assume the inverse in H^+) parameters to determine if the alteration in $Paco_2$ is the result of a primary respiratory disturbance or a compensatory response to a metabolic acid-base abnormality.

Pao_2:   Partial pressure of oxygen in the arteries. The Pao_2 determines the usable gas, that is, oxygen that is free to diffuse across the capillary and cell wall to oxygenate the tissue. The presence of hypoxemia (Pao_2 <80 mm Hg) or the inability of the cells to extract oxygen from the blood can lead to anoxic metabolism, resulting in lactic acid production and metabolic acidosis. Pao_2 normally declines in the older adult. Pao_2 is always evaluated in relationship to Fio_2; that is, the higher the oxygen percent that is delivered to the lungs, the higher the oxygen in the blood should be.

Saturation (Sao_2):   Measures the degree to which hemoglobin is saturated by oxygen. Hemoglobin is the primary transporter of oxygen and supplies a reservoir (reserve) of oxygen for cellular use. Oxygen must be in a dissolved state to diffuse across the cell wall. Saturation and desaturation reflect the uptake of oxygen at the lungs and the download of oxygen at the tissues. It can be affected by changes in metabolism, temperature, pH, and $Paco_2$. When the Pao_2 falls to <60 mm Hg, there is a large drop in saturation. *Pulse oximetry* (Spo_2) can be used to monitor arterial oxygen saturation and thus determine oxygenation status. This noninvasive monitoring technique frequently is used in critical care areas, operating rooms, and emergency departments. Spo_2 should be correlated with Sao_2 (or oxyhemoglobin) via ABGs with the initiation of oximetry. It is vital to remember that pulse oximetry is a close correlate to Sao_2 but the measure of true oxyhemoglobin requires an ABG. To evaluate the tissue utilization of oxygen, a comparison of post-cellular saturation of Hgb is necessary. This evaluation requires a right heart catheter that resides in the pulmonary artery. These mixed venous blood gases are drawn intermittently or measured continuously from the distal tip of the pulmonary artery catheter. A blood sample taken from this site ensures complete mixing of blood returned from all parts of the body. Mixed venous oxygen saturation (Svo_2) may provide an early indication of perfusion failure or increased tissue demands for oxygen, reflected by a decreased saturation of Hgb. If the saturation of mixed venous Hgb is normal or high but the patient has evidence of lactic acidemia, the cells may be unable to utilize the oxygen. Mixed venous saturation numbers must always be correlated with tissue indicators of hypoxia, base deficit, serum bicarbonate, and lactic acidemia.

Base excess or deficit: Indicates, in general terms, the amount of blood buffer present. Reflects the tissue and renal presence or absence of acid. As the proportion of acid rises, the relative amount of base decreases (and vice versa). Abnormally high values (>+2) reflect alkalosis; low values (≤2) reflect acidosis.

Serum bicarbonate: Serum HCO_3^- is the major renal component of acid-base regulation. It is generated or excreted by the kidneys in direct proportion to the amount of circulating acid to maintain a normal acid-base environment. Decreased HCO_3^- levels (<22 mEq/L) signify an increase in circulating metabolic acid and are indicative of metabolic acidosis (seen infrequently as a compensatory mechanism for respiratory alkalosis); elevated HCO_3^- levels (>26 mEq/L) reflect decreasing circulating metabolic acids and are seen as metabolic alkalosis. Metabolic alkalosis occurs either as a primary metabolic disorder or as a compensatory alteration in response to respiratory acidosis. If bicarbonate changes, acid changes in the opposite direction. To determine the cause of bicarbonate changes, problem or compensation, the relationship to pH must be evaluated. pH will respond to the presence or absence of acid, and the directional relationship reflects the system that is problematic. For example, if bicarbonate is down, the inverse metabolic acid H^+ is increased and therefore the pH is down, If pH is inside of range, there must be respiratory compensation, signified by a low $Paco_2$. If pH is outside of range, there is either no or inadequate respiratory compensation at this time.

Step-by-step guide to ABG analysis
A systematic analysis is critical to the accurate interpretation of ABG values.
Step 1:   Determine if pH is perfect (7.40). If it is not perfect, determine the direction (up or down) Then determine if it is in the range of normal (7.35 to 7.45). If it is abnormal, identify whether it is on the acidotic (<7.35) or alkalotic (>7.45) side of normal.
Step 2:   Check $Paco_2$ for perfect levels (40 mm Hg). If not perfect, determine the direction (up or down). Then determine if it is in the range of normal (35 to 45). If abnormal, identify whether it is on the acidotic (>45) or alkalotic (<35) side of normal. If changes in the $Paco_2$ caused a change from perfect pH, the change in pH will be in the opposite direction of the $Paco_2$. If the change in pH is inside range but not perfect and the $Paco_2$ has traveled in the opposite direction, respiratory acid is the problem. This determines whether the primary problem is respiratory (involving $Paco_2$) or metabolic (involving H^+ but reflected by bicarbonate) in nature.
Step 3:   Check bicarbonate and base for perfect levels (24 and 0 respectively). If not perfect, determine the direction (up or down). Then determine if it is in the range of normal (22 to 26 and +2 to −2 respectively). If the values are abnormal, relate the two values to metabolic acid (H^+). If bicarbonate and base are down, metabolic acid is increased. If bicarbonate and base are in excess, metabolic acid is decreased. If changes in the metabolic acid (determined by the change in bicarbonate and base) caused a change from perfect pH, the change in pH will be in the opposite direction of the metabolic acid, but the same as the buffer. If the change in pH is inside range but not perfect and the metabolic acid has traveled in the opposite direction, metabolic acid is the problem. This determines whether the primary problem is respiratory (involving $Paco_2$) or metabolic (involving H^+ but reflected by bicarbonate) in nature.
Step 4:   If both $Paco_2$ and HCO_3^- are abnormal, the value that deviates the most from normal suggests the primary disturbance responsible for the altered pH. A mixed metabolic-respiratory disturbance or compensatory elements may be present.
Step 5:   Check Pao_2 and oxygen saturation to determine whether they are decreased, normal, or increased. Decreased Pao_2 and O_2 saturation can lead to

lactic acidosis and may signal the need for increased concentrations of oxygen. Conversely, high Pao_2 may be indicative of the need to decrease delivered concentrations of oxygen.

Arteriovenous oxygen content difference: $C(a-v)o_2$

The difference between the arterial oxygen content and the venous oxygen content reflects the tissue extraction of oxygen. This difference increases when ventricular performance is impaired. Simultaneous analysis of arterial and pulmonary artery blood sampling provides an accurate and reliable index of ventricular function.

CARING FOR ADULTS WITH ACID-BASE IMBALANCES

ACUTE RESPIRATORY ACIDOSIS

Pathophysiology

Respiratory acidosis (hypercapnia) occurs secondary to alveolar hypoventilation and results in an elevated $Paco_2$. $Paco_2$ derangements are direct reflections of the degree of ventilatory function or dysfunction. The degree to which the increased $Paco_2$ alters the pH depends on the rapidity of onset and the body's ability to compensate through the blood buffer and renal systems. The acidemia may develop rapidly because of the delay (hours to days) before renal compensation occurs. Acute rises in $Paco_2$ precipitate a rise in extracellular buffering systems (primarily hemoglobin and proteins) even before renal compensation occurs, but the extracellular rise is not sufficient to maintain a normal pH in the presence of an elevated $Paco_2$. The most common causes of acute respiratory acidosis are sudden respiratory failure from a depressed respiratory center (drugs or cerebral injury) or a catastrophic event, such as cardiac arrest.

Assessment

History and risk factors

Acute respiratory disease.

Overdose of drugs: Oversedation with drugs that cause respiratory center depression.

Chest wall trauma: Flail chest, pneumothorax.

CNS trauma/lesions: Can lead to depression of respiratory center.

Asphyxiation: Mechanical obstruction, anaphylaxis.

Impaired respiratory muscles: Can occur with hypokalemia, hyperkalemia, poliomyelitis, Guillain-Barré syndrome.

Iatrogenic: Inappropriate mechanical ventilation (increased dead space, insufficient rate or volume).

Clinical presentation: Dyspnea, tachypnea, nausea, vomiting, headache, fine tremors, asterixis, and restlessness and confusion leading to lethargy and coma. The restlessness and confusion are early signs that may be subtle but are very important indicators.

Physical assessment: Increased heart and respiratory rates, diminished or absent breath sound, may have asymmetric chest expansion, hypotension, and diaphoresis. Severe hypercapnia may cause cerebral vasodilation, resulting in increased intracranial pressure (IICP). Another finding may be dilated conjunctival and facial blood vessels.

Monitoring parameters: Presence of ventricular dysrhythmias; IICP.

Diagnostic tests

ABG analysis: Aids in diagnosis and determination of severity of respiratory acidosis. $Paco_2$ will be >45 mm Hg and pH will be <7.35 (if acute). If the patient is breathing room air, hypoxemia always will be present to some degree with increased $Paco_2$.

Serum bicarbonate: Initially, HCO_3^- values will be normal (22-26 mEq/L) unless a mixed disorder is present.

Serum electrolyte levels: Usually not altered; depend on cause of respiratory acidosis.
Chest x-ray: Determines presence of underlying respiratory disease.
Drug screen: Determines presence and quantity of drug if patient is suspected of taking an overdose.

Collaborative management
Restoration of effective alveolar ventilation: Accomplished by supporting respiratory function. If $Paco_2$ is >50-60 mm Hg, Pao_2 is ≤50 mm Hg, and clinical signs of ventilatory failure (e.g., confusion, lethargy) are present, the patient usually requires intubation and mechanical ventilation. The primary mechanism to treat respiratory acidosis is to increase the tidal volume and/or the respiratory rate. Generally, use of bicarbonate is avoided because of the risk of alkalosis when the respiratory disturbance has been corrected. Although a life-threatening pH must be corrected to an acceptable level promptly, a normal pH is not the immediate goal.
Treatment of underlying disorder.

Nursing diagnoses and interventions
Nursing diagnoses and interventions are specific to the pathophysiologic process. See appropriate section(s) in this and other chapters for diagnoses such as **Impaired gas exchange, Ineffective airway clearance,** and **Activity intolerance.**

CHRONIC RESPIRATORY ACIDOSIS (COMPENSATED)
Pathophysiology
This disorder occurs in pulmonary diseases in which effective alveolar ventilation is decreased. For CO_2 to be removed from the blood, the partial pressure of CO_2 in the alveoli must be less than that in the blood. In air-trapping syndrome or profound hypoventilation states, the alveolar concentration of CO_2 will limit the removal of CO_2 from the blood. Over time, the amount of CO_2 eliminated is less than the amount generated and thus $Paco_2$ levels increase. Chronic hypercapnia occurs with chronic obstructive pulmonary disorders (e.g., chronic emphysema and bronchitis, cystic fibrosis), restrictive disorders (e.g., pneumothorax, hemothorax, pickwickian syndrome), neuromuscular abnormalities (myasthenia gravis, Guillain-Barré, amyotrophic lateral sclerosis), and respiratory center depression (e.g., brain tumor, stroke, bleed, head injury). In patients with a chronic lung disease, a near-normal pH can be seen if renal function is normal, even if the $Paco_2$ is as high as 60 mm Hg. Chronic compensation from the kidney (retention and generation of serum HCO_3^- >26 mEq/L and an increase in renal excretion of metabolic acid) occurs and maintains an acceptable acid-base environment, which results in a near-normal pH level. Patients with chronic lung disease can experience acute rises in $Paco_2$ or lose their metabolic compensation (increased production of metabolic acid or loss of renal function) secondary to superimposed disease states such as pneumonia, hypermetabolic cellular hypoxia, or renal dysfunction. If the chronic compensatory mechanisms in place (e.g., elevated HCO_3^-) are inadequate to meet the sudden increase in $Paco_2$ or if the circulation of metabolic acids increases, decompensation may occur with a resultant decrease in pH.

Assessment
History and risk factors
Chronic obstructive pulmonary disease (COPD): Predominantly emphysema and bronchitis; cystic fibrosis.
Extreme obesity: Pickwickian syndrome.
Acute respiratory infection in a patient with COPD.
Exposure to pulmonary toxins: Occupational risk; pollution.

Clinical presentation: If the $Paco_2$ does not exceed the body's ability to compensate, no specific findings will be noted. If $Paco_2$ rises rapidly, the following may occur: dyspnea, asterixis, agitation, and insomnia progressing to somnolence and coma. The progression of symptoms may be subtle. Therefore thorough assessment and evaluation are important.

Physical assessment: Tachypnea, cyanosis (depending on the underlying disorder). Severe hypercapnia ($Paco_2$ >70 mm Hg) may cause cerebral vasodilation resulting in increased ICP, papilledema, and dilated conjunctival and facial blood vessels. Depending on the underlying pathophysiologic process, edema may be present secondary to right ventricular failure.

Monitoring parameters: Supraventricular tachycardia and ventricular tachycardia are common if an acute exacerbation is present.

Diagnostic tests

ABG values: Data necessary for determining the diagnosis and severity of respiratory acidosis. Although the $Paco_2$ will be elevated, the pH level will be near normal, although on the acidic (low) side of normal except in patients who are also experiencing an acute pulmonary disorder or metabolic problem superimposed on chronic hypercapnia (e.g., pneumonia). If the $Paco_2$ has increased abruptly from baseline value, a pH value lower than normal may be seen.

Serum electrolyte levels: Serum HCO_3^- is especially helpful in determining the level of metabolic compensation that has occurred (e.g., HCO_3^- increased with a near-normal pH value if fully compensated). This information is particularly useful in identifying "mixed" acid-base disturbances because the HCO_3^- is expected to be elevated in chronic respiratory acidosis. If the HCO_3^- is normal or low, this could be diagnostic of a second pathologic process (e.g., metabolic acidosis) concurrent with the first.

Chest x-ray: Determines extent of underlying pulmonary disease and identifies further pathologic changes that may be responsible in acute exacerbation (e.g., pneumonia).

ECG: Isoelectric P wave and an isoelectric QRS complex in lead I in a middle-age or older adult suggest chronic bronchitis or emphysema.

Sputum culture: Determines presence of pathogens causing an acute exacerbation of a chronic pulmonary disease (e.g., pneumonia) present in a patient with COPD.

Collaborative management

Oxygen therapy: Used cautiously in patients with chronic CO_2 retention for whom hypoxemia, rather than hypercapnia, stimulates ventilation. Patient may require intubation and mechanical ventilation for stupor and coma precipitated by oxygen if the drive to breathe is eliminated by high concentrations of oxygen. Continuous pulse oximetry may be used for close monitoring of oxygen delivery and to help ensure maintenance of oxygen saturation within acceptable range (e.g., 90%-92%).

Pharmacotherapy: Bronchodilators and antibiotics as indicated. Narcotics and sedatives can depress the respiratory center and are avoided unless intubation and mechanical ventilation are in place.

IV fluids: Maintain adequate hydration for mobilizing pulmonary secretions.

Chest physiotherapy: Aids in expectoration of sputum. Includes postural drainage if hypersecretions are present. Assess patient closely during this procedure because it may be poorly tolerated, especially the postural drainage component.

Nursing diagnoses and interventions

Impaired gas exchange related to alveolar-capillary membrane changes secondary to pulmonary tissue destruction

Desired outcome: Within 24 h of initiation of treatment, patient has adequate gas exchange as evidenced by $Paco_2$, pH, and Sao_2 normal or within 10% of patient's baseline.

- Monitor serial ABG results to assess patient's response to therapy. Consult physician for significant findings: increasing $Paco_2$ and decreasing pH, Pao_2, and Sao_2 values.
- Monitor oxygen saturation via pulse oximetry (Spo_2). Compare Spo_2 with Sao_2 values to assess reliability. Watch Spo_2 closely, especially when changing Fio_2 or to evaluate patient's response to treatment (e.g., repositioning, chest physiotherapy).
- Assess and document patient's respiratory status: respiratory rate and rhythm, exertional effort, and breath sounds. Compare pretreatment findings with posttreatment (e.g., oxygen therapy, physiotherapy, medications) findings for evidence of improvement.
- Assess and document patient's LOC. If $Paco_2$ increases, be alert to subtle, progressive changes in mental status. A common progression is agitation→insomnia→somnolence→coma. To avoid a comatose state caused by rising CO_2 levels, always evaluate the arousability of a patient with elevated $Paco_2$ who appears to be sleeping. Consult physician if patient is difficult to arouse.
- Ensure appropriate delivery of prescribed oxygen therapy. Assess patient's respiratory status after every change in Fio_2. Patients with chronic CO_2 retention may be very sensitive to increases in Fio_2, resulting in depressed ventilatory drive. If patient requires mechanical ventilation, be aware of the importance of maintaining the compensated acid-base status. If the $Paco_2$ is rapidly decreased by excessive mechanical ventilation, a severe metabolic alkalosis (posthypercapnic metabolic alkalosis) could develop. The sudden onset of metabolic alkalosis may lead to hypocalcemia, which can result in tetany (see "Hypocalcemia," p. 654). Severe alkalosis also can precipitate cardiac dysrhythmias.
- Assess for presence of bowel sounds, and monitor for GI distention, which can impede movement of the diaphragm and restrict ventilatory effort further.
- Assess for presence of symmetric lung expansion and normal resonance of lung fields. Hyperresonance and asymmetry indicate pneumothorax; dullness and asymmetry indicate solid tissue or fluid occupation of lung or pleural space (hemothorax, pleural effusion, hyperplasia).
- In patient without intubation, encourage use of pursed-lip breathing (inhalation through nose, with slow exhalation through pursed lips), which helps airways to remain open and allows for better air excursion. Optimally, this technique will diminish air entrapment in the lungs and make respiratory effort more efficient.

ACUTE RESPIRATORY ALKALOSIS (HYPOCAPNIA)

Pathophysiology

Respiratory alkalosis occurs as a result of an increase in the rate of alveolar ventilation (alveolar hyperventilation). It is defined as $Paco_2$ <35 mm Hg. Acute alveolar hyperventilation results most frequently from anxiety and is commonly referred to as *hyperventilation syndrome*. In addition, numerous physiologic disorders that cause hypoxemia (e.g., early acute respiratory distress syndrome, pneumonia, pulmonary edema, pulmonary emboli) can cause acute hypocapnia. If the underlying condition worsens, respiratory acidosis can occur as the exchange of CO_2 is impaired. Because CO_2 is 20 times more diffusible than O_2 across the alveolar membrane, hypoxemia is the first abnormality noted in many pulmonary diseases. Hypocapnia will result in increased pH. The rise in pH is modified to a small degree by intracellular buffering. To compensate for increased CO_2 loss and the resultant base excess, hydrogen ions are released from tissue buffers, which in turn lowers the plasma

HCO_3^- concentration. Whenever hydrogen ions are released from tissue, potassium will enter the cell and the result may be hypokalemia. Renal compensation for the respiratory alkalosis is not clinically apparent for hours; maximal compensation is not seen for days. Acute respiratory alkalosis can progress to chronic respiratory alkalosis if it persists for >6 h and renal compensation occurs.

Assessment
History and risk factors
Anxiety: Patient is often unaware of hyperventilation.
Acute hypoxemia: Pulmonary disorders (e.g., pneumonia, pulmonary edema, pulmonary thromboembolism) and extremely high altitudes (e.g., >6500 ft) may result in hypoxemia, which stimulates the ventilatory effort, causing respiratory alkalosis. Tissue acidosis (e.g., systemic inflammation, sepsis, DKA, lactic acidemia) will stimulate the respiratory effort, resulting in respiratory alkalosis.
Hypermetabolic states: Fever; sepsis, pain, agitation.
Salicylate intoxication.
Excessive mechanical ventilation: Increased tidal volume or RR.
CNS trauma: That which results in damage to respiratory center.
Clinical presentation: Lightheadedness, anxiety, paresthesias (especially of the fingers), circumoral numbness. In extreme alkalosis, confusion, tetany, syncope, and seizures may occur.
Physical assessment: Increased rate and depth of respirations (hyperventilation).
Monitoring parameters: Cardiac dysrhythmias.

Diagnostic tests
ABG values: Pa_{CO_2} <35 mm Hg and pH >7.45 will be present. A decreased Pa_{O_2}, along with the clinical picture (e.g., pneumonia, pulmonary edema, pulmonary embolism), may help diagnose cause of the respiratory alkalosis.
Serum electrolyte levels: HCO_3^- will be decreased 2 mEq/L for each 10 mm Hg drop in Pa_{CO_2} as a result of H^+ release from nonbicarbonate buffers and tissues.

- *Sodium* and *potassium* may be decreased slightly (potassium will shift from the extracellular space to the intracellular space in exchange for H^+).
- *Serum calcium* may be decreased because of increased calcium and bicarbonate binding. Signs of hypocalcemia include muscle cramps, hyperactive reflexes, carpal spasm, tetany, and convulsions.
- *Serum phosphorus* may decrease (<2.5 mg/dl), especially with salicylate intoxication and sepsis, because the alkalosis causes increased uptake of phosphorus by the cells. No symptoms occur, and treatment usually is not required unless a preexisting phosphorus deficit is present.

ECG: Detects cardiac dysrhythmias, which may occur with alkalosis.

Collaborative management
Treatment of underlying disorder.
Reassurance or sedation: If anxiety is the cause of decreased Pa_{CO_2}. If symptoms are severe, it may be necessary for patient to rebreathe exhaled air via a paper bag.
Oxygen therapy: If hypoxemia is the causative factor, increase FiO_2. If increases in FiO_2 do not result in resolution of hypoxemia and the patient does not have acute restrictive disorders, increase PEEP with circuit PEEP (dialed at ventilator) or mechanical PEEP (prolonged inspiratory time, high frequency ventilation).
Adjustments to mechanical ventilators: Settings are checked and adjustments made to ventilatory parameters in response to ABG results that signal

hypocapnia. Respiratory rate and/or volume are decreased, and dead space is added, if necessary, by attaching extra tubing to the mechanical ventilator circuitry.

Pharmacotherapy: Sedatives and tranquilizers may be given for anxiety-induced respiratory alkalosis.

Nursing diagnoses and interventions
Ineffective breathing pattern related to anxiety
Desired outcome: Within 4 h of initiating treatment, patient's breathing pattern is effective as evidenced by a state of eupnea; $Paco_2$ $\geq$35 mm Hg; and pH $\leq$7.45.

- To help alleviate anxiety, reassure patient that a staff member will remain with him or her.
- Encourage patient to breathe slowly. Pace patient's breathing pattern by having him or her mimic your own breathing pattern.
- Monitor patient's cardiac rhythm. Consult physician for new or increased dysrhythmias. With acute respiratory alkalosis, even a modest alkalosis can precipitate dysrhythmias in a patient with a preexisting heart disease who is also taking inotropic drugs (see Appendix 7). In part, this is caused by the hypokalemia that occurs with alkalosis.
- Administer sedatives or tranquilizers as prescribed. Assess and document effectiveness.
- Have patient rebreathe into a paper bag as indicated.
- Ensure that patient rests undisturbed after his or her breathing pattern has stabilized. Hyperventilation can result in fatigue.

Note: Hyperventilation may lead to hypocalcemic tetany despite a normal or near-normal calcium level because of increased binding of calcium.

CHRONIC RESPIRATORY ALKALOSIS

Pathophysiology
Chronic respiratory alkalosis is a state of chronic hypocapnia caused by stimulation of the respiratory center. The decreased $Paco_2$ stimulates the renal compensatory response and results in a proportionate decrease in plasma bicarbonate until a new, steady state is reached. Maximal renal compensatory response requires several days to occur and can result in a normal or near-normal pH. Chronic respiratory alkalosis is not commonly seen in acutely ill patients, but when present it can signal a poor prognosis.

Assessment
History and risk factors
Cerebral disease: Tumor, encephalitis, stroke.
Chronic hepatic insufficiency: A sustained respiratory alkalosis with this diagnosis has a poor prognosis.
Restrictive lung diseases: Interstitial pulmonary fibrosis. Respiratory alkalosis continues throughout the course of the disease. A normal $Paco_2$ followed by increased $Paco_2$ occurs in the terminal stage of the disease.
Pregnancy.
Chronic hypoxia: Adaptation to high altitude, cyanotic heart disease, lung disease resulting in decreased compliance (e.g., fibrosis).
Clinical presentation: Individuals with chronic respiratory alkalosis usually are free of symptoms.

Physical assessment: Increased respiratory rate and depth.
Diagnostic tests
ABG values: $Paco_2$ will be <35 mm Hg, with a near-normal or normal pH; Pao_2 may be decreased if hypoxemia is the causative factor.
Serum electrolyte levels: Probably will be normal, with the exception of plasma HCO_3^-, which will decrease as renal compensation occurs.
Phosphate levels: Hypophosphatemia (as low as 0.5 mg/dl) may be seen with intense hyperventilation. Alkalosis causes increased uptake of phosphate by the cells.

Collaborative management
Treatment of underlying cause.
Oxygen therapy: If hypoxemia is present and identified as causative factor in respiratory alkalosis.

Nursing diagnoses and interventions
Nursing diagnoses and interventions are specific to the pathophysiologic process. See appropriate medical disorders and nursing diagnoses in this and other chapters.

ACUTE METABOLIC ACIDOSIS
Pathophysiology
Metabolic acidosis is caused by a primary increase in metabolic acids and/or a decrease in plasma bicarbonate, as reflected by a serum HCO_3^- of <22 mEq/L with a pH <7.4. The decrease in serum HCO_3^- is caused by one of the following mechanisms: (1) increase in the concentration of H^+ in the form of nonvolatile acids (e.g., ketoacidosis associated with diabetes and alcoholism, lactic acidosis); (2) loss of alkali (e.g., severe diarrhea, intestinal malabsorption); and (3) decreased acid excretion by the kidneys (e.g., acute and chronic renal failure). The decrease in pH stimulates respirations. Attempts to compensate occur rapidly, as manifested by lowering of the $Paco_2$, which may be reduced to as much as 10-15 mm Hg. The most important mechanism for ridding the body of excess H^+ is the increase in acid excretion by the kidneys. Nonvolatile acids, however, may accumulate more rapidly than they can be neutralized by the body's buffers, compensated for by the respiratory system, or excreted by the kidneys. As the nonvolatile acid H^+ increases, it will displace the intracellular potassium, resulting in a serum hyperkalemia but a cellular hypokalemia. Abnormal substrate metabolism increases H^+.

The two most common forms of abnormal metabolism are lipolyis, which produces ketones and results in ketoacidosis, and anoxia at the cellular level, in which the cells fail to convert lactate to pyruvate, resulting in lactic acidemia. If a patient has a lactate level >2 mmol/L and the patient has no tissue opening (surgery, wounds, trauma), tissue hypoxia should be suspected. Patients who do have a tissue opening and a lactate level >4 mmol/L should be investigated for tissue hypoxia. Lactic acidosis is considered to be present when lactate is elevated, base and bicarbonate are in deficit, and the patient has anion gap acidosis. Frequently, in early lactic acidemia, patients will have a normal but slightly or moderately decreased pH with respiratory compensation (low $Paco_2$). Lactic acid levels, or serum lactate levels, indicate the presence of lactate. Lactate normal concentration is about 1-2 mmol/L.

Assessment
History and risk factors
Ketoacidosis: Diabetes mellitus, alcoholism, starvation.
Lactic acidosis: Respiratory or circulatory failure, drugs and toxins, hereditary disorders, septic shock. Lactic acidosis can be associated with other disease

states, such as leukemia, pancreatitis, bacterial infection, and uncontrolled diabetes mellitus.

Renal disease: Acute renal failure, renal tubular acidosis.

Poisonings and drug toxicity: Salicylates, methanol, ethylene glycol, ammonium chloride.

Loss of alkali: Draining wounds (e.g., pancreatic fistulas), diarrhea, ureterostomy.

Clinical presentation: Findings vary, depending on underlying disease states and the severity of the acid-base disturbance and speed with which it developed. There may be changes in LOC that range from fatigue and confusion to stupor and coma.

Physical assessment: Tachycardia (until pH <7, then bradycardia), decreased BP, tachypnea leading to alveolar hyperventilation (Kussmaul respirations), dysrhythmias, and shock state. With mild to moderate acidosis the skin will be cold and clammy, whereas with severe acidosis it will be flushed, warm, and dry. Mild metabolic acidosis (HCO_3^- 15-18 mEq/L) may result in no symptoms, whereas with a pH <7.2 symptoms will develop.

Monitoring parameters: A waveform suggestive of hyperkalemia (prolonged PR interval, widened QRS, and peaked T waves) may occur.

Diagnostic tests

ABG values: Determine pH (usually <7.35) and degree of respiratory compensation as reflected by $Paco_2$, which usually is <35 mm Hg.

Serum bicarbonate: Determines presence of metabolic acidosis (HCO_3^- <22 mEq/L, signifying a significant increase in H^+).

Serum electrolyte levels: Elevated potassium (K^+ >5 mEq/L) may be present as the H^+ moves into the cells to be buffered and the K^+ moves out of the cells to maintain electroneutrality. Hyperkalemia related to metabolic acidosis occurs most frequently in renal failure and diabetic ketoacidosis. If the K^+ is normal or low in the presence of metabolic acidosis, this signals low body stores of K^+ or profound hypokalemia.

To help identify the cause of metabolic acidosis, an analysis of serum electrolytes to detect anion gap may be helpful. Anion gap reflects unmeasurable anions (H^+) present in plasma and is calculated by subtracting the sum of chloride and sodium bicarbonate from plasma sodium concentration

$$Anion\ gap = Na^+ - (Cl^- + HCO_3^-)$$

Normal anion gap is 12 ($\pm$ 2) mEq/L. Normal anion gap acidosis results from direct loss of HCO_3^- (e.g., diarrhea, renal tubular acidosis, pancreatic fistulas) or the addition of chloride-containing acids (e.g., ammonium chloride, hydrochloric acid), some hyperalimentation fluids, and oral calcium chloride. An increased anion gap acidosis >12-14 mEq/L results from accumulation of nonvolatile acids (acids from lactic acidosis, DKA, renal failure, salicylate and methanol toxicity). Nongap acidosis occurs with hyperchloremia.

ECG: Detects dysrhythmias, which may be caused by acidosis or hyperkalemia. Changes seen with hyperkalemia include peaked T waves, depressed ST segment, decreased size of R waves, decreased or absent P waves, and widened QRS complex. Ventricular fibrillation also may occur with metabolic acidosis.

Collaborative management

Sodium bicarbonate ($NaHCO_3$):   May be indicated when arterial pH is $\leq$7.2. The usual mode of delivery is IV drip: 2-3 ampules (44.5 mEq/ampule) in 1000 ml D_5W, although $NaHCO_3$ may be given IV push in emergencies. Deficit should be calculated and replaced accordingly. Concentration depends on severity of the acidosis and presence of any serum sodium disorders. $NaHCO_3$ must be given very cautiously to avoid metabolic alkalosis and pulmonary edema as a result of the sodium load.

Potassium replacement: Usually, serum hyperkalemia is present, but an intracellular potassium deficit may be present. If a potassium deficit exists (K^+ <3.5), it must be corrected before $NaHCO_3$ is administered, because when the acidosis is corrected, the potassium shifts back to intracellular spaces. This shift in K^+ could result in serum hypokalemia with serious consequences, such as cardiac irritability with fatal dysrhythmias and generalized muscle weakness. See "Hypokalemia," p. 649, for more information.

Mechanical ventilation: If mechanical ventilation is required on the basis of ABG results and clinical signs, it is important that the patient's compensatory hyperventilation be allowed to continue to prevent acidosis from becoming more severe. Therefore the respiratory rate on the ventilator should not be set lower than the rate at which patient has been breathing spontaneously, and the tidal volume should be large enough to maintain compensatory hyperventilation until the underlying disorder can be resolved.

Treatment of underlying disorder

Diabetic ketoacidosis: Insulin and fluids. If acidosis is severe (with a pH of <7.1 or HCO_3^- 6-8 mEq/L), judicious administration of $NaHCO_3$ may be necessary.

Alcoholism-related ketoacidosis: Glucose and saline.

Diarrhea: Usually occurs in association with other fluid and electrolyte disturbances; correction addresses concurrent imbalances.

Acute renal failure: Hemodialysis or peritoneal dialysis to maintain an adequate level of plasma HCO_3^-.

Renal tubular acidosis: May require modest amounts (<100 mEq/day) of bicarbonate.

Poisoning and drug toxicity: Treatment depends on drug ingested or infused. Hemodialysis or peritoneal dialysis may be necessary.

Lactic acidosis: Correction of underlying disorder related to hypoxia and/or hypoperfusion. Mortality associated with lactic acidosis is high. Unless pH is life threatening, treatment with $NaHCO_3$ generally is not indicated and may actually be harmful.

Nursing diagnoses and interventions

Nursing diagnoses and interventions are specific to the pathophysiologic process. See **Altered oral mucous membrane** in other sections of this text. Also see nursing diagnoses and interventions in "Mechanical Ventilation," p. 17; "Psychosocial Support," p. 83; "Psychosocial Support for the Patient's Family and Significant Others," p. 95; "Acute Renal Failure," p. 371; and "Diabetic Ketoacidosis," p. 470.

CHRONIC METABOLIC ACIDOSIS

Pathophysiology

Most often, chronic metabolic acidosis is seen with chronic renal failure in which the kidneys' ability to excrete acids (endogenous and exogenous) is exceeded by acid production and ingestion. The acidosis usually is mild in the initial stage, with HCO_3^- 18-22 mEq/L and a pH of 7.35. Treatment is indicated when serum HCO_3^- levels reach 15 mEq/L. Respiratory compensation occurs but only to a limited degree. A modest decrease in $Paco_2$ will be noted on ABG values. If the patient suffers a respiratory failure state, acidosis will become profound.

Assessment

History and risk factors: Chronic renal failure, renal tubular acidosis, loss of alkaline fluid (e.g., with diarrhea or pancreatic or biliary drainage) for >3-5 days.

Clinical presentation: Usually the process leading to chronic metabolic acidosis is gradual and the patient is symptom free until serum HCO_3^- is ≤15 mEq/L. Fatigue, malaise, and anorexia may be present in relation to the underlying disease.

Diagnostic tests
ABG values: $Paco_2$ will be <35 mm Hg; pH will be <7.35.
Serum bicarbonate: Will be <22 mEq/L (usually 18-21 mEq/L). With severe acidosis, it will be <15 mEq/L.
Serum electrolyte levels: Serum calcium level is checked before treatment of acidosis is initiated to prevent tetany induced by hypocalcemia (caused by a decrease in ionized calcium). Serum phosphorus level is evaluated to determine presence of hyperphosphatemia, a common complication of chronic renal failure. Serum potassium level should be monitored after acidosis has been corrected to detect hypokalemia, inasmuch as potassium shifts back into the cells after correction of the acidosis.

Collaborative management
Alkalizing agents: For serum HCO_3^- levels <15 mEq/L, oral alkalis are administered ($NaHCO_3$ tablets or sodium citrate and citric acid oral solution [Shohl solution]). They are used cautiously to prevent fluid overload and tetany caused by hypocalcemia.

> *Caution:* Be alert to the possibility of pulmonary edema if bicarbonate is administered parenterally to patients with renal insufficiency or cardiovascular disorders.

Oral phosphates: Given if hypophosphatemia is present (not common with chronic renal failure) but may result from overuse of phosphate binders given to treat hyperphosphatemia (very common with chronic renal failure).
Hemodialysis or peritoneal dialysis: If indicated by chronic renal failure or other disease processes (see p. 395).

Nursing diagnoses and interventions
Nursing diagnoses and interventions are specific to the underlying pathophysiologic process. See other sections of this text, particularly Chapter 5.

ACUTE METABOLIC ALKALOSIS
Pathophysiology
Acute metabolic alkalosis results in an elevated serum HCO_3^- (up to 45-50 mEq/L) as a result of H^+ loss or excess alkali intake. A compensatory increase in $Paco_2$ (up to 50-60 mm Hg) will be seen. Respiratory compensation is very limited because of the hypoxemia, which develops as a result of decreased alveolar ventilation. The major causes of this disturbance are loss of gastric acid from vomiting or gastric suction, diuretic therapy, posthypercapnic alkalosis (which occurs when chronic CO_2 retention is corrected rapidly), and excessive $NaHCO_3$ administration (i.e., overcorrection of a metabolic acidosis). Even when the causative factors have been removed, the alkalosis will be maintained until volume and electrolyte disturbances that are contributing to the alkalosis have been corrected. Severe alkalosis (pH >7.6) is associated with high morbidity and mortality. The body can tolerate a greater degree of acidosis than alkalosis.

Assessment
History and risk factors
Clinical circumstances associated with volume/chloride depletion:　　Vomiting or gastric drainage; cystic fibrosis in hot weather when excessive chloride and sodium losses are not replaced.

Diuretic use:　　Usually a mild metabolic alkalosis will occur with diuretic use. The alkalosis will be more severe if using a potent diuretic (i.e., furosemide), especially in patients on sodium-restricted diets.

Posthypercapnic alkalosis:　　May occur after rapid correction of chronic hypercapnia.

Excessive alkali intake.

Clinical presentation:　　Muscular weakness, neuromuscular instability, and hyporeflexia because of accompanying hypokalemia. Decrease in GI tract motility may result in an ileus. Severe alkalosis can result in apathy, confusion, and stupor. Seizures may occur.

Physical assessment:　　Decreased respiratory rate and depth, periods of apnea, tachycardia (atrial or ventricular).

Monitoring parameters:　　Atrial-ventricular dysrhythmias as a result of cardiac irritability secondary to hypokalemia; prolonged QT interval.

Diagnostic tests
ABG values:　　Determine severity of alkalosis and response to therapy.

Serum bicarbonate levels:　　Values will be elevated to >26 mEq/L.

Serum electrolyte levels:　　Usually, serum potassium will be low (<4 mEq/L) as will serum chloride (<95 mEq/L).

Urinalysis:　　Urine chloride levels can help identify the cause of the metabolic alkalosis. Urine chloride level will be <15 mEq/L if hypovolemia and hypochloremia are present and >20 mEq/L with excess retained HCO_3^-. This test is not reliable if diuretics are used within the previous 12 h.

ECG findings:　　To assess for dysrhythmias, especially if profound hypokalemia or alkalosis is present.

Collaborative management
Management will depend on the underlying disorder. Mild or moderate metabolic alkalosis usually does not require specific therapeutic interventions.

Saline infusion:　　Normal saline infusion may correct volume (chloride) deficit in patients with gastric alkalosis because of gastric losses. Metabolic alkalosis is difficult to correct if hypovolemia and chloride deficit are not corrected.

Potassium chloride (KCl):　　Indicated for patients with low potassium levels. KCl is preferred over other potassium salts because chloride losses can be replaced simultaneously.

Sodium and potassium chloride:　　Effective for posthypercapnic alkalosis, which occurs when chronic CO_2 retention is corrected rapidly (e.g., via mechanical ventilation). If adequate amounts of chloride and potassium are not available, renal excretion of excess HCO_3^- is impaired and metabolic alkalosis continues.

Cautious IV administration of isotonic hydrochloride solution, ammonium chloride, or arginine hydrochloride:　　May be warranted if severe metabolic alkalosis (pH >7.6 and HCO_3^- >40-45 mEq/L) exist, especially if chloride or potassium salts are contraindicated. The medication is delivered via continuous IV infusion at a slow rate, with frequent monitoring of IV insertion site for signs of infiltration. Ammonium chloride and arginine hydrochloride may be dangerous to patients with renal or hepatic failure.

Nursing diagnoses and interventions
Nursing diagnoses and interventions are specific to the underlying pathophysiologic process. See Chapter 5, particularly.

CHRONIC METABOLIC ALKALOSIS

Pathophysiology
Chronic metabolic alkalosis results in a pH >7.45 and HCO_3^- >26 mEq/L. $Paco_2$ will be elevated (>45 mm Hg) to compensate for the loss of H^+ or excess serum HCO_3^-. The three clinical situations in which this can occur are: (1) abnormalities in the kidneys' excretion of HCO_3^- related to a mineralocorticoid effect; (2) loss of H^+ through the GI tract; and (3) long-term diuretic therapy, especially the thiazides and furosemide.

Assessment
History and risk factors
Diuretic use: Thiazide diuretics cause a loss of chloride, potassium, and hydrogen ions. Massive depletion of potassium stores with loss of up to 1000 mEq, which is one third of total body potassium, may occur, causing profound hypokalemia (K^+ ≤2.0 mEq/L).
Hyperadrenocorticism: Cushing syndrome, primary aldosteronism. This is not a chloride deficit but a chronic loss of potassium, which can lead to total body depletion of potassium with profound hypokalemia (K^+ ≤2.0 mEq/L).
Chronic vomiting or chronic GI losses through GI suction.
Milk-alkali syndrome: An infrequent cause of metabolic alkalosis.
Hypercalcemic nephropathy and alkalosis: Develop as a result of excessive intake of absorbable alkali (antacids containing calcium carbonate).
Clinical presentation: Patient may be free of symptoms. With severe potassium depletion and profound alkalosis, patient may experience weakness, neuromuscular instability, and decrease in GI tract motility, which can result in ileus.
Monitoring parameters: Frequent PVCs or U waves with hypokalemia and alkalosis.

Diagnostic tests
ABG values: Determine severity of acid-base imbalance. $Paco_2$ will be increased (>45 mm Hg), and pH will be >7.4.
Serum bicarbonate levels: Will be >26 mEq/L.
Serum electrolyte levels: Usually potassium will be profoundly low (may be ≤2 mEq/L). Chloride may be <95 mEq/L. Magnesium may be <1.5 mEq/L in both renal system abnormalities.

Collaborative management
The goal is to correct the underlying acid-base disorder via the following interventions.
Fluid management: If volume depletion exists, normal saline infusions are given.
Potassium replacement: If a chloride deficit also is present, KCl is the drug of choice. If a chloride deficit does not exist, other potassium salts are acceptable.
IV potassium: If the patient is undergoing cardiac monitoring, up to 20 mEq/h of KCl is given for serious hypokalemia. Concentrated doses of KCl (>40 mEq/L) require administration through a central venous line because of blood vessel irritation.
Oral potassium: Tastes very unpleasant; 15 mEq/glass is all most patients can tolerate, with a maximum daily dose of 60-80 mEq. Slow-release potassium tablets are an acceptable form of KCl. All forms of KCl may be irritating to gastric mucosa.
Dietary: Normal diet contains 3 g or 75 mEq of potassium but not in the form of KCl. Dietary supplementation of potassium is not effective if a concurrent chloride deficit also is present.

Potassium-sparing diuretics: May be added to treatment if thiazide diuretics are the cause of hypokalemia and metabolic alkalosis.
Identify and correct cause of hyperadrenocorticism.

Nursing diagnoses and interventions
Nursing diagnoses and interventions are specific to the underlying pathophysiologic process. See Chapter 5 for examples.

Bibliography

American College of Chest Physicians/Society of Critical Care Medicine Consensus Conference Committee: Definitions for sepsis and organ failure and guidelines for the use of innovative therapies in sepsis, *Crit Care Med* 20(6):864-874, 1992.

Baue AE et al: Systemic inflammatory response syndrome (SIRS), multiple organ dysfunction syndrome (MODS), multiple organ failure (MOF): are we winning the battle? *Shock* 10(2):79-89, 1998.

Brown M, Hess R: Managing latex allergy in the cardiac surgical patient, *Crit Care Nurs Q* 21(1):8-15, 1998.

Carroll K et al: Nonpharmacologic approaches to substance abuse treatment, *Med Clin North Am* 81(4):927-944, 1997.

Coupey S: Barbiturates, *Pediatr Rev* 18(8):260-264, 1997.

Cunningham J: Ecstasy-induced rhabdomyolysis and its role in the development of acute renal failure, *Intensive Care Nurs* 13(4):216-223, 1997.

Dahlen K et al: Acute lung failure induced by tricyclic antidepressants, *Toxicol Appl Pharmacol* 146(2):309-316, 1997.

Deftos LJ: Hypercalcemia: mechanism, differential diagnosis and remedies, *Postgrad Med* 100(6):119-126, 1996.

Dellinger RP: Current therapy for sepsis, *Infect Dis Clin North Am* 13(2):495-507, 1999.

Dunne J et al: Practice parameter for the assessment and treatment of children and adolescents with substance use disorders, *J Am Acad Child Adolesc Psychiatry* 36(10):140S-156S, 1997.

Faist E, Kim C: Therapeutic immunomodulary approaches for the control of systemic inflammatory response syndrome and the prevention of sepsis, *New Horiz* 6(suppl 2):S97-S102, 1998.

Fraser CL, Arieff AI: Epidemiology, pathophysiology, and management of hyponatremic encephalopathy, *Am J Med* 102:67-77, 1997.

Fried LF, Palevsky PM: Hyponatremia and hypernatremia, *Med Clin North Am* 81(3):585-609, 1997.

Gorman M et al: What do you do when your patient uses illicit drugs? *Am J Nurs* 98(3):54, 1998.

Greenberg A: Hyperkalemia: treatment options, *Semin Nephrol* 18(1):46-57, 1998.

Gross P et al: The treatment of severe hyponatremia, *Kidney Int* 53(64):S6-S11, 1998.

Halperin ML, Goldstein MB: *Fluid, electrolyte and acid-base physiology*, ed 3, Philadelphia, 1999, Saunders.

Harvey MA: Systemic inflammatory response syndrome and multiorgan dysfunction syndrome. In Kinney MR et al: *AACN clinical reference for critical care nursing,* ed 4, St Louis, 1998, Mosby.

Harwood S: ActionStat, *Nursing* 2:33, 1997.

Hazinski MF: Mediator-specific therapies for the systemic inflammatory response syndrome, sepsis, severe sepsis, and septic shock, *Crit Care Clin Nurs North Am* 6(2):309-319, 1994.

Hoffman R et al: Evaluation of the patient with chest pain after cocaine use, *Crit Care Clin* 13(4):809-828, 1997.

Hollander J et al: Predictors of coronary artery disease in patients with cocaine-associated myocardial infarction. Cocaine-Associated Myocardial Infarction (CAMI) Study Group, *Am J Med* 102(2):158-163, 1997.

Horne MM, Heitz UE, Swearingen PL: *Pocket guide to fluids and electrolytes,* ed 3, St Louis, 1997, Mosby.

Kalant H et al: Opium revisted: a brief review of its nature, composition, non-medical use and relative risk, *Addiction* 92(3):267-277, 1997.

Keen J et al: *Mosby's critical care and emergency drug reference,* ed 2, St Louis, 1996, Mosby.

Kokko JP, Tannen RL: *Fluids and electrolytes,* ed 3, Philadelphia, 1996, Saunders.

Lauro R, Karp BI: Myelinolysis after correction of hyponatremia, *Ann Intern Med* 126(1):57-62, 1997.

Liebelt E et al: Serial electrocardiogram changes in acute tricyclic antidepressant overdose, *Crit Care Med* 25(10):1721-1726, 1997.

Lundberg JS et al: Septic shock: an analysis of outcomes for patients with onset on hospital wards versus intensive care units, *Crit Care Med* 26(6):1020-1024, 1998.

Malek N: Acute salicylate overdose, *Hosp Pract (Off Ed)* 33(6):46, 1998.

Mandal AK: Hypokalemia and hyperkalemia, *Med Clin North Am* 81(3):611-639, 1997.

Marino PL: *The ICU book,* ed 2, Baltimore, 1998, Williams & Wilkins.

Mayo-Smith M et al: Pharmacological management of alcohol withdrawal: a meta-analysis and evidenced-based practice guideline, *JAMA* 278(2):144-151, 1997.

McDonough J: Emergency! Acetaminophen overdose, *Am J Nurs* 93(3):52, 1998.

McGeary T: Fatal reaction, *Nurs Times* 93(34):26-28, 1997.

Miller PR et al: Systemic inflammatory response syndrome in the trauma intensive care unit: who is infected? *J Trauma* 47(6):1004-1008, 1999.

Mitchell I et al: Earlier identification of patients at risk from acetaminophen-induced acute liver failure, *Crit Care Med* 26(2):279-284, 1998.

Moriyama S et al: Evaluation of oxygen consumption and resting energy expenditure in critically ill patients with systemic inflammatory response syndrome, *Crit Care Med* 27(10):2133-2136, 1999.

Muelleman RL, Lindzon RD, Silvers WS: Allergy, hypersensitivity, and anaphylaxis. In Rosen P, Barkin R, editors: *Emergency medicine: concepts and clinical practice*, ed 4, St Louis, 1998, Mosby.

O'Connor P et al: Rapid and ultrarapid opioid detoxification techniques, *JAMA* 279(3):229-234, 1998.

Osborn H et al: New-onset bronchospasm or recrudescence of asthma associated with cocaine abuse, *Acad Emerg Med* 4(7):689-692, 1997.

Palevsky PM: Hypernatremia, *Semin Nephrol* 18(1):20-30, 1998.

Perazella MA, Mahnessmith RL: Hyperkalemia in the elderly, *J Gen Intern Med* 12:646-656, 1997.

Preston RA: *Acid-base, fluids and electrolytes made ridiculously simple*, Miami, 1997, MedMaster.

Rauen C, Munro N: Shock. In Kinney MR et al: *AACN clinical reference for critical care nursing,* ed 4, St Louis, 1998, Mosby.

Rohaly-Davis J, Johnston K: Hematologic emergencies in the intensive care unit, *Crit Care Nur Q* 18(4):35-43, 1996.

Schrier RW, editor: *Renal and electrolyte disorders*, ed 5, Philadelphia, 1997, Lippincott-Raven.

Secor VH: The inflammatory response in critical illness, *Crit Care Clin North Am* 6(2):251-264, 1994.

Sporer K: Clinical course of crack cocaine body stuffers, *Ann Emerg Med* 29(5):596-601, 1997.

Stanley M: Sepsis in the elderly, *Crit Care Nurs Clin North Am* 8(1):1-6, 1996.

Stein M et al: Women and substance abuse, *Med Clin North Am* 81(4):979-998, 1997.

Stiesmeyer J: Drug overdose. In Keen J, editor: *Mosby's critical care nursing consultant,* St Louis, 1997, Mosby.

Sulkowski J et al: Acute mental status changes, *AACN Clin Issues* 8(3):319-334, 1997.

Talmor M, Hydo L, Barie PS: Relationship of systemic inflammatory response syndrome to organ dysfunction, length of stay, and mortality in critical surgical illness: effect of intensive care unit resuscitation, *Arch Surg* 134(1):81-87, 1999.

Verbalis JG: Adaption to acute and chronic hyponatremia: implications for symptomatology, diagnosis, and therapy, *Semin Nephrol* 18(1):3-19, 1998.

Whang R: Clinical disorders of magnesium metabolism, *Compre Ther* 23(3):168-173, 1997.

White V: ActionStat. Aspirin overdose, *Nursing* 28(4):33, 1998.

Zafonte RD, Mann NR: Cerebral salt wasting syndrome in brain injury patients: a potential cause of hyponatremia, *Arch Phys Med Rehabil* 78:540-542, 1997.

Zimmerman P: Emergency! Tricyclic antidepressant overdose, *Am J Nurs* 97(10):39, 1997.

The American Heart Association's Advanced Cardiac Life Support (ACLS) Algorithms

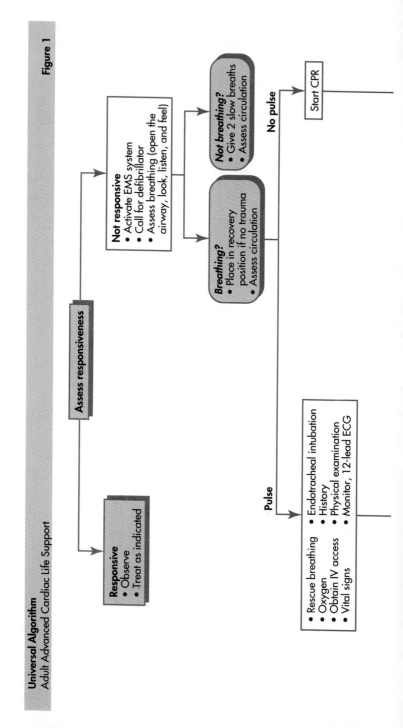

Universal Algorithm
Adult Advanced Cardiac Life Support

Figure 1

Assess responsiveness

Responsive
• Observe
• Treat as indicated

Not responsive
• Activate EMS system
• Call for defibrillator
• Assess breathing (open the airway, look, listen, and feel)

Breathing?
• Place in recovery position if no trauma
• Assess circulation

Not breathing?
• Give 2 slow breaths
• Assess circulation

No pulse → Start CPR

Pulse

• Rescue breathing   • Endotracheal intubation
• Oxygen   • History
• Obtain IV access   • Physical examination
• Vital signs   • Monitor, 12-lead ECG

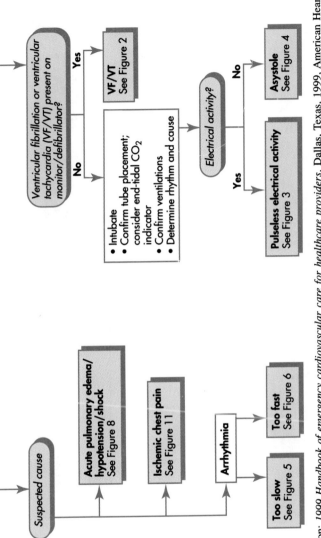

From American Heart Association: *1999 Handbook of emergency cardiovascular care for healthcare providers*, Dallas, Texas, 1999, American Heart Association.

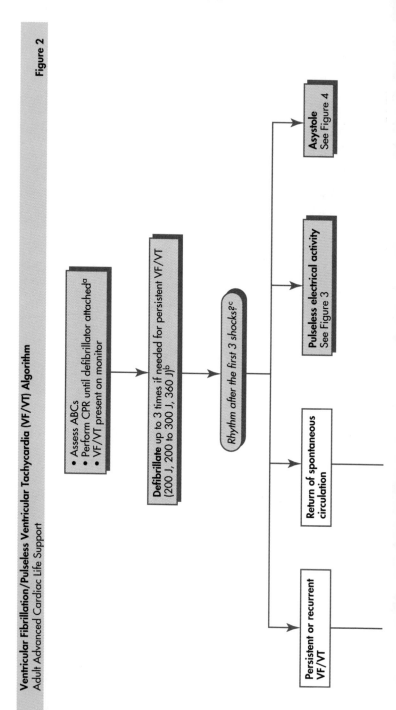

Ventricular Fibrillation/Pulseless Ventricular Tachycardia (VF/VT) Algorithm
Adult Advanced Cardiac Life Support

Figure 2

- Assess ABCs
- Perform CPR until defibrillator attached[a]
- VF/VT present on monitor

Defibrillate up to 3 times if needed for persistent VF/VT
(200 J, 200 to 300 J, 360 J)[b]

Rhythm after the first 3 shocks?[c]

Persistent or recurrent VF/VT

Return of spontaneous circulation

Pulseless electrical activity
See Figure 3

Asystole
See Figure 4

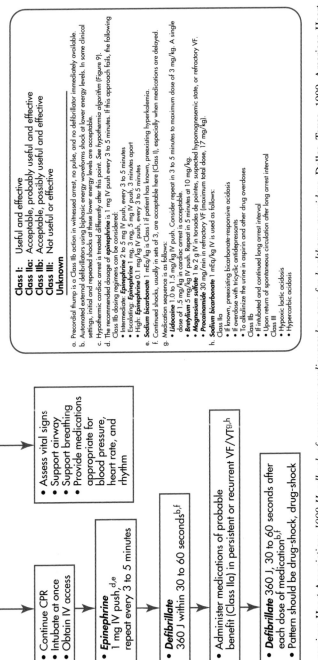

- Continue CPR
- Intubate at once
- Obtain IV access

- *Epinephrine*
  1 mg IV push,[d,e]
  repeat every 3 to 5 minutes

- *Defibrillate*
  360 J within 30 to 60 seconds[b,f]

- Administer medications of probable benefit (Class IIa) in persistent or recurrent VF/VT[g,h]

- *Defibrillate* 360 J, 30 to 60 seconds after each dose of medication[b,f]
- Pattern should be drug-shock, drug-shock

- Assess vital signs
- Support airway
- Support breathing
- Provide medications appropriate for blood pressure, heart rate, and rhythm

Class I: Useful and effective
Class IIa: Acceptable, probably useful and effective
Class IIb: Acceptable, possibly useful and effective
Class III: Not useful or effective
Unknown

a. Precordial thump is a Class IIb action in witnessed arrest, no pulse, and no defibrillator immediately available.
b. Automated external defibrillators using biphasic energy waveforms shock at lower energy levels. In some clinical settings, initial and repeated shocks of these lower energy levels are acceptable.
c. Hypothermic cardiac arrest is treated differently after this point. See hypothermia algorithm (Figure 9).
d. The recommended dosage of *epinephrine* is 1 mg IV push every 3 to 5 minutes. If this approach fails, the following Class IIb dosing regimens can be considered:
   - Intermediate: *Epinephrine* 2 to 5 mg IV push, every 3 to 5 minutes
   - Escalating: *Epinephrine* 1 mg, 3 mg, 5 mg IV push, 3 minutes apart
   - High: *Epinephrine* 0.1 mg/kg IV push, every 3 to 5 minutes
e. *Sodium bicarbonate* 1 mEq/kg is Class I if patient has known, preexisting hyperkalemia.
f. Continued shocks, usually in sets of 3, are acceptable here (Class I), especially when medications are delayed.
g. Medication sequence is as follows:
   - *Lidocaine* 1.0 to 1.5 mg/kg IV push. Consider repeat in 3 to 5 minutes to maximum dose of 3 mg/kg. A single dose of 1.5 mg/kg in cardiac arrest is acceptable.
   - *Bretylium* 5 mg/kg IV push. Repeat in 5 minutes at 10 mg/kg.
   - *Magnesium sulfate* 1 to 2 g IV in torsades de pointes, suspected hypomagnesemic state, or refractory VF.
   - *Procainamide* 30 mg/min in refractory VF (maximum total dose, 17 mg/kg).
h. *Sodium bicarbonate* 1 mEq/kg IV is used as follows:
   Class IIa
   - If known, preexisting bicarbonate-responsive acidosis
   - If overdose with tricyclic antidepressants
   - To alkalinize the urine in aspirin and other drug overdoses
   Class IIb
   - If intubated and continued long arrest interval
   - Upon return of spontaneous circulation after long arrest interval
   Class III
   - Hypoxic lactic acidosis
   - Hypercarbic acidosis

From American Heart Association: *1999 Handbook of emergency cardiovascular care for healthcare providers*, Dallas, Texas, 1999, American Heart Association.

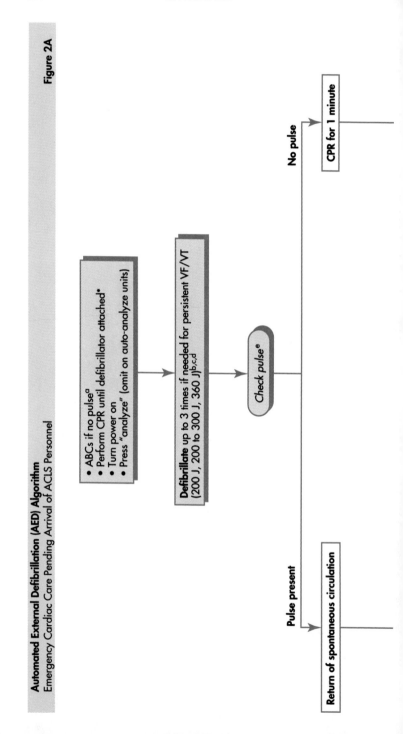

Automated External Defibrillation (AED) Algorithm
Emergency Cardiac Care Pending Arrival of ACLS Personnel

Figure 2A

- ABCs if no pulse[a]
- Perform CPR until defibrillator attached*
- Turn power on
- Press "analyze" (omit on auto-analyze units)

Defibrillate up to 3 times if needed for persistent VF/VT
(200 J, 200 to 300 J, 360 J)[b,c,d]

Check *pulse*[e]

Pulse present

Return of spontaneous circulation

No pulse

CPR for 1 minute

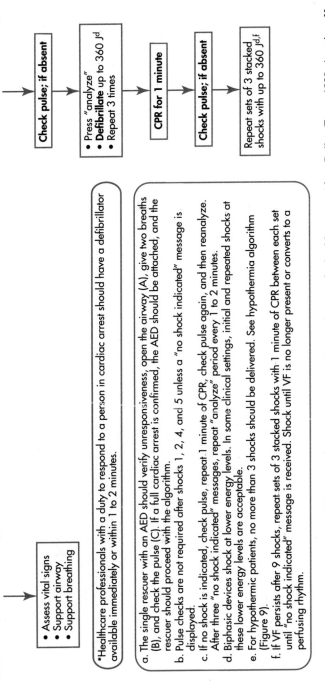

Check pulse; if absent

- Press "analyze"
- **Defibrillate** up to 360 J^d
- Repeat 3 times

CPR for 1 minute

Check pulse; if absent

Repeat sets of 3 stacked shocks with up to 360 J^{d,f}

- Assess vital signs
- Support airway
- Support breathing

*Healthcare professionals with a duty to respond to a person in cardiac arrest should have a defibrillator available immediately or within 1 to 2 minutes.

a. The single rescuer with an AED should verify unresponsiveness, open the airway (A), give two breaths (B), and check the pulse (C). If a full cardiac arrest is confirmed, the AED should be attached, and the rescuer should proceed with the algorithm.

b. Pulse checks are not required after shocks 1, 2, 4, and 5 unless a "no shock indicated" message is displayed.

c. If no shock is indicated, check pulse, repeat 1 minute of CPR, check pulse again, and then reanalyze. After three "no shock indicated" messages, repeat "analyze" period every 1 to 2 minutes.

d. Biphasic devices shock at lower energy levels. In some clinical settings, initial and repeated shocks at these lower energy levels are acceptable.

e. For hypothermic patients, no more than 3 shocks should be delivered. See hypothermia algorithm (Figure 9).

f. If VF persists after 9 shocks, repeat sets of 3 stacked shocks with 1 minute of CPR between each set until "no shock indicated" message is received. Shock until VF is no longer present or converts to a perfusing rhythm.

From American Heart Association: *1999 Handbook of emergency cardiovascular care for healthcare providers*, Dallas, Texas, 1999, American Heart Association.

Pulseless Electrical Activity Algorithm
Adult Advanced Cardiac Life Support

Figure 3

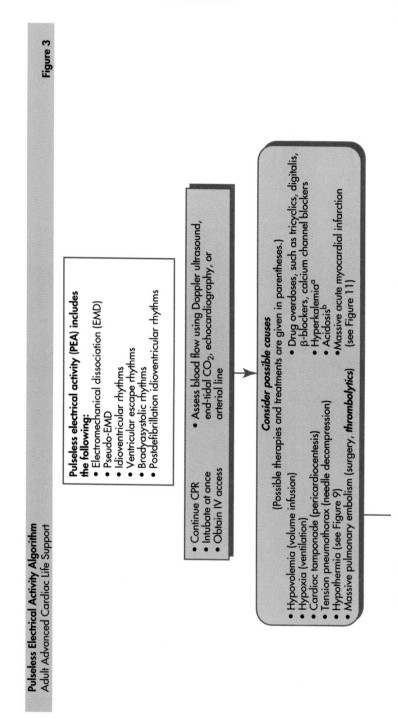

Pulseless electrical activity (PEA) includes the following:
- Electromechanical dissociation (EMD)
- Pseudo-EMD
- Idioventricular rhythms
- Ventricular escape rhythms
- Bradyasystolic rhythms
- Postdefibrillation idioventricular rhythms

- Continue CPR
- Intubate at once
- Obtain IV access

- Assess blood flow using Doppler ultrasound, end-tidal CO_2, or arterial line

Consider possible causes
(Possible therapies and treatments are given in parentheses.)

- Hypovolemia (volume infusion)
- Hypoxia (ventilation)
- Cardiac tamponade (pericardiocentesis)
- Tension pneumothorax (needle decompression)
- Hypothermia (see Figure 9)
- Massive pulmonary embolism (surgery, *thrombolytics*)

- Drug overdoses, such as tricyclics, digitalis, β-blockers, calcium channel blockers
- Hyperkalemia[a]
- Acidosis[b]
- Massive acute myocardial infarction (see Figure 11)

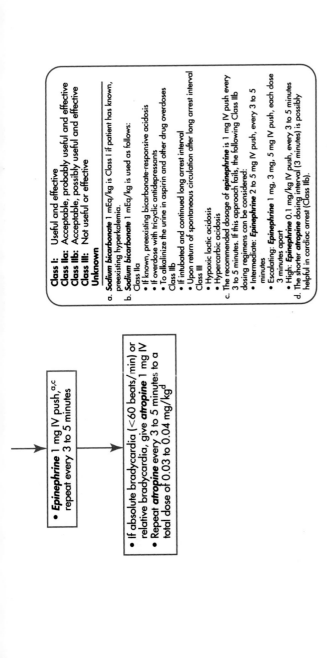

- **Epinephrine** 1 mg IV push,[a,c] repeat every 3 to 5 minutes

---

- If absolute bradycardia (<60 beats/min) or relative bradycardia, give **atropine** 1 mg IV
- Repeat **atropine** every 3 to 5 minutes to a total dose of 0.03 to 0.04 mg/kg[d]

Class I: Useful and effective
Class IIa: Acceptable, probably useful and effective
Class IIb: Acceptable, possibly useful and effective
Class III: Not useful or effective
Unknown

a. **Sodium bicarbonate** 1 mEq/kg is Class I if patient has known, preexisting hyperkalemia.
b. **Sodium bicarbonate** 1 mEq/kg is used as follows:
Class IIa
 • If known, preexisting bicarbonate-responsive acidosis
 • If overdose with tricyclic antidepressants
 • To alkalinize the urine in aspirin and other drug overdoses
Class IIb
 • If intubated and continued long arrest interval
 • Upon return of spontaneous circulation after long arrest interval
Class III
 • Hypoxic lactic acidosis
 • Hypercarbic acidosis
c. The recommended dosage of **epinephrine** is 1 mg IV push every 3 to 5 minutes. If this approach fails, the following Class IIb dosing regimens can be considered:
 • Intermediate: **Epinephrine** 2 to 5 mg IV push, every 3 to 5 minutes
 • Escalating: **Epinephrine** 1 mg, 3 mg, 5 mg IV push, each dose 3 minutes apart
 • High: **Epinephrine** 0.1 mg/kg IV push, every 3 to 5 minutes
d. The shorter **atropine** dosing interval (3 minutes) is possibly helpful in cardiac arrest (Class IIb).

From American Heart Association: *1999 Handbook of emergency cardiovascular care for healthcare providers*, Dallas, Texas, 1999, American Heart Association.

Asystole Algorithm
Adult Advanced Cardiac Life Support

Figure 4

- Continue CPR
- Intubate at once
- Obtain IV access
- Confirm asystole in more than one lead

Consider possible causes
- Hypoxia
- Hyperkalemia
- Hypokalemia
- Preexisting acidosis
- Drug overdose
- Hypothermia

Consider immediate transcutaneous pacing[a]

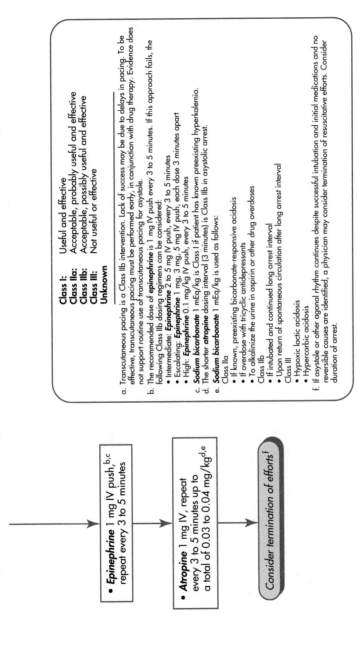

Class I: Useful and effective
Class IIa: Acceptable, probably useful and effective
Class IIb: Acceptable, possibly useful and effective
Class III: Not useful or effective
Unknown

a. Transcutaneous pacing is a Class IIb intervention. Lack of success may be due to delays in pacing. To be effective, transcutaneous pacing must be performed early, in conjunction with drug therapy. Evidence does not support routine use of transcutaneous pacing for asystole.

b. The recommended dose of *epinephrine* is 1 mg IV push every 3 to 5 minutes. If this approach fails, the following Class IIb dosing regimens can be considered:
  • Intermediate: *Epinephrine* 2 to 5 mg IV push, every 3 to 5 minutes
  • Escalating: *Epinephrine* 1 mg, 3 mg, 5 mg IV push, each dose 3 minutes apart
  • High: *Epinephrine* 0.1 mg/kg IV push, every 3 to 5 minutes

c. *Sodium bicarbonate* 1 mEq/kg is Class I if patient has known preexisting hyperkalemia.

d. The shorter *atropine* dosing interval (3 minutes) is Class IIb in asystolic arrest.

e. *Sodium bicarbonate* 1 mEq/kg is used as follows:
  Class IIa
  • If known, preexisting bicarbonate-responsive acidosis
  • If overdose with tricyclic antidepressants
  • To alkalinize the urine in aspirin or other drug overdoses
  Class IIb
  • If intubated and continued long arrest interval
  • Upon return of spontaneous circulation after long arrest interval
  Class III
  • Hypoxic lactic acidosis
  • Hypercarbic acidosis

f. If asystole or other agonal rhythm continues despite successful intubation and initial medications and no reversible causes are identified, a physician may consider termination of resuscitative efforts. Consider duration of arrest.

• *Epinephrine* 1 mg IV push,[b,c] repeat every 3 to 5 minutes

• *Atropine* 1 mg IV, repeat every 3 to 5 minutes up to a total of 0.03 to 0.04 mg/kg[d,e]

Consider termination of efforts[f]

From American Heart Association: *1999 Handbook of emergency cardiovascular care for healthcare providers*, Dallas, Texas, 1999, American Heart Association.

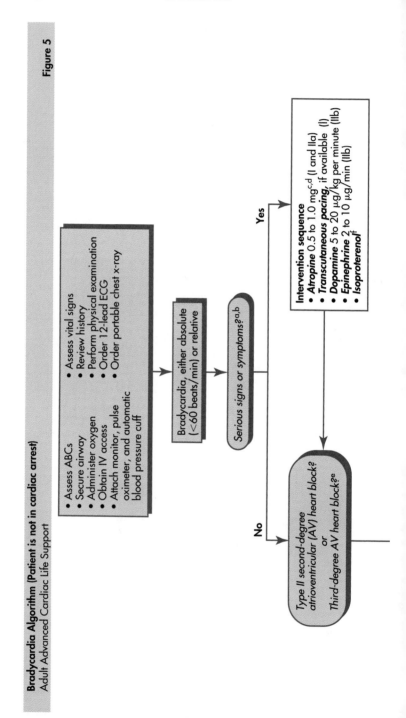

Bradycardia Algorithm (Patient is not in cardiac arrest)
Adult Advanced Cardiac Life Support

Figure 5

No

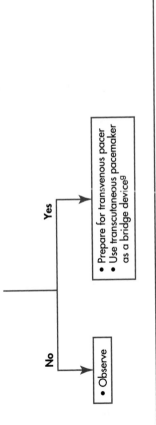

• Observe

Yes

• Prepare for transvenous pacer
• Use transcutaneous pacemaker as a bridge device[g]

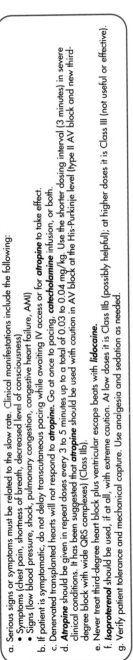

a. Serious signs or symptoms must be related to the slow rate. Clinical manifestations include the following:
  • Symptoms (chest pain, shortness of breath, decreased level of consciousness)
  • Signs (low blood pressure, shock, pulmonary congestion, congestive heart failure, AMI)

b. If patient is symptomatic, do not delay transcutaneous pacing while awaiting IV access or for *atropine* to take effect.

c. Denervated transplanted hearts will not respond to *atropine*. Go at once to pacing, *catecholamine* infusion, or both.

d. *Atropine* should be given in repeat doses every 3 to 5 minutes up to a total of 0.03 to 0.04 mg/kg. Use the shorter dosing interval (3 minutes) in severe clinical conditions. It has been suggested that *atropine* should be used with caution in AV block at the His-Purkinje level (type II AV block and new third-degree block with wide QRS complexes) (Class IIb).

e. Never treat third-degree heart block plus ventricular escape beats with *lidocaine.*

f. *Isoproterenol* should be used, if at all, with extreme caution. At low doses it is Class IIb (possibly helpful); at higher doses it is Class III (not useful or effective).

g. Verify patient tolerance and mechanical capture. Use analgesia and sedation as needed.

From American Heart Association: *1999 Handbook of emergency cardiovascular care for healthcare providers*, Dallas, Texas, 1999, American Heart Association.

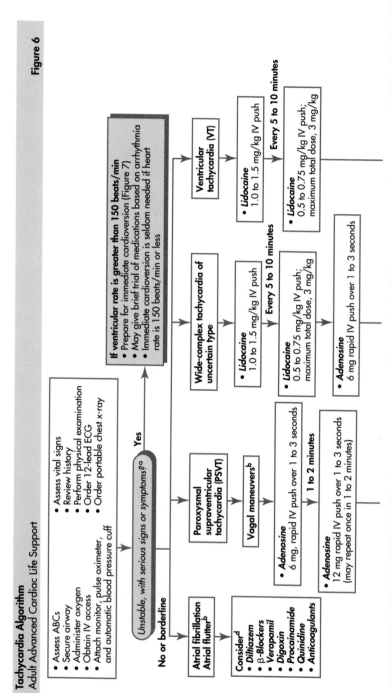

Tachycardia Algorithm
Adult Advanced Cardiac Life Support

Figure 6

From American Heart Association: *1999 Handbook of emergency cardiovascular care for healthcare providers*, Dallas, Texas, 1999, American Heart Association.

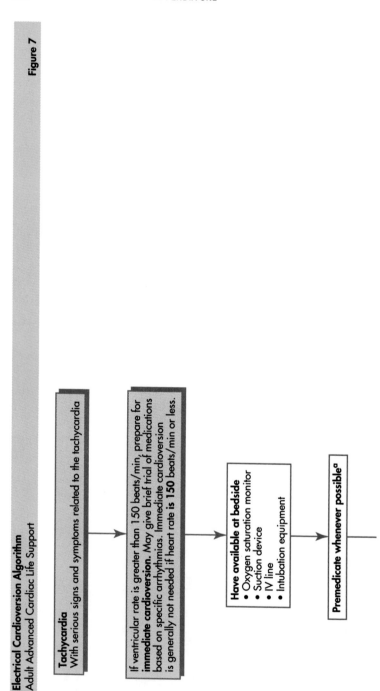

Electrical Cardioversion Algorithm
Adult Advanced Cardiac Life Support

Figure 7

Tachycardia
With serious signs and symptoms related to the tachycardia

If ventricular rate is greater than 150 beats/min, prepare for **immediate cardioversion.** May give brief trial of medications based on specific arrhythmias. Immediate cardioversion is generally not needed if heart rate is **150 beats/min or less.**

Have available at bedside
• Oxygen saturation monitor
• Suction device
• IV line
• Intubation equipment

Premedicate whenever possible[a]

Synchronized cardioversion[b,c]
- Ventricular tachycardia (VT)[d]
- Paroxysmal supraventricular tachycardia[e]
- Atrial fibrillation
- Atrial flutter[e]

— 100 J, 200 J, 300 J, 360 J

a. Effective regimens have included a sedative (eg, *diazepam, midazolam, barbiturates, etomidate, ketamine, methohexital*) with or without an analgesic agent (e.g., *fentanyl, morphine, meperidine*). Many experts recommend anesthesia if service is readily available.

b. Note possible need to resynchronize after each cardioversion.

c. If delays in synchronization occur and clinical condition is critical, go to immediate unsynchronized shocks.

d. Treat polymorphic VT (irregular form and rate) like ventricular fibrillation: see ventricular fibrillation/pulseless ventricular tachycardia algorithm (Figure 2).

e. Paroxysmal supraventricular tachycardia and atrial flutter often respond to lower enegy levels (start with 50 J).

From American Heart Association: *1999 Handbook of emergency cardiovascular care for healthcare providers*, Dallas, Texas, 1999, American Heart Association.

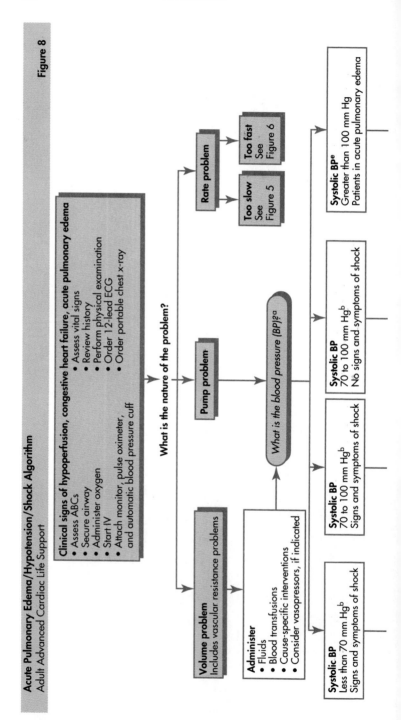

Acute Pulmonary Edema/Hypotension/Shock Algorithm
Adult Advanced Cardiac Life Support

Figure 8

Clinical signs of hypoperfusion, congestive heart failure, acute pulmonary edema
- Assess ABCs
- Secure airway
- Administer oxygen
- Start IV
- Attach monitor, pulse oximeter, and automatic blood pressure cuff
- Assess vital signs
- Review history
- Perform physical examination
- Order 12-lead ECG
- Order portable chest x-ray

What is the nature of the problem?

Volume problem
Includes vascular resistance problems

Pump problem

Rate problem

Too slow See Figure 5

Too fast See Figure 6

Administer
- Fluids
- Blood transfusions
- Cause-specific interventions
- Consider vasopressors, if indicated

What is the blood pressure (BP)?[a]

Systolic BP[b]
Less than 70 mm Hg
Signs and symptoms of shock

Systolic BP[b]
70 to 100 mm Hg
Signs and symptoms of shock

Systolic BP[b]
70 to 100 mm Hg
No signs and symptoms of shock

Systolic BP[e]
Greater than 100 mm Hg
Patients in acute pulmonary edema

Consider
- **Norepinephrine**
  0.5 to 30 μg/min IV
  or
- **Dopamine**
  5 to 20 μg/kg
  per minute

Dopaminec
2.5 to 20 μg/kg per
minute IV (Add
norepinephrine if
dopamine dose is
greater than 20 μg/kg
per minute.)

Dobutamined
2 to 20 μg/kg
per minute IV

- **Nitroglycerin:** Start 10 to 20 μg/min IV (Use
  if ischemia persists and BP remains elevated.
  Titrate to effect.) and/or
- **Nitroprusside** 0.1 to 5.0 μg/kg per minute IV

Consider
Further actions, especially if the patient is in acute pulmonary edema

First-line actions
- **Furosemide**
  IV 0.5 to 1.0 mg/kg
- **Morphine** IV 1 to 3 mg
- **Nitroglycerin** sublingual
- **Oxygen/** intubation as
  needed

Second-line actions
- **Nitroglycerin** IV if BP >100 mm Hg
- **Nitroprusside** IV if BP >100 mm Hg
- **Dopamine** if BP <100 mm Hg
- **Dobutamine** if BP >100 mm Hg
- Positive end-expiratory pressure (PEEP)
- Continuous positive airway pressure (CPAP)

Third-line actions
- **Amrinone** 0.75 mg/kg, then 5 to 15 μg/kg per minute (if other
  drugs fail)
- **Aminophylline** 5 mg/kg (if wheezing)
- **Thrombolytic** therapy (if not in shock)
- **Digoxin** (if atrial fibrillation, supraventricular tachycardias)
- Angioplasty (if drugs fail)
- Intra-aortic balloon pump (bridge to surgery)
- Surgical interventions (repair/replace valves, cardiac-assist
  devices, coronary artery bypass grafts, heart transplant)

a. Base patient management after this point on invasive hemodynamic monitoring if possible. Guidelines
presume clinical signs of hypoperfusion.
b. Fluid IV bolus of 250 to 500 mL normal saline should be tried. If no response, consider sympathomimetics.
c. Move to **dopamine** and stop **norepinephrine** when BP improves. Avoid **dopamine** (consider **dobutamine**)
if no signs of hypoperfusion.
d. Add **dopamine** (and avoid **dobutamine**) if systolic BP drops below 90 mm Hg.
e. Consider **nitroglycerin** if initial blood pressures are in this range; reduces preload in patients with acute
pulmonary edema.

From American Heart Association: *1999 Handbook of emergency cardiovascular care for healthcare providers,* Dallas, Texas, 1999, American Heart
Association.

Hypothermia Algorithm
Adult Advanced Cardiac Life Support

Figure 9

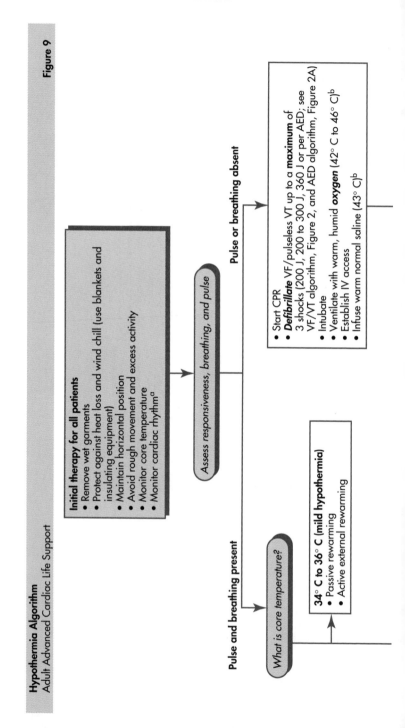

Initial therapy for all patients
- Remove wet garments
- Protect against heat loss and wind chill (use blankets and insulating equipment)
- Maintain horizontal position
- Avoid rough movement and excess activity
- Monitor core temperature
- Monitor cardiac rhythm[a]

Assess responsiveness, breathing, and pulse

Pulse and breathing present

Pulse or breathing absent

- Start CPR
- **Defibrillate** VF/pulseless VT up to a **maximum** of 3 shocks (200 J, 200 to 300 J, 360 J or per AED; see VF/VT algorithm, Figure 2, and AED algorithm, Figure 2A)
- Intubate
- Ventilate with warm, humid *oxygen* (42° C to 46° C)[b]
- Establish IV access
- Infuse warm normal saline (43° C)[b]

What is core temperature?

34° C to 36° C (mild hypothermia)
- Passive rewarming
- Active external rewarming

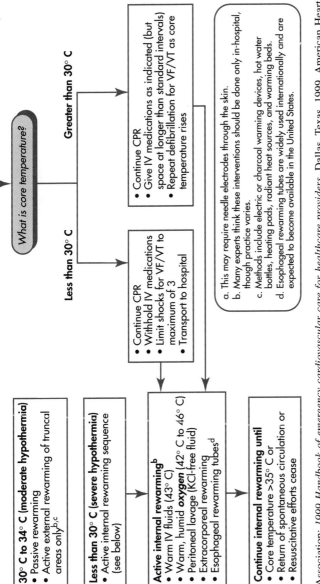

What is core temperature?

Less than 30° C

- Continue CPR
- Withhold IV medications
- Limit shocks for VF/VT to maximum of 3
- Transport to hospital

Greater than 30° C

- Continue CPR
- Give IV medications as indicated (but space at longer than standard intervals)
- Repeat defibrillation for VF/VT as core temperature rises

30° C to 34° C (moderate hypothermia)
- Passive rewarming
- Active external rewarming of truncal areas only[b,c]

Less than 30° C (severe hypothermia)
- Active internal rewarming sequence (see below)

Active internal rewarming[b]
- Warm IV fluids (43° C)
- Warm, humid **oxygen** (42° C to 46° C)
- Peritoneal lavage (KCl-free fluid)
- Extracorporeal rewarming
- Esophageal rewarming tubes[d]

Continue internal rewarming until
- Core temperature >35° C or
- Return of spontaneous circulation or
- Resuscitative efforts cease

a. This may require needle electrodes through the skin.
b. Many experts think these interventions should be done only in-hospital, though practice varies.
c. Methods include electric or charcoal warming devices, hot water bottles, heating pads, radiant heat sources, and warming beds.
d. Esophageal rewarming tubes are widely used internationally and are expected to become available in the United States.

From American Heart Association: *1999 Handbook of emergency cardiovascular care for healthcare providers*, Dallas, Texas, 1999, American Heart Association.

Figure 11

Ischemic Chest Pain Algorithm (Update)*
Adult Advanced Cardiac Life Support

1 Chest pain: Pain suggestive of ischemia

2 Immediate assessment (<10 minutes)
- Vital signs with automatic or standard BP cuff
- Oxygen saturation
- Obtain IV access
- Obtain 12-lead ECG (physician reviews)
- Brief, targeted history and physical exam; focus on eligibility for thrombolytic therapy
- Initial serum cardiac marker levels
- Initial electrolyte and coagulation studies
- Portable chest x-ray (<30 minutes)

3 Immediate general treatment
- Oxygen at 4 L/min
- Aspirin 160 to 325 mg
- Nitroglycerin SL or spray
- Morphine IV (if pain not relieved with nitroglycerin)

Memory aid: "MONA" greets all patients

4 Much of the immediate assessment and treatment ("MONA") is appropriately performed by the EMS system, including the initial 12-lead ECG and review for thrombolytic therapy indications.

5 Assess initial 12-lead ECG

21 Nondiagnostic ECG: absence of changes in ST segment or T waves

22 Meets criteria for unstable or new-onset angina?

13 ST depression or T-wave inversion: ECG strongly suspicious for ischemia

14 Consider adjunctive treatments
(as indicated; no contraindications)
- Heparin (UFH/LMWH)
- Aspirin 160 to 325 mg qd
- Glycoprotein IIb/IIIa receptor inhibitors
- Nitroglycerin IV

Yes

6 ST elevation or new or presumably new BBB: strongly suspicious for injury

7 Consider adjunctive treatments
(as indicated; no reperfusion delay)
- β-Blockers IV
- Nitroglycerin IV
- Heparin IV (especially with t-PA)
- ACE inhibitors

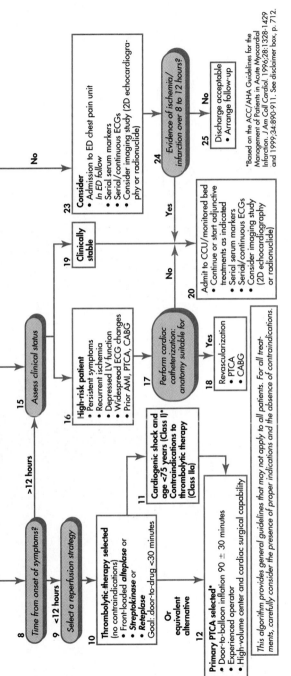

8 Time from onset of symptoms?

>12 hours → No

9 <12 hours

Select a reperfusion strategy

10 Thrombolytic therapy selected (no contraindications)
• Front-loaded *alteplase* or
• *Streptokinase* or
• *Reteplase*
Goal: door-to-drug <30 minutes

Or
equivalent
alternative

11 Cardiogenic shock and age <75 years (Class I)*
Contraindications to thrombolytic therapy (Class IIa)

12 Primary PTCA selected*
• Door-to-balloon inflation 90 ± 30 minutes
• Experienced operator
• High-volume center and cardiac surgical capability

This algorithm provides general guidelines that may not apply to all patients. For all treatments, carefully consider the presence of proper indications and the absence of contraindications.

15 Assess clinical status

16 High-risk patient
• Persistent symptoms
• Recurrent ischemia
• Depressed LV function
• Widespread ECG changes
• Prior AMI, PTCA, CABG

17 Perform cardiac catheterization: anatomy suitable for

18 Yes → Revascularization
• PTCA
• CABG

No

19 Clinically stable

20 Admit to CCU/monitored bed
• Continue or start adjunctive treatments as indicated
• Serial serum markers
• Serial/continuous ECGs
• Consider imaging study (2D echocardiography or radionuclide)

No → (from 8, >12 hours)

23 Consider
• Admission to ED chest pain unit
In ED follow
• Serial serum markers
• Serial/continuous ECGs
• Consider imaging study (2D echocardiography or radionuclide)

24 Evidence of ischemia/infarction over 8 to 12 hours?

Yes → (to 20)

25 No → Discharge acceptable
• Arrange follow-up

Based on the ACC/AHA Guidelines for the Management of Patients in Acute Myocardial Infarction. J Am Coll Cardiol. 1996;28:1328-1429 and 1999;34:890-911. See disclaimer box, p. 712.

From American Heart Association: *1999 Handbook of emergency cardiovascular care for healthcare providers,* Dallas, Texas, 1999, American Heart Association.

Disclaimer Box

This section contains recommendations from the third report of the American College of Cardiology/American Heart Association Task Force on Practice Guidelines (Committee on Management of Acute Myocardial Infarction). It represents the work of Thomas Ryan, MD, and his committee and was published in *J Am Coll Cardiol,* 1999;34:890-911, and *Circulation,* 1999;100:1016-1030 (executive summary). It is available on both the ACC and AHA websites.

The ECC guidelines presented here are interim guidelines. They include several recommendations not yet reviewed in the AHA ECC evidence evaluation process. Healthcare providers working under medical authority should check with that authority for any necessary changes in protocol.

Heart and Breath Sounds

Assessing Heart Sounds

Sound	Auscultation site	Timing	Pitch	Clinical occurrence	End-piece/patient position
S_1 (M_1 T_1)	Apex	Beginning of systole	High	Closing of mitral and tricuspid valves; normal sound	Diaphragm/patient supine
S_1 split	Apex	Beginning of systole	High	Ventricles contracting at different times because of electrical or mechanical problems (e.g., longer time span between M_1 T_1, caused by right bundle-branch heart block, or reversal [T_1, M_1] caused by mitral stenosis)	Same as S_1
S_2 (A_2 P_2)	A_2 at second ICS, RSB; P_2 at second ICS, LSB	End of systole	High	Closing of aortic and pulmonic valves; normal sound	Diaphragm/patient supine
S_2 physiologic split	Second ICS, LSB	End of systole	High	Accentuated by inspiration; disappears on expiration. Sound that corresponds with the respiratory cycle because of normal delay in closure of pulmonic valve during inspiration. It is accentuated during exercise or in individuals with thin chest walls; heard most often in children and young adults	Same as S_2
S_2 persistent (wide) split	Second ICS, LSB	End of systole	High	Heard throughout the respiratory cycle; caused by late closure of pulmonic valve or early closure of aortic valve. Occurs in atrial septal defect, right ventricular failure, pulmonic stenosis, hypertension, or right bundle-branch heart block	Same as S_2

S_2 paradoxic (reversed) split (P_2 A_2)	Second ICS, LSB	End of systole	High	Because of delayed left ventricular systole, the aortic valve closes after the pulmonic valve rather than before it. (Normally during expiration the two sounds merge.) Causes may include left bundle-branch heart block, aortic stenosis, severe left ventricular failure, MI, and severe hypertension	Same as S_2
S_2 fixed split	Second ICS, LSB	End of systole	High	Heard with equal intensity during inspiration and expiration because of split of pulmonic and aortic components, which are unaffected by blood volume or respiratory changes. May be heard in pulmonary stenosis or atrial septal defect	Same as S_2
S_3 (ventricular gallop)	Apex	Early in diastole just after S_2	Dull, low	Early and rapid filling of ventricle, as in early ventricular failure, heart failure. Common in children, during last trimester of pregnancy, and possibly in healthy adults >50 yr of age	Bell/patient in left lateral or supine position
S_4 (atrial gallop)	Apex	Late in diastole just before S_1	Low	Atrium filling against increased resistance of stiff ventricle, as in heart failure, coronary artery disease, cardiomyopathy, pulmonary artery hypertension, ventricular failure. May be normal in infants, children, and athletes	Same as S_3

ICS, Intercostal space; *LSB,* left sternal border; *RSB,* right sternal border; *MI,* myocardial infarction.

Commonly Occurring Heart Murmurs

Type	Timing	Pitch	Quality	Auscultation site	Radiation
Pulmonic stenosis	Systolic ejection	Medium-high	Harsh	Second ICS, LSB	Toward left shoulder, back
Aortic stenosis	Midsystolic	Medium-high	Harsh	Second ICS, RSB	Toward carotid arteries
Ventricular septal defect	Late systolic	High	Blowing	Fourth ICS, LSB	Toward RSB
Mitral insufficiency	Holosystolic	High	Blowing	Fifth-sixth ICS, left MCL	Toward left axilla
Tricuspid insufficiency	Holosystolic	High	Blowing	Fourth ICS, LSB	Toward apex
Aortic insufficiency	Early diastolic	High	Blowing	Second ICS, RSB	Toward sternum
Pulmonary insufficiency	Early diastolic	High	Blowing	Second ICS, LSB	Toward sternum
Mitral stenosis	Mid-late diastolic	Low	Rumbling	Fifth ICS, left MCL	Usually none
Tricuspid stenosis	Mid-late diastolic	Low	Rumbling	Fourth ICS, LSB	Usually none

ICS, Intercostal space; *LSB,* left sternal border; *MCL,* midclavicular line; *RSB,* right sternal border.

Assessing Normal Breath Sounds

Type	Normal site	Duration	Characteristics
Vesicular	Peripheral lung	I > E	Soft and swishing sounds. Abnormal when heard over the large airways
Bronchial	Trachea and bronchi	E > I	Louder, coarser, and of longer duration than vesicular. Abnormal if heard over peripheral lung
Bronchovesicular	Sternal border of major bronchi	E = I	Moderate in pitch and intensity. Abnormal if heard over peripheral lung

I, Inspiration; *E*, expiration.

Assessing Adventitious Breath Sounds

Type	Waveform	Characteristics	Possible clinical condition
Coarse crackle		Discontinuous, explosive, interrupted. Loud; low in pitch	Pulmonary edema, pneumonia in resolution stage
Fine crackle		Discontinuous, explosive, interrupted. Less loud than coarse crackles, lower in pitch, and of shorter duration	Interstitial lung disease; heart failure; atelectasis
Wheeze		Continuous, of long duration, high pitched, musical, hissing	Narrowing of airway; bronchial asthma; COPD
Rhonchus		Continuous, of long duration, low pitched, snoring	Production of sputum (usually cleared or lessened by coughing or suctioning)
Pleural friction rub		Grating, rasping noise	Rubbing together of inflamed parietal linings; loss of normal pleural lubrication

COPD, Chronic obstructive pulmonary disease.

Assessing Respiratory Patterns

Type	Waveform	Characteristics	Possible clinical condition
Eupnea		Normal rate and rhythm for adults and teenagers (12-20 breaths/min)	Normal pattern while awake
Bradypnea		Decreased rate (<12 breaths/min); regular rhythm	Normal sleep pattern; opiate or alcohol use; tumor; metabolic disorder
Tachypnea		Rapid rate (>20 breaths/min); hypoventilation or hyperventilation	Fever; restrictive respiratory disorders; pulmonary emboli
Hyperpnea		Depth of respirations greater than normal	Meeting increased metabolic demand (e.g., sepsis, MODS, SIRS, and exercise)
Apnea		Cessation of breathing; may be intermittent	Intermittent with CNS disturbances or drug intoxication; obstructed airway; respiratory arrest if it persists
Kussmaul		Deep, rapid (>20 breaths/min), sighing, labored	Renal failure, DKA, sepsis, shock
Cheyne-Stokes		Alternating patterns of apnea (10-20 sec) with periods of deep and rapid breathing. Lesions located bilaterally and deep within cerebral hemispheres	Heart failure, opiate or hypnotic overdose, thyrotoxicosis, dissecting aneurysm, subarachnoid hemorrhage, IICP, aortic valve disorders; may be normal in older adults during sleep
Central neurogenic hyperventilation		Rapid (>20 breaths/min), deep, regular. Lesions of midbrain or upper pons thought to be source of pattern	Primary injury (ischemia, infarction, space-occupying lesion); secondary injury (IICP, metabolic disorders; drug overdose)

MODS, Multiple organ dysfunction syndrome; *SIRS,* systemic inflammatory response syndrome; *CNS,* central nervous system; *DKA,* diabetic ketoacidosis; *IICP,* increased intracranial pressure.

Continued

Assessing Respiratory Patterns—cont'd

Type	Waveform	Characteristics	Possible clinical condition
Apneustic		Deep, prolonged inspiration, followed by 20-30 sec pause and short expiration. Lesion located in lower pons	Anoxia, meningitis, basilar artery occlusion
Cluster		Irregular breaths occurring in clusters with periods of apnea. Overall pattern irregular. Lesion located in lower pons or upper medulla	Primary and secondary neurologic injury may produce this respiratory pattern
Ataxic (Biot)		Irregular deep or shallow breaths. No discernible pattern. Lesion located in medulla	Primary and secondary neurologic injury may produce this respiratory pattern

Glasgow Coma Scale

Parameter	Patient response	Score
Best eye opening response (record "C" if eyes closed due to swelling)	Spontaneously	4
	To speech	3
	To pain	2
	No response	1
Best motor response (record best upper limb response to painful stimuli)	Obeys verbal command	6
	Localizes pain	5
	Flexion—withdrawal	4
	Flexion—abnormal	3
	Extension—abnormal	2
	No response	1
Best verbal response (record "E" if endotracheal tube is in place or "T" if tracheostomy tube is in place)	Conversation—oriented × 3	5
	Conversation—confused	4
	Speech—inappropriate	3
	Sounds—incomprehensible	2
	No response	1

Total score	Interpretation
15	Normal
13-15	Minor head injury
9-12	Moderate head injury
3-8	Severe head injury
≤7	Coma
3	Deep coma or brain death

Cranial Nerves: Functions and Dysfunctions

Cranial nerve	Type	Functions	Dysfunctions
I Olfactory	Sensory	Smell	Anosmia
II Optic	Sensory	Sight	Blindness
		Visual acuity	Visual field deficits
		Visual fields	
		Fundus	
III Oculomotor	Motor	Pupillary constriction	Ptosis, diplopia, pupillary dilation, strabismus
		Elevation of upper eyelid	
		Extraocular movements	
IV Trochlear	Motor	Downward and inward movement of eye	Diplopia, visual disturbances with downward gaze
V Trigeminal	Sensory and motor	*Sensory:* Facial, scalp, anterior two thirds of tongue, lips, teeth, proprioception for mastication, corneal reflex	Loss of corneal reflex
		Motor: Temporal and masseter muscles (jaw clenching and lateral movement for mastication)	Paresis or paralysis of muscles of mastication, decreased facial sensation
VI Abducens	Motor	Lateral eye movement	Eye will not move laterally
VII Facial	Sensory and motor	*Sensory:* Taste in anterior two thirds of tongue, proprioception for face and scalp	Loss of taste in anterior two thirds of tongue
		Motor: Facial expression, lacrimal and salivary glands	Paresis or paralysis of facial muscles, facial droop, loss of glandular secretions

VIII Acoustic	Sensory	*Cochlear division:* Hearing *Vestibular division:* Balance	Tinnitus, deafness Vertigo, nystagmus
IX Glossopharyngeal	Sensory and motor	*Sensory:* Taste in posterior one third of tongue; pain, touch, heat, cold in tongue, tonsils, soft palate, and pharynx *Motor:* Elevation of the soft palate, movement of pharynx, secretion and vasodilation of parotid glands for saliva; gag reflex	Loss of taste, pain, touch, heat, and cold in posterior one third of tongue, tonsils, and soft palate. Paresis or paralysis of soft palate and pharynx, dysphagia, dysarthria, hoarseness, loss of gag reflex
X Vagus	Sensory and motor	*Sensory:* Muscles of pharynx, larynx, esophagus, thoracic and abdominal viscera; external ear, mucous membranes of larynx, trachea, esophagus, thoracic and abdominal viscera; lungs (stretch receptors), aortic bodies (chemoreceptors), respiratory/GI tract (pain receptors) *Motor:* Muscles of pharynx, larynx, esophagus, thoracic and abdominal viscera; respiratory/GI tract (smooth muscle), pacemaker and cardiac atrial muscle	Similar to dysfunction of glossopharyngeal Loss of gag reflex and difficulty swallowing
XI Spinal accessory	Motor	Sternocleidomastoid and trapezius muscles	Paresis or paralysis of sternocleidomastoid and trapezius muscles Inability to turn head or shrug shoulders
XII Hypoglossal	Motor	Tongue movement	Paresis or paralysis of the tongue

Major Deep Tendon (Muscle-Stretch) Reflexes

Reflex	Innervation	Examination technique	Normal response
Biceps	C5, C6	Arm partially flexed at elbow, palm down. Place thumb or finger on biceps tendon. Strike finger with reflex hammer	Contraction of biceps muscle Flexion at elbow
Triceps	C6, C7	Arm flexed at elbow, palm toward body, arm pulled slightly across body. Strike triceps tendon with reflex hammer above elbow	Contraction of triceps muscle Extension of arm at elbow
Brachioradialis	C5, C6	Hand resting on abdomen, palm slightly pronated. Strike radius with reflex hammer 3-5 cm above wrist	Contraction of brachioradialis muscle Flexion and supination of forearm
Achilles (ankle jerk)	S1, S2	Leg flexed at knee, dorsiflex the foot. Strike Achilles tendon with reflex hammer	Plantar flexion of foot
Quadriceps (knee jerk)	L3, L4	Leg flexed at knee. Strike patellar tendon with reflex hammer	Contraction of quadriceps muscle. Extension of knee

Grading of Deep Tendon Reflexes

Scale (0 to 4+)	Interpretation
4+	Very brisk, hyperactive, repetitive, rhythmic flexion and extension (clonus); indicative of disease
3+	Brisker than average; may be normal for certain individuals or may indicate disease
2+	Average/normal
1+	Diminished response or low normal
0	No response

Major Superficial (Cutaneous) Reflexes

Reflex	Innervation	Examination technique	Normal response
Abdominals Above/upper Below/lower	T8, T9, T10 T10, T11, T12	Using tongue blade or wooden end of cotton-tipped applicator, lightly stroke abdomen in each quadrant, outer to inner direction, toward umbilicus	Contraction of abdominal muscles Umbilicus deviates (pulls) toward the stimulus
Bulbocavernous (male)	S3, S4	Pinch glans penis or apply pressure over bulbocavernous muscle behind scrotum	Scrotum will elevate toward the body
Corneal	Cranial nerves V and VII	Using wisp of cotton, lightly touch cornea	Eyelids will quickly close
Cremasteric (male)	L1, L2	Lightly stroke inner aspect of thigh	Testicle on side stroked will elevate
Gag	Cranial nerves IX and X	Using tongue blade, lightly touch posterior pharynx	Gagging or retching
Perianal	S3, S4, S5	Stroke tissue surrounding anus with blunt instrument, or examine rectum by gently inserting gloved finger	Anal puckering with external stimuli. Tightening of anal sphincter with internal examination

Inotropic and Vasoactive Agents

Inotropics/vasoactives

Agent	Effects				Dosage	Nursing implications
	(Preload)		(Afterload)			
	HR	PAWP	SVR	Contractility		
Dopamine hydrochloride (Intropin)	—↑	—↓	—	↑↑	Low dose 1-2 µg/kg/min	Affect cardiac contractility and vascular resistance
	—	—	↑↑	—	Moderate dose 2-10 µg/kg/min	Major effect is increasing urine output; may potentiate effect of diuretics
					High dose >10 µg/kg/min	
Dobutamine (Dobutrex)	—↑	—↓	—↓	↑↑	2.5-10 µg/kg/min	Can cause tissue necrosis and sloughing if infiltration occurs
Isoproterenol (Isuprel)	↑↑	—↓	↓↓	↑↑	2-10 µg/min	Overall effect is improved CO; may cause tachycardia and dysrhythmias as side effects. Significant increase in myocardial oxygen consumption; can produce ventricular tachycardia and fibrillation
Norepinephrine (Levophed)	↓↑	↑	↑↑↑	↑	2-12 µg/min	Contraindicated when hypotension occurs secondary to hypovolemia. Can cause tissue necrosis and sloughing if infiltration occurs. Increased myocardial oxygen demand without increased coronary artery flow can cause myocardial ischemia and infarction
Epinephrine	↑↑	↑	↓↑	↑↑	0.5-1 mg for cardiac arrest 1-4 µg/min for inotropic support	May induce ventricular ectopy

Drug	HR	CO	SVR	PAWP	IV dose	Comments
Amrinone lactate (Inocor)	—↑	↓	↓	↑	2-20 µg/kg/min	Can exacerbate myocardial ischemia
Vasopressors						
Methoxamine hydrochloride (Vasoxyl)	—	↑	↑↑	—	3-5 mg	Main effect is vasoconstriction of peripheral blood vessels. Used rarely; may increase myocardial oxygen demand
Phenylephrine (Neo-Synephrine)	—	↑	↑↑	—	0.1-0.5 mg	May cause dysrhythmias or trigger reflex bradycardia
Vasodilators						
Sodium nitroprusside (Nipride)	—↑	↓	↓↓	—	Starting dose of 0.5-0.8 µg/kg/min; titrate up to 10 µg/kg/min	Main effect is dilation of arterial and/or venous beds. Drug is photosensitive; keep infusion container protected from light. Thiocyanate (a metabolite of nitroprusside) toxicity can occur after 72 h. Monitor thiocyanate levels daily, being alert to levels >10 mg/dl and for signs of metabolic acidosis (see p. 680)
Nitroglycerin (Tridil, Nitrostat)	—↑	↓↓	↓	—	Starting dose of 0.5 µg/kg/min; titrate up to 200 µg/kg/min	Absorbed by standard plastic IV tubing. Use special polyvinyl chloride tubing. Ensure that the drug is diluted for IV use

—, No effect; ↑, minimal effect; ↑↑, moderate effect; ↑↑↑, major effect; *HR*, heart rate; *PAWP*, pulmonary artery wedge pressure; *SVR*, systemic vascular resistance; *CO*, cardiac output; *IV*, intravenous.

Infection Prevention and Control

For several decades, infection prevention and control have focused on the use of barriers (e.g., gloves, gowns, masks, eye protection) to interrupt transmission of organisms among and between patients and health care workers. These barriers are a major component of various systems of isolation precautions.

Systems of Isolation Precautions

Five different systems of isolation precautions commonly have been used in hospitals. The Centers for Disease Control and Prevention (CDC) revised its guidelines for isolation precautions in 1996 to meet the following objectives: (1) to be epidemiologically sound; (2) to recognize the importance of all body fluids, secretions, and excretions in the transmission of nosocomial pathogens; (3) to ensure adequate precautions for infections transmitted by the airborne, droplet, and contact routes of transmission; (4) to be as simple and user friendly as possible; and (5) to use new terms to avoid confusion with existing infection control and isolation systems. The 1996 guidelines contain two tiers of precautions (Table A8-1):

- **Standard Precautions,** which are designed for the care of all patients in hospitals regardless of their diagnosis or presumed infection status
- **Transmission-Based Precautions,** which are used for patients known to be or suspected of being infected or colonized with epidemiologically important pathogens that can be transmitted by airborne or droplet transmission or by contact with dry skin or contaminated surfaces.

The 1996 guidelines replace the 1983 guidelines for isolation precautions in hospitals, which offered three options: a *category-specific* system, a *disease-specific* system, and a *hospital-designed* system. Body Substance Isolation (BSI) is a hospital-designed system that has been adopted by many hospitals in the United States and elsewhere. In 1987-1988, the CDC introduced Universal Precautions to reduce health care workers' risk of being exposed to bloodborne pathogens. The 1996 Standard Precautions system synthesizes the major features of Universal Precautions and Body Substance Isolation and applies to (1) blood; (2) all body fluids, secretions, and excretions, except sweat, regardless of whether they contain visible blood; (3) nonintact skin; and (4) mucous membranes. Standard Precautions are designed to reduce the risk of transmission of microorganisms from both recognized and unrecognized sources of infection in hospitals.

The 1996 Transmission-Based Precautions are designed for patients documented to be or suspected of being infected or colonized with organisms transmitted by the airborne route, by droplets, and by organisms that are epidemiologically important. Transmission-Based Precautions replace the 1983 category-specific and disease-specific systems.

Text continued on p. 742

TABLE A 8 - 1 Recommendations for Isolation Precautions in Hospitals

	Standard Precautions	Transmission-Based Precautions: Airborne	Transmission-Based Precautions: Droplet	Transmission-Based Precautions: Contact
When to use	All patients	Use in addition to Standard Precautions for patients known to be or suspected of being infected with microorganisms transmitted by airborne droplet nuclei (≤5 µm) of evaporated droplets containing microorganisms that can remain suspended in the air and can be widely dispersed by air currents	Use in addition to Standard Precautions for patients known to be or suspected of being infected with microorganisms transmitted by droplets (>5 µm) that can be generated during coughing, sneezing, talking, or performance of procedures	Use in addition to Standard Precautions for specified patients known to be or suspected of being infected or colonized with epidemiologically important microorganisms that can be transmitted by direct contact with patient, such as occurs during patient care activities, or by indirect contact, such as touching surfaces or equipment in patient's environment
Hand washing	Wash hands after touching blood, body fluids, secretions, excretions, and contaminated items, regardless of whether gloves are worn; wash hands immediately after gloves are removed, between patient contacts, and to prevent transfer of microorganisms to other patients or environment; use plain (nonantimicrobial) soap for routine hand washing			Wash hands with an antimicrobial agent or a waterless antiseptic agent

Gloves	Wear nonsterile gloves when touching blood, body fluids, secretions, excretions, and contaminated items; put on clean gloves just before touching mucous membranes and nonintact skin; remove gloves promptly after use, before touching noncontaminated items or environmental surfaces, and before going to another patient; wash hands immediately to avoid transfer of microorganisms to other patients or environment		In addition to glove use as described in Standard Precautions, wear gloves when entering the room and during patient care; change gloves after contact with infective material (e.g., fecal material, wound drainage). After glove removal and hand washing, do not touch items in room
Mask, eye protection, face shield	Wear mask and eye protection or face shield to protect mucous membranes of eyes, nose, and mouth during procedures and patient care activities likely to generate splashes or sprays	Wear respiratory protection, such as particulate respirator mask, when entering room of patient known to have or suspected of having tuberculosis	Wear a mask when working within 3 ft of patient

Modified from Garner JS: CDC guideline for isolation precautions in hospitals, *Infect Control Hosp Epidemiol* 17:53-80, 1996.

Continued

TABLE A8-1   Recommendations for Isolation Precautions in Hospitals—cont'd

	Standard Precautions	Transmission-Based Precautions: Airborne	Transmission-Based Precautions: Droplet	Transmission-Based Precautions: Contact
Mask, eye protection, face shield—cont'd		Do not enter room of patient known to have or suspected of having measles (rubeola) or varicella (chickenpox) if susceptible to these infections		
Gown	Wear clean, nonsterile gown to protect skin and prevent soiling of clothing during procedures and patient care activities likely to generate splashes or sprays of blood, body fluids, secretions, or excretions, or to cause soiling of clothing; remove gown promptly when tasks are completed; wash hands			Wear clean, nonsterile gown when entering room if substantial contact is anticipated with patient, surfaces, or items in environment; wear gown when entering room if patient is incontinent or has diarrhea, an ileostomy, colostomy, or uncontained wound drainage; remove gown carefully when tasks are completed; wash hands
Patient care equipment	Handle used patient care equipment in manner that prevents skin and mucous membrane exposures, contamination of clothing, and environmental soiling			When possible, dedicate use of noncritical patient care equipment to a single patient to avoid sharing among patients;

Linen	Handle, transport, and process used linen in manner that prevents skin and mucous membrane exposure, contamination of clothing, and environmental soiling		if common equipment or items must be shared, adequately clean and disinfect them between uses
Patient placement	Place patient who contaminates environment or who does not (or cannot) assist in maintaining appropriate hygiene or environmental control in private room, if possible; consult infection control professionals for other alternatives	Place patient in private room that has (1) monitored negative air pressure in relation to surrounding areas, (2) 6-12 air exchanges per hour, and (3) appropriate discharge of air outdoors or monitored high-efficiency filtration of room air before air is circulated to other areas of the hospital; keep room door closed when patient is in room	Place patient in private room; when a private room is not available, cohort* infected patients or maintain spatial separation of at least 3 ft between infected patient and other patients and visitors; consult infection control professional for other alternatives	Place patient in private room; when a private room is not available, cohort* infected patients; consult infection control professionals for selection of suitable roommates or other alternatives

Continued

Modified from Garner JS: CDC guideline for isolation precautions in hospitals, *Infect Control Hosp Epidemiol* 17:53-80, 1996.

Cohorting is a term used when patients share a room if infected by the same microorganism, provided they are not infected with other potentially transmissible microorganisms and the likelihood of reinfection with the same organism is minimal. Cohorting is used when there is a shortage of private rooms and may be useful during outbreaks.

TABLE A8-1 Recommendations for Isolation Precautions in Hospitals—cont'd

	Standard Precautions	Transmission-Based Precautions: Airborne	Transmission-Based Precautions: Droplet	Transmission-Based Precautions: Contact
Patient placement—cont'd		When a private room is not available, patient may be placed in room with another patient who has an active infection with the same microorganism; consult infection control professionals for alternatives		
Patient transport		Limit movement and transport of patient from room to essential purposes only; if transport or movement is necessary, minimize patient dispersal of droplet nuclei by placing surgical mask on patient if possible	Limit movement and transport of patient from room to essential purposes only; if transport or movement is necessary, minimize patient dispersal of droplets by placing surgical mask on patient if possible	Limit movement and transport of patient from room to essential purposes only; if transport is necessary, ensure that precautions are maintained to minimize contamination of environmental surfaces or equipment
Environmental control	Ensure that hospital has adequate procedures for routine care, cleaning, and disinfection of environment and patient care items			Ensure that patient care items, bedside equipment, and frequently touched surfaces receive daily cleaning

Occupational Safety and Health Administration (OSHA) Bloodborne Pathogens Standard (1991)	Take care to prevent injuries when using needles, scalpels, and other sharp instruments or devices; when handling sharp instruments after procedures; when cleaning used instruments; and when disposing of used needles
	Never recap used needles or otherwise manipulate them using both hands or use any other technique that involves directing the point of a needle toward any part of the body
	Use either one-handed "scoop" technique or mechanical device designed for holding needle sheath if recapping is required by procedure
	Do not remove used needles from disposable syringes by hand; do not bend, break, or manipulate used needles by hand
	Place used sharps in appropriate puncture-resistant containers located as close as practical to location of use
	Use mouthpieces, resuscitation bags, or other ventilation devices as an alternative to mouth-to-mouth resuscitation methods in areas where need is predictable

Modified from Garner JS: CDC guideline for isolation precautions in hospitals, *Infect Control Hosp Epidemiol* 17:53-80, 1996.

Thus, beginning in 1996, all hospitals are encouraged to review and consider adoption of Standard Precautions and Transmission-Based Precautions and discontinue use of the older forms of isolation precautions. As always, the CDC offers hospitals the option of modifying the recommendations according to their needs and circumstances and as directed by federal, state, or local regulations. For example, the Occupational Safety and Health Administration's (OSHA) Bloodborne Pathogens Standard (1991) is still operable, and all facilities are required to comply with its provisions. The CDC's 1996 Standard Precautions incorporate all requirements of the OSHA Bloodborne Pathogens Standard.

Isolation Precautions for Patients With Pulmonary or Laryngeal Tuberculosis

In response to the increasing incidence of pulmonary tuberculosis (TB) in the United States, the CDC in 1990 published guidelines for preventing the transmission of TB in the health care setting. These guidelines were revised in 1994. A component of these guidelines is Airborne Precautions for persons diagnosed with or suspected of having pulmonary or laryngeal tuberculosis that can be transmitted to others via the airborne route. These guidelines focus on early identification and treatment of persons with a diagnosis or suspected diagnosis of active tuberculosis. In addition, the CDC defined requirements for special ventilation and use of masks that provide better filtration and a tighter fit than standard surgical masks. Masks of this type are called *particulate respirators (PRs)* and were originally developed for industrial use to protect workers from dust, fumes, and other hazardous substances that could affect the respiratory tract. The efficacy of PRs in protecting susceptible persons from infection with TB has not been demonstrated; however, research is in progress. Meanwhile, OSHA is in the process of developing a Tuberculosis Control Standard for health care settings that will include requirements for risk assessment, special ventilation, PRs, skin testing programs, exposure management, training programs, and other elements similar to those of OSHA's Bloodborne Pathogens Standard of 1991. The proposed OSHA Control Standards are being evaluated, with the expectation that a final Standard will be forthcoming in the year 2000.

Management of Devices and Procedures to Reduce Risk of Nosocomial Infection

Use of barriers is but one of many strategies that can reduce the risk of nosocomial infection among patients and personnel. In fact, studies from the CDC show that significant gains can be made in reducing infection risks by focusing on the management of devices and procedures frequently used in patient care. For example, many patients need intravascular devices that deliver therapeutic medications, but they are put at risk for site infections and bacteremias when these devices are used. It is well known that rotating the access site at appropriate intervals reduces these risks to the patient, and catheter materials that are more "vein friendly" also reduce trauma to the vascular system. In addition, use of needles to deliver medications and fluids to patients through these intravascular devices can put the health care worker at risk for puncture injury. Needleless or needle-free IV access devices now are used to access line ports, making it unnecessary to use needles once the intravascular catheter has entered the vascular system. Thus the use of newer and safer intravascular devices and procedures can benefit both the patient and health care worker by reducing their risk of nosocomial infection. Research studies of interventions to reduce nosocomial infection risks are published in general and specialty journals and presented at professional meetings each year. Infection control practitioners and hospital epidemiologists use these studies to make recommendations about changes in nursing and medical practice. The Joint Commission on Accreditation of Healthcare Organizations (JCAHO) requires that all accredited facilities have a person qualified to provide infection surveillance, prevention, and control services. The national associations for these professionals are the Association for Professionals in Infection Control and Epidemiology, Inc. (APIC), which publishes the *American Journal of Infection Control,* and the Society for Healthcare Epidemiology of America (SHEA), which publishes the journal *Infection Control and Hospital Epidemiology.*

Bibliography

Association for Professionals in Infection Control and Epidemiology, Inc.: *APIC infection control and applied epidemiology: principles and practice,* St Louis, 1996, Mosby.

Bennett JV, Brachman PS, editors: *Hospital infections,* ed 4, Boston, 1998, Little, Brown.

Centers for Disease Control: Guideline for isolation precautions in hospitals, *Infect Control* 4:245-325, 1983.

Centers for Disease Control: Recommendations for prevention of HIV transmissions in health-care settings, *MMWR Morb Mortal Wkly Rep* 36(suppl 2):1-18, 1987.

Centers for Disease Control: Update: Universal Precautions for prevention of transmission of human immunodeficiency virus and other bloodborne pathogens in health-care settings, *MMWR Morb Mortal Wkly Rep* 37:377-388, 1988.

Centers for Disease Control and Prevention: Guidelines for preventing the transmission of tuberculosis in health-care settings, with special focus on HIV-related issues, *MMWR Morb Mortal Wkly Rep* 39(no. RR-1-17), 1990.

Centers for Disease Control and Prevention: Guidelines for preventing the transmission of *Mycobacterium tuberculosis* in health-care facilities, *MMWR Morb Mortal Wkly Rep* 43(no. RR-13):1-133, 1994.

Centers for Disease Control and Prevention: Guideline for isolation precautions in hospitals, *Infect Control* 17:53-80, 1996.

Department of Labor, Occupational Safety and Health Administration: Occupational exposure to bloodborne pathogens; final rule, 29 CFR part 1910:1030, *Federal Register* 56:64003-64182, Dec 6, 1991.

Jackson MM: Infection prevention and control, *Crit Care Nurs Clin North Am* 4(3):401-409, 1992.

Jackson MM, Lynch P: Infection control: too much or too little? *Am J Nurs* 84:208-210, 1984.

Jackson MM, Lynch P: In search of a rational approach, *Am J Nurs* 90(10):65-73, 1990.

Jackson MM, Lynch P: An attempt to make an issue less murky: a comparison of four systems for infection precautions, *Infect Control Hosp Epidemiol* 12:448-450, 1991.

Jackson MM, Lynch P: Development of a numeric health care worker risk-assessment scale to evaluate potential for blood-borne pathogen exposures, *Am J Infect Control* 23(1):13-21, 1995.

Jackson MM et al: Why not treat all body substances as infectious? *Am J Nurs* 87:1137-1139, 1987.

Lynch P et al: Implementing and evaluating a system of generic infection precautions: body substance isolation, *Am J Infect Control* 18:1-12, 1990.

Lynch P et al: Rethinking the role of isolation practices in the prevention of nosocomial infections, *Ann Intern Med* 107:243-246, 1987.

Martone WJ, Garner JS, editors: Proceedings of the Third Decennial International Conference on Nosocomial Infections, *Am J Med* 91(3B):1-333, 1991.

Mayhall DG, editor: *Hospital epidemiology and infection control,* ed 2, Philadelphia, 1999, Lippincott Williams & Wilkins.

Pugliese G, Lynch P, Jackson MM, editors: *Universal Precautions: policies, procedures, and resources,* Chicago, 1990, American Hospital Publishing.

Wenzel RP: *Prevention and control of nosocomial infections,* ed 3, Philadelphia, 1997, Lippincott Williams & Wilkins.

Abbreviations Used in This Manual

AACN: American Association of Critical Care Nurses
AAL: anterior axillary line
ABA: American Burn Association
ABG: arterial blood gas
ACC: American College of Cardiology
ACE: angiotensin-converting enzyme
ACh: acetylcholine
AChR: acetylcholine receptors
ACLS: advanced cardiac life support
ACS: abdominal compartment syndrome
ACT: activated clotting time
AD: autonomic dysreflexia
ADA: American Diabetes Association
ADH: antidiuretic hormone
ADL: activity of daily living
AED: automatic external defibrillator
AEG: atrial electrogram
AF: atrial fibrillation
AHA: American Heart Association
AIDS: acquired immunodeficiency syndrome
AIS: acute ischemic stroke
ALP: alkaline phosphatase
ALT: alanine aminotransferase
AM: akinetic mutism
AMA: American Medical Association
AMI: acute myocardial infarct
ANA: American Nurses Association
ANP: atrial natriuretic peptide
APAS: antiphospholipid antibody syndrome
APSAC: anisoylated plasminogen streptokinase activator complex
aPTT: activated partial thromboplastin time
ARDS: acute respiratory distress syndrome
ARF: acute respiratory failure; acute renal failure
ARS: adjective rating scale
ASA: acetylsalicylic acid (aspirin)
ASO: antistreptolysin O
AST: aspartate aminotransferase
AT: antithrombin
AT_1: receptor antagonist
ATGAM: antithymocyte gamma globulin
atm: atmosphere (standard)
ATN: acute tubular necrosis
ATP: adenosine triphosphate

AV: atrioventricular; arteriovenous
AVM: arteriovenous malformation
BAL: bronchoalveolar lavage
BEE: basal energy expenditure
BMI: body mass index
BP: blood pressure
bpm: beats per minute
BS: bowel sounds
BSA: body surface area
BUN: blood urea nitrogen
C: centigrade
CABG: coronary artery bypass grafting
CAD: coronary artery disease
CAPD: continuous ambulatory peritoneal dialysis
CASHD: coronary atherosclerotic heart disease
CAVH: continuous arteriovenous hemofiltration
CBC: complete blood cell count
CBF: cerebral blood flow
CD: Cotrel-Dubousset
CDC: Centers for Disease Control and Prevention
CDI: central diabetes insipidus
CHF: congestive heart failure
CI: cardiac index
CIE: counterimmunoelectrophoresis
CK: creatine kinase
CK-MB: creatine kinase–myocardial band
CM: cardiomyopathy
CMV: cytomegalovirus; controlled mechanical ventilation
CNS: central nervous system
CO: cardiac output; carbon monoxide
CO_2: carbon dioxide
COPD: chronic obstructive pulmonary disease
CPAP: continuous positive airway pressure
CPK: creatine phosphokinase
CPP: cerebral perfusion pressure; coronary perfusion pressure
C&S: culture and sensitivities
CSF: cerebrospinal fluid
CT: computed tomography
cTnI: cardiac troponin I
CVA: cerebrovascular accident; costovertebral angle
CVC: central venous catheter
CVP: central venous pressure
CVVH: continuous venovenous hemofiltration
CXR: chest x-ray
CyA: cyclosporine
DAI: diffuse axonal injury
DCM: dilated cardiomyopathy
DFI: diffusion weighted imaging (or DWI)
DI: diabetes insipidus
DIC: disseminated intravascular coagulation
DKA: diabetic ketoacidosis
DM: diabetes mellitus
DNR: do not resuscitate
Do_2: oxygen delivery
DOE: dyspnea on exertion
DPAHC: durable power of attorney for health care
DPL: diagnostic peritoneal lavage

DTR: deep tendon reflex
DVT: deep vein thrombosis
EACA: epsilon- (ε-) aminocaproic acid
EBV: Epstein-Barr virus
ECG: electrocardiogram
ECHO: electrocardiography
EEG: electroencephalogram
EFA: Epilepsy Foundation of America
ELISA: enzyme-linked immunosorbent assay
EMI: electromagnetic interference
EPS: electrophysiologic studies
ESR: erythrocyte sedimentation rate
ET: endotracheal
ETCO$_2$: end-tidal carbon dioxide
ETOH: alcohol
ETT: endotracheal tube
F: Fahrenheit
FDP: fibrin degradation product
FEF: forced expiratory flow
FEV: forced expiratory volume
FHF: fulminant hepatic failure
fr: French
FRC: functional residual capacity
FSP: fibrin split product
FVC: forced vital capacity
GABA: gamma- (γ-) amniobutyric
GBS: Guillain-Barré syndrome
GCS: Glasgow coma scale
GERD: gastroesophageal reflux disease
GI: gastrointestinal
GKI: glucose-potassium-insulin
G6PD: glucose-6-phosphate dehydrogenase
GU: genitourinary
HAT: heparin-associated thrombocytopenia
HCM: hypertrophic cardiomyopathy
Hct: hematocrit
HDL: high-density lipoprotein
HELLP: hemolysis, elevated liver enzymes, low platelet count
Hgb: hemoglobin
HHNS: hyperglycemic hyperosmolar nonketotic syndrome
HITT: heparin-induced thrombocytopenia thrombosis
HIV: human immunodeficiency virus
HOB: head of bed
HR: heart rate
HRS: hepatorenal syndrome
HSV: herpes simplex virus
HUS: hemolytic-uremic syndrome
HVPG: hepatic venous pressure gradient
HVWP: hepatic vein wedge pressure
IABP: intraaortic balloon pump
IAP: intraabdominal pressure
ICA: internal cerebral artery
ICD: implantable cardioverter-defibrillator
ICH: intracerebral hematoma
ICP: intracranial pressure
ICS: intercostal space
ICU: intensive care unit

IE: infective endocarditis
I/E: inspiration/expiration
IER: in expected range
IgG: immunoglobulin G
IHSS: idiopathic hypertrophic subaortic stenosis
IICP: increased intracranial pressure
IM: intramuscular
INR: international normalized ratio
I&O: intake and output
IPD: intermittent peritoneal dialysis; intracranial pressure dynamics
IPPB: intermittent positive-pressure breathing
IRV: inverse ratio ventilation
ITP: idiopathic thrombocytopenic purpura
IV: intravenous
IVP: intravenous pyelogram
JNC VI: Joint National Committee VI
JT: junctional tachycardia
JVD: jugular vein distention
kcal: kilocalorie
KCl: potassium (K^+) chloride
kg: kilogram
KUB: kidney, ureter, bladder
L: liter; lumbar
LAD: left anterior descending (coronary artery)
LAP: left atrial pressure
LDH: lactate dehydrogenase; also abbreviated LD
LDL: low-density lipoprotein
LIS: locked-in-syndrome
LMW: low molecular weight
LOC: level of consciousness
LOS: length of stay
LP: lumbar puncture
LR: lactated Ringer's
LUQ: left upper quadrant
LUT: lower urinary tract
LV: left ventricular
LVEDP: left ventricular end-diastolic pressure
LVH: left ventricular hypertrophy
m: meter
MAP: mean arterial pressure
MCA: middle cerebral artery
MCL: modified chest lead; midclavicular line
MCS: minimally conscious state
MCT: medium-chain triglycerides
MCV: mean corpuscular volume
MG: myasthenia gravis
MI: myocardial infarction
MODS: multiple organ dysfunction syndrome
mOsm: milliosmole
MPAP: mean pulmonary artery pressure; also abbreviated PAM
MRA: magnetic resonance arteriogram
MRI: magnetic resonance imaging
MS: multiple sclerosis
MSO$_4$: morphine sulfate
MUGA scan: multiple-gated acquisition scan
Na/Na$^+$: sodium
NaCl: sodium chloride/saline

NCV: nerve conduction velocity
NDI: nephrogenic diabetes insipidus
NG: nasogastric
NHO: National Hospice Organization
nl: normal
NMBA: neuromuscular blocking agent(s)
NPO: nothing by mouth
NRS: numeric rating scale
NSAID: nonsteroidal antiinflammatory drug
NTG: nitroglycerin
OT: occupational therapist
OTC: over the counter
PA: pulmonary artery
PAC: premature atrial complexes
PAD: pulmonary artery diastolic
PAP: pulmonary artery pressure/positive airway pressure
PASG: pneumatic antishock garment
PAT: paroxysmal atrial tachycardia
PAW: pulmonary artery wedge
PAWP: pulmonary artery wedge pressure
PBV: percutaneous balloon valvuloplasty
PCA: patient-controlled analgesia
PE: pulmonary embolus
PEEP: positive end-expiratory pressure
PEG: percutaneous endoscopic gastrostomy
PET: positron emission tomography
PJC: premature junctional complexes
PK: pyruvate kinase
PMI: point of maximal impulse
PN: parenteral nutrition
PND: paroxysmal nocturnal dsypnea
PO: by mouth
PPF: plasma protein fraction
PRA: panel-reactive antibody
PRBCs: packed red blood cells
PSB: protected specimen brush
PSV: pressure support ventilation
PT: physical therapy; physical therapist; prothrombin time
PTCA: percutaneous transluminal coronary angioplasty
PTH: parathyroid hormone
PTT: partial thromboplastin time
PVC: premature ventricular complex, peripheral venous catheter
PVR: pulmonary vascular resistance
PWI: perfusion weighted imaging
RAP: right atrial pressure
RBC: red blood cell
RCM: restrictive cardiomyopathy
RDA: Recommended Daily Allowance; Recommended Dietary Allowance
rHuEPO: recombinant human erythropoietin
RLA: Rancho Los Amigos
ROM: range of motion
RPE: rate perceived exertion
RR: respiratory rate
RRT: renal replacement therapy
rt-PA: recombinant tissue plasminogen activator
RV: right ventricle
RVP: right ventricular pressure

SA: status asthmaticus
SAH: subarachnoid hemorrhage
SAS: subarachnoid space
SBP: systolic blood pressure
SCI: spinal cord injury
SGOT: serum glutamic oxaloacetic acid transaminase
SGPT: serum glutamic pyruvic transaminase
SIADH: syndrome of inappropriate antidiuretic hormone
SIMV: synchronized intermittent mandatory ventilation
SIRS: systemic inflammatory response syndrome
Sjo$_2$: jugular venous oxygen saturation
SOB: shortness of breath
SQ: subcutaneous; also abbreviated *SC*
SS: sensory stimulation
STSG: split-thickness skin graft
SV: stroke volume
Svo$_2$: mixed venous oxygen saturation
SVR: systemic vascular resistance
TBSA: total body surface area
TCD: transcranial Doppler
TE: thrombotic emboli
TEA: tranexamic acid
TEC: transluminal extraction catheterization
TEE: total energy expenditure; transesophageal echocardiography
TENS: transcutaneous electrical nerve stimulation
TIA: transient ischemic attack
TIBC: total iron-binding capacity
TIPS/TIPSS: transjugular intrahepatic portal-systemic shunt
TMP: transmembrane pressure
TNA: total nutrient admixtures
TNF: tumor necrosis factor
TOF: train-of-four
TPA: tissue plasminogen activator
TPN: total parenteral nutrition
TSF: triceps skinfold thickness
UF: ultrafiltration
URI: upper respiratory infection
UTI: urinary tract infection
VAD: venous access device; ventricular assist device
VAS: visual analog scale
VC: vital capacity
VEDP: ventricular end-diastolic pressure
VF: ventricular fibrillation
VLDL: very-low-density lipoprotein
VMA: vanillylmandelic acid
Vo$_2$: oxygen consumption
VS: vital signs/vegetative state
VSD: ventricular septal defect
VT: ventricular tachycardia
WBC: white blood cell
WNL: within normal limits

Index